Pediatric Considerations

PROCEDURES

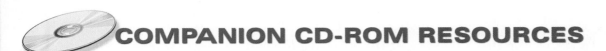

COMPANION CD-ROM RESOURCES

NCLEX®-STYLE REVIEW QUESTIONS for each chapter

ANIMATIONS

Patient Noncompliance
Receptor Interaction
Agonists/Antagonists
Comparison of Drug Absorption by Route of Administration
Bioavailability of Oral Drugs
Passive Diffusion
Drug Movement Through the Body
Distribution: Fat- vs. Water-Soluble Drugs
The Effect of Protein Binding When the Volume of Distribution Is Large
The Effect of Protein Binding When the Volume of Distribution Is Small
Phase I and Phase II Biotransformation Reactions
Sites of Drug Metabolism: First-Pass Metabolism in the Liver
Cytochrome P-450 Drug Metabolism
Enzyme Induction: Examples of CYP Inducers
Enzyme Inhibition: Examples of CYP Inhibitors
Drug-Drug Interaction: Displacement of Drug from Binding Proteins When the V_d Is Low
Effect of Food on Drug Absorption: Gastric Emptying with Digoxin
Effect of Drugs on Nutrient Absorption
Normal Electrophysiology
Renin-Angiotensin in Control of Blood Pressure

VIDEO CLIPS

Right Medication
Right Time
Right Dose
Right Patient
Right Route
Documentation
Oral Medication
Rectal Suppositories
Medication from Ampule
Medication from Vial
Intradermal Medications
Subcutaneous Injections
Intramuscular Injections
Initiating a Peripheral IV
Topical Medications
Measured Ointment
Transdermal Patch
Ear Drops
Eye Drops
Metered-Dose Inhaler

AUDIO PRONUNCIATION GUIDE

TOP 200 PRESCRIPTION DRUGS

DRUG DOSAGE CALCULATORS

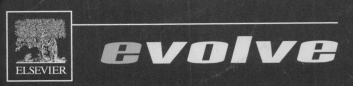

To access your Student Resources, visit the web address below:

http://evolve.elsevier.com/Edmunds/LPN/

Evolve Student Learning Resources for **Edmunds:** *Introduction to Clinical Pharmacology,* **Fifth Edition**, offer the following features:

- **WebLinks**
  An exciting resource that lets you link to hundreds of websites carefully chosen to supplement the content of the textbook. The WebLinks are regularly updated, with new ones added as they develop.

- **Top 200 Drugs**
  by number of U.S. prescriptions dispensed

- **Sign-up page for the** *Elsevier ePharmacology Update* **newsletter**
  An informative, full-color quarterly newsletter written by Evelyn Salerno, PharmD, the *Elsevier ePharmacology Update* provides current and well-documented information on new drugs, drug warnings, medication errors, and more. Available to students and instructors.

The CD-ROM included with every copy of
Introduction to Clinical Pharmacology,
**Fifth Edition, offers learning tools for study and review,
animations, video clips, an audio pronunciation guide, and more!**

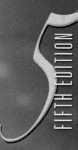

FIFTH EDITION

INTRODUCTION TO CLINICAL PHARMACOLOGY

Marilyn Winterton Edmunds, PhD, ANP/GNP

Adjunct Faculty
Johns Hopkins University
School of Nursing
Baltimore, Maryland

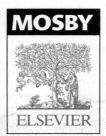

MOSBY

ELSEVIER

11830 Westline Industrial Drive
St. Louis, Missouri 63146

INTRODUCTION TO CLINICAL PHARMACOLOGY,
FIFTH EDITION

ISBN-13 978-0-323-02875-2
ISBN-10 0-323-02875-6

ISBN-13   978-0-323-02875-2
ISBN-10   0-323-02875-6

Executive Publisher: Barbara Nelson Cullen
Acquisitions Editor: Lee Henderson
Associate Developmental Editors: Laura Chu, Catherine Ott
Publishing Services Manager: Deborah L. Vogel
Senior Project Manager: Deon Lee
Design Manager: Teresa McBryan

Printed in Canada

Last digit is the print number: 9 8 7 6 5 4 3 2

Contributors & Reviewers

CONTRIBUTORS

RAQUEL T. BRAITHWAITE, BA, RN, BSN
Nurse Consultant
Columbia, Maryland
Legal Aspects (in Chapter 3), Medication Administration Equipment (in Chapter 10)

LINDA FLUHARTY, RN, MSN
Associate Professor
Ivy Tech State College
Indianapolis, Indiana
Drug Calculation Review Questions and Answers

KAREN ODLE IPPOLITO, BSN, MSN, FNP
Instructor, Nursing Science
San Joaquin Delta College
Stockton, California
Dimensional Analysis (in Chapter 9), Drug Calculation Review Questions and Answers

ELAINE T. PRINCEVALLI, RN, BSN, MS
Instructor, Practical Nurse Education Program
State of Connecticut Department of Education
Hamden, Connecticut
Critical Thinking Questions and Answers

REVIEWERS

MARILYN J. BARKLEY, RN, MSN, CNS, CLCP
Akron School of Practical Nursing
Akron, Ohio

JUDITH LYNN BARTELS, RN, BSN
Butler Technology and Career Development Schools
Hamilton, Ohio

GAIL G. BOEHME, BA, TESOL CERTIFICATION
Formerly, Santa Barbara City College
Santa Barbara, California

DONNA W. BOHMFALK, RN, MSN
Galveston College
Galveston, Texas

KAREN SUE CAMPBELL, RN, BSN
Butler Technology and Career Development Schools
Fairfield Township, Ohio
Fort Hamilton Hospital
Hamilton, Ohio

PATRICIA CLOWERS, MSN, APRN-BC
East Mississippi Community College
Mayhew, Mississippi

GWEN DALIDA, RNC, BSN
South Texas College
McAllen, Texas

LISA K. HAWTHORNE, RN, MSN, PHN, DSD
Maric College, San Diego Campus
San Diego, California

KAREN ODLE IPPOLITO, BSN, MSN, FNP
San Joaquin Delta College
Stockton, California

VIRGINIA MARIE KIMMETH-BUELL, RN, MSN, ACNP, CCRN
Trinity Valley Community College
Palestine, Texas

PATRICIA A. KNECHT, RN, MSN
Center for Arts & Technology
Coatesville, Pennsylvania

AUDREY MCGUINEA, MSN, MED
Cuyahoga Community College
Cleveland, Ohio

JANET TOMPKINS MCMAHON, RN, MSN
Pennsylvania College of Technology
Williamsport, Pennsylvania

KATHLEEN A. PAVALKIS, RN, MA, MSN
Middlesex County Vocational-Technical Schools
East Brunswick, New Jersey

MARY RUSSO, RN, MSN
Lincoln Land Community College
Jacksonville, Illinois

LYNDI C. SHADBOLT, RN, MS, BSN
Amarillo College
Amarillo, Texas

BEVERLEY D. TURNER, RN, MA
Desert Career College
Palm Springs, California

MICHAEL A. VITALE JR, BS PHARM, PHARMD, RPH
Clinical Pharmacist
Philadelphia, Pennsylvania

LEEANN H. ZERR, BS, PA, LVN
Maric College, San Diego Campus
San Diego, California

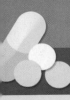

Introduction to Clinical Pharmacology is a basic guide for nursing students beginning the study of pharmacology. The fifth edition boasts a new emphasis on health literacy, making the text more readable and accessible to LPN/LVN and ESL students. Up-to-date information on drugs, procedures, regulations, and issues provides a strong platform of essential knowledge for the safe, effective administration of drugs.

Every effort has been made to incorporate into this edition the excellent suggestions of the nurses and students who used and evaluated the text. Two new chapters reflect the latest trends and developments in both drugs and drug therapy. **Chapter 2, Patient Teaching and Health Literacy,** reinforces that the patient's knowledge is as key as the nurse's knowledge to the success of drug therapy. **Chapter 17, Medications for Pain Management,** responds to growing interest in pain management with discussions of popular medications and their issues. Chapter 9, Calculating Drug Dosages, now includes a discussion of dimensional analysis with detailed examples, and new Drug Calculation Review questions at the ends of selected chapters help students reinforce necessary math skills. A vibrant full-color design and illustration program gives the text a fresh, current look with an open, readable format.

We have revised this fifth edition specifically for those individuals in LPN/LVN programs. Among this group of students are many who are returning to school after raising a family or changing from another career. For many LPN/LVN students, English is a second language. Using new literacy information, the text has been rewritten using the concepts of "clear communication." This style avoids unnecessary medical jargon and complicated words when simple terms are better. Pharmacology is a complex discipline. In learning about this subject, a balance has to be made between using simple terms and using medical and pharmacological words that nurses will hear and see and must master if they are to be seen as well prepared. We have used shorter sentences, simpler terminology, and shorter paragraphs to make the book less intimidating and more engaging to students.

ORGANIZATION AND STANDARD FEATURES

Pharmacology is a science: there are both right answers and wrong answers. Accuracy and precision are extremely important. In fact, nurses are legally responsible and accountable for how they administer drugs. The science of medication administration for nurses is outlined in **Unit One: General Principles of Pharmacology.** This unit stresses the nursing process, the importance of working with patients to assess medication needs and actions, and the differences among many types of medications. It also discusses establishing patient trust, teaching the patient or family about drugs and how to take them appropriately, and evaluating patient responses to drugs. **Unit Two: Principles of Medication Administration** emphasizes precision—the precision required in dosage calculations. This unit includes review chapters on mathematical principles, equivalents, and drug dosage calculations. Medication administration throughout the lifespan and in health promotion and disease prevention is also included. **Unit Three: Drug Groups** briefly outlines essential information on 14 specific groups of medications.

Each chapter begins with **Objectives** to guide students through the chapter content. A list of **Key Terms** provides a quick review of terminology. The terms appear in color at first mention and are briefly defined in the text, with complete definitions in the Glossary. New to this edition are simple phonetic pronunciations and page number references. Terms that were assigned pronunciations were selected because they are either (1) difficult medical, nursing, or scientific terms; or (2) words that may be difficult for students with limited proficiency in English to pronounce. Each chapter ends with a list of **Key Points** correlated with the objectives, which serve as a useful chapter review. **Critical Thinking Questions** help promote higher level thinking skills while reinforcing the Key Points. Suggested answers to the Critical Thinking Questions are located in the Instructor's Resource Manual.

Unit One provides a **solid grounding** in the nursing process, the importance of patient teaching in the success of drug treatment, legal considerations, and cultural and lifespan issues. Content includes cultural considerations, genetics, and spirituality and religion. Women's health issues are further addressed with new appendices on the drug risk categories for pregnant women and nursing mothers.

Unit Two provides a **comprehensive unit on Mathematics and Calculations,** allowing students to review the mathematical concepts necessary for understanding pharmacology. The content is also limited to what is most essential; numerous equivalencies and other mathematical reference features are included for student review or reference to help students learn and retain basic mathematical skills. Every attempt has been made to present a systematic approach to solving mathematical problems. New material on dimensional analysis has been added to this edition. Numerous sample problems, which are solved in a logical step-by-step approach, provide students with concrete examples of how to work problems. The unit concludes with medication administration, providing step-by-step **Procedure boxes** with clear instructions and illustrations for various routes of drug administration. Selected chapters in Units Two and Three contain new **Drug Calculation Questions** for additional practice. Answers to the calculation problems are in the back of the book.

Unit Three uses a **consistent, practical format** to help the student develop logical thinking skills in preparing and administering medications. Drugs are grouped by their therapeutic class within body system chapters, allowing students to learn quickly by making generalizations about similar drugs in a class. A brief review of anatomy begins each chapter. Each **drug class** is presented in a consistent format: its action, uses, adverse reactions, and drug interactions, as well as the highlighted section **Nursing Implications and Patient Teaching.** Content in this especially important section is organized by the nursing process: **Assessment, Diagnosis, Planning, Implementation, Evaluation,** and **Patient and Family Teaching.** Integrated **Case Studies** require the student to use information not only from the chapter, but also from previous chapters, in answering the questions posed about the cases. Suggested answers to the Case Studies can be found in the Instructor's Resource Manual.

We realize the importance of differentiating between what the student must learn from reading a pharmacology text and what kind of material to include strictly for reference. Because educators continually stress the nursing students' need for both in a pharmacology textbook, we have retained the book's unique format, which meets both of these needs: **narrative content** deals exclusively with major drug groups, whereas all the information related to specific drugs appears in **reference tables.** Using this approach, the student is not overwhelmed with extensive reading material but at the same time has ready access to generic names, trade names, forms, and dosages for individual drugs. We have marked trade name drugs available only in Canada with a maple leaf symbol as a reference for the many Canadian educators and students who also use this text.

SPECIAL FEATURES

- **Clinical Goldmines** throughout the text identify the important knowledge that will aid nurses in giving particular drugs.
- **Clinical Landmines** point to critical information, warnings, or adverse effects that nurses must know if they are to safely administer or monitor the drug.
- **Memory Joggers** restate key points from anatomy, physiology, or pharmacology that are important for the nurse to understand and that provide foundational information for drug use. In the math chapters, they also break up the text and remind the student of basic principles or reinforce what has just been learned.

- **Pediatric Considerations** draw attention to informati[on] that would be especially important to remember in givi[ng] a specific medication to a child.
- **Geriatric Considerations** identify special vulnerabiliti[es] of the older patient.
- **Complementary and Alternative Therapies** boxes hig[h]light special considerations for herbal therapies, includi[ng] drug interactions.

STUDENT ANCILLARY PACKAGE

For the first time, supplemental student learning aids inclu[de] a **Companion CD-ROM** and companion **Evolve Resource[s]** website.

Companion CD-ROM

- Approximately 250 interactive **NCLEX®-style review que[s]**tions
- **Animations** illustrating basic pharmacology principles
- **Videos** demonstrating medication administration tec[h]niques
- **Audio Pronunciation Guide** of over 150 key terms
- **Top 200 Drugs** by number of U.S. prescriptions dispens[ed] with audio pronunciations of generic drug names
- Online **Drug Calculators** providing additional reinforc[e]ment of math skills

Evolve Resources Website

- **WebLinks** supplementing the content of the text wi[th] online resources
- *Elsevier ePharmacology Update* **newsletter signup** pr[o]viding current and well-documented information on ne[w] drugs, drug warnings, medication errors, and more
- **Top 200 Drugs** by number of U.S. prescriptions dispens[ed] with audio pronunciations of generic drug names

Study Guide

The printed Study Guide includes new study hints for ES[L] students, worksheets, review sheets and case studies, the T[op] 200 Drugs, FDA Pregnancy Ratings, and an explanation [of] how to read/use drug labels.

INSTRUCTOR ANCILLARY PACKAGE

Instructors may choose the ancillary format with which the[y] are most comfortable:

- A printed *Instructor's Resource Manual* includes Tips f[or] Teaching English as a Second Language (ESL) student[s,] resources to use in teaching or learning material, revie[w] sheets for mathematics and calculations concepts, classroo[m] activities aligned with applicable sections of chapter outlines, reproducible quizzes, suggested answers to the textbook's Critical Thinking Questions, and the answer key to the companion Study Guide with suggested answers to the textbook's Case Studies. A selection of valuable Internet addresses is included with each chapter to help the student obtain the most recent information about new products as they become available.

The *Instructor's Electronic Resource* CD-ROM offers the complete Instructor's Resource Manual in addition to a unique Electronic Image Collection with approximately 200 images and a Computerized Test Bank with 400 NCLEX®-format questions.

The *Evolve* website offers to the instructor the Student Resources mentioned previously, as well as the complete Instructor's Resource Manual, Electronic Image Collection, Test Bank, and *Mosby's Nursing Pharmacology PowerPoint Collection.*

The *Lesson Plan Manual,* an exciting new instructor's resource from Elsevier's **TEACH (Total Education and Curriculum Help)** program, is based on learning objectives for each chapter in the textbook and provides a road map to help instructors link and integrate all the parts of the educational package. This for-sale manual is customized for *Introduction to Clinical Pharmacology* and provides the ultimate tool for busy new LPN/LVN instructors or instructors who want to revitalize their classroom presentations.

othing teaches the nurse more about pharmacology than tually giving medications to a patient. To develop mastery of this content, the nursing student should approach each encounter with a patient as an opportunity to learn. The nurse should accept it as a personal challenge to learn about each medication ordered for a patient under his or her care and to understand why the medication is given. Completing medication cards and personalizing the information to a specific patient are valuable strategies in learning about medications. Because pharmacology is a rapidly changing and dynamic field, it is suggested that the student be exposed early on to other drug information such as package inserts or current drug handbooks. Although every attempt is made to include new drugs, new products appear all the time, and the nurse will need to learn how to obtain this information. Students should be encouraged to develop the habit of seeking up-to-date and timely information to supplement this book and to provide specific details that cannot be covered in a textbook.

In working with patients, the nursing student will quickly learn that giving medications is one of the most challenging parts of the nursing role. A nurse who develops the knowledge and skills needed to correctly give medications will be noticed and recognized with respect by both patients and colleagues in the health care system. Both the responsibilities and the personal rewards are great.

The author and publisher sincerely hope this book helps the student understand the basic concepts and procedures in giving medications. We welcome your suggestions or comments on *Introduction to Clinical Pharmacology,* Fifth Edition, so that we may continue to provide a clear and useful discussion of introductory pharmacology in future editions.

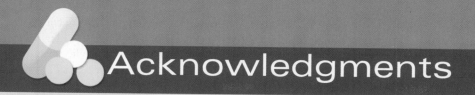

Acknowledgments

Writing a pharmacology text is like running a race that never ends. There are always new drugs arriving on the market and new information available about old products. The available information is endless, and it is a real challenge to try to acquire enough knowledge to be a safe practitioner.

I wish to acknowledge my personal stimulation from the many students who have asked challenging questions throughout my years as a teacher and the support of my professional colleagues. I am grateful for the help of the Elsevier editorial, production, and design staff. Acquisitions Editor Lee Henderson and Associate Developmental Editors Laura Chu and Cathy Ott provided ongoing editorial guidance and support. Deon Lee, Senior Project Manager, smoothly directed the manuscript through the production process. Megan Westerfeld, Copy Editor, offered a sharp eye and constructive suggestions. Teresa McBryan, Design Manager, created a beautiful new full-color design for this edition, and Joseph Selby, Multimedia Producer, helped enhance the ancillary package with a new Companion CD and companion Evolve website.

Several educators have lent their knowledge and experti to this edition: Karen Ippolito, Linda Fluharty, and Raqu Braithwaite all made valuable contributions to help keep t text fresh and current. Elaine Princevalli revised and updat the Critical Thinking questions that appear at the end of ea chapter, as well as the answers to these questions for t Instructor's Electronic Resource CD. Kathleen Nacos-Bur and Sandra Cooper have written new interactive study a review questions for each chapter for the Companion CD, a Donna Hubbard has revised and updated the Computerize Test Bank. Thanks are also due to Gail Boehme for her inp as a reviewer in helping to make the text more accessible English as a Second Language students and to Michael A. Vita Jr for his assistance in ensuring the clinical accuracy of the te and its accompanying Study Guide.

As always, I owe a special debt of gratitude to my famil who is so important in my life and who supports me in a the things in which I get involved.

MARILYN WINTERTON EDMUNDS, PhD, ANP/GN

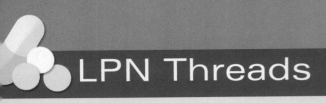

LPN Threads

roduction to Clinical Pharmacology, Fifth Edition, shares
ne features and design elements with other LPN titles on the
evier list. The purpose of these LPN Threads is to make it eas-
for students and instructors to use the variety of books
quired by the relatively brief and demanding LPN curriculum.
The shared features in *Introduction to Clinical Pharmacology,*
th Edition, include the following:

A **reading level evaluation** performed on every manuscript chapter during the book's development to increase
the consistency among chapters and to make the reading
easy to understand

Cover and internal **design similarities;** the colorful,
student-friendly design encourages reading and learning of
this core content

Numbered lists of **Objectives** that begin each chapter

Key Terms with phonetic pronunciations and page number references at the beginning of each chapter; the key
terms are in color the first time they appear in the chapter

A bulleted list of **Key Concepts** at the end of each chapter

A **Bibliography** list at the end of the text

A **Glossary** at the end of the text

And for instructors. . .

- A **Computerized Test Bank** with the following categories
  of information: Topic, Step of the Nursing Process,
  Objective, Cognitive Level, NCLEX® Category of Client
  Need, Correct Answer, Rationale, and Text Page Reference
- A **PowerPoint slide presentation** on the companion Evolve
  website
- **Tips for teaching English as a Second Language (ESL)
  students** in the Instructor's Resource Manual

In addition to content and design threads, these LPN textbooks benefit from the advice and input of the Elsevier LPN
Advisory Board.

LPN Advisory Board

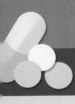

To the Student

Designed with the student in mind, *Introduction to Clinical Pharmacology,* Fifth Edition, will help you learn basic pharmacology with its visually appealing and easy-to-use format. Here are some of the numerous special features that will help you understand and apply the material.

COMPANION CD-ROM

The Companion CD-ROM packaged in your copy of *Introduction to Clinical Pharmacology,* Fifth Edition, contains the following sections: NCLEX® review and study questions, an audio pronunciation guide of Key Terms, a list of the Top 200 U.S. Prescriptions with audio pronunciations of generic drug names, animations illustrating principles of pharmacology, video clips demonstrating medication administration techniques, and online drug calculators. Using these resources as you study can help you master the material in this book.

Chapters open with numbered **Objectives** and **Key Terms** with pronunciations.

New Chapter on Pain Management discusses popular pain medications and their issues.

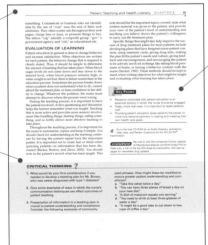

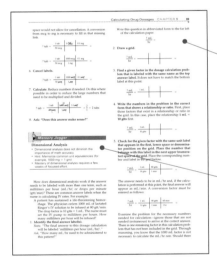

New Dimensional Analysis content in Chapter 9 strengthens your drug calculation skills with detailed examples.

Memory Joggers restate key points from anatomy, physiology, or pharmacology.

Clinical Goldmines highlight and reinforce important knowledge.

New Chapter on Patient Education emphasizes the importance of health literacy.

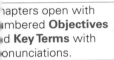

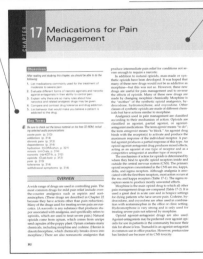

Critical Thinking Questions at the end of each chapter help you develop problem-solving skills. Answers are provided in the IRM.

End-of-chapter **Key Points** summarize chapter topics.

Clinical Landmines point to critical information, warnings, and adverse effects.

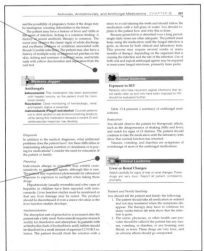

Complementary and Alternative Therapies boxes
highlight popular herbal supplements and their potential interactions with commonly used drugs.

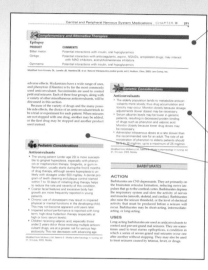

Considerations boxes offer tips and warnings on adverse drug interactions common in children and older adults.

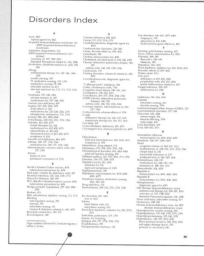

A **Disorders Index,** in addition to the General Index, lists drugs by the disorders for which they are used.

Case Studies help you apply drug information to clinical practice.

Step-by-step **Procedure boxes** give clear instructions and illustrations for routes of drug administration.

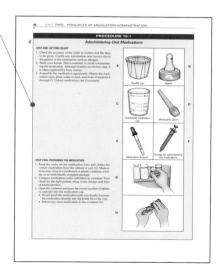

Drug Calculation Questions at the end of selected chapters in Units Two and Three sharpen your math skills. Answers are provided at the back of the book.

Evolve Resources
Be sure to consult the new Evolve website
(http://evolve.elsevier.com/Edmunds/LPN/)
For web activities and signup page for the
Elsevier ePharmacology Update newsletter

THE TOP 50 PRESCRIPTIONS
BY NUMBER OF U.S. PRESCRIPTIONS DISPENSED

BRAND NAME	MANUFACTURER	GENERIC NAME
Hydrocodone w/APAP*	Various†	hydrocodone w/APAP
Lipitor	Pfizer US Pharm	atorvastatin
Lisinopril	Various	lisinopril
Atenolol	Various	atenolol
Synthroid	Abbott	levothyroxine
Amoxicillin	Various	amoxicillin
Hydrochlorothiazide	Various	hydrochlorothiazide
Zithromax	Pfizer US Pharm	azithromycin
Furosemide	Various	furosemide
Norvasc	Pfizer US Pharm	amlodipine
Toprol-XL	AstraZeneca	metoprolol tartrate
Alprazolam	Various	alprazolam
Albuterol	Various	albuterol
Zoloft	Pfizer US Pharm	sertraline
Zocor	MSD	simvastatin
Metformin	Various	metformin
Ibuprofen	Various	ibuprofen
Triamterene w/HCTZ	Various	triamterene/HCTZ
Ambien	Sanofi	zolpidem
Cephalexin	Various	cephalexin
Nexium	AstraZeneca	esomeprazole
Prevacid	Tap Pharm	lansoprazole
Lexapro	Forest Pharm	escitalopram
Prednisone	Various	prednisone
Zyrtec	Pfizer US Pharm	cetirizine
Singulair	MSD	montelukast
Celebrex **(FDA advisory issued December 2004)**	Pharmacia Upjohn	celecoxib
Fluoxetine HCL	Various	fluoxetine
Fosamax	MSD	alendronate
Metoprolol Tartrate	Various	metoprolol tartrate
Premarin	Wyeth Pharm	conjugated estrogens
Levoxyl	Monarch Pharm	levothyroxine
Lorazepam	Various	lorazepam
Allegra	Aventis	fexofenadine
Plavix	BMS Primary Care	clopidogrel
Effexor XR	Wyeth Pharm	venlafaxine
Potassium Chloride	Various	potassium chloride
Protonix	Wyeth Pharm	pantoprazole
Propoxyphene NAP w/APAP	Various	propoxyphene N/APAP
Advair Diskus	GlaxoSmithKline	salmeterol/fluticasone
Warfarin Sodium	Barr	warfarin
Acetaminophen w/Codeine	Various	acetaminophen/codeine
Clonazepam	Various	clonazepam
Neurontin	Pfizer US Pharm	gabapentin
Flonase	Allen & Hanburys	fluticasone
Amitriptyline HCL	Various	amitriptyline
Ranitidine HCL	Various	ranitidine
Trazodone HCL	Various	trazodone
Naproxen **(FDA alert issued December 2004)**	Various	naproxen
Amox TR-Potassium Clavulanate	Various	amoxicillin/potassium clavulanate

For 2004. Based on more than 3 billion prescriptions: Data furnished by NDC Health.

*Hydrocodone w/APAP = 92.7 million prescriptions

Lipitor = 69.8 million prescriptions

Lisinopril = 46.2 million prescriptions

Atenolol = 44.2 million prescriptions

Synthroid = 44.1 million prescriptions

†When manufacturer listed = *Various:* the data for two or more generic manufacturers have been combined.

Contents

CONTENTS

INTRODUCTION TO CLINICAL PHARMACOLOGY

CHAPTER 1

The Nursing Process

After reading and studying this chapter, you should be able to do the following:

1. List the five steps of the nursing process.
2. Discuss how the nursing process is used in administering medications.
3. Identify subjective and objective data.
4. List specific nursing activities related to assessing, diagnosing, planning, implementing, and evaluating the patient's response to medications.

Key Terms

Be sure to check out the bonus material on the free CD-ROM, including selected audio pronunciations.

assessment (ă-SĔS-mĕnt, p. 1)
auscultation (ăw-skŭl-TĀ-shŭn, p. 2)
database (DĀT-ă-bās, p. 2)
diagnosis (dī-ăg-NŌ-sĭs, p. 3)
evaluation (ĭ-văl-ū-Ā-shŭn, p. 7)
implementation (ĭm-plĕ-mĕn-TĀ-shŭn, p. 5)
inspection (ĭn-SPĔK-shŭn, p. 2)
nursing process (p. 1)
objective data (ŏb-JĔK-tĭv DĀT-ă, p. 2)
palpation (păl-PĀ-shŭn, p. 2)
percussion (pĕr-KŬ-shŭn, p. 2)
six "rights" of medication administration (mĕd-ĭ-KĀ-shŭn ăd-mĭn-ĭ-STRĀ-shŭn, p. 5)
subjective data (sŭb-JĔK-tĭv DĀT-ă, p. 2)
therapeutic effects (thĕr-ă-PŪ-tĭk, p. 7)

STEPS OF THE NURSING PROCESS

Nursing actions are specific tasks that are done on purpose, and are not done without thinking about them. A plan that helps guide the nurse's work in logical steps has been used for years and is known as the **nursing process.** The nursing process consists of the following five major steps:

1. Assessment
2. Diagnosis
3. Planning
4. Implementation
5. Evaluation

All of these steps are followed when you are giving medications to patients. The nursing process is shown in Figure 1-1.

Registered nurses (RNs) have both the knowledge and the authority they need to carry out all of the steps of the nursing process. Their nursing actions do not require a legal order, so the RNs are acting independently. Licensed practical nurses/licensed vocational nurses (LPNs/LVNs) do not have the same type of authority when they work with patients. Although LPNs/LVNs may be dependent on the RNs they work with in the planning and evaluation steps of the nursing process, they might be more independent as they collect data (assessment step) or help with the care of the patient (implementation step). For example, RNs are allowed to interview the patient and do a physical examination of the patient's body, but LPNs/LVNs also collect information as they work with patients. It is usually the LPN/LVN who takes vital signs, checks response to medications and treatments, and collects data about symptoms the patient is having. RNs and LPNs/LVNs both also carry out medication or treatment orders written by health care providers. (Doctors are not the only ones who write orders anymore. You may work with nurse practitioners, physician assistants, or other types of health care providers who have this legal responsibility.)

As you grow in the LPN/LVN role and gain more experience, you will learn more complex skills that help you with the nursing process. LPNs/LVNs are often given jobs with greater responsibility as they show that they can do the work. In nursing homes and extended-care facilities, you may have opportunities to be a charge nurse and to manage the patient care under the supervision of the RN. So, it is important to master all parts of the nursing process.

ASSESSMENT

An RN has been legally assigned as the staff member who must perform the initial assessment for each patient. However, the LPN/LVN is often asked to assist with part of this task. You will help in carrying out the nursing plan and continuing to collect data.

Assessment involves looking and listening carefully! It is a process that helps you gather information about the patient, the patient's problem, and anything that

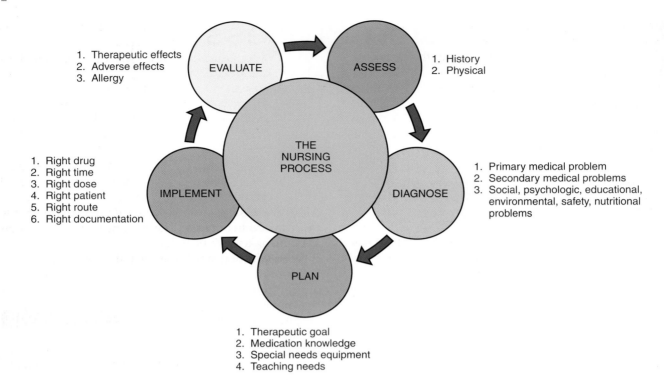

1. Therapeutic effects
2. Adverse effects
3. Allergy

1. History
2. Physical

1. Right drug
2. Right time
3. Right dose
4. Right patient
5. Right route
6. Right documentation

1. Primary medical problem
2. Secondary medical problems
3. Social, psychologic, educational, environmental, safety, nutritional problems

1. Therapeutic goal
2. Medication knowledge
3. Special needs equipment
4. Teaching needs

EVALUATE   ASSESS   IMPLEMENT   THE NURSING PROCESS   DIAGNOSE   PLAN

FIGURE **1-1** The nursing process.

may have an influence on the choice of drug to be given to the patient for this problem. This step of the nursing process is very important because it gives you initial information you must start with as you begin to make a **database,** or record, from which all other nursing process plans develop. Assessment means getting information by talking to the patient, looking at old records, or reviewing information that the patient may bring with her. When the patient is admitted to the hospital, you will want to question her carefully about any current health problems as well as any history of illnesses, surgery, and medications she has taken both now and in the past. This information is important for all team members to know and helps everyone plan the patient's care. Information in the patient's history often directs the nurse and the physician to look for certain physical signs of illness that may be present.

Information you gather through assessment falls into two groups: subjective data and objective data. **Subjective data,** or information given by the patient or family, includes the concerns or symptoms felt by the patient. Examples of subjective data include:
- The chief problem of the patient (in the patient's own words)
- The detailed history of the present illness
- The medical history of the patient
- The family medical history
- Social information: the patient's job, education level, and cultural background
- A review of problems found in different body systems

Some patient problems are more subjective than others. For example, if a patient reports pain in the abdomen, you must accept the patient's word that the pain is present. The nurse cannot see, hear, or feel the patient's abdominal pain—that is why it is subjective. A patient may state that he has trouble breathing. Although you may observe his rapid breathing, the degree of difficulty he has cannot be measured. This trouble with breathing is what the patient is feeling; the nurse cannot see or measure this. Information is subjective if you have to rely on the patient's words or if the symptoms cannot be felt by anyone other than the patient. In such cases, you would report, "The patient states that . . . "

Objective data are obtained when the health care provider gives the patient a physical examination. It also comes from documents that patients may bring with them, such as old laboratory results, electrocardiogram (ECG) printouts, or x-rays, or from information you gather during the physical examination. Vital signs (respiratory rate, pulse, blood pressure, weight, height, temperature); physical findings you can see during careful **inspection** (close observation), **palpation** (feeling), **percussion** (detecting differences in vibrations through the skin), and **auscultation** (listening with the stethoscope); and the results of recent laboratory tests and diagnostic procedures all give you objective data.

It is especially important to obtain subjective and objective assessment data when the patient is first seen or on admission to the hospital. This provides initial, or baseline, information that can be used to determine how ill the patient may be. Assessment is done during the entire time the patient is being cared for to determine if the patient is getting better with the treatment that has been ordered.

The nurse may not always be the one gathering the subjective and objective data; however, the nurse and everyone else on the health care team should learn whatever information they can from the chart, the physician, the family, or other team members, and use that information to plan the patient's care. Understanding the difference between subjective and objective information will help you in reporting, or charting, the information. For example, if the patient reports pain (subjective information), your notes should say, "The patient complains of pain" rather than "The patient has pain" because you cannot really know if what the patient is feeling is actually pain or only discomfort. Much of your job in assessing will be in reporting data that you collect to the RN. As you learn more skills, or work in places such as nursing homes where you may have more responsibility, you will play a bigger role in assessing the patient. But, as an LPN/LPN, you are not responsible for collecting all data.

How big a part you play in assessing the patient is defined by your state nurse practice act, which lists what LPNs/LVNs may and may not do. In some states, it may be possible for an LPN/LVN to perform partial or full assessment only in such areas as personal care or support services. In other states, it may be possible for you to collect most of the patient assessment information and then have an RN review the data, decide what the patient needs, and help develop the plan for care.

Factors to Consider in Assessing the Patient

Certain information is very helpful in planning drug therapy. The nursing assessment at the time of the patient's admission to the hospital should take special note of the drug history. You must talk to the patient, who is the first or primary source, but sometimes you also have to talk to a patient's relatives, or get old medical records, ECG results, or laboratory reports (secondary sources). Sometimes your nursing books or the Internet (tertiary sources) may also provide helpful information about a specific disease, medication, or procedure.

When asking about the patient's drug history, the nurse makes assessments in the following areas:
1. Symptoms, signs, or diseases that explain the patient's need for medication (such as high blood glucose levels, high blood pressure, or pain)
2. Current (and sometimes past) use of all medications and drugs:
   - All prescription medications (patients often forget to mention birth control pills in this category)
   - Over-the-counter medications such as aspirin, vitamins, laxatives, cold and sinus preparations, and antacids

- Street drugs used for recreational purposes (such as marijuana or cocaine)
- Alternative therapies such as herbal medicines or aromatherapy
3. Any problems with drug therapy:
   - Allergies: What is the patient's response to a medicine to which he believes he is allergic? Does it represent a true allergy? An adverse effect? A common side effect?
   - Diseases that may prohibit or limit use of some medications (such as sickle cell anemia, G6PD deficiency, migraine headaches, or angina)

You will also be assessing changes in patient status that may influence drug therapy during the entire time the patient is in the hospital. This is how you will know if the medication is helping the patient or not.

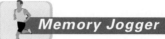

Memory Jogger

Nursing Assessment

Assessment means learning as much as you can about your patients and their problems.

DIAGNOSIS

Once the assessment information has been collected, the LPN/LVN and other health care team members must make a **diagnosis** (a conclusion about what the patient's problems are). The physician will decide the medical diagnoses. The RN will identify the nursing diagnoses. The hospital where you work may use the formal nursing diagnosis system developed by the North American Nursing Diagnosis Association (NANDA) that allows RNs to share a common language and a common way of describing a patient's condition. However, many hospitals do not recognize or use this system. In either case, you will come to some decisions about the status of the patient, or about how sick she is and how carefully you will need to watch her. You will make your own decisions about some of the following questions:
- What are the major problems of this patient? (Think about the problem that led to the patient coming to the hospital.)
- How sick is this patient?
- What procedures or medications will this patient require?
- What special knowledge or equipment is required in giving these medications?
- What special concerns or cultural beliefs does the patient have?
- How much does this patient understand about her medicine?

The answers to these questions help you set the goals of nursing care, and will tell you how closely you will need to work with the patient and what types of patient education will be needed. Getting accurate answers to these questions may be harder with children, elderly patients, or people whose language or culture is different from yours. However, just as a physician must have the correct diagnosis if he is to prescribe the right treatment, the nurse must find the correct answers to these questions to be able to plan the best care for the patient.

PLANNING

Based on the data you find, the medical and nursing diagnoses are made, goals are set, and care plans are written. As a member of the health care team, the LPN/LVN will be able to help with the planning step. As you help the RN plan the care for each patient you see, the plan will become easier to write. Nursing plans involve two groups of people: the nurses and the patient. Patient goals help the patient learn about a medication and how to use it properly. Nursing goals help the nurse plan what equipment or procedures are needed to give the medication. Using the information about the patient's history, medical and social problems, and risk factors, and about how ill the patient may be, both types of plans can be prepared. The patient-focused care plan will include any medications that will be given on either a short-term or a long-term basis. For example, goals may be written to apply ointments or patches, or for showing the patient how he can give himself an aerosol nebulizer treatment. Nursing goals may include deciding how to rotate the injection site for drugs that require repeated injections (such as insulin), or teaching the patient about specific side effects of medications that he might develop and when they should be reported.

As you write a list of the patient's problems, you may find that the problems are related. For example, a patient who cannot see very well may have a risk of falling down in an unfamiliar hospital setting. The importance of problems may also shift as the patient's condition changes. For this reason, what you do for the patient may change according to the patient's changing needs.

Factors to Think About in Planning to Give a Medication

Planning to give a medication involves four steps:
1. Decide the reason or goal for each medication to be given. (That is, what is this drug supposed to do for the patient?)
2. Learn specific information about the medication:
   * The desired action of the drug
   * Side effects that may develop
   * The usual dosage, route, and frequency
   * Situations in which the drug should not be given (contraindications)
   * Drug interactions (What is the influence of another drug given at the same time?)
3. Plan for special storage or procedures, techniques, or equipment needs.

4. Develop a teaching plan for the patient:
   * What the patient needs to know about the medication's action and side effects
   * What the patient needs to know about the administration of the medication
   * What the patient needs to report to the nurse or physician about the medication or her response

The most important step in planning is to collect and use information about the patient (his physical condition, cultural background, and expectations) and the medication. This step requires knowledge of the patient and the drug he is taking, plus your common sense and professional judgment.

Once the medication is ordered by the health care provider, the nurse must verify that the order is accurate. This is usually done by checking the medication chart, medication card, or computer medication record with the physician's original order. You will need to learn and follow the procedures of the agency where you work when checking medications. This step of checking must be done each time the medication is given. In this way, errors resulting from changes can be avoided.

The nurse must also compare the information known about the drug with the specific drug order to determine whether the drug and the dosage ordered seem correct. You should learn the patient's diagnosis to understand why the medication is being given. No part of the order or the reason for giving the medication should be unclear. Any questions about whether a drug is appropriate or safe for that patient should be answered before the medication is given. You must use good judgment in carrying out the medication order. If you decide that (1) any part of the order is incorrect or unclear, (2) the patient's condition would be made worse by the medication, (3) the physician may not have had all the information she needed about the patient when she planned the therapy, or (4) there has been a change in the patient's condition so that there is a question about whether the medication should be given, the medication should be withheld (not be given) until the question can be answered and the physician is called. If you believe there is a problem with the medication order and the physician cannot be contacted or does not change the order under question, you should notify the head nurse and the nursing supervisor as soon as possible. Most hospitals have clear policies about whom to contact, how to report this problem, and what to do next.

Memory Jogger

Medication Orders

Make certain you understand each part of the medication order.

The planning step of the nursing process is also the time to do the following:

1. Get any special equipment you need to give the medication (such as intravenous [IV] infusion bottles, tuberculin syringes, or nebulizers).
2. Review any special procedures you will need to give the medicine (such as the Z-track injection technique or the IV push policy).
3. Decide what you will need to tell the patient.

All this information can be written on the nursing care plan or in the Kardex file so that other team members can see the plan.

IMPLEMENTATION

Implementation involves following the care plan and giving the medicine accurately to the patient. This step of the nursing process requires that the nurse learn the needed information about each patient and about each drug ordered. It is your job to understand why each medication is ordered, to know about the drug's actions, and to know how to safely administer it. For example, if you add an antibiotic solution to an IV line, you need to know about the proper equipment, aseptic technique, rate of flow, and reactions with the drugs already in the IV solution, as well as how to flush the line after therapy has ended. Implementation also may require you to do specific nursing tasks before giving the medication. For example, you may take the patient's pulse before giving digitalis to make sure it may be given safely. Implementation also means that you will watch for any changes in the patient's status that may make it unwise to give the medication. For example, if a patient receiving antibiotics says she has an itchy rash on her chest and arms, you will withhold the next dose of the antibiotic until you have called the patient's physician to report the rash.

There are **six "rights" of medication administration** that the nurse must always keep in mind. You must give the right drug, at the right time, in the right dose, to the right patient, by the right route, and use the right documentation to record that the dose has been given.

Memory Jogger

The Six "Rights" of Administering a Medication

1. The right drug
2. The right time
3. The right dose
4. The right patient
5. The right route
6. The right documentation

The Right Drug

Many drug names are hard to remember and difficult to read. Also, many drugs have names that sound or look nearly the same as the names of other drugs. It is important to carefully check the spelling of the name and the dose of each medication before any drug is given. For example, digitoxin and digoxin are both cardiotonic drugs (increase the contractions of the heart), but they are quite different in dosage and duration of action. It is also easy to get confused when a medication is ordered by a trade name (such as Valium), but the pharmacy sends up the medication labeled with the generic name (diazepam). You must not assume that the correct medication has been sent without checking a reliable book or calling the pharmacy.

The drug may come in a unit-dose system package or as a prescription filled for one person, or the medication may be taken from a unit's stock. However it comes, you must read the drug label at least three times:

1. Before taking the drug from the unit dose cart or shelf
2. Before preparing or measuring the prescribed dose of medication
3. Before putting the medication back on the shelf or just before opening the medication at the time you give it to the patient

The Right Time

The drug order should say when the medication is to be given. Hospitals have policies that tell you what time drugs will be given when they are ordered (such as "every 4 hours"). You must be familiar with hospital policy and use only standard abbreviations in recording the drugs that are given (see Chapter 3 for information on standard abbreviations). To be effective in the body, many drugs must be given exactly on schedule day and night to keep the level of medication constant in the body. Other medications may only need to be given during the day.

You will also need to plan around other patient activities when you give medications. For example, if a patient is taking an anticoagulant to thin the blood and prolong the clotting time (to decrease the risk of blood clots), the medication must be given at the same time every day, and a blood test to measure the clotting time should also be taken at the same time every day and just before the next scheduled dose. Patients with infections need to have specimens taken for culture before starting antibiotic therapy. Patients undergoing evaluation of thyroid function need to have blood tests for those functions done before having gallbladder x-ray studies, which involve the use of chemicals that may confuse thyroid function study results or make them inaccurate.

Medications are usually given when there is the best chance for absorption and the least risk for side effects. This may mean that some medications should be given when the patient's stomach is empty, and others should be given with food. Some medications require that the patient not eat certain foods. (For example, imipramine has special dietary restrictions.) Others do not mix well with alcohol. (For example, metronidazole [Flagyl] causes a disulfiram reaction [see Chapter 18] if taken with alcohol.) When a patient is taking several medications, you must check to make sure the drugs do not interfere with each other. For example, some antibiotics interfere with the action of birth control pills, so a woman taking both could get pregnant if she does not use another form of contraception.

Finally, one-time-only, as-needed ("prn"), or emergency medications are especially important to check. The nurse must be certain that no one else has already given the medication and that the appropriate time interval for giving the drug has elapsed. Narcotics are often ordered as "stat" (given within a few minutes of the order) or prn medications. You will need to note on the patient's chart that you have given a narcotic so that it is clear whether or not the patient has already been given the medication.

Box 1-1 lists the main factors to remember in giving medication at the right time.

The Right Dose

The amount of medicine to be given is usually ordered for the "average" patient. A patient who is old, who has severe weight loss as a result of illness, or who is small or very obese may require changes in the usual dosages. Pediatric patients often have doses ordered depending on how much they weigh. Geriatric, or elderly, patients may be very sensitive to many medications and may require a change in dosage. If patients have other diseases or poor liver or kidney function, this may make changes in dosage necessary. Patients who have nausea or vomiting may be unable to take oral medications. Also, the physician may order the correct dosage of the medication when treatment begins, but changes in the patient's status may require that you go back to the physician to have the dose altered.

| Box 1-1 | *Factors to Think About in Giving Medication at the Right Time* |

- Understand and follow the rules of your hospital regarding the times to give scheduled drugs.
- Follow drug treatment guides to achieve the best drug absorption and to limit chances for drug interactions with other drugs. Give medications as ordered to help keep blood levels constant.
- Plan drug therapy keeping in mind other diagnostic and laboratory testing plans.
- Be especially careful in giving prn or stat medications to avoid the risk of overdosing the patient (giving too much medicine).

Giving the correct dosage of a medication also requires that you use the proper equipment (for example, insulin must be measured in an insulin syringe), the proper drug form (oral or rectal, water or oil base, scored tablets or coated capsules), and the proper concentration (0.25 mg or 2.5 mg) and that you accurately calculate the right drug dosage. Most hospitals and clinics have rules that require two nurses to check any medication dosage that must be calculated, particularly for medications such as narcotics, heparin, insulin, or IV medications.

The Right Patient

Although it seems like common sense to make certain the right patient gets the medication, errors may occur on a busy hospital unit. Four groups of patients are most at risk for errors: the pediatric patient, the geriatric patient, the non–English-speaking patient, and the very confused or critically ill patient. The common factor among these four groups is that it might be hard for them to tell the nurse who they are. They also may not understand what you are asking or that a drug is being given to them. The identification bracelets (name bands) that some patients wear may have been removed for tests or when blood was drawn and not replaced. You must be especially careful with children because they enjoy hiding, changing beds, answering to another name, and so on. Each patient should be asked his name as you check the identification bracelet. In a hospital, medications should never be given to a patient who is not wearing an identification bracelet. Nursing homes may present a special challenge for a nurse who does not know the patients well because these patients usually do not wear identification bracelets, and they may be confused or unable to answer to their name.

The Right Route

The drug order should also state how the drug should be given (route of drug administration). The nurse must never change routes without getting a new order from the physician. Although many drugs may be given by different routes, the dose is often different for each route.

The oral route is usually the route that everyone prefers if the patient is oriented (awake and able to understand). In some cases, faster delivery or a higher blood level of a drug is needed, so the medication may be given intravenously (IV) or intramuscularly (IM). There may be special precautions for medications given through these routes (such as how fast they can be given or in what dosage). Some injections should be given into the subcutaneous tissue rather than IM. Because of these differences, you would need to know how to give an injection in several different places on the body. Also, some drugs are very painful if given IM, so giving them IV is better.

When drugs to help breathing are ordered, you need to find out whether the aerosol nebulizer is to be used through the nose or the mouth. You must teach the patient the way to use the nebulizer so that the medication goes into the lungs. You will also need to teach patients how to correctly use eye drops, eardrops, ointments, lotions, shampoos, and rectal or vaginal medications.

The Right Documentation (Record Keeping)

A note about how and when you gave the drug should be made on the patient's chart as soon as possible after the drug is given. In an emergency or when a drug is only used once or twice, this is very important. Rules at your agency may require that the chart note of IM medications also include where on the body you gave the injection and any complaints made by the patient at the time of the injection. The chart note should always list the drug given, the dose, and the time it was actually given (not the time it was supposed to be given). In some offices or clinics where immunizations are given, the policy may require that the lot number listed on the bottle be recorded in the patient's chart. Progress notes should include a note about the patient's response to the medication. Any complaints or adverse effects should be noted in the chart and reported to the head nurse and the physician. When you make notes in the patient's chart about medications, you should never record medications that were not given or record them before they are given.

It must be stressed that you must never give medication prepared by another nurse. Even when you are very busy, when there is an emergency, or when you are interrupted, you cannot assume that all the "rights" are followed unless the person who prepares the medication is the one who gives the medication. Sometimes, a physician will ask you to prepare the medication for the physician to give. You may then prepare the medication, but you should go with the physician to see that the medication is given as ordered. You should also write in the notes that the physician gave the medication.

Following the rules of your hospital, using common sense, and being accurate and ethical will reduce the risk of medication error. Should an error be made, talking about it honestly and taking quick action to correct any damage are especially important to protect the patient from harm.

EVALUATION

Evaluation is the process of looking at what happens when the care plan is implemented. Evaluation requires the nurse to watch for the patient's response to a drug, noting both expected and unexpected findings. When antipyretic medications (drugs that reduce fever) are given, you need to take the patient's temperature to see if the medication reduced the fever. When antiarrhythmic agents are given to make the patient's heartbeat more regular, taking the pulse will help show how the patient responded to the medication.

Evaluation of what happens when you administer a drug helps the health care team decide whether to continue the same drug or make a change. Gathering such information is also a part of the continuing assessment of a patient during care. Thus the nursing process may be seen as a circle (see Figure 1-1). For example, taking the patient's temperature is part of the evaluation step of the nursing process, but it may also be part of the assessment step when you notice that the patient's temperature is still high, and that the patient needs more medication, a cooling bath, or some other treatment.

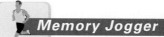

Memory Jogger

Evaluate Response to Medication
It is important to watch the patient and look for any adverse reactions, side effects, or allergic responses.

Factors to Think About in Evaluating Response to Medication

The nurse checks for two types of responses to drug therapy: therapeutic effects and adverse effects.

Therapeutic effects are seen when the drug does what it was supposed to do. If you understand why the medication is being given (the therapeutic goal of the drug), you will be able to decide whether or not that goal is being met. For example, if the patient's blood glucose is high and regular insulin is given, you should see a lower blood glucose level when the blood level is measured in 1 to 2 hours.

Adverse or side effects are seen when patients do not respond to their medications in the way they should or develop new signs or symptoms. For example, a patient with pneumonia may be given penicillin. Although this antibiotic may be working to control the infection, the patient may develop a rash, which may mean that she has an allergy to the medicine, and the penicillin must be stopped. A patient getting an anticoagulant to thin the blood must be closely watched for signs of bleeding or bruising that would indicate overdosage or overresponse to the medication. Sometimes, side effects such as nausea or vomiting may be stopped by decreasing the dosage or by giving the medication with food. Telling the physician about whether the side effects are mild or severe helps the physician decide whether the patient should keep taking the drug or it should be stopped.

Because the nurse is the health care provider who is most often with the patient, he is in an important position to notice the patient's response to drug therapy. Carefully and repeatedly evaluating the patient and writing down the findings in the patient's chart are especially important in the care of the hospitalized patient.

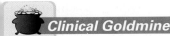

Clinical Goldmine

Critical Decision Points in Administering Drugs

- Assess the patient and clearly understand why the patient is getting that medication.
- Prepare the medication to be given (for example, check labels, prepare injections, observe proper aseptic technique with needles and syringes).
- Accurately calculate dosages.
- Administer the medication (with proper injection technique, aids to help swallowing, materials needed for topical creams).
- Record the medications given.
- Watch the patient's reaction and evaluate his response.
- Educate the patient about his medications.

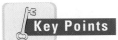

Key Points

- The nursing process is a logical process that helps you give good care to the patient and avoid making mistakes.
- The nursing process involves assessing the patient, making a nursing decision or diagnosis about what is required, planning to give medications, implementing the correct procedures, and evaluating the patient's response. These steps will become habit as you gain greater skill and experience.
- For new nurses, the nursing process gives you a safe and standard way to do things when you are learning many new and important skills.

Go to the free CD-ROM for an Audio Glossary, animations, video clips, and Review Questions for the NCLEX-PN® Examination.

evolve Be sure to visit the companion Evolve website at http://evolve.elsevier.com/Edmunds/LPN/ for WebLinks, a link to the top 200 drugs by prescription, and sign-up pages for newsletter drug updates.

CRITICAL THINKING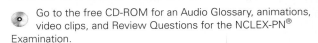

1. Identify each of the following as either objective (O) or subjective (S) information:
   a. The patient complains of pain in the abdomen.
   b. The nurse takes the patient's blood pressure and determines that it is too high.
   c. The nurse counts rapid respirations and retractions of the chest, notices cyanosis of the skin, and concludes that the patient is short of breath.
   d. After palpating the patient's abdomen, the nurse reports that it is tender to the touch.
   e. The patient complains of being "too fat."
   f. Four-year-old Sean's thermometer registers a temperature of 102° F.
   g. After weighing Mr. Tracy this morning, the nurse reports that he has gained 2 pounds in 6 days.
   h. Ms. Jackson says that almost every day she has trouble breathing or "catching" her breath.
   i. A 50-year-old female patient asks for aspirin, saying she is getting "hot flashes."
   j. Mr. Clark tells the nurse, "My heart is really pounding!"

2. You are assigned to give medications to eight different patients this morning. Write a paragraph describing the step-by-step procedure you would use to ensure that you are observing the six rights of drug administration.

3. Describe four things a nurse might do for a patient taking morphine that would fall under the category of assessment.

4. What is the difference between planning and evaluation in drug administration? Are they sometimes the same thing? Give examples of each.

5. What would you do if one of your patients refused a prescribed medication?

6. Why does the nurse have to keep repeating assessment of the patient receiving medications?

7. Identify three areas of assessment necessary in completing a patient's drug history.

2 Patient Teaching and Health Literacy

After reading and studying this chapter, you should be able to do the following:

1. List some of the problems that patients have when they cannot read or understand health instructions.
2. Identify the common causes of patient medication errors.
3. Describe the process of teaching patients about medications.

Key Terms

Be sure to check out the bonus material on the free CD-ROM, including selected audio pronunciations.

compliant (kŏm-PLĪ-ănt, p. 9)
concordance (kŭn-KŌR-dăns, p. 9)
health disparity (dĭs-PĂR-ĭ-tē, p. 10)
health literacy (p. 10)
literacy (LĬT-ĕr-ă-sē, p. 10)
noncompliant (NŎN-kŏm-plī-ănt, p. 9)

OVERVIEW

One of the basic tasks of the nursing role is the teaching of patients. If patients are to have success in taking their drugs, they must learn information about the drugs themselves and how to take the drugs properly. Patients are not always willing or ready to learn, so the nurse must learn new skills to talk to patients effectively. This can be very difficult sometimes when patients do not speak English, or have poor reading or writing skills.

The reason we teach patients about their diseases, their drugs, and what to expect when they take the drugs is to help patients improve their health. Patients who do not clearly understand basic health information have less ability to carry out the treatment plan. Patients who are unable to carry out the treatment plan, for whatever reason, have greater risk of not getting well or having problems.

COMPLIANCE, NONCOMPLIANCE, AND CONCORDANCE

Often a patient is said to be **compliant** when she follows a prescribed plan of care and **noncompliant** when she does not follow the plan. However, these terms are no longer preferred. A term that does not judge the patient is **concordance**: when the nurse, patient, family, and pharmacist work together as a team to reduce problems with taking drugs (MarketLetter, 1997).

There are two basic reasons a patient has difficulty meeting treatment goals:

1. The patient does not understand what she should do.
2. The patient understands what she should do but fails to do it:
   - She may not believe that she needs to carry out the plan.
   - She believes she should do something but fails to carry out the plan.
   - She believes she should do something but does not have money, time, or ability to do it.

When you teach the patient, you should have some ability to discuss both of these reasons, with the goal of helping the patient make informed decisions about taking her drugs. (See Chapter 5 for further discussion of factors contributing to problems with following treatment plans, including cultural and life span considerations.)

COMMUNICATING WITH THE PATIENT

In the busy health care setting, it is often difficult to find time to talk with patients. In addition, many of our patients are from different countries or cultures, and may have different languages and beliefs that affect their ability to understand or talk about their health. Many nurses also are from different countries and cultures. This means that their beliefs about what is important or harmful may not be the same. Even words used by both patient and nurse might have different meanings to each.

Although speaking clearly to patients is important, much of the teaching that patients need will be given in writing. Thus, how and what is written is very important if we wish to send the right message.

We say that a person is literate when he has the ability to read, write, and speak in English, to do math, and to solve problems at the level necessary to function on the job and in society. Over the last 10 years, research has shown that many people in the United States do not have the basic level of **literacy** to allow them to do these tasks. This is a far bigger problem than anyone realized. In 1993, the National Adult Literacy Study reported that 40 million adult Americans scored at level 1, the lowest of five levels of literacy, and another 50 million scored at level 2. People are placed in these two lowest levels if they have trouble finding pieces of information or numbers in a long text, putting many pieces of information together into one story, or finding two or more numbers in a chart and doing a math problem. These levels are roughly equal to being able to read at about the fifth grade level.

Low literacy also limits a person's ability to deal with the health care setting, which over the years has become more complex and which uses written materials that are even more difficult than those used in everyday life. In the past, the average reading level of the information about health care that is given to patients was at the 11th to 14th grade level, but the average person's reading level has been found to be much lower. Even patients who read at the college level have been found to prefer medical information written at the seventh grade level. Recent research suggests that written information given to most patients should be written at the fifth to the seventh grade level if we wish to make it more likely that the information will be understood. This will be a challenge.

We have also learned that many patients do not have high levels of **health literacy**—the ability to understand and use information that is important in keeping them healthy. This may mean they cannot read a prescription to learn how many pills they should take, they cannot figure out when their next appointment is, or they cannot read a map to help them get where they need to go. It often means that they cannot read the information that nurses or doctors send home with them that tells them about their disease, the medicines they are taking, and important things they need to know. Thus, they often do not have the information they need to help them get well or stay well.

Although there may be large numbers of people in the United States with low literacy, certain groups may have more problems than others. People who are elderly, belong to some races or ethnic backgrounds, live in certain areas of the country, have a low income level, or are in prison may have a lower literacy level. The reason these individuals may have low literacy levels is usually that they have not been able to stay in school and get an education.

It makes sense that individuals who have low literacy levels often have poor health outcomes. Their inability to read and write puts them at higher risk for disease and disability. This situation is called **health disparity.** Unfortunately, such individuals might die from a disease several years before someone else simply because of this difference in ability to read and write.

Because of these factors, it is clear that there is no more important teaching than that which nurses give to the patient about his disease and its drug treatment. This teaching is a big factor in whether the drug therapy that is ordered will be effective. Patient difficulty with treatment plans is a major problem that health care workers must face. Good, careful teaching of the patient should help reduce such problems. This is very true when medications are involved because this information is usually complex and often given in writing.

THE PROCESS OF PATIENT EDUCATION

ASSESSMENT OF PATIENT EDUCATION NEEDS

The fact that a nurse knows that a patient needs information does not mean that the patient is aware of that need, or in fact, expects to learn from the nurse. Patient education has to involve both teacher and learner and is not effective if one or the other is not ready to be involved. A study that examined what patients want to know about their prescriptions (Morris et al., 1987) found that patients showed one of four types of behavior when seeking drug information, as shown in Table 2-1. This study suggests that patients go to the person they feel is the best source of information or with whom they feel most comfortable.

Some studies have found differences between the information that clinicians see as important and the information patients want. It may be particularly difficult to discuss some of the serious side effects that might be caused by a drug. Nurses may not want to discuss some of these effects for fear of scaring patients from taking their drugs. However, research has shown just the opposite result with many patients. Patients who are given more information are better able to correctly recognize side effects should they occur (Carter, 1992).

More emphasis is being placed on the use of computers both in learning the needs of patients and in meeting those needs. Whereas many first believed that computers would not be useful for people with poor literacy skills, the research findings show the opposite. Computers are being used to conduct health surveys and have been shown to result in more honest reports of certain health behaviors and to be accepted by people with poor literacy skills (Slater et al., 1994). A few

Table 2-1	*Behaviors of People Seeking Drug Information*	
CLASSIFICATION	PERCENTAGE	CHARACTERISTICS
Uninformed	34%	This group tended to be older, was less likely to have received written or verbal counseling from a provider or pharmacist, and did not seem to recognize the results of improper drug use.
Rely on physician	40%	This group took information as given from the physician and was most likely to get prescriptions filled at chain pharmacies.
Rely on pharmacist	19%	This was the youngest group; they got information at the pharmacy and saw few barriers to getting information.
Questioners	7%	This group included those who were more likely to receive information from books or magazines. They required clear information about specific questions and appeared to be the most difficult group to satisfy.

Modified from Morris LA, et al: A segmentational analysis of prescription drug information seeking, *Med Care* 25:953-64, 1987.

years ago, a study found that patients might actually be more comfortable revealing personal information on a computer than to a human being—even though they know the information will be seen later by health care workers.

The important items to include in the patient teaching process include the following:

1. Assess the patient's specific needs to learn. Often the nurse may wish to provide information about a new treatment plan or medication, or the patient may ask direct questions. Teaching materials should then be written that take into account the specific needs of the patient, including her knowledge, reading ability, beliefs, and experiences.

2. Assess the patient's willingness to learn. This requires getting to know the patient and talking with him about his interest in learning. The patient must see a need for the patient education he receives.

3. Together, the patient and nurse decide what needs to be taught. This information should be written down as objectives that can be measured (that is, you can determine when they are met). For example, the objective "Learn about adverse reactions of the medication" is not measurable. The objective "List 5 possible adverse reactions" is measurable.

4. Select a teaching method: verbal instructions, written materials, audiovisual materials, or a combination of methods. The method and pace of the teaching must be designed for each patient, recognizing the differences in the ways that people learn and the rate at which they learn (Rankin, 2001). Different teaching skills may be needed at different times for the same patient. Teaching should be carried out in small amounts over several meetings.

5. Have the patient repeat information back, show a procedure, or follow through on a behavior to determine how well she has learned the material. Giving feedback comments to the patient helps her realize what she has learned or identify areas in which she still needs help. Giving verbal praise, being excited about good compliance, or showing support for a change in behavior may be the most effective type of feedback for patients. Negative or fear-arousing comments may also be effective, but must be used rarely and cautiously. Removing blocks to compliance with the treatment plan helps get the patient to cooperate. This may be done by giving the patient special pill containers, making changes in the time medicines are taken to fit in with the patient's activities, or getting the patient drug samples or coupons to reduce costs.

6. Remembering to use a variety of teaching methods is more effective than using one single teaching method.

PREPARING A TEACHING PLAN

The patient's need for information is based on the patient's disease, the treatment plan, and the patient-nurse relationship. When a patient is first diagnosed with a problem, education must start with what has gone wrong and what is likely to happen. It is only when the patient understands what has happened to him that he can move on to consideration of what to do about it.

As patients begin any therapy, there is a good deal of information that needs to be shared regarding what they think, what they expect, and any choices they might have. For example, starting the patient on a new medication requires a lot of teaching. It is clearly not possible to provide all of the information the patient might need in one teaching session. Instead, you need to have a plan in mind for the things that need to be covered, and this plan needs to be shared with the patient (Carter, 1992) (Box 2-1). Additional teaching will be required when drugs are changed or the dosage or schedule is altered, or when changes in patient condition warrant further adjustment in therapy. Therefore, teaching becomes specific to what the patient requires, but it is always given in quantities that the patient can handle.

Box 2-1 | *Key Information for Patients Receiving Medications*

- Drug name (generic and brand)
- Intended use and expected action
- Route, dosage form, dosage, and specific administration schedule (hours of day to take)
- Special directions for storage or preparation of medication
- Special directions for administration of medication
- Common side effects
- What the patient should do if there are side effects
- Possible drug-drug, drug-food, or drug-alcohol interactions
- Information about getting a prescription refill
- Action to be taken if the patient misses taking a dose
- Special precautions when taking medication (driving, actions requiring alertness)
- Other information particular to the patient or drug
- When to return to the health care provider
- How the patient will know that the drug is doing what it should do

Data from Carter BL: Patient education and chronic disease monitoring. In Herfindal ER, Gourley DR, Hart LL, editors: *Clinical pharmacy and therapeutics,* ed 5, Baltimore, 1992, Williams & Wilkins; and Selby MR: *An in-depth study of educational strategies for increased patient compliance with medications,* unpublished scholarly paper written to meet graduation requirement, University of Maryland at Baltimore, School of Nursing, 1983.

Informed consent is something we assume in the process of giving a medication to a patient. The nurse shares a legal obligation with other health care providers to make certain that the patient understands her condition, the treatment, and the risks and benefits of the treatment plans. The law requires that the amount and type of information provided to the patient be "reasonable." It is up to the nurse who is given the task of teaching the patient to determine what is reasonable for a specific patient to understand, and the nurse may be held legally responsible if he fails to teach the patient this information.

In the clinic or hospital, teaching often happens in response to a patient's question, and the nurse may need to respond quickly without time to prepare, plan, or consider overall what the patient needs to know. Using scientific or nursing language or jargon, giving too much technical detail, or being vague all waste the teaching effort. Although it is impossible to avoid answering questions even if they take you by surprise, it is important for you to also write a plan that will cover what will be taught, how it will be taught, and how you will know when the patient has learned the material.

The nurse should write specific objectives to guide teaching. The objectives must state the new behaviors that will occur because of changes in the patient's thinking or understanding. The best objectives are clearly stated by describing the desired performance and what makes it adequate. Specific goals help clarify for patients what they are to do. For example, "Blood pressure will decrease to the diastolic reading of less than 90 mm Hg within 3 months" is a specific, measurable goal based on national guidelines. As patients and nurses create objectives together, the nurse has a chance to evaluate the patient's knowledge, understanding, and general desire to change behavior.

IMPLEMENTING THE TEACHING PLAN

Both the content of patient education and the process of patient education are important to think about in planning the specific teaching-learning objectives. Many patients are feeling fear when they first learn about their diagnosis. Stress and anxiety increase the confusion they often feel and interfere with their ability to learn.

In order to avoid creating more stress for the patient, teaching needs to be given in a systematic manner. It needs to be provided in a timely way and in a quiet and unhurried setting that gives the patient a chance to ask questions. It is hard to find a setting like that in today's busy health care system. Research has suggested that people are able to remember three major things that they are taught in any one session. Also, they generally remember those three things in the order in which they are presented. If you keep this in mind when developing a teaching plan, you can set aside small periods of time to use for teaching a few, very specific things. At future visits, you can review the information presented in an earlier session to find out how much the patient remembers before you move on to the next phase of teaching that has been planned.

Researchers have made a special effort to determine ways that nurses can help increase medication compliance. The results of this research encourage the nurse to use a variety of ways to give patients information about their medications. Some of these methods include telling patients the necessary information, reviewing written instructions with them, and using audiovisual aids such as audiotapes, videotapes, CD-ROMs, or computer teaching systems that may use animation, color, music, and action figures to help the patient learn the information.

Verbal Education

Verbal education is often direct teaching, with the nurse telling the patient information and then giving the patient a chance to ask questions. Patients with chronic diseases such as diabetes or hypertension who have extensive needs for teaching may also be brought together in small groups for part of their teaching experiences.

Written Information

Written information can include special labels for prescription bottles, materials inserted in the drug package, or special materials or booklets that are prepared to accompany the medicine. Preprinted instructions about medicines are available from manufacturers, pharmacy associations or some medical associations, and private companies. Written information may also be created by the nurse, hospital, or clinic, or may come from a professional group such as the Arthritis Foundation or the Asthma and Allergy Foundation of America.

Many books and preprinted patient information materials are already available from commercial sources (Box 2-2). With the growing use of the Internet, information about new products is widely available and often may be downloaded by the nurse to create high-quality handouts that may be changed as necessary for specific patients. In fact, the problem is not in finding patient teaching materials, but in evaluating their quality and how they may be used. Many publications are written at far too high a grade level for the general reading ability of many patients, and thus are not very helpful.

Box 2-2 | *Patient Teaching Resources*

Many of the best texts in this area are very old but are still currently available through commercial sources.

Allen LV, Berardi RR: *Handbook of nonprescription drugs: an interactive approach to self-care,* ed 13, Washington, DC, 2002, American Pharmaceutical Association.

Andrus MR, Roth MT: Health literacy: a review, *Pharmacotherapy* 22(3): 282-302, 2002.

Baker DW, Gazmararian JA, Sudano J et al: Health literacy and performance on the Mini-Mental State Examination, *Aging Ment Health* 6(1):22-9, 2002.

Barker LR, Burton JR, Zieve PD et al: *Principles of ambulatory medicine,* ed 6, Baltimore, 2002, Lippincott, Williams & Wilkins.

Canobbio MM: *Mosby's handbook of patient teaching,* ed 2, St Louis, 2000, Mosby.

Carter BL: Patient education and chronic disease monitoring, In Herfindal ER, Gourley DR, Hart LL, editors: *Clinical pharmacy and therapeutics,* ed 5, Baltimore, 1992, William & Wilkins.

Cramer JA, Spiker B, editors: *Patient compliance in medical practice and clinical trials,* New York, 1991, Raven Press.

Culbertson VL, Arthur TG, Rhodes PJ, Rhodes RS: Consumer preferences for verbal and written medication information, *Drug Intell Clin Pharm* 22(5): 390-6, 1988.

Doak CC, Doak LG, Root JH: *Teaching patients with low literacy skills,* ed 2, Philadelphia, 1996, JB Lippincott.

Ferri FF: *Ferri's patient teaching guides.* St. Louis, 1999, Mosby.

Gannon W, Hildebrandt E: A winning combination: women, literacy, and participation in health care, *Health Care Women Int* 23(6-7):754-60, 2002.

Gausman Benson J, Forman WB: Comprehension of written health care information in an affluent geriatric retirement community: use of the Test of Functional Health Literacy, *Gerontology* 48(2):93-7, 2002.

Griffith HW: *Instructions for patients* (Spanish version), ed 5, Philadelphia, 1997, WB Saunders.

Haworth K: *Patient teaching made incredibly easy,* Springhouse, Pa, 1998, Springhouse Publishing.

Kalichman SC, Benotsch EG, Weinhardt L et al: Health-related Internet use, coping, social support, and health indicators in people living with HIV/AIDS: preliminary results from a community survey, *Health Psychol* 22(1):111-6, 2001.

McKenry LM: *Mosby's pharmacology patient teaching guides,* St Louis, 1999, Mosby.

Moore SW: *Griffith's instructions for patients,* ed 7, Philadelphia, 2005, WB Saunders.

Rankin SH, Stallings KD, London F: *Patient education in health and illness,* ed 5, Philadelphia, 2005, Lippincott, Williams & Wilkins.

Redman BK: *The practice of patient education,* ed 9, St Louis, 2001, Mosby.

Sackett DL, Haynes RB, Guyatt GH, Tugwell P: Helping patients follow the treatments you prescribe. In *Clinical epidemiology: a basic science for clinical medicine,* Boston, 1991, Little, Brown.

Schmitt B: *Instructions for pediatric patients,* ed 2, Philadelphia, 1998, WB Saunders.

Sodeman W, Sodeman T: *Instructions for geriatric patients,* ed 3, Philadelphia, 2005, WB Saunders.

Springhouse: *Patient teaching reference manual,* ed 2, Philadelphia, 2001, Lippincott, Williams & Wilkins.

Steckel SB: *Patient contracting,* Norwalk, Conn, 1982, Appleton-Century-Crofts.

Teaching patients with acute conditions, Springhouse, Pa, 1992, Springhouse.

Teaching patients with chronic conditions, Springhouse, PA, 1992, Springhouse.

U.S. Pharmacopeial Convention: *Advice for the patient* (USP DI Vol II), Rockville, Md, 2002, Author. (Yearly, with monthly updates. For information call 800-227-8772.)

U.S. Pharmacopeial Convention: *Patient education leaflets* (USP DI), Rockville, MD, 2002, Author. (Yearly, with monthly updates or as USP Leaflet Diskette, a software product. For information call 800-227-8772.)

To write your own materials or to determine if published handouts are something you want to use for your patients, you should keep the following principles in mind:

- Be sure that the goals of the handout are stated in the material.
- Limit the content to one or two objectives. State what the patient will learn and do after reading the information.
- Emphasize the desired behavior rather than the medical facts.
- Use clear headings, lots of white space, and photographs or realistic illustrations to attract the patient's attention and tell the message.
- Always use common words and not medical words. Use familiar words.
- Develop materials that involve the patient: Ask patients to do, write, say, or show something to demonstrate their understanding.
- Whenever possible, prepare materials with the help of patients who have low health literacy skills. Their comments will help you make the information more appropriate.
- Limit the number of three-syllable words in the handout to decrease the grade level of writing. To aid understanding, write short, simple sentences without complex grammar.

Particular attention should be paid to making sure to include the major facts that each patient should know about his medications. The handout should be short; teaching has been shown to be most successful when the information is on no more than one page, front and back. When possible, the material should be presented in lists rather than in paragraphs. Key items or warnings should be highlighted with bullets or symbols. The content should be specific and written in words that will be familiar to the patient. The print size should be fairly large (at least 14 points) if elderly patients will use the material.

If only one handout will be used for all patients receiving a given drug, the readability should be below the eighth grade level—preferably at the fourth grade level. Or, two or three handouts at different ability levels could be written for each drug. Many computer software programs have a way to determine how difficult material is to read. Keeping sentences short and choosing simple words makes it much easier to develop reading materials at a simple and basic reading level. In some locations, handouts may be needed in several languages.

Audiovisual Resources

Audiovisual programs such as slide-tape programs, videocassettes, and CD-ROMs are also available for patient teaching. Some patients will be able to use the Internet to collect information, and this allows patients to select what they want and download it for future reference.

Television ads that are created by drug companies for patients are called direct-to-consumer advertising. Patients may have many questions or inaccurate information because they have seen these ads. When patients raise questions because of these ads, this is a good opportunity for you to assess what they know and to provide correct information.

Research has shown that a combination of spoken and written information, or talking to the patient along with showing audiovisual aids, is usually better than only giving the patient written materials. This is very important for patients with new prescriptions (Culbertson et al., 1988). Giving only written information does not help in meeting the patient's needs.

Nurse and Patient Use of the Internet

One of the biggest challenges for health care workers is finding up-to-date information to use in teaching. Textbooks and journal articles may be years or months old before being printed. New information is available every day. Thus, it is required that the nurse-teacher make certain she is giving the latest information. This task is easier than it has been in the past because of the Internet. The Internet is becoming a source of up-to-date health information, not only for nurses, but for patients as well. Many Internet sites meet the needs of both.

A number of sites offer directions for using the Internet. They range from The Internet Learning Tree and Beginners Central, which focus on the basics, to the more advanced Internet Web Text Index (Table 2-2).

Although many business websites have accurate information, others may be more interested in selling

Table 2-2 | *Websites That Offer Information for Navigating the Web*

WEBSITE	URL ADDRESS
Beginners Central	*www.northernwebs.com/bc*
The HelpWeb	*www.imagescape.com/helpweb*
The Internet Learning Tree	*www.walthowe.com/navnet/*
Internet Web Text Index	*www.december.com/web/text*
Too Old for Computers?	*web.pdx.edu/~psu01435/tooold.html*
Welcome to Folks Online	*www.folksonline.com*

something. Commercial or business sites are identifiable by the use of "com" near the end of their web addresses. They often scatter ads throughout their web pages, charge fees or dues, or promote things to buy. The letters "org" identify a nonprofit group, "gov" a government agency, and "edu" an educational site.

EVALUATION OF LEARNING

Patient education in general is done to change behavior and increase satisfaction. When objectives are written for each patient, the behavior change that is required is clearly stated. Thus, it should be simple to determine the amount of learning that has taken place. When blood sugar levels do not come down and stay down to the desired level, when blood pressure remains high, or when weight is not lost, there is failure somewhere in the education process. Sometimes the process breaks down when a patient does not understand what to do, cannot afford the treatment plan, or loses confidence in her ability to change. Whatever the problem, the nurse must attempt to discover where the process went wrong.

During the teaching process, it is important to have the patient involved. Active questioning and discussion helps the learner remember what was taught. Teaching that is more active and provides more sensory involvement (like handling things, hearing things, eating something, and so forth) allows more effective learning to take place.

Throughout the teaching process, it is important for the nurse to summarize, repeat, and keep it simple. You should check for understanding as the teaching continues by having the patient repeat back the important points. It is important not to create fear or stress when quizzing patients on information that has been discussed (Barker, Burton, and Zieve, 2002). You should note in the patient's record what has been taught. This note should list the important topics covered, state what written material was given to the patient, and provide your view of the patient's level of understanding and anything you believe shows the patient's willingness to carry out the treatment plan.

Specific things that might also help improve the success of drug treatment plans for most patients include developing plans that have frequent nurse-patient contacts, using reminder cards, giving drug tests, making the plan fit the patient's needs and culture, giving feedback and encouragement, and encouraging the patient to be actively involved in things like taking blood pressures at home, or having a behavior contract with the nurse (Steckel, 1982). These methods should be kept in mind when writing objectives for what might be taught and evaluating what learning has taken place.

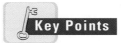
Key Points

- Research concludes that patient education is an essential activity in which the nurse should be engaged.
- Today, more than ever, it is important to teach patients well.
- Providing patient education gives patients the power to more fully become partners in making and meeting their own health care goals.

Go to the free CD-ROM for an Audio Glossary, animations, video clips, and Review Questions for the NCLEX-PN® Examination.

evolve   Be sure to visit the companion Evolve website at http://evolve.elsevier.com/Edmunds/LPN/ for WebLinks, a link to the top 200 drugs by prescription, and sign-up pages for newsletter drug updates.

CRITICAL THINKING ❓

1. What would be your first consideration if you needed to develop a teaching plan for Mr. Brown, who was newly diagnosed with type 1 diabetes?

2. Give some examples of ways in which the nurse's communication techniques can affect outcomes of patient teaching.

3. Presentation of information in a teaching plan is crucial to patient understanding and compliance. Consider the following examples of commonly used phrases. How might these be modified to ensure greater patient understanding and compliance?
   a. "Take this tablet twice a day."
   b. "You can have three pieces of bread a day on your new diet."
   c. "A dish of macaroni equals one serving."
   d. "You need to drink at least three glasses of water a day."
   e. "It might be a good idea to cut down to two cups of coffee a day."

3 Legal Aspects Affecting the Administration of Medications

Objectives

After reading and studying this chapter, you should be able to do the following:

1. List the names of major federal laws about drugs and drug use.
2. Explain what is meant by "scheduled drugs" or "controlled substances" and give examples of drugs in the different schedules.
3. List rules of states and agencies that affect how nurses give drugs.
4. Explain how the nurse is responsible for controlled substances.
5. List what information is included in a medication order or prescription.
6. Define and give examples of the four different types of medication orders.
7. Describe the differences between authority, responsibility, and accountability.
8. List what you need to do if you make a medication error.

Key Terms

Be sure to check out the bonus material on the free CD-ROM, including selected audio pronunciations.

controlled substances (p. 16)
delegation (dĕl-ĕ-GĀ-shŭn, p. 20)
engineering controls (ĕn-jĭn-ĔR-ĭng, p. 28)
legal responsibility (p. 20)
nurse practice act (p. 20)
over-the-counter (OTC) medications (mĕd-ĭ-KĀ-shŭnz, p. 16)
physical dependence (FĬZ-ĭ-kăl, p. 18)
prescription, or legend, drugs (prĭ-SKRĬP-shŭn, p. 16)
problem-oriented medical record (POMR) (p. 22)
professional responsibility (p. 20)
psychologic dependence (sī-kō-LŌJ-ĭk, p. 18)
scheduled drugs (p. 16)

PHARMACOLOGY AND REGULATIONS

Nurses who give medications have three levels of rules to follow:

1. Federal laws, which describe rules that control how certain drugs may be given
2. State laws and regulations, or rules, which say who may prescribe, dispense (give a supply), and administer or give medications, and the process to be used
3. Individual hospital or agency rules, which may include other guidelines or policies about how and when drugs are given and the records that must be kept about use of the drug

FEDERAL LEGISLATION

Laws passed by Congress try to make medications as safe as possible for patients to take and to make sure that the drug does what it claims to do (effectiveness). Congress created the Food and Drug Administration (FDA) to watch over the testing, approval, and marketing of new drugs. Many laws have been passed to control drugs that might easily be abused and are dangerous. Table 3-1 lists some of the major federal drug laws that have been passed.

Federal laws created three drug categories in the United States:

1. **Controlled substances,** which include major pain killers (narcotics) and some sedatives or tranquilizers that can only be prescribed by someone with a special license
2. **Prescription, or legend, drugs** such as antibiotics and oral contraceptives
3. **Over-the-counter (OTC) medications,** which patients may buy without a prescription

Controlled Substances

The greatest number of regulations are written for controlled substances because they are so commonly abused. After the Controlled Substances Act of 1970 classed these medications into five "schedules," they became known as **scheduled drugs.** The degree of control, the record keeping required, the order forms, and other regulations are different for each of these five classes. Table 3-2 describes the five drug schedules, with examples of medications in each category. Sometimes the drugs are moved from one class to another if it is clear that they have become more or less of a problem.

Table 3-1 *Summary of Major Federal Drug Legislation*

TITLE OF LEGISLATION	YEAR	DESCRIPTION OF LEGISLATION
Harrison Narcotic Act	1914	Limited the indiscriminate use of addictive drugs. Regulated the importation, manufacture, sale, and use of opium, cocaine, and their compounds and derivatives. Amended many times and finally repealed and replaced by the Controlled Substances Act in 1970.
Federal Food, Drug and Cosmetic Act	1938	Authorized the Food and Drug Administration of the Department of Health and Human Services to determine the safety of drugs before marketing, to determine labeling specifications, and to ensure that advertising claims are met.
Durham-Humphrey Amendment	1951	Restricts the number of prescriptions that can be refilled.
Kefauver-Harris Amendments	1962	Provides greater control and surveillance of clinical testing and distribution of investigational drugs. A product must be proven to be both safe and effective before it may be released for sale.
Comprehensive Drug Abuse Prevention and Control Act (Controlled Substances Act)	1970	Composite law that repealed almost 50 other laws. Designed to improve the administration and regulation of manufacturing, distributing, and dispensing of controlled drugs. The Drug Enforcement Administration (DEA) was created to enforce the Controlled Substances Act, gather intelligence, train investigators, and conduct research on potentially dangerous drugs and drug abuse.
Needlestick Safety and Prevention Act	2001	Requires hospitals to have programs to prevent needlestick injuries, document them when they occur, and purchase safe equipment regardless of cost.

Table 3-2 *Controlled Substance Schedule*

SCHEDULE	POTENTIAL FOR ABUSE	COMMENTS AND EXAMPLES
I	High	No currently accepted medical use in the United States. Lack of accepted safety for use under medical supervision. *Examples:* hashish, heroin, lysergic acid diethylamide (LSD), marijuana, peyote, 2,5-demethoxy-4-methamphetamine (STP).
II	High	Abuse potential that may lead to severe psychologic or physical dependence. *Examples:* amphetamines, meperidine, methadone, methaqualone, morphine, pentobarbital, oxycodone (Percocet), secobarbital.
III	High but less than I or II	Abuse potential that may lead to moderate or low physical dependence or high psychologic dependence. *Examples:* glutethimide (Doriden), aspirin with codeine (Empirin with codeine), aspirin with butalbital and caffeine (Fiorinal), methyprylon (Noludar), paregoric, acetaminophen with codeine (Tylenol with Codeine).
IV	Low compared with III	Abuse potential that may lead to limited physical or psychologic dependence. *Examples:* lorazepam (Ativan), diazepam (Valium).
V	Low compared with IV	Abuse potential that may lead to limited physical or psychologic dependence. *Examples:* diphenoxylate with atropine sulfate (Lomotil), guaifenesin with codeine sulfate (Robitussin A-C).

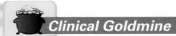

Clinical Goldmine

Dependence

Physical dependence refers to the physiologic need for a medication to relieve shaking, pain, or other symptoms. **Psychologic dependence,** on the other hand, refers to anxiety, stress, or tension that is felt if the patient does not have the medication. One type of dependency often leads to the other; they are often found together in the same individual.

Federal and state laws make it a crime for anyone to possess controlled substances without a prescription. Each state has a practice act that lists which health care providers may dispense and write prescriptions for controlled substances. Pharmacists usually dispense the medications; physicians, dentists, osteopaths, nurse practitioners, physician assistants, and sometimes nurse-midwives may write prescriptions. Licensed practical nurses or licensed vocational nurses (LPNs/LVNs) may give controlled substances to a patient only under the direction of a health care provider who is licensed to administer or prescribe these drugs. Student nurses work under the delegated authority of the registered nurse (RN). The RN is responsible for any errors that might be made.

Nurses may not have controlled substances in their possession unless one of the following conditions is met:
- The nurse is giving them to the patient for whom they are ordered.
- The nurse is the person who has been chosen to be in control of the supply of medications of a ward or department.
- The nurse is the patient for whom a physician has prescribed the medication.

Each state and health care agency has rules that cover the ordering, receiving, storing, and record keeping of controlled substances. All scheduled or controlled drugs must be counted every 8 hours. Records must be kept for every pill or ampule. Agency policy will decide which nurses will be held responsible for handing over the control of these medications from one shift to the next and for how medications will be counted and checked. All controlled substances ordered for a patient but not used while she is in the hospital go back to the pharmacy when the patient is discharged.

In a time when drug abuse is so common, the nurse who has responsibility for the controlled substances must remain alert. Abuse is not limited to patients. Some health care professionals may not be able to resist such a large supply of medication and will seek to hide the theft of a patient's medication. Things that might cause suspicion include a pattern in which a nurse says he drops or spills medications a lot and records that

show that patients got large or frequent doses of medications on certain shifts but the patients report no relief from pain. In these cases, you might wonder if the patients are really getting the medication.

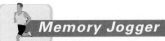

Memory Jogger

Federal Regulations

The nurse must know federal rules about giving medication.

The rules that govern controlled substances are very clear and very strict. Breaking the rules is very serious. If it is found that you have violated the Controlled Substance laws, you may be punished by a fine, a prison sentence, or both. A nurse with a drug abuse problem will lose her nursing license and may have a hard time getting it back. Nurses who do not report their suspicion that other nurses may be breaking the rules risk their own jobs. In most states, the state nursing association has a program to help nurses who have drug abuse or other problems that affect their ability to carry out their nursing duties.

Prescription, or Legend, Drugs

The FDA has decided that many drugs are so dangerous that their use must be carefully controlled. Access to these drugs is provided by a few health care professionals (physicians, dentists, and nurse practitioners). This control is through a written prescription or order that must be written before the drug may be given. Prescription drugs make up most of the medications the nurse will be giving to patients in a hospital. Prescription drugs are carefully tested before they are put on the market. The drugs have been shown to be safe and effective. However, even though much may be known about a particular medication, each patient is different and may have a somewhat different reaction to the drug. Pediatric patients, elderly patients, and critically ill patients may be weak and be more likely to have problems taking a drug. The nurse must be alert and watch for signs that the drug is working the way it should, as well as for adverse reactions that may develop. Because the patient often gets several drugs at the same time, the interaction among the drugs may make it hard to tell how each drug affects the patient. Although a lot of research about drugs has been done, many drugs have not been tested to see if they are safe and effective for children.

The Omnibus Budget Reconciliation Acts of 1989, 1990, and 1991 placed further controls on drugs for Medicare or older patients. More and more, insurance or government groups who pay for drugs limit the types and numbers of drugs that may be ordered to those on a preferred drug list. Because new or brand-name drugs usually cost more, the preferred drug list may require the use of cheaper generic drugs to control costs.

Over-the-Counter Medications

The FDA has also found that many drugs do not need a prescription and may be easily purchased at a drugstore or pharmacy. These drugs often come in a low dosage, and they have low risk to the patient. Warning labels and special information supplied with these drugs make them safer for the average buyer. These drugs also have low risk for abuse. They are used to treat many common human illnesses: colds, allergies, headaches, burns, constipation, upset stomach, and so on. These drugs are often the first thing patients try before they go to the doctor. Although OTC medications are widely available, they are not without risk. Like all drugs, some may produce adverse effects in some patients. They may also have "hidden" chemicals such as caffeine or stimulants that may produce problems if taken with other drugs. Talking to patients about the use of OTC medications is very important for patients who are already taking many prescription drugs. New federal laws for labeling of these products will make more information available about the drug and make it easier for the patient to understand.

Many OTC drugs are also given in the hospital for minor problems that patients may have. Although these medications do not require a prescription for purchase, a physician's order is required before they may be given in the hospital. In fact, without an order, a patient in a hospital cannot take even his own OTC medicines that he brought with him to the hospital.

In recent years, many people have become interested in herbal products. Research shows that most people will try an herbal product at some time in their lives. Health food stores, grocery stores, and pharmacies all carry some of these products. Some people take these herbal products instead of their prescription drugs, and some use them along with their prescription drugs. Although research may someday find that these products are safe and effective, at present these herbal products are not regulated, standardized, or tested for safety and effectiveness. Because the federal government considers herbal products to be supplements rather than drugs, there are no regulations to control how they are made. There is no way to know if one leaf that is ground up and made into a pill will work the same as another leaf that is ground up. Also, you cannot easily tell how much of the herbal product is in each pill, or even if each pill in a bottle contains the same amount of the product. Because research on these products is only beginning, little is known about side effects, and it is even hard to tell if some of them actually have the intended effect. Finally, adverse effects may occur when a patient takes herbal products and prescription drugs at the same time. You must be careful in what you say to patients about these herbal products because very little is known about them.

Because of the high cost of drugs in the United States, some patients try to buy drugs from other countries where they both cost less and are easier to buy—usually in Mexico or Canada. Although this may be good for patients, in some cases, there is a risk that the drugs may not be pure, may not be the drugs that patients believe they are buying, or may even be dangerous. Drugs that originate in China or India often look like real drugs but may be fake. It is hard to know if the drugs that are sold in other countries or over the Internet are real or not. At this time, buying drugs in other countries and bringing them into the United States is not legal. The FDA is opposed to patients being able to get drugs that cannot be proven to meet high U.S. standards.

Because drug companies often sell their drugs to other countries at a cheaper rate than in the United States, there is growing interest by many groups in getting more drugs from Canada in a way that can assure they are pure. Many nurses and patients in Canada or along the U.S.-Canadian border must deal with Canadian drug regulations and classifications that are different from those in the United States; some specific information is provided in the next section.

CANADIAN DRUG LEGISLATION

The Canadian Health Protection Branch of the Department of National Health and Welfare is like our FDA of the U.S. Department of Health and Human Services. This branch is responsible for the administration and enforcement of federal legislation such as the Food and Drugs Act, the Proprietary or Patent Medicine Act, and the Controlled Drugs and Substances Act. These acts, together with provincial acts and regulations that cover the sale of poisons and drugs and those that cover the health care professions, are designed to protect the Canadian consumer from health hazards; misleading ads about drugs, cosmetics, and devices; and impure food and drugs. The Canadian Food and Drugs Act divides drugs into various categories. Regulations covering the various categories or schedules of drugs differ from those in the United States. There are three major classes of drugs under the Food and Drugs Act: nonprescription drugs, prescription drugs, and restricted drugs.

The laws within the Canadian Food and Drugs Act allow the government to withdraw from the market drugs found to be toxic. New drugs put on the market must be shown to be effective and safe in human clinical studies to the satisfaction of the manufacturer and the government.*

---

*For more specific information, the nurse can obtain a copy of *Health Protection and Drug Laws* from Supply and Services Canada, Canadian Government Publishing, Ottawa, Canada, K1A 0S9.

The Proprietary or Patent Medicine Act provides for a class of products that may be sold to the general public by anyone. The drug formula is not found in the official drug manuals or printed on the label. The formulas for all such proprietary (trade secret) nonpharmacologic drugs must be registered and have a license under the Proprietary or Patent Medicine Act. The nurse needs to be aware of this act in the case of possible drug interactions.

The Canadian Controlled Drugs and Substances Act covers the possession, sale, manufacture, production, and distribution of narcotics in Canada. Only authorized persons may have narcotics in their possession. All persons authorized to be in possession of a narcotic must keep a record of the names and quantities of all narcotics dispensed, and they must ensure the safekeeping of all narcotics. The law covering this act is enforced by the Royal Canadian Mounted Police. Nurses are in violation of this act if they are guilty of illegal possession of narcotics.

OTC drugs are regulated in Canada by the Canadian Food and Drugs Act. These drugs can be purchased without a prescription, but there are rules about the package, label, and dispensing of the drug. The nurse needs to be aware of the risks these medications have, and watch for possible adverse effects and interactions with other drugs. OTC drugs that are available in Canada differ from those available in the United States.

STATE LAW AND HEALTH CARE AGENCY POLICIES

Although many regulations about giving medications come from federal laws, the details about who may actually give medications are determined by each state. This authority is spelled out for nurses in the **nurse practice act** of each state, which describes who can be called a nurse and what they can and cannot do. These rules vary from state to state and have changed over the years to reflect the increased responsibility many nurses have for giving medications. The authority to administer medications is clearly specified for LPNs/LVNs, RNs, and nurse practitioners in the state nurse practice act. This is a privilege given to those nurses who are named by law to administer medications, and can document their educational preparation to do so. These nurses must also show the willingness to accept **professional responsibility** for administering drugs appropriately, ethically, and to the best of their ability. This means they also accept **legal responsibility** for good judgment and actions while carrying out professional duties.

Because of the differences of practice in different states, each nurse must learn what is legal with regard to medications, and make sure that they and others follow all the rules. Because people in our society tend to move so much, it is especially important for nurses to know what is in the nurse practice act as they move from state to state and accept different nursing positions and jobs. Using computers for ordering drugs, record keeping, and even advising patients (telemedicine) makes it possible for doctors and nurses in one state to be involved in health care for patients in different states. Because of the differences among states in what is allowed, a national nursing license may one day be granted. Today, some states recognize the license of the nurse in another state through a nursing agreement called a Compact.

Memory Jogger

State Nurse Practice Act
You must understand how your state nurse practice act describes your drug administration responsibilities.

State rules about nursing practice often list minimum standards of practice. Therefore, agency or institutional policies and guidelines may be more specific or restrictive than state nurse practice acts. Agency employers should provide:
1. Written policy statements regarding
   - Educational preparation of nurses administering medications
   - Agency or institutional policies nurses must follow
2. Orientation to particular policies, procedures, and record-keeping rules

When you accept employment in an institution, it implies you are willing to obey set policies or procedures and to take part in revising and changing them as needed.

Sometimes the nurse must meet very formal rules in order to give medications. It may be an agency's policy to require employment for a certain period of time, completion of special orientation and training sessions, and passing a probation period in order to administer medications. Although the nurse may have the legal authority to give medications, this action is valid only when the nurse has a valid medication order signed by an authorized prescriber.

All nurses have legal responsibility for what they do. What they can and cannot do is listed in the nurse practice act of the state. Some RNs have expanded their clinical practice to include tasks that only doctors performed in the past, and LPNs/LVNs in some settings perform tasks that were once completed only by RNs. These trends are likely to continue because of efforts to cut overall health care costs. The changes in who does what are legally linked to the term *delegation*.

Delegation is when the responsibility for performing a task is passed from one person to another, but the accountability for what happens, or the outcome, remains with the original person. The person who delegates a task to someone else must have the authority to do so, and the person to whom it is delegated must also have the authority to perform that task. RNs now often delegate many of their tasks, including giving medications, to an LPN/LVN. For example, if the LPN/LVN has the educational preparation, clinical experience, and agency authority to give medications, then the RN may delegate this task to her. The RN still retains accountability for making sure that the LPN/LVN is able to perform the task correctly, whereas the LPN/LVN is responsible for what she does. In some settings, an LPN/LVN may direct the work of other LPNs/LVNs or unlicensed personnel such as nurse's aides. The LPN/LVN in this situation would remain accountable and responsible for assigning tasks to the nurse's aide or other LPN/LVN, and the aide or other LPN/LVN is responsible for the care that is actually delivered. This principle is also true for the student nurse. The student in an RN or LPN/LVN program is held to the same standard of practice as the graduate. The student works under delegated responsibility from the RN, but the RN maintains accountability.

Although there are many formal regulations for giving medications, there are also some requirements to give medications that are less formal and rely on the judgment and knowledge of the nurse. The agency expects the nurse to carry out the steps of the nursing process and, in fact, holds the nurse responsible for good assessment, diagnosis, planning, implementation, and evaluation of the patient as the nurse gives the medication. The nurse will be held responsible if he fails to perform every step well.

Thus the nursing process is not just a helpful system that you might want to think about when giving medications. There is a professional and an implied legal requirement that you use this process. *You must understand information about the patient:* symptoms, diagnosis, and why the medication is to be given. You must also know other information about the patient's past medical history, allergies, risk factors, and reaction to medications or any information that contraindicates (forbids) giving the drug. *You must know about the medication itself:* the dosage, the route of administration, the expected response, and adverse reactions. Knowledge about other medications is also mandatory, because you must watch for possible drug interactions. *You must understand the procedure:* how, when, and where the medication is to be given, and equipment or special techniques needed. You must monitor the patient's response after the medication is given, record the information about the drug that was given, and report promptly to the RN or physician any unexpected results. Finally, you must use every chance you have to teach the patient and the family the information they need to know for continued and safe administration of this medication.

Patient Charts

The patient's chart is a legal record. It is the major source of information about the patient and the care she receives while in the hospital. It provides a central place where all members of the health care team record information about the patient and her treatment. The physician or other health care provider describes the patient's condition on admission, determines the diagnosis, and provides orders to identify or resolve the patient's problems. The nurse records the assessment of the patient's condition, the implementation of basic nursing procedures, the patient's response, and the progress in completing the diagnostic and therapeutic plans. The chart belongs to the hospital. It is not the property of the patient, the nurse, or the physician. It is the legal record of the patient's stay in the hospital. It is kept after the patient has been discharged, and is often used for billing, insurance, and auditing activities; in medical or nursing research; and to provide information if the patient should be admitted again. In cases of court action or lawsuits, the chart may be used by lawyers as evidence. It is especially important that you write meaningful and accurate information in a complete and readable manner.

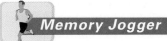

Memory Jogger

The Patient's Chart

Look at and understand the different parts of the patient's chart.

Health care is delivered in many different places in this country and around the world. Some agencies and countries have few resources and care is very limited. Others have the latest computers and treatment systems. As a nurse, you will probably work in places with different resources throughout your career. For example, you may work in an agency that has the latest computerized medication system installed in each patient's bedroom, or in a nursing home that has no medication recording system. If you have the chance to practice in another country, you will find that, although the tasks that nurses perform for patients are often the same, there may be different ways of carrying out nursing activities. You should learn the basics about nursing activities related to giving medications and then adjust that knowledge to the setting in which you practice. Some of the basics include the following:

- The nurse is responsible for checking that the medication order is correct. This may mean you need to check the order you have (in a medication Kardex or drug system) against the original order in the patient's chart.

- The nurse must record the drug administration information. Every agency has its own order sheets and recording forms for the patient's chart. Agency policy will tell you what information is to be placed in each section. Although there is a variety of forms, certain things are traditionally part of every chart. These parts are listed in Box 3-1.
- Many hospitals use the chart format called the **problem-oriented medical record (POMR)**. The POMR uses a list of numbered patient problems as an index to the chart. The way the notes are written in the chart also helps make information easy to find.

Kardex

The Kardex is a flip-file card system that has important information from the patient summary form and the physician's orders. It is regularly updated and changed to reflect current orders. This format keeps important information about the patient easily available for all team members. In the past, all tests, medications, and treatment orders were listed here, along with the nursing care plan. Some agencies still require use of a medication card for each drug to be given to the patient (Figure 3-1). More commonly, when a unit-dose system is used, individual medication cards are not needed because all medications are listed in the Kardex or medication profile sheet (Figure 3-2). Some computerized dispensing systems create their own separate patient medication forms as drugs are dispensed. The Kardex card is thrown away when the patient is discharged. It is not a legal document and serves no further purpose.

Drug Distribution Systems

Each agency has its own way of ordering and administering medications. There are four commonly used systems to distribute medications to the nurse:
1. The floor or ward stock system
2. The individual prescription order system
3. The unit-dose system
4. The computerized or automated dispensing system
These four systems are described in Box 3-2.

Narcotics Control Systems

Both federal and state laws, as well as agency policies, are very clear about how controlled substances are handled in the hospital. These procedures are nearly identical from hospital to hospital. The primary goal of all regulations and policies is to verify and account for all controlled substances. When controlled substances, particularly narcotics, are ordered from the pharmacy, they come in single-dose unit or prefilled syringes and are attached to a special inventory sheet. The nurse receiving the order must inspect the medication and return to the pharmacy a signed record stating that all the medication ordered was received and that it was

in acceptable condition. As each medication is used, it must be accounted for on the inventory sheet by the nurse giving the medication.

The use of controlled substances is carefully monitored on the hospital unit. Medication is stored in a special locked cabinet. The key to this cabinet is carried by the head nurse or by a medication nurse. This individual has the legal responsibility for the use and recording of all the controlled substance medications during that shift, whether or not they give all the medications.

When a controlled substance is ordered for a patient, the nurse responsible for giving the medication first checks the order and verifies the dosage and the last time the medication was given before obtaining the key to the cabinet. The nurse must sign out all medications he or she administered during the shift. The inventory report form is completed before the drug is removed from the cabinet. This report indicates the patient's name, date, drug, dosage, and the signature of the nurse giving the medication. If a dose is ordered that is smaller than that provided (so that some medication must be discarded), or if the medication is accidentally dropped, contaminated, spilled, or otherwise made unusable and unreturnable, two nurses must sign the inventory report and describe the situation. The medication given should be noted in the patient's chart, and there should also be a follow-up note about the patient's response to the medication.

At the end of each shift, the responsibility for all controlled substances and the key to the controlled substances cabinet are transferred to another nurse from the new shift. The contents of the locked cabinet are counted together by one nurse from each shift. The numbers of each ampule, tablet, and prefilled syringe in the cabinet must match the numbers listed on the inventory report form. Sealed packages are kept sealed. Opened packages of medications must be individually inspected and counted. Prefilled syringes must be examined to make sure they all have the same color, the same fluid levels, and the same amounts of air within them. Both nurses must sign the inventory report saying that the records and inventory are accurate at that time.

Occasionally, the inventory and the report do not agree. Any errors in the number of remaining doses and the number listed in the inventory report must be explained. All nurses having access to the key must be asked about medication they have given. Steps must be retraced to see if someone forgot to record any medication. Patient charts might also be checked to see if medication was given that was not signed for on the inventory report. If errors in the report cannot be found, both the pharmacy and the nursing service office must be notified. If the error is large, the hospital administrator and security police are usually contacted.

You can see that the nurse with the key has a lot of responsibility in watching over the controlled drugs on

Box 3-1 | *Parts of the Problem-Oriented Medical Record Patient Chart*

SUMMARY SHEET

The summary sheet is the standard hospital information form that gives basic information about the patient: name, address, date of birth, sex, marital status, nearest relative, employer, insurance carrier or payment arrangements, religion, date and time of admission, admission diagnoses, and attending physician. It may also contain information about allergies, past diagnoses or admissions, and the patient's occupation. A summary of surgeries, diagnoses, and the date and time of discharge may also be added when the patient leaves.

HISTORY AND PHYSICAL EXAMINATION

On admission, a comprehensive history and a physical examination are completed by the physician. The nurse admitting the patient may also conduct a nursing history and a physical examination to supplement the physician's report. All findings are listed, and the problem list is constructed from this information.

PROBLEM LIST

The problem list contains all the symptoms, signs, problems, and diagnoses that have been identified. New problems are added as indicated. The list is numbered, and dates are given for when each problem began and when it was detected. All further entries in the chart that relate to a given problem would use the problem number.

PHYSICIAN'S ORDERS

All procedures and treatments are ordered on the physician's order form. These orders include general care (activity level, diet, vital signs), diagnostic and laboratory tests (blood work, x-ray studies), and medications and treatments (hot packs, dressings, physical therapy).

PROGRESS NOTES

The progress notes section contains observations made by health care workers about the patient. Physicians' and nurses' notes are written in a SOAP format: Subjective information, Objective findings, Assessment of problem, and Plan of care. (Some hospitals put physicians' and nurses' notes into separate sections.)

GRAPHIC RECORD

The graphic record section contains forms for recording vital signs, fluid intake and output, and treatments. In some hospitals, medications are also recorded in this section. In other hospitals, medications are kept in a separate medication Kardex and are not part of the chart until the patient is discharged.

LABORATORY TESTS

All laboratory test results are recorded either on a single sheet as separate entries as they are received by the unit, or as sequential entries or summaries updated by computers. (If a patient is critically ill, charts may be developed to show all laboratory test results in one place so any changes can be easily seen.) These are often called "flow charts." Results of electrocardiograms (ECGs), electroencephalograms (EEGs), x-ray studies, or other tests may be placed here, or there may be another section for other diagnostic reports.

CONSULTATIONS

When other specialists are asked to evaluate the patient, the summary of their findings and recommendations is placed in this section.

the nursing unit. This nurse is usually a very mature person, often the head nurse or a nurse who has been with the hospital for some time and who has shown he can be trusted. It is the duty of this nurse to give the key only to other nurses authorized to administer controlled substances. Keys are never given to physicians

Name _____ Room _____

Drug _____

Dosage _____

Time_____

Date _____ Initials _____

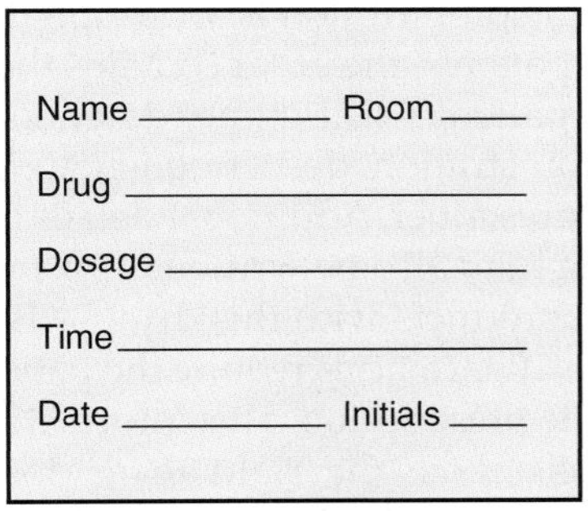

FIGURE **3-1** Example of a medication card.

or any other health care worker. (Sometimes a physician will want to give the medication, but the nurse should get the medication and sign the inventory report.) The nurse in charge of controlled substances should be able to monitor all activity with the controlled drugs on a daily basis so that, if a pattern develops, changes from normal are easily seen. On a hospital unit that has many patients coming from surgery, use of narcotics for these patients will be high soon after surgery but should taper off within 2 to 3 days. If a patient continues to need large or frequent doses or needs narcotics for longer than other patients with the same condition, the nurse in charge of these drugs should be suspicious. Nurses who always "drop," "spill," or give smaller doses of medications than normal should also be watched thoughtfully to learn whether or not there is a problem. Any activity that causes concern relating to controlled substances should be noted by the head nurse. Sometimes, patterns do not become evident until they are examined over a period of months.

MEDICATION KARDEX

PRN MEDICATIONS

Order date initials	Expir. date	Medication dose/frequency/route	Doses given
			Date
			Time
			Initials
			Date
			Time
			Initials
			Date
			Time
			Initials
			Date
			Time
			Initials
			Date
			Time
			Initials
			Date
			Time
			Initials
			Date
			Time
			Initials
			Date
			Time
			Initials
			Date
			Time
			Initials
			Date
			Time
			Initials
			Date
			Time
			Initials

IM Injection Site Code
1. Rt. posterior gluteal
2. Lt. posterior gluteal
3. Rt. anterior gluteal
4. Lt. anterior gluteal
5. Rt. anterolateral thigh
6. Lt. anterolateral thigh
7. Rt. deltoid
8. Lt. deltoid

Indicate the number of the site used with each IM dose given.

Record site with time.

Signatures/Initials

ALLERGIES ______ DIAGNOSIS ______

ROOM NO. ______ NAME ______ DOCTOR ______ AGE ______

FIGURE **3-2** Example of a medication Kardex.

Memory Jogger

Controlled Substances

Always be sure to verify orders for and account for all controlled substances.

The Drug Order

Both state law and agency policy require that all medications given in hospitals must be ordered by licensed health care providers acting within their areas of professional training. This generally restricts prescriptive authority (the authority to write an order or prescription for medication) to physicians, dentists, and, in some states, nurse practitioners, nurse-midwives, nurse anesthetists, and physician assistants. Prescriptions for a hospitalized patient are written on the order form in the patient's chart. Sometimes, the order is on a tear-off sheet that can be sent directly to the pharmacy to obtain the medication. Other times, the order must be transcribed, or rewritten, by the nurse or unit secretary onto a special pharmacy order form.

Prescriptions for patients leaving the hospital are written on regular prescription pads and taken to a pharmacy or drugstore to get the medication (Figure 3-3).

Whether the prescription is for hospitalized or nonhospitalized patients, the order contains the same information: the patient's full name, date, name of drug, route of administration, dose, frequency, duration, and signature of prescriber. Additional details about how to give the drug may also be written: "Take with meals," "Avoid milk products with this drug," "Do not refill," "Please label." Pharmacies require the patient's age and address on the prescription. This information may help the pharmacist give the right drug dosage for the patient (if he is a child or older adult) or verify the patient's identity.

Box 3-2   *Common Drug Distribution Systems*

FLOOR OR WARD STOCK SYSTEM

In the floor or ward stock system, all frequently used medications (except potentially dangerous or controlled substances) are stocked in large containers at the nursing station. This system is usually used in small hospitals, in nursing homes with no pharmacist, or where there are no direct charges to patients for the medications (such as in most government hospitals); it is also used in some emergency rooms. Medication is taken from each container as needed for each patient.

Advantages
- Few inpatient prescription orders
- Minimal return of medications
- Ready availability of medications

Disadvantages
- Increased potential for medication errors
- Potential for use of medication by hospital personnel
- Potential for unnoticed drug deterioration
- Potential for increased number of expired drugs that may be difficult to detect
- Storage and space problems
- Lack of review of medication order by pharmacist

INDIVIDUAL PRESCRIPTION ORDER SYSTEM

In the individual prescription order system, medication orders are sent to the pharmacy, which issues an individual box or bottle for each drug. The container may hold a 3- to 5-day supply of the drug. Medications are stored in a cabinet at the nursing station. They are arranged either alphabetically by drug name or according to the patient's room number. Medication is taken from each container by the nurse as needed and distributed to the patient.

Advantages
- Review of prescription by both pharmacist and nurse before administration
- Less chance for deterioration of the drug or for drug misuse
- Smaller total drug inventories needed
- Medication frequently available for stat or prn usage
- Easy charging and billing mechanisms

Disadvantages
- Frequent need to return or discard unused medications
- Complex ordering, preparing, administering, controlling, and recording systems required

UNIT-DOSE SYSTEM

Single-unit packages of drugs are dispensed to fill each dosage requirement as ordered. Each package is clearly labeled and is often dispensed by the pharmacy into drawers assigned to individual patients in a special medication cart or an individual patient drug cabinet near the patient's room. (This is known as a "nurse service" format.) Every 24 hours, the pharmacist refills this cart or cabinet with all the medications required for the patient for 1 day. This is the safest and most economical method of drug distribution in use today.

Advantages
- Little nursing time is required for preparation of medications.
- A better use is made of pharmacist skills and knowledge, because the pharmacist has greater information about the patient and is able to evaluate each order for contraindications or drug interactions.
- Errors are reduced, because no drug calculations by the nurse are required.
- There is little waste or misuse of medication because only small doses are dispensed.
- Credit can be given for unused drugs because medication packages have not been opened.

Disadvantages
- Nurses must administer a medication prepared by someone else, which may occasionally lead to an error.
- Delays in starting medications may occur if no stock is on the hospital unit.
- This system requires the presence of a pharmacist(s) at the hospital, which may not be possible or may be very expensive in some areas.

COMPUTERIZED OR AUTOMATED DISPENSING SYSTEM

Medication orders are sent to the pharmacy, where medication is loaded into an automated drug dispensing system (e.g., Sure-Med, PYXIS). The stocked cart with the proper medications is delivered to the hospital unit. When the medication is to be administered, the nurse enters the patient's name and the drug needed, and that drug is dispensed and automatically entered into the computerized drug administration record. The cart then goes back to the pharmacy for refill.

Advantages
- It reduces time for nurses.
- Medication is automatically recorded at the time of delivery.
- Tight control over medication is possible.

Disadvantages
- It is costly, because it requires a pharmacist and special equipment.
- The nurse is highly dependent on pharmacist accuracy.

NOTE: All of these systems are in use today in the different places that nurses may be working.

```
DEA # _____

              ROBERT GOODFELLOW, M.D.
              SARAH BOCK, R.N., A.N.P.
            MARILYN EDWARDS, R.N., A.N.P.-C.
             THICK FOREST PROFESSIONAL CENTER
               THUNDER MILLS VILLAGE CENTER
                    3333 TRELLIS LANE
                  ST. GEORGE, MD  21043
    _____

    Name _____

    ADDRESS _____  DATE _____

    R




    [ ]  Label

    Refill _____ times PRN NR

    _____ M.D.
    To ensure brand name dispensing, prescriber must write 'Dispense As Written' on
    the prescription.
```

FIGURE **3-3** Example of a prescription pad order form.

Memory Jogger

Institutional Regulations
You must learn agency rules about giving medications.

In emergencies or when the physician is not in the hospital, the physician might give the nurse either a verbal order or an order over the telephone. All agencies have policies about these types of orders. The hospital decides who may take these orders—usually the RN. The nurse taking the order is responsible for writing the order on the order form in the chart, including both the name of the nurse and the name of the doctor. The physician must then cosign this order, usually within 24 hours, for the order to be valid.

Medication orders may be classed into one of four types of orders:
1. The standing order
2. The emergency or "stat" order
3. The single order
4. The as-needed or "prn" order

The agency's policy clearly defines each of these types of orders and how they are carried out. Some agencies have also created a "now" order classification. A "now" order is different than a "stat" order, in that the nurse has 1.5 hours to give the medication, unlike the "stat" order that must be given within minutes. The general definition of each type of order and examples of each are presented in Table 3-3. Table 3-4 lists common abbreviations used in pharmacology, which the nurse must memorize.

In an effort to cut down on medication errors, the Joint Commission on Accreditation of Healthcare Organizations (JCAHO), the agency that accredits hospitals, has discouraged health care workers from using any abbreviations that might lead to confusion. Many abbreviations that were used in the past (such as "hs" for nighttime, "cc" for cubic centimeter, and "Q.D." and "Q.O.D." for daily and every other day) are now not used in hospitals that wish to maintain their accreditation. Table 3-5 lists the minimum abbreviations that must be included on each accredited organization's Do Not Use list as of January 1, 2004.

Table 3-3 | Types of Medication Orders

DESCRIPTION	EXAMPLE
STANDING ORDER	
Indicates that the drug is to be administered until discontinued, or for a certain number of doses; hospital policy dictates that most standing orders expire after a certain number of days and that a renewal order must be written by the physician before the drug may be continued.	"Amoxicillin trihydrate 500 mg PO × 10 days." "Ibuprofen 600 mg PO q6h."
STAT ORDER	
One-time order to be given immediately.	"Lidocaine 50 mg IV push stat."
SINGLE ORDER	
One-time order to be given at specified time.	"Meperidine 100 mg IM 8 AM preoperatively."
PRN ORDER	
Given as needed based on nurse's judgment of safety and patient need.	"Docusate calcium 100 mg PO at bedtime prn constipation."

Table 3-4 | Common Abbreviations Used in Pharmacology

ABBREVIATION	DEFINITION	ABBREVIATION	DEFINITION
ac	before meals	on	every night
ad lib	as desired	oz	ounce
AM	before noon	pc‹	after meals
bid	twice a day	PM•	after noon
c̄	with	PO	by mouth
cap	capsule	PR	per rectum
comp	compound	prn	as required
D	give	q	every
D	day	qh	every hour
dil	dilute	q2h	every 2 hours
div	divide	qid*	four times daily
dos	dose	Rx	take
dr	drain	S	mark
elix	elixir	s̄	without
ext	extract	sig	write on the label
fl	fluid	ss	one half
gm	gram	stat	immediately
gr	grain	sub-Q*	subcutaneous
gt (gtt)	drop(s)	tab	tablet
h	hour	tid	three times a day
IM	intramuscular	tr	tincture
IV	intravascular	ung	ointment
m	minim	ʒ*	dram
od*	every day	℥*	ounce
oh	every hour		

*To reduce potential medication errors, the Institute of Safe Medication Practices recommends that this abbreviation not be used.

Table 3-5 | *JCAHO Minimum Do-Not-Use List of Abbreviations*

ABBREVIATION	POTENTIAL PROBLEM	PREFERRED TERM
U (for unit)	Mistaken as zero, four, or cc	Write *unit*
IU (for international unit)	Mistaken as IV (intravenous) or 10 (ten)	Write *international unit*
Q.D., Q.O.D., Q.I.D. (Latin abbreviations for once daily, every other day, and 4 times daily)	Mistaken for each other The period after the "Q" can be mistaken for an "I," and the "O" can be mistaken for "I"	Write *daily, every other day,* and *4 times daily*
Trailing zero (X.0 mg) *(Note: prohibited only for medication-related notations)* Lack of leading zero (X mg)	Decimal point is missed	Never write a zero by itself after a decimal point (X mg), and always use a zero before a decimal point (0.X mg)
MS, MSO$_4$, MgSO$_4$	Confused for one another Can mean morphine sulfate or magnesium sulfate	Write *morphine sulfate* or *magnesium sulfate*

From the Joint Commission on Accreditation of Healthcare Organizations, 2003.

MEDICATION ERRORS

Despite the best rules and procedures, medication errors sometimes occur in busy hospitals. Procedures differ about what to do when a medication error is made. However, there are some guidelines that everyone accepts. When it is discovered that an error has been made, the nurse should immediately check the patient. Does the error pose a risk to the patient's condition (for example, giving too large a dose of insulin)? If so, the physician should be notified promptly, and any orders the physician gives must be followed. Every effort should be made to watch the patient's condition through measuring vital signs, drawing blood for tests, or any other method ordered by the physician. The nurse should also notify her nursing supervisor, record in the patient's chart exactly what happened, and fill out any other reports as required by the agency. Whether the error is a problem for the nurse is often related to what happens to the patient. How and why the error was made and how it might be avoided in the future will be determined. If the nurse was careless or negligent, she may be held legally liable for any adverse consequences to the patient. Although almost every nurse has made one medication error, repeated errors will not be ignored.

The Institute of Medicine (IOM) issued a report in 2000 about the number of errors made in medical care. As detailed in the IOM report, estimates from 1991 and 1999 suggest that adverse events, which include medical errors, occur in 3% to 4% of patients. The IOM report and other studies estimate that the costs of medical errors in the United States, including lost income, disability, and need for additional health care, may be between $17 billion and $136.8 billion or more annually. These costs are from a variety of drug-related problems, including patient compliance issues and medical or medication errors. Unfortunately, the IOM estimates that more than half of the adverse medical events occurring each year are attributable to medical errors that could be prevented.

Because of this report, most agencies have tightened up ways to report and follow up on medication errors. Nurses should make every effort to obtain the most recent agency policies in this area.

LEGISLATION TO PROTECT HEALTH CARE WORKERS

Because patients have infections that may place nurses at risk, care must be taken to protect nurses. One of the most dangerous things nurses do is to recap the needle of a syringe that has been used in the injection of a sick patient. This frequently leads to nurses accidentally sticking themselves. In 2001, the Needlestick Safety and Prevention Act became federal law. The object of the law is to prevent exposure in hospitals to blood-borne pathogens such as hepatitis B, hepatitis C, and human immunodeficiency virus (HIV). The law requires hospitals to follow the guidelines in the Occupational Safety and Health Administration (OSHA) Bloodborne Pathogens Standard. As part of this standard, health care institutions must have a written plan spelling out their efforts to cut the risk of needlestick injuries. In addition, employers are required to provide the safest equipment available, regardless of cost. Such equipment includes products with **engineering controls,** which are built-in safety features to reduce risk. When selecting products, management is to seek the input of end users (nurses)— those providing direct patient care. If a needlestick injury does occur, it is to be carefully recorded in a needlestick injury log. The exposure control plan, selection of safety products, and needlestick injury log must be reviewed at least every year. Many states have chosen to pass "tougher" laws, but at a minimum, every state law must meet the OSHA standard.

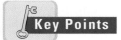

Key Points

- The nurse's authority to administer medications has grown slowly over time out of complex federal, state, and agency policies.
- These policies describe not only general procedures and rules but also very specific responsibilities of the nurse who administers medications.

- The nurse is legally required to exercise judgment and responsibility in carrying out these tasks.
- The nurse may delegate authority to others who are authorized to administer medications but keeps the responsibility for that delegation.

Go to the free CD-ROM for an Audio Glossary, animations, video clips, and Review Questions for the NCLEX-PN® Examination.

evolve Be sure to visit the companion Evolve website at http://evolve.elsevier.com/Edmunds/LPN/ for WebLinks, a link to the top 200 drugs by prescription, and sign-up pages for newsletter drug updates.

CRITICAL THINKING ?

1. Identify three levels of regulations the nurse must adhere to in giving medicines.

2. What is the major focus of each of the different forms of drug legislation?

3. Identify three categories of "scheduled" drugs and define the sort of drug that fits into each schedule.

4. Research the nurse practice act in your state. Discuss at least three of your findings with the rest of the class.

5. Interview nurses in your practice setting to discover institutional policy regarding drug administration. Share your findings with the class. If you are in a hospital setting, do some agency regulations apply more frequently to specific types of floor nurses?

6. Explain the difference between a drug order form, a prescription, and a verbal order. What does the nurse do in response to each of these items?

7. Identify the difference between standing, stat, NOW, single, and prn orders.

8. Assume that it is your responsibility to take inventory of the narcotic box at the end of your shift. What should you do if you discover that an injectable narcotic is missing (i.e., the count does not match the written inventory report)?

9. What are three important things you should do if you discover you have made a medication error?

10. What should you do if you do not understand a physician's medication order?

Foundations and Principles of Pharmacology

Objectives

After reading and studying this chapter, you should be able to do the following:

1. Define the key words used in pharmacology and about giving drugs.
2. Explain the differences between the chemical, generic, official, and brand names of medicines.
3. Describe the four basic physiologic processes that affect medications in the body.
4. List the basic types of drug actions.
5. Discuss the differences between side effects and adverse effects.

Key Terms

Be sure to check out the bonus material on the free CD-ROM, including selected audio pronunciations.

absorption (ăb-SŎRP-shŭn, p. 32)
additive effect (ĂD-ĭ-tĭv, p. 36)
adverse reactions (ăd-VŬRS, p. 34)
agonists (ĂG-ō-nĭsts, p. 31)
allergy (ĂL-ĕr-jē, p. 35)
anaphylactic reaction (ăn-ă-fĭ-LĂK-tĭk, p. 35)
antagonistic effect (ăn-tăg-ō-NĬS-tĭk, p. 36)
antagonists (ăn-TĂG-ō-nĭsts, p. 31)
bioequivalent (BĪ-ō-ĭ-KWĬV-ĭ-lent, p. 35)
biotransformation (BĪ-ō-trăns-fŏr-MĀ-shŭn, p. 33)
chemical name (KĔM-ĭ-kăl, p. 31)
desired action (p. 34)
displacement (p. 36)
distribution (dĭs-trĭ-BŪ-shŭn, p. 33)
drug interaction (ĭn-tĕr-ĂK-shŭn, p. 35)
enteral (route) (ĔN-tĕr-ăl, p. 33)
excretion (ĕks-KRĒ-shŭn, p. 33)
first-pass (effect) (p. 33)
generic name (jĕn-ĔR-ĭk, p. 30)
half-life (p. 34)
hepatotoxic (hĕp-ă-tō-TŎK-sĭk, p. 34)
hypersensitivity (hī-pĕr-sĕn-sĭ-TĬV-ĭ-tē, p. 35)
idiosyncratic response (ĭd-ē-ō-sĭn-KRĂ-tĭk, p. 34)
incompatibility (p. 36)
interference (p. 36)
nephrotoxic (nĕf-rō-TŎK-sĭk, p. 34)
official name (p. 31)
parenteral (route) (pĕ-RĔN-tĕr-ăl, p. 33)
partial agonists (PĂR-shăl ĂG-ō-nĭsts, p. 31)

percutaneous (route) (pĕr-kū-TĀ-nē-ŭs, p. 33)
pharmacodynamics (FĂRM-ă-kō-dī-NĂM-ĭks, p. 30)
pharmacokinetics (FĂRM-ă-kō-kĭ-NĔT-ĭks, p. 30)
pharmacotherapeutics (FĂRM-ă-kō-thĕr-ă-PŪ-tĭks, p. 30)
receptor site (rē-SĔP-tŏr, p. 31)
side effects (p. 34)
solubility (sŏl-ū-BĬL-ĭ-tē, p. 32)
synergistic effect (sĭn-ĕr-JĬS-tĭk, p. 36)
trade name (p. 31)

OVERVIEW

This chapter provides an overview of very basic information from chemistry, physics, anatomy, and physiology that explains the action of drugs in the body (**pharmacokinetics,** or what the body does to the drug). It also covers basic information on the effects of drugs on the functions of the body (**pharmacodynamics,** or what the drug does to the body). This information is vital in order to understand **pharmacotherapeutics,** or the use of drugs in the treatment of disease (Box 4-1).

DRUG NAMES

Medications have several different names that may be confusing when you are first learning to work with drugs. It is very important to know the various names of a medication so that the wrong drug is not given to a patient. Sometimes a medication is ordered by one name for the drug and the pharmacist labels it with another name for the same drug. For example, Valium (trade name) is the same as diazepam (generic name). It is important to know whether the medication is the same or a different drug.

The most common drug name that is used is the **generic name.** This is the name drug manufacturer uses for a drug, and it is the same in all countries. It is the name given to a drug before there is an official name, or when the drug has been available for many years and more than one company makes the drug. Examples would be digitalis and tetracycline. The American Pharmaceutical Association, the American Medical

> **Box 4-1** *Key Words Used in Pharmacology and Drug Administration*
>
> **Drug** comes from the Dutch word *droog*, which means "dry." For centuries, most drugs used for treating health problems came from dried plants.
> **Medicines** are those drugs used in the prevention or treatment of diseases.
> **Pharmacology** deals with the study of drugs and the action of drugs on living organisms. It comes from the Greek words *pharmakon*, which means "drugs," and *logos*, which means "science."
> **Therapeutic regimen** refers to all the methods to be used for treatment of disease. In addition to drug therapy, this may include plans for special diets; use of hot packs, whirlpools, or ultraviolet lights; and counseling, biofeedback, or psychotherapy.

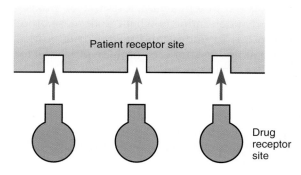

FIGURE **4-1** Drug receptor sites.

Association, and the U.S. Adopted Names Council assign generic names. Generic names are not capitalized when written. An example would be celecombix.

Another common drug name is the **trade name,** or brand name. This name is often followed by the symbol ®, which indicates that the name is registered to a specific drug maker or owner and no one else can use it. This is the drug name used in advertisements and other marketing, and it is often descriptive, easy to spell, or catchy sounding so that prescribers will remember it easily and will be more likely to use it. The first letter of the trade name, and sometimes other letters, are capitalized. Examples of trade names are Dimetapp, Lanoxin, and Pen-Vee K.

Chemical names are often the most difficult to remember because they include the chemicals that make up the drug. These names are usually long and hyphenated, and they describe the atomic or molecular structure. An example would be ethyl 1-methyl-4-phenylisonipecotate hydrochloride, the chemical name for meperidine (Demerol).

The final type of name is the **official name,** which the name is given by the Food and Drug Administration (FDA). Sometimes this name is similar to the brand or chemical name. The first letter of the official name is also capitalized. An example would be Ethacrynic acid.

TYPES OF DRUG ACTIONS

DRUG ATTACHMENT

Drugs take part in chemical reactions that change the way the body acts. They do this most commonly when the medication forms a chemical bond at a specific site in the body called a **receptor site** (Figure 4-1). The chemical reactions between a drug and a receptor site are possible only when the receptor site and the drug can fit together like pieces of a jigsaw puzzle or a key fitting into a lock. If the drug fits the receptor site well, the chemical response is generally good. Some drugs attach at the receptor site and activate the receptor, producing an action similar to that of the body's own chemicals. These drugs are called **agonists.**

Some drugs attach to the receptor site but produce only a small chemical response. These drugs are called **partial agonists.** Other drugs attach at the receptor site but then produce no new chemical reaction. However, they prevent the activation of the receptor, stopping other chemical reactions from occurring. These drugs are called **antagonists.** Some partial agonists and antagonists are able to compete with other chemicals or drugs that are already bonded to a receptor site and replace them. The Memory Jogger box summarizes the various types of receptor site activity.

> *Memory Jogger*
>
> **Drug Receptor Sites**
> ***Agonist:*** Drug attaches at receptor site and activates the receptor; the drug has an action similar to the body's own chemicals, and the chemical response is usually good.
> ***Antagonist:*** Drug attaches at drug receptor site, but then remains chemically inactive; no chemical drug response is produced but the drug prevents activation of the receptor.
> ***Partial agonist:*** Drug attaches at drug receptor site, but only a slight chemical action is produced.

BASIC DRUG PROCESSES

Drugs must be changed chemically in the body to become usable. There are four basic processes involved in drug utilization in the body. These processes are absorption, distribution, metabolism, and excretion.

Drugs have different characteristics, or pharmaco-kinetics, that determine to what extent these processes will be used. To understand how a drug works, the nurse must understand each of these processes for the specific drug being given.

The Process of Absorption

Absorption involves the way a drug enters the body and passes into the body fluids and tissues. Absorption takes place through processes of diffusion, filtration, and osmosis. These mechanisms of absorption are more fully described in Box 4-2. How fast the drug is absorbed into the body through these processes depends on the solubility of the drug, the route of administration, and the degree of blood flow through the tissue where the medication is found.

All medication must be dissolved in body fluid before it can enter body tissues. The ability of the medication to dissolve is called **solubility.** In order to achieve the best possible drug action, sometimes the medication must be dissolved quickly; at other times it should be dissolved slowly. Solubility of the drug is

---

| Box 4-2 | *Mechanisms Involved in Absorption* |

DIFFUSION

Diffusion is the tendency of the molecules of a substance (gaseous, liquid, or solid) to move from a region of high concentration to one of lower concentration.

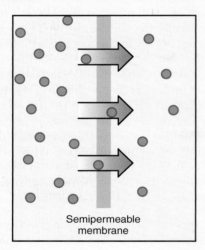

Semipermeable membrane

OSMOSIS

Osmosis is the diffusion of fluid through a semipermeable membrane; the flow is primarily from the less dense solution to the more dense solution.

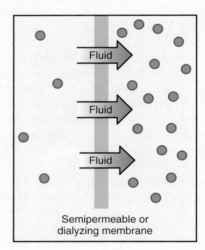

Semipermeable or dialyzing membrane

FILTRATION

Filtration is the passage of a substance through a filter or through a material that prevents passage of certain molecules.

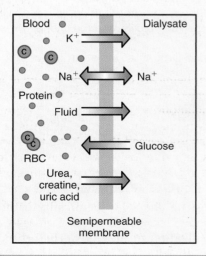

Semipermeable membrane

often controlled by the form of the medication; for example, solutions are more soluble than capsules because a liquid is absorbed faster than a tablet, which must dissolve. An injection with an oil base must be chemically changed before absorption can take place, and this holds the drug in the tissues longer, which may be the desired action. When the patient takes water with a tablet, it not only helps in swallowing but also helps dissolve the medication and increase its solubility.

The route of administration also influences absorption. The most common medication routes are **enteral** (directly into the gastrointestinal [GI] tract through oral, nasogastric tube, or rectal administration); **parenteral** (directly into dermal, subcutaneous, or intramuscular tissue, epidurally into the cerebrospinal fluid, or into the bloodstream through intravenous [IV] injections); and **percutaneous** (through topical [skin], sublingual [under the tongue], buccal [against the cheek], or inhalation [breathing] administration).

In areas where the blood flow through tissues is very high, medication will be rapidly absorbed. Examples of this include placing a nitroglycerin tablet under the tongue right next to blood vessels or spraying steroids into the nose and lungs through a nebulizer. Medications injected IV into the bloodstream have the fastest action. Oral or rectal medications usually take much longer because they must dissolve and diffuse across the barrier tissue in the GI tract (the gastric mucosa) in order to be carried to the body tissues where they will have their action.

The Process of Distribution

Once the medication is absorbed, it must travel throughout the body. The term **distribution** refers to the ways that drugs move by means of circulating body fluids to their sites of action in the body. The bloodstream and lymphatic system usually carry the drug throughout the whole body. The organs that have the biggest blood supply receive the medication faster, and areas of skin and fat receive the medication more slowly. Some drugs do not pass well through cell membranes with very small passages, such as those covering the placenta and the brain. These are referred to as *placental* and *blood-brain barriers*, although the *barrier* is not a complete barrier because some drugs and some conditions make it possible for drugs to easily pass through these areas. The various types of tissues, including bone, fat, and muscle, do not absorb equal amounts of the drug. Thus the distribution is different for different drugs.

The chemical properties of a drug also affect how the drug is distributed. Some chemicals bind together with proteins, such as albumin (found in the blood plasma), which serve as carriers giving a ride to drugs that are not easily dissolved. For this reason, some drugs are a complex (more than one part), with part of the chemicals bound to the protein and part of the chemicals free to flow or diffuse into the tissues. The ratio of bound chemical compared to free chemical remains the same in the blood. As more of the free chemical diffuses into the tissues, more of the bound chemical becomes unlocked and thus also available to diffuse.

Some medications are attracted to tissues other than the target receptor sites. For example, medications that dissolve easily in lipids (fats) prefer adipose, or fat, tissue, and stores of the medication may build up in these areas. As the medication moving throughout the body binds at the receptor sites, more of the medication stored in adipose tissue will gradually be given up by those cells. Thus a drug that can be stored in the fat cells may remain in the body for a long time while it is slowly released.

The Process of Metabolism

Once the medication is absorbed and distributed in the body, the body's enzymes use it in chemical reactions through the process of metabolism. Some drugs that are breathed into the lungs or injected into the tissue may go directly into the bloodstream and be carried quickly to the site of action. But many medications have to be broken down into smaller usable parts, primarily in the liver, through a series of complex chemical reactions until they become chemically inactive. This process is called **biotransformation.** When most of a medicine goes very quickly to the liver, a lot of the medication is inactivated on its "**first pass**" through the liver before it can be distributed to other parts of the body. That is why some medicines are given sublingually or IV; otherwise, patients do not get the amount of medication they require. (For example, only 1 mg of propranolol is required IV, but 40 mg are required when the drug is given by mouth.)

Genetic differences in the enzyme pathways in the liver also explain why people respond differently to a drug—whether they are tolerant of the drug and seem to need larger doses, or whether they are sensitive to the drug and only need a small dose. These enzyme pathways, known as the cytochrome P-450 system, play an important role in the adverse drug reactions patients may have when taking several drugs at the same time or when there are drug-food interactions.

The Process of Excretion or Elimination

All inactive chemicals, chemical by-products, and waste (often referred to as *metabolites*) finally break down through metabolism and are removed from the body through the process of **excretion.** Fibrous or insoluble waste is usually passed through the GI tract as feces. Chemicals that may be made water soluble are dissolved and filtered out as they pass through the kidneys, and then lost in the urine. Some chemicals are exhaled from the lungs through breathing or lost through evaporation from the skin during sweating. Very small amounts of medication may also escape in tears, saliva, or milk of breastfeeding mothers.

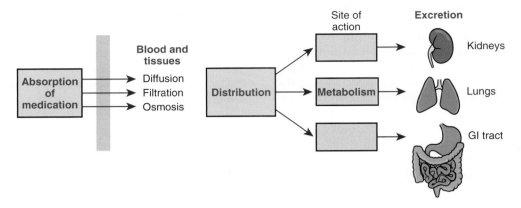

FIGURE **4-2** Processes of absorption, distribution, metabolism, and excretion.

The major processes involved in drug utilization in the body are shown in Figure 4-2. These four major processes are basic for you to understand how medications are used in the body.

Half-Life. Some drugs enter and leave the body very quickly; other drugs remain for a long time. The standard method of describing how long it takes to metabolize and excrete a drug is the **half-life,** or the time it takes the body to remove 50% of the drug from the body. Because the rates of metabolism and excretion are usually the same for most people, the half-life helps explain the dose (how much medicine should be taken), the frequency (how often it should be taken), and the duration (how long it will last) for different drugs. If a drug has a long half-life, it may need to be taken only once a day. If a person takes too much medication with a long half-life, this may cause a serious problem because the action of the drug lasts for such a long time. If the half-life of a drug is short, such as for many antibiotics, the person must take frequent doses to keep the correct level in the blood. If a person's liver or kidneys do not function correctly, medications may not be properly metabolized or excreted, and this would mean that higher doses of the medication will circulate for a longer time and produce symptoms of overdosage. Therefore, the function of the kidney and the liver will be watched by doing repeated renal and hepatic tests.

BASICS OF DRUG ACTION

When a drug is given to a patient, it is usually possible to predict the chemical reaction that will be seen. However, because each patient is different, some unexpected chemical reactions are also seen. With each patient, giving a medication is somewhat of an experiment, and the patient must be watched closely to see how she will react to the medication.

The expected response of the medication is called the **desired action.** This is when the medication does what

is desired and the therapeutic goal is reached (for example, meperidine [Demerol] relieves pain).

Because a medication may influence many body systems at the same time, the effect of the medication is often not restricted to the desired action. Other actions may also take place, which are called side effects or adverse reactions. **Side effects** are usually seen as mild but annoying responses to the medication. **Adverse reactions,** or adverse effects, usually imply more severe symptoms or problems that develop because of the drug. Some adverse effects may require the patient to be hospitalized or may even pose a risk to his life. Because a lot of testing is required for each drug before it can be sold, most side effects and adverse reactions that might occur are known. Some side effects, such as drowsiness, may go away after the patient takes the medication for a time. Certain side effects, such as nausea, may be stopped if the dosage is reduced. Some side effects are such a problem that the medication must be changed or stopped. An example of this might be insomnia (inability to sleep) or making the patient pass out. Certainly, if adverse effects such as damage to the kidney (**nephrotoxic** drug) or liver (**hepatotoxic** drug) damage or bleeding develops, the medication must be stopped.

Occasionally a patient may have a drug reaction that is a surprise. Strange, unique, or unpredicted responses are called **idiosyncratic responses.** These reactions may be the result of missing or defective metabolic enzymes caused by a genetic or hormonal variation. They often produce either an unexpected result, such as pain or bleeding, or an overresponse to the drug. These types of reactions are usually rare. One type of idiosyncratic response is called a *paradoxic response.* In this situation, the patient's reaction may be just the opposite of what would be expected. For example, pseudoephedrine hydrochloride, a common chemical found in decongestants for children, usually produces sedation or drowsiness as a side effect. However, some children respond with insomnia and tachycardia (rapid heartbeat) and are overly stimulated.

A second type of unexpected reaction is an increased reaction to a drug (**hypersensitivity**) or a sensitivity caused by antibody response to a drug (**allergy**). Some medications (sulfa products, aspirin, penicillin) and some conditions (asthma) are more likely to produce allergic reactions than others. Allergic reactions usually occur when an individual has taken the drug and her body has developed antibodies to it. When the patient takes the drug again, the antigen-antibody reaction produces hives, rash, itching, or swelling of the skin. This type of allergic reaction is very common, so you should ask all patients about whether they have ever had a drug reaction. Patients with an allergy to one medication may be more likely to develop an allergy to another medication, but individuals may also develop a reaction to medications that they have taken before without problems.

Occasionally, the allergic reaction is so severe that the patient has trouble breathing and his heart may stop. This life-threatening response is called an **anaphylactic reaction.** A patient who has a mild allergic reaction to a medication is much more likely to develop the more severe anaphylactic reaction if the medication is given again. An anaphylactic reaction is a true medical emergency because the patient may suffer paralysis of the diaphragm and swelling of the oropharynx, so he cannot breathe. Patients who have anaphylactic reactions should always be warned about their allergy so they will not take the drug again, and they should wear a Medic Alert bracelet or necklace or carry identification about their allergy.

Patients often confuse allergy with side effects—both of which may produce unpleasant symptoms. If a patient says she has an allergy to a drug, make sure you understand how she reacted to the drug. If the patient had nausea or stomach pain when taking aspirin, that is a side effect, but not an allergy. If the patient reported sedation when taking an antihypertensive medication, that is also not an allergy.

The common responses to medications are listed in Box 4-3.

BIOEQUIVALENCE

After a new drug enters the market, a patent protects the financial interest of the drug developer for some time, usually 17 years, by prohibiting other companies from producing that drug. After that time, other companies may file an application to produce the same drug under a generic name. Brand-name drugs are usually more expensive than generic drugs because the manufacturer of the brand-name drug is attempting to recover the huge sums of money invested in research and development of the drug. Thus generic products are often seen as cost-effective.

Drug products that are considered to be identical with respect to their active ingredients are known as *generic equivalents*. However, slight differences in processing or formulation may mean that the action of the

---

| Box 4-3 | *Common Responses to Medications* |

DESIRED EFFECT

When the desired effect takes place, the therapeutic goal is achieved. The drug does what it is supposed to do. An example would be temperature reduction after taking aspirin.

SIDE EFFECT

Side effects are mild but annoying responses to medication. An example would be stomach pain caused by aspirin.

ADVERSE EFFECT

Adverse effects are more severe symptoms or problems that arise because of the medication. An example would be that the patient might develop severe gastric bleeding from an ulcer caused by aspirin.

DIOSYNCRATIC RESPONSE

Idiosyncratic responses are strange, unique, or unpredicted reactions. An example would be blood in the urine caused by aspirin. This is rare.

PARADOXIC REACTION

Paradoxic reactions are reactions that are the opposite of what would be expected.

ALLERGIC RESPONSE

An allergic response is an antigen-antibody reaction. The body develops hives, rashes, itching, or swelling of the skin. A rash or shortness of breath is occasionally seen in patients allergic to aspirin.

ANAPHYLACTIC RESPONSE

An anaphylactic response is a severe form of allergic reaction that is life-threatening. The patient develops severe shortness of breath, may stop breathing, or may have cardiac collapse.

---

generic drug in the body is slightly different from that of the brand-name product. These differences most commonly result in variations in absorption, distribution, or metabolism. Thus what product the patient actually purchases when a prescription is written for a drug may vary according to what specific brand the pharmacist dispenses. Some products are chemically identical, and thus **bioequivalent.** Some products vary dramatically, and thus the medication that is dispensed should not be changed from what the prescriber has written. This may be particularly important for some cardiac or antiseizure medications.

DRUG INTERACTIONS

When one drug changes the action of another drug, a **drug interaction** is present. These reactions often take place during the process of metabolism (or biotransformation) in the liver and are a result of the cytochrome

P-450 enzyme pathways each person inherits. The actions of many drugs may be altered when they are taken with other drugs; these drugs include many antidepressants, theophylline, warfarin, cimetidine, ciprofloxacin, isoniazid, ketoconazole, phenytoin, tolbutamide, zafirlukast, phenobarbital, rifampin, codeine, and morphine. Some medications are given together on purpose because the drug interactions are helpful. For example, probenecid is given with penicillin to increase the amount of penicillin that is absorbed, which is important in treating venereal disease. Other drug interactions produce adverse effects. For example, some antibiotics make birth control pills less effective, thus placing a woman at risk for pregnancy.

Several types of effects are seen with drug interactions (Box 4-4). When two drugs are given together and the combined effect of the drugs is equal to either that of the most active drug, or the sum of the effects of the individual drugs, an **additive effect** is seen. If one drug interferes with the action of another drug, it is described as an **antagonistic effect.** At times, one drug may replace another drug at a receptor site, increasing the effect of the first drug. This is called **displacement.** Sometimes **incompatibility** occurs when drugs do not mix well chemically. Attempts to mix them together in a syringe may cause a chemical

reaction so that neither of the drugs can be given. **Interference** is seen when one drug promotes the rapid excretion of another drug, thus reducing its activity. Finally, if the effect of two drugs taken at the same time is greater than the sum of the effects of each drug given alone, the drugs have a **synergistic effect.** This is often seen when individuals are exposed to pollutants and toxins. *Potentiation* is one type of synergistic effect in which a drug that might produce only a small effect by itself produces a larger effect when given with another specific drug.

Food, Alcohol, and Drug Interactions

Food, alcohol, and most medications taken by mouth must travel through the liver for chemical changes before they can be used by the body. Thus the risk for drug interaction with food or alcohol is high. When taken together, food or alcohol and drugs may alter the body's ability to use a particular food or drug. Part of these interactions may be due to activation of the P-450 enzyme system or competition for receptor sites. Monoamine oxidase inhibitors (MAOIs) are some of the drugs most noted for drug-food interactions, because they cannot be taken with aged cheese or many processed foods. Information that each patient should know about possible drug interactions includes the following:

- Cigarette smoking can decrease the effect of medication or create other problems with some drugs by increasing metabolism.
- Caffeine, which is found in coffee, tea, some soft drinks, chocolate, and some medications, can also affect the action of some drugs.
- Medication should never be taken during pregnancy without the advice of the health care provider.
- If the patient has any problem related to medication, he should call his health care provider or a pharmacist immediately.

Alcohol-Medication Interactions. The amount of alcohol use is very high in the U.S. population. It has been estimated that about 70% of adults consume alcohol at least occasionally, and up to 10% of people may drink daily. Many patients may not be aware that alcohol is one of the products that reacts most commonly with drugs. The extent to which a dose of medicine reaches its site of action is called *availability.* Alcohol can influence whether a drug is effective or not by changing its availability.

In an alert from the National Institute on Alcohol Abuse and Alcoholism,* it was estimated that alcohol-medication interactions may be a factor in at least 25% of all emergency room admissions. An unknown number of

---

| Box 4-4 | *Common Drug Interactions* |

ADDITIVE EFFECT

When two drugs are given together, the combined effect of the drugs is equal to either that of the single more active component of the mixture or the sum of the effects of the individual drugs.

ANTAGONISTIC EFFECT

An antagonistic effect takes place when one drug interferes with the action of another drug.

DISPLACEMENT

Displacement takes place when one drug replaces another at the drug receptor site, increasing the effect of the first drug.

INCOMPATIBILITY

Incompatibility occurs when two drugs mixed together in a syringe produce a chemical reaction so they cannot be given.

INTERFERENCE

Interference occurs when one drug promotes the rapid excretion of another, thus reducing its activity.

SYNERGISTIC EFFECT

A synergistic effect takes place when the effect of two drugs taken at the same time is greater than the sum of the effects of each drug given alone.

---

*Alcohol-medication interactions, *Alcohol Alert*, No. 27 (PH 355), Washington, DC, January 1995, National Institute on Alcohol Abuse and Alcoholism.

less serious interactions go unrecognized and un-recorded. One group of individuals at high risk for alcohol-drug interactions is older adults, who take 25% to 30% of all prescription medications and also frequently drink alcohol. Elderly individuals are more likely to suffer medication side effects compared with younger persons, and these effects tend to be more severe with advancing age.

Table 4-1 provides information about food-drug-alcohol interactions that you should tell patients.

Table 4-1 *Specific Food-Alcohol-Drug Interactions by Drug Category*

MEDICATION CATEGORY	COMMON MEDICATION EXAMPLES	INTERACTIONS AND INSTRUCTIONS TO GIVE PATIENTS
DRUGS FOR PAIN		
Analgesics-antipyretics— Used to relieve pain and reduce fever.	Acetaminophen (Tylenol, Tempra)	Take on an empty stomach for more rapid relief because food may slow the body's absorption of the drug. Avoid alcohol because this can increase the risk of liver damage or GI bleeding.
Analgesics-narcotics— Used to suppress cough and relieve pain; often with ASA or acetaminophen.	Codeine with aspirin; codeine with acetaminophen (Tylenol #2, #3, #4); morphine (Roxanol, MS Contin); oxycodone with acetaminophen (Percocet, Roxicet); meperidine (Demerol); hydrocodone with acetaminophen (Vicodin, Lorcet)	Avoid alcohol because it increases the sedative effect of these medications. Take with meals, small snacks, or milk because these medications may cause stomach upset. Use caution when motor skills are required.
RESPIRATORY TRACT DRUGS		
Antihistamines—Used to relieve or prevent symptoms of colds, hay fever, and other types of allergy. They act to limit or block histamine.	Brompheniramine (Dimetane, Bromphen, chlorpheniramine/Chlor-Trimeton, Teldrin); diphenhydramine (Benadryl, Banophen); clemastine (Tavist); fexofenadine (Allegra); loratadine (Claritin); cetirizine (Zyrtec)	Avoid alcohol because antihistamines combined with alcohol may cause drowsiness and slowed reactions. Take prescription antihistamines on an empty stomach to increase their effectiveness.
Bronchodilators—Used to treat the symptoms of bronchial asthma, chronic bronchitis, and emphysema. These medicines relieve wheezing, SOB, and dyspnea. They work by opening the air passages of the lungs.	Theophylline (Slo-bid, Theo-Dur, Theo-Dur 24, Uniphyl); albuterol (Ventolin, Proventil, Combivent); epinephrine (Primatene Mist)	Avoid eating or drinking large amounts of foods or beverages that contain caffeine because both bronchodilators and caffeine stimulate the central nervous system. High-fat meals may increase the amount of theophylline in the body, whereas high-carbohydrate meals may decrease it. The effect of food on theophylline products varies. Many over-the-counter cold remedies contain aspirin in combination with other active ingredients.
ANTIINFLAMMATORY AND ANTIALLERGIC DRUGS		
Aspirin—Used to reduce pain, fever, and inflammation.	Aspirin (Bayer, Ecotrin)	Because aspirin can cause stomach irritation, avoid alcohol. To avoid stomach upset, take with food. Do not take with fruit juice. Buffered aspirin or enteric-coated aspirin may also reduce GI bleeding.
Corticosteroids—Used to provide relief to inflamed areas. Lessen swelling, redness, itching, and allergic reactions.	Methylprednisolone (Medrol); prednisone (Deltasone); prednisolone (Pediapred, Prelone); cortisone acetate (Cortef)	Take with food or milk to decrease GI distress. Avoid alcohol because both alcohol and corticosteroids can cause stomach irritation. Also avoid foods high in sodium (salt). Check labels on food packages for sodium. Take with food to prevent stomach upset.

Table 4-1	*Specific Food-Alcohol-Drug Interactions by Drug Category—cont'd*	
MEDICATION CATEGORY	**COMMON MEDICATION EXAMPLES**	**INTERACTIONS AND INSTRUCTIONS TO GIVE PATIENTS**
ANTIINFLAMMATORY AND ANTIALLERGIC DRUGS—cont'd		
NSAIDs—Used to relieve pain and reduce inflammation and fever.	Ibuprofen (Advil, Motrin); naproxen (Anaprox, Aleve, Naprosyn); ketoprofen (Orudis); nabumetone (Relafen)	These drugs should be taken with food or milk because they can irritate the stomach. Avoid taking these medications with those foods or alcoholic beverages that tend to bother the stomach.
DRUGS FOR BONE AND JOINT DISORDERS		
Indomethacin—Used to reduce pain, swelling, stiffness, joint pain, and fever in certain types of arthritis and gout.	Indomethacin (Indocin)	This drug should be taken with food because it can irritate the stomach. Avoid taking the medication with the kinds of foods or alcoholic beverages that tend to irritate the stomach.
Piroxicam—used to reduce pain, swelling, stiffness, joint pain, and fever in certain types of arthritis.	Piroxicam (Feldene)	This medication should be taken with a light snack because it can cause stomach irritation. Avoid alcohol because it can add to the possibility of stomach upset.
DIURETICS		
Use to eliminate water, sodium, and chloride.	Furosemide (Lasix); hydrochlorothiazide (Esidrix, HydroDIURIL); triamterene (Dyrenium); bumetanide (Bumex); metolazone (Zaroxolyn); triamterene + hydrochlorothiazide (Dyazide, Maxzide)	Diuretics vary in their interactions with nutrients. Loss of potassium, calcium, and magnesium occurs with some diuretics. May require potassium supplement. With some diuretics, potassium loss is less significant.
DRUGS FOR THE HEART, BLOOD VESSELS, AND BLOOD		
Nitrates—Used to relax veins and arteries to reduce work of the heart.	Nitroglycerin (Nitro-Bid, Nitro-Dur, Transderm-Nitro); isosorbide dinitrate (Isordil, Sorbitrate)	Use of sodium (salt) should be restricted for medication to be effective. Use with alcohol may drastically lower blood pressure. Check labels on food packages for sodium.
Antihypertensives—Used to relax blood vessels, increase the supply of blood and oxygen to the heart, and lessen the heart's workload. May regulate heartbeat.	*Beta blockers:* atenolol (Tenormin); metoprolol (Lopressor); propranolol (Inderal); nadolol (Corgard) *ACE inhibitors:* captopril (Capoten); enalapril (Vasotec); lisinopril (Prinivil, Zestril); quinapril (Accupril); moexipril (Univasc)	*Beta blockers:* Use of sodium (salt) should be restricted for medication to be effective. Check labels on food packages for sodium. Alcohol and propranolol in combination may dramatically lower blood pressure. *ACE inhibitors:* Food can decrease absorption. ACE inhibitors may increase the amount of potassium. Avoid eating large amounts of foods high in potassium.
Anticoagulants—Used to prolong clotting of the blood.	Warfarin (Coumadin)	Moderation in consumption of foods high in vitamin K is recommended because vitamin K produces blood-clotting substances. Such foods include beef liver, green leafy vegetables (spinach), cabbage, cauliflower, brussels sprouts, potatoes, vegetable oil, and egg yolk. High doses of vitamin E (400 international units or more) may prolong clotting time.
Antihyperlipidemics—HMG-CoA reductase inhibitors, or "statins," used to lower cholesterol.	Atorvastatin (Lipitor); fluvastatin (Lescol); lovastatin (Mevacor); pravastatin (Pravachol); simvastatin (Zocor)	Mevacor should be taken with the evening meal to enhance absorption. Avoid large amounts of alcohol because it may increase risk of liver damage.

Table 4-1 | *Specific Food-Alcohol-Drug Interactions by Drug Category—cont'd*

MEDICATION CATEGORY	COMMON MEDICATION EXAMPLES	INTERACTIONS AND INSTRUCTIONS TO GIVE PATIENTS
ANTIINFECTIVES		
Cephalosporins	Cefaclor (Ceclor, Ceclor CD); cefadroxil (Duricef); cefixime (Suprax); cefprozil (Cefzil); cephalexin (Keflex, Keftab)	Take on an empty stomach 1 hr before or 2 hr after meals. Can be taken with food if severe GI upset occurs.
Macrolides—Used to treat skin, ear infections.	Erythromycin (E-Mycin, Ery-Tab, Eryc); erythromycin + sulfisoxazole (Pediazole); azithromycin (Zithromax); clarithromycin (Biaxin)	Macrolides vary in their reactions with food. Avoid acidic fruit juices, citrus fruits, or acidic beverages, such as cola drinks because these antibiotics are acid labile (acid reduces absorption). Take on an empty stomach 1 hr before or 2 hr after meals.
Methenamine—Used in treating urinary tract infections.	Mandelamine, Urex	Cranberries, plums, prunes, and their juices help the action of this drug. Avoid citrus fruits and citrus juices. Eat foods with protein, but avoid dairy products.
Metronidazole—Used to treat intestinal and genital infections caused by bacteria and parasites.	Flagyl	Avoid using any form of alcohol while taking this drug, or severe prolonged vomiting and other symptoms may develop (antebuse-reaction).
Penicillins—Used to treat a wide variety of infections.	Amoxicillin (Trimox, Amoxil); ampicillin (Principen, Omnipen); penicillin V (Veetids)	Amoxicillin and bacampicillin may be taken with food; however, absorption of other types of penicillins is reduced when taken with food. Avoid acidic fruit juices, citrus fruits, or acidic beverages, such as cola drinks, because the penicillins are acid labile (acid reduces absorption). Take on an empty stomach 1 hr before or 2 hr after meals.
Quinolones	Ciprofloxacin (Cipro); levofloxacin (Levaquin); ofloxacin (Floxin); trovafloxacin (Trovan)	Take on an empty stomach 1 hr before or 2 hr after meals. Can be taken with food if severe GI upset occurs. Avoid calcium-containing products, vitamins and minerals containing iron, and antacids because they significantly decrease drug concentrations. Taking with caffeine products may increase caffeine levels and produce excitability and nervousness.
Sulfonamides—Used to treat stomach and urinary infections.	Sulfamethoxazole + trimethoprim (Bactrim, Septra)	Avoid alcohol because the combination may cause nausea. Take on an empty stomach, if possible.
Tetracyclines—Used to treat a wide variety of infections.	Tetracycline (Achromycin, Sumycin); doxycycline (Vibramycin); minocycline (Minocin)	These drugs should not be taken within 2 hr of eating dairy products such as milk, ice cream, yogurt or cheese, or taking calcium or iron supplements. Calcium forms a complex with the drug, resulting in reduced absorption of the antibiotic. Take 1 hr before meals or 2 hr after.
Antifungals	Fluconazole (Diflucan); griseofulvin (Grifulvin); ketoconazole (Nizoral); itraconazole (Sporanox)	Avoid taking these medications with dairy products or antacids. Avoid drinking alcohol or using medications or food that contain alcohol for at least 3 days after taking ketoconazole. It may produce a disulfiram-type reaction.

Continued

Table 4-1 | *Specific Food-Alcohol-Drug Interactions by Drug Category—cont'd*

MEDICATION CATEGORY	COMMON MEDICATION EXAMPLES	INTERACTIONS AND INSTRUCTIONS TO GIVE PATIENTS
DRUGS FOR PSYCHIATRIC PROBLEMS		
Antianxiety drugs	Lorazepam (Ativan); diazepam (Valium); alprazolam (Xanax)	Use with caffeine may cause excitability, nervousness, and hyperactivity and lessen the antianxiety effect. Use with alcohol may impair mental and motor functions.
Antidepressants	Paroxetine (Paxil), sertraline (Zoloft), fluoxetine (Prozac)	Avoid concurrent use with alcohol. These medications can be taken with or without food.
Lithium carbonate—regulates changes in chemical levels in the brain.	Various names	Follow the dietary and fluid intake instructions of the health care provider to avoid very serious toxic reactions.
MAO inhibitors—antidepressant	Phenelzine (Nardil); tranylcypromine (Parnate)	A very dangerous, potentially fatal interaction can occur with foods containing tyramine, a chemical in alcoholic beverages, particularly wine, and in many foods such as hard cheeses, chocolate, beef or chicken livers, sour cream, yogurt, raisins, bananas, avocados, soy sauce, yeast extract, meat tenderizers, sausages, and anchovies. Patient may develop severe headache, nosebleed, chest pain, photosensitivity, or severe hypertension with hypertensive crisis.
Sedative-hypnotics	Various names	Do not use alcohol with any sleep medications because oversedation occurs.
ANTACIDS, ANTIULCER MEDICATIONS, AND HISTAMINE BLOCKERS		
Work to reduce acid in the stomach.	Cimetidine (Tagamet); famotidine (Pepcid); ranitidine (Zantac); nizatidine (Axid)	Follow specific diets given by health care provider. Avoid large amounts of caffeine; dairy products such as milk or cream may increase acid secretion. If calcium carbonate is used as a calcium supplement, avoid bran and whole-grain breads or cereals that reduce absorption of calcium.
LAXATIVES		
Stimulate intestine, soften stool, add bulk or fluid to stool.	Various names	Excessive use of laxatives can cause loss of essential vitamins and minerals, and may require replenishment of potassium, sodium, and other nutrients through diet. Mineral oil can cause poor absorption of vitamins A, D, E, and K, and calcium. Take 2 hr before eating food.

Modified from *Food & drug interactions,* Washington, DC, 1999, National Consumers League (see http://www.nclnet.org.); McKenry LM, Salerno E: *Mosby's pharmacology in nursing,* ed 21, St Louis, 2003, Mosby.
ACE, Angiotensin-converting enzyme; *GI,* gastrointestinal; *HMG-CoA,* 3-hydroxy-3-methylglutaryl coenzyme A; *NSAIDs,* nonsteroidal antiinflammatory drugs; *SOB,* shortness of breath; *ASA,* acetylsalicylic acid; *MAO,* monoamine oxidase.

Drug Effects on Laboratory Tests and Blood Substances. Although medications exert a therapeutic effect in the body, they may also have effects on various natural substances in the blood, or they may alter the results of some laboratory tests. For example, the drug may increase the blood glucose level or affect the clotting time. Nurses should be aware of these changes as they look at the results of laboratory tests and try to monitor the action of a drug.

Chronotherapy. Research has shown that certain drugs are more effective at different times of the day, and that drug treatment may work best when it is linked to the normal human circadian rhythm (a repetitive cycle based on a 24-hour clock). The circadian clock controls rhythms in endocrine gland secretion, metabolic processes, and behavioral activity. Certain diseases, such as asthma, angina, diabetes mellitus, and hypertension, get better or worse throughout the day according to the circadian cycle. Chronotherapy is a process that attempts to time the peak of drug action so that it occurs when that action is most needed by the body. For example, secretion of catecholamines increases early in the morning as the patient awakens. Catecholamines cause an increase in heart rate, contractile force, cardiac output, and systolic blood pressure and may place enough stress on a weak heart to cause a heart attack. Antihypertensive medications, which work to reduce these effects, must be at a high level during this period of time. So, it is important that the patient's drug treatment program be designed to achieve this timing.

PATIENT VARIABLES AFFECTING DRUG USE

Special knowledge and sometimes special medications are required for neonates, small children, adults, and elderly patients. Women who are pregnant have special risks when they take any type of medication. People of different cultures also have different attitudes about medication use. All of these factors are important for the nurse to know and may affect the nursing care plan in giving medications to these individuals. (These variables are discussed in greater detail in Chapters 5 and 6.)

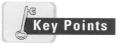
Key Points

- As you prepare to administer medications, you must be aware of the pharmacologic actions of each drug.
- You must learn about the absorption, distribution, metabolism, and excretion actions of each drug.
- The information gained through assessment of the patient and the nurse's knowledge about the expected patient response, side effects, adverse effects, and drug interactions become the foundation for the diagnosis, planning, implementation, and evaluation of the patient's response to the medication.

Go to the free CD-ROM for an Audio Glossary, animations, video clips, and Review Questions for the NCLEX-PN® Examination.

evolve Be sure to visit the companion Evolve website at http://evolve.elsevier.com/Edmunds/LPN/ for WebLinks, a link to the top 200 drugs by prescription, and sign-up pages for newsletter drug updates.

CRITICAL THINKING ?

1. Using the *Physician's Desk Reference, Mosby's Drug Consult,* or drug package inserts from a pharmacy, complete the following chart, identifying the appropriate names for each drug:

Generic Name	Chemical Name	Official Name	Brand Name
phenobarbital	_____	_____	_____
metronidazole	_____	_____	_____
Keflex	_____	_____	_____
albuterol	_____	_____	_____
Valium	_____	_____	_____

2. Sometimes the brand-name version of a drug is more expensive than a generic version of the same drug. Can you always substitute a generic drug for a brand-name version? Explain.

3. To get an idea of the range of chemical reactions that can be involved with a single drug, take these steps:
   a. Pick a drug from the index of this text, look it up, and describe each of the following actions or reactions as it applies to the drug you have chosen to investigate: adverse reaction; anaphylactic reaction; desired action; drug interaction; side effect
   b. What did you learn about the differences in these effects or reactions? For instance, what is the difference between a side effect and an adverse reaction?
   c. Now, if time permits, repeat this exercise with another drug of your choice.

4. Choose a drug. In the second column of the following table, define the physiologic processes listed in the first column. In the third column, describe how the drug you chose is absorbed, distributed, metabolized, and excreted.

Drug: _____

Process	Definition	Action
Absorption		
Distribution		
Metabolism		
Excretion		

5. Referring to the information you gathered in Question 4, what factors may affect these processes? Why?

6. Using Unit Three as your resource, work with a partner to find examples of each of the following types of drug interactions:

   Displacement

   Incompatibility

   Interference

7. The patient states that he is "allergic to codeine." When the nurse inquires further, the patient reports that he became severely constipated when he took codeine. Is this a drug allergy?

Lifespan and Cultural Modifications

After reading and studying this chapter, you should be able to do the following:

1. Identify specific considerations in giving medications to pediatric, pregnant, breastfeeding, or elderly patients.
2. Identify special considerations that should be taken in providing care to individuals from different cultures.
3. Describe specific nursing behaviors that assist in helping patients succeed with their medication plans.

Key Terms

Be sure to check out the bonus material on the free CD-ROM, including selected audio pronunciations.

adolescence (ăd-ō-LĔS-ĕns, p. 43)
culture (p. 52)
geriatric (jĕr-ē-ĂT-rĭk, p. 46)
infants (p. 44)
neonates (NĒ-ō-nāts, p. 43)
noncompliance (NŌN-cŏm-PLĪ-ăns, p. 54)
pediatric (pē-dē-ĂT-rĭks, p. 45)
regimen (RĔJ-ĭ-mĕn, p. 48)
teratogenic (TĔR-ă-tō-JĔN-ĭk, p. 49)

OVERVIEW

You are preparing to learn how to give medications to patients as part of their treatment. There are many differences in the medications that your patients will take, but there are differences in the patients as well. For example, small infants cannot take the same medications as adults. Elderly patients may have many diseases and require multiple drugs; the risk for problems is increased with the addition of each new product to the treatment plan. How can the information you learn help you in dealing with patients from birth to death?

Patient variables, or differences such as age, weight, and other diseases a patient may have or medications she may be taking at the same time, affect how a drug acts in the body. Many cultural and even religious beliefs may influence whether a patient is willing to take medication. Helping your patient understand the importance of taking her medication, and how to take it properly, is one of the biggest challenges you will face. You must learn about your patients' backgrounds and the things that are important to them if you are to assist them in getting well.

PATIENT FACTORS THAT MAY AFFECT DRUG ACTION

A lot of research is conducted on drugs before they can be sold, and much information is gathered on each new drug. Standards have been set up by the U.S. Food and Drug Administration (FDA) that require the drug company to provide certain information to people who may prescribe, administer, or take the drug. This information includes a description of the therapeutic response, side effects, and adverse effects of the drug, and a list of other drugs that may interact with this drug. This information is printed by the manufacturer on a slip of paper inserted into the product container (the "product package insert" or PPI).

General factors that influence drug activity help the nurse figure out what the response to the medication should be. Some of these patient factors or variables are listed in Box 5-1.

SPECIAL CONSIDERATIONS IN THE PEDIATRIC PATIENT

The changes that occur as the child grows from birth to **adolescence** (12 to 16 years of age) have a profound impact on drug action and effect. Some changes are obvious, but subtle changes in the response to drugs occur throughout the growth and developmental cycle.

The term *children* covers a very broad category from neonates to 16-year-old adolescents. Very clear changes in drug effects on **neonates** (less than 1 month of age) are the result of their small body mass, low body fat content, high body water volume, and increased membrane (for example, the skin or the blood-brain barrier) permeability. Immediately after birth, several factors influence drug absorption: no gastric acid is present to help break down drugs, no intestinal bacteria or enzyme function is present to metabolize a drug, and the gastrointestinal (GI) transit time (the time it takes for a drug to move through the stomach and intestines) is slow.

Box 5-1 | *Patient Variables Influencing Drug Action*

BODY WEIGHT

An overweight individual requires a larger dosage. An underweight individual requires a smaller dosage.

AGE

Infants and children require smaller dosages because they have smaller fat and total water content, immature enzyme systems, reduced kidney function, and variation in circulating blood proteins.

Elderly individuals may require smaller dosages because of changes in cellular composition and functioning throughout the body (especially in the liver and kidney), the presence of several disease processes, and the necessity for many medications.

ILLNESS

The type of pathologic process influences body processes. Nephrotic syndrome, dehydration, malabsorption, or malnutrition may cause changes in blood volume and protein composition. Kidney disease produces changes in blood and electrolyte concentrations. Liver disease leads to decreased metabolism of some drugs and foods. Hyperthyroidism may produce a higher metabolic rate, which increases drug metabolism. A patient in shock may have reduced circulation with delays in drug distribution in tissues.

PREGNANCY AND BREASTFEEDING

Many drugs are contraindicated during pregnancy because of the teratogenic effect on the fetus. Medications may also be passed to the child through breast milk. Thus, no pregnant or breastfeeding mother should take any medications without contacting her health care provider. The Food and Drug Administration requires that all drug manufacturers supply published information regarding the safety of drugs when taken during pregnancy.

GENETICS

The genetic makeup of each individual influences such factors as the cytochrome P-450 enzyme system of metabolism in the liver, as well as patient intolerance to some medications. For example, atropine is contraindicated in patients with angle-closure glaucoma, anesthetic agents may precipitate sickle cell anemia crisis, and salicylates may trigger Crigler-Najjar syndrome.

CUMULATIVE DRUG EFFECTS

A drug may reach a higher level than needed because it is administered too often, the dosage is too high, or other drugs or chemicals (such as alcohol) that increase the effect of the drug are taken at the same time. The drug may accumulate in a high concentration and produce side effects.

INDIVIDUAL PSYCHOLOGY

The patient's attitude about drug acceptability and effectiveness is important. Some patients can be given a placebo, which is made of an inert or ineffective substance, that can be as effective as real medication in certain cases. Other patients develop tolerance or a need for an increased dosage over time to produce the same effects. This is often a symptom of psychologic dependence.

DEPENDENCE

An individual may develop both a physical and a psychological need for a drug, usually a controlled substance. This may also be termed *addiction* or *habituation*.

The systems in the liver that are used to deactivate drugs are immature, and even the immaturity of the kidney and renal excretion system adds to the speed with which a drug might be eliminated in the neonate.

In **infants** (1 month to 12 to 24 months of age) and young children, the decrease in total body water, increase in body mass, decrease in membrane permeability, and changes in body fat produce less obvious changes in drug response. The infant has a high metabolic rate and a rapid turnover of body water, which result in relatively higher fluid, calorie, and drug dosage requirements per kilogram of body weight than those of the adolescent. Growth and development or maturation of drug-metabolizing systems and the development of the urinary tract also results in changes in drug response.

Absorption

Drug absorption in infants and children follows the same basic principles as in adults. However, three factors tend to be especially important in children. First, the physiologic status of the infant or child determines the blood flow at the site of intramuscular (IM) or subcutaneous drug administration. Factors that may reduce blood flow to muscular or subcutaneous tissues include cardiovascular shock, vasoconstriction caused by sympathomimetic agents, or heart failure. In these conditions, there would be reduced absorption of any drugs injected IM or into subcutaneous tissues. In premature infants with little muscle mass, the blood supply to these areas and the resulting absorption are very irregular. In older children, the size of and circulation in the muscles affects how rapidly a medication is absorbed.

There is more rapid absorption from the deltoid muscle than from the vastus lateralis muscle, and the slowest absorption is from the gluteal muscles.

The instability or immaturity of different body processes in premature infants compared with older children and adults is a second influence on drug absorption from IM sites. For example, toxic drug levels may occur if the blood supply to IM or subcutaneous tissues suddenly increases, leading to greater absorption of medication, and increasing the amount of the drug entering the blood. With some drugs, there is only a small difference between the level of drug that is helpful and the level of drug that is toxic and harmful. We say that these drugs have a *narrow therapeutic margin.* Examples of these drugs would be anticonvulsants, cardiac glycosides, and aminoglycoside antibiotics. With these drugs, it would be easy for an infant to get too much medicine when absorption is variable.

A final factor in drug absorption is that the skin of premature and newborn infants has a greater ability to absorb some chemicals because of its greater hydration. That is, the outside stratum corneum of the epidermal barrier in the skill may allow more fluid to enter because the system is not well developed. The transdermal route may be used with some infants to reduce the unpredictability of some medications that are usually given orally or IM (for example, theophylline). However, transdermal dosage patches available for sale are not intended for pediatric patients and would deliver doses much higher than what is needed for infants and children. Instead, rubbing the drug into the skin, putting the drug in an oil base, and using an occlusive dressing (covering the skin on which the drug is placed by wrapping the area in plastic wrap) may increase the absorption of topical products.

Distribution

Drug distribution is determined by two factors: (1) the chemical properties of the drug itself (for example, the molecular weight), which do not vary; and (2) the physiologic factors specific to the patient, including total body water, extracellular water, protein binding, and pathologic conditions modifying physiologic function, all of which vary widely in different patient populations.

Metabolism

The biotransformation of drugs in the body into usable substances involves chemical reactions that convert a drug to an inactive or less active compound. In general, drug metabolism in infants is much slower than that in older children and adults. Because most drug metabolism takes place in the liver, the fact that the levels of cytochrome P-450 enzymes of infants are only 50% to 70% of adult values is important in treatment of children. The amounts vary for the different enzymes, but the ability to increase production of all enzymes continues until the third or fourth year of life.

Because neonates have a decreased ability to metabolize drugs, they may be at increased risk for adverse effects as a result of slow clearance rates and prolonged half-lives, particularly when drugs must be given over long periods of time.

Excretion

As with metabolism, the growth and maturity of the child's organs has an important effect on the child's ability to excrete the end products of the drug reactions. Problems caused by the incomplete development of the renal excretion system, including glomerular filtration, tubular secretion, and tubular reabsorption, are slowly resolved as the child develops prior to birth. However, this system may still be very immature at birth and may only slowly develop to normal over the first year of life.

This process of normal development has implications for drug clearance, particularly of common drugs such as penicillin, aminoglycosides, and digoxin, for which clearance rates may fall to 17% to 34% of the adult clearance rate. If a child is sick enough to require these drugs, his or her glomerular filtration rate (GFR) may not improve as predicted during the first weeks and months of life. This means that adjustments must be made in dosage and dosing schedules. The child will also require more careful monitoring, and dosages should be determined based on plasma drug levels determined at intervals throughout the course of therapy.

The growth spurt and the increase in adrenal steroid and sex hormone (estrogen in girls, androgens in both sexes) levels that occur before puberty affect drug response in children who are near puberty and in adolescents. The increase in male muscle mass, increase in female body fat, and stability of the body temperature in both sexes also affect adolescent drug response.

These facts about the drug-metabolizing system in **pediatric** patients (infants through adolescents) are important to remember in looking at a child's sensitivity to medication. For example, infants and children require a total daily digoxin dose that is approximately twice that of an adult on a basis of the ratio of weight to dose. It is thought that this increased requirement for digoxin is the result of a greater binding strength of the child's developing myocardial digoxin receptors for digitalis derivatives. Variations in the development of drug receptors may make a neonate very sensitive to anesthetics such as curare but resistant to other anesthetics such as succinylcholine.

Adverse Reactions

The risk for drug-drug interactions and adverse effects is increased in very ill children and infants. Children may be exposed to drugs in three major ways: (1) transplacentally, when the drug is given to the mother during pregnancy and delivery; (2) by direct administration of the drug to the child; and (3) by swallowing of the drug in breast milk after the drug is given to a nursing mother. Fetal exposure to drugs through the placenta and neonatal exposure through breast milk share a common characteristic: these are the only stages in life in which one is exposed to and affected by drugs administered to another person, the mother.

The number of adverse reactions in pediatric patients is unknown. Because young children are vulnerable, their diseases are often complex, their drug therapy is often complicated, and adverse drug reactions are unavoidable or hard to assess. However, studies have generally found that rates of adverse reactions in children are equal to those in adults. The rate may be as high as 5.8% of drugs administered to children, although the rate is higher if the child is hospitalized rather than at home. Adverse drug reactions may have a profound immediate, delayed, or long-term impact on the child's neurologic and somatic development.

With younger children, it may be difficult to tell whether the child is having an adverse reaction, is just experiencing symptoms of the underlying illness, or is having a paradoxical reaction to a drug (for example, hyperactive behavior with antihistamines or chloral hydrate, and sleepiness with stimulants such as Ritalin). Over-the-counter preparations (particularly antihistamines and adrenergic drugs found in various cough syrups, cold remedies, decongestants, and nose drops) may also provoke adverse reactions in pediatric patients. A broad spectrum of reactions may be seen, varying from minor hypersensitivity reactions to more serious problems including alterations in growth, damage to anatomic or physiologic systems, and numerous other problems.

Children are not just small adults who require a proportionally smaller dose of medication. Although we know that children do respond differently to drugs, very little research has been conducted to determine the safety and efficacy of many specific drugs when used in children. It has only been since 1996 that the FDA has required drug companies to label all medications with specific information related to their use in different pediatric age groups. In many cases, the information gathered during research on a drug used in an adult population may be safely extended to pediatric patients. But in some cases, the FDA has required companies to file additional information about their products when used with pediatric patients. Very frequently, nurses find that drugs are labeled with "safety for use in infants and children not determined" when they look for pediatric information about a drug. Thus all drug use in very young children should be approached with caution because of their more immature metabolic and elimination systems. Toxic effects may develop more quickly and stay around longer, so special dosages are required (see Chapter 9).

SPECIAL CONSIDERATIONS IN THE GERIATRIC PATIENT

Elderly patients also react differently to drugs. Medications are absorbed, metabolized, and excreted more slowly and less completely in older adults. In **geriatric** (older adult and elderly) persons, problems with medications are often due to a lack of understanding of the way drugs are processed in the aging body and the body's changed response to drugs. To further complicate matters, people age differently and their individual body systems may also age at different rates.

Absorption

The overall importance of changes in the absorption of drugs with aging is not completely clear. There may be some delay in the absorption process. Physiologic changes that affect the GI tract include a reduction in acid output so there is a more alkaline environment, which may affect drugs that require an acid medium for absorption. Reductions in blood flow, enzyme activity, gastric emptying, and bowel motility may increase the delay in absorption of some drugs, although they probably have little if any effect on the extent of absorption. Compounds such as iron, calcium, and certain vitamins that depend on active transport mechanisms, and thus the delivery of oxygen, for absorption may be affected by the decreased blood flow in the aging patient's GI tract.

Distribution

The distribution of drugs in the body may also be affected by the aging process and is linked to the chemical makeup of the agent involved. There is a decline in total body water and lean body mass with aging that may result in less movement or distribution of water-soluble drugs into some tissues. If the dose of these drugs is not changed, the patient may develop higher serum concentrations, leading to an increased effect or toxicity. Thus the usual rule is to start drugs using a low dose and then increase the dose slowly in elderly patients. Drugs that are distributed into body water or lean body mass include digoxin, cimetidine, lithium, gentamicin, meperidine, phenytoin, and theophylline.

The distribution of fat-soluble drugs may also be changed by the aging process. With aging, there is usually a decrease in lean body mass but an increase in total body fat. Thus, lipid-soluble drugs may be stored in larger amounts in fat tissues and thus remain in the body for a longer time. Diazepam, chlordiazepoxide, flurazepam, thiopental, antipsychotics, and some antidepressants are lipid-soluble drugs that may require a lower dose and slow increases if used in the elderly population.

Another important concern that may exist with elderly patients is a decrease in serum proteins such as albumin. Albumin is the most common protein that binds to various acidic drugs, and a large decrease in albumin may result in a greater amount of unbound drug that may circulate freely. Highly protein-bound drugs that tend to bind quickly to albumin include phenytoin, warfarin, naproxen, theophylline, phenobarbital, and some antidepressants.

Metabolism

The effect of aging on liver function is difficult to determine because there is no good marker for measuring liver, or hepatic, function. Overall, a decrease in liver mass occurs with age, along with a reduction in hepatic blood flow. The result of lowered hepatic blood flow may be seen with drugs that are mostly broken down the first time they go through the liver (high first-pass metabolism). The extent to which these drugs are metabolized depends on how fast they go through the liver. When blood flow is reduced, as may occur with aging, less of the drug is metabolized, so increased amounts of the active form may remain the blood.

In an aging liver, there may also be changes in the specific pathways or phases of metabolism during which certain chemical and molecular changes occur to prepare the drug for metabolism. During phase I metabolism, drugs are generally made more water soluble so they may be excreted in the urine. Because of age-related changes in this process, drugs that are metabolized by phase I pathways may have decreased or unchanged clearance, so the drug may stay in the body and not be eliminated. Drugs that undergo phase I metabolism include diazepam, flurazepam, chlordiazepoxide, piroxicam, quinidine, and barbiturates. Such drugs should be used with caution and at lower doses in elderly patients, and the nurse must observe these patients carefully for adverse effects. If possible, these drugs should be avoided and other drugs that are metabolized differently (phase II metabolism) should be used. No changes with aging have been reported with drugs that are metabolized by phase II metabolic processes, including conjugation acetylation, sulfonation, and glucuronidation.

Drugs that are metabolized by the liver may have reduced metabolism because of other changes in the liver and also because of the influence of other diseases. The aging liver often gets smaller, has less blood flow, is affected by changes in nutritional status, and may become overloaded with fluid from diseases such as chronic heart failure. These factors may result in a loss of "hepatic reserve," or the liver's ability to handle all the different chemicals it must process. In this situation, the patient may have more risk of adverse effects when drugs are added to the existing treatment plan.

The important point in terms of giving medications to elderly patients is to use greater care in treating each patient individually and adjust the dose downward, if necessary.

Excretion

Kidney, or renal, function is the single most important factor that causes adverse drug reactions. Studies show that renal function varies with aging. Biologic changes in the aging kidney include decreases in the number of nephrons; decreases in renal blood flow, glomerular filtration, and tubular secretion rate; and an increase in the number of damaged glomeruli. In addition, damage to the arterial walls of blood vessels and lowered cardiac output reduce the amount of blood that flows to the kidneys by 40% to 50% between the ages of 25 and 65. The result of these changes may be a decrease in excretion of creatinine, which is reported to decrease 10% for each decade (10 years) after age 40 years.

Creatinine is a muscle by-product, and almost all of it is removed by the kidney, making it an excellent marker to measure kidney function (or renal clearance). A drug's creatinine clearance rate is the amount of blood from which a drug is cleared per unit of time. Although creatinine clearance is used to measure renal function, it is important to note that it is only an estimate. A number of formulas can be used to determine the creatinine clearance rate, but the results may not be very accurate. Creatinine clearance can be assessed more accurately by collecting urine for 24 hours and directly measuring the amount of creatinine in it, although this may be difficult to do. However, any method of estimating creatinine clearance may not be accurate in elderly patients, who have very little muscle mass and produce very little creatinine. In addition to the normal slowing of kidney function that may occur with aging and may be made worse by disease, problems leading to dehydration can also affect renal function and make the decision about how much drug to give the elderly patient even more complex.

The important factors to remember when caring for elderly patients who are taking drugs that will be excreted from the kidneys is to treat these patients individually, use the best creatinine clearance estimates that you can make, and use low doses or longer intervals between doses when you suspect that some kidney damage might be present. Drugs that depend on the kidneys for elimination include many antibiotics, some antivirals, antineoplastics, antifungals, analgesics, and many cardiac drugs.

Other kidney changes that occur with aging include a decrease in the ability of the kidney to remove only chemicals and not fluid (renal concentrating ability) and a tendency for the kidney to hold onto sodium (sodium conservation), which may affect patients on high-dose diuretics.

Adverse Reactions

Many older adults with chronic illnesses are required to take medications daily. These drugs are helpful in controlling disease, but they also present a very real hazard to elderly patients. About 90% of older adults have adverse reactions to drugs, and 20% of these reactions require hospitalization. As many as 30,000 people may die each year as a result of adverse drug reactions.

Because many elderly patients take several drugs, interactions among these different drugs may also cause problems for them. These patients may see several specialists, each of whom may prescribe different medications. If the specialists don't know about all the different drugs that a patient may be taking at the same time, the patient may be at risk from combining drugs that have adverse interactions with each other.

All drugs have some risk or hazard, but the medications most dangerous to the elderly patient are tranquilizers, sedatives, and other drugs that alter the mind and change what the patient thinks he sees, or may cause the patient to become dizzy or lose his balance. Diuretics and cardiac drugs such as digitalis also pose special dangers and must be given with caution and careful observation of how the patient responds. Elderly patients may become dehydrated easily, thus allowing the amount of drug in the blood to increase. This places them at greater risk for side effects and toxicity with normal dosages. Results of research show that there is also a high rate of alcohol use among many older people who either live at home or live in nursing homes. Thus we are now becoming aware that drug-alcohol interactions are a serious concern in this age group.

Laboratory tests should be ordered regularly to look at kidney and liver function, and the nurse should look for side effects and signs of toxicity at every visit. If you notice signs or symptoms of toxic reactions or adverse effects of drugs, or behavior that might be a side effect, you should report this immediately to the registered nurse. These signs and symptoms include changes in level of mental function, increased fatigue, restlessness, irritability, depression, weakness, dizziness, headache, and disorientation. These problems may interfere with appetite, balance, and energy, leading to dehydration, weight loss, falls, and immobility (not being able to move around). It is important to see that these often mild symptoms may be caused by drugs and should not simply be ignored as "typical" elderly behavior.

Patient Teaching Considerations

You must be sure that older persons are taught how to take their prescription medications and about the danger of taking nonprescription drugs at the same time. Failure of elderly patients to follow their medication plan, or **regimen,** may be caused by a number of factors. The cost of the drug, difficulty in getting it from a pharmacy, poor memory, lack of desire to take the drug regularly, depression, and feelings of being overwhelmed by the responsibility to take care of themselves all contribute to elderly patients failing to follow their medication regimen. In some cases, arthritis or another disease that causes physical disability may make it difficult for older adults to open bottle lids or use an inhaler. Poor eyesight may make it hard to draw up insulin or read the dose accurately. Many older patients also diagnose each other's health problems and share medications, which may make it very difficult for you to evaluate the effects of prescribed medications in a particular patient.

WOMEN'S HEALTH ISSUES

There are some drugs that are only taken by women because of the differences in their bodies from men. These include drugs to treat female genital tract infections and supplements used during the childbearing years. Other drugs taken by women may either prepare them for pregnancy, prevent pregnancy, or help their bodies recover from the loss of fertility-related hormones as a result of aging. Some women take these drugs faithfully, some take them only part of the time, and many women never have the chance to take the medications because of lack of information or money. But all of these medications may influence the woman's quality of life.

One of the biggest problems women have faced, particularly with the increase in diets high in refined sugars, is recurrent vaginal *Candida* infection. Newer antifungal medications have cut the treatment time for vaginal fungal infections from 7 days to 1 or 2 days. Although these products were only used by women, now men with acquired immunodeficiency syndrome (AIDS) are also using these medications to treat the opportunistic infections that often occur in patients with reduced immunity.

There is now a great deal of scientific data showing that eating more foods high in folate (citrus fruits, cereals, leafy greens, and whole grains) or taking a multivitamin that has folic acid protects against birth defects such as neural tube defect, spina bifida, and anencephaly. Folic acid may also reduce the risk of heart disease and stroke.

Iron supplements have long been known to be helpful for patients who suffer from anemia resulting from blood loss. Thus women of childbearing age are often placed on iron supplements. Most menopausal women would probably also benefit from a multivitamin containing 10 mg of iron or less.

Although oral contraceptive pills (OCPs) do not reduce the patient's risk of getting a sexually transmitted disease, their use has cut both the birth rate and the abortion rate. For older women, the risks associated with taking OCPs are less than those of pregnancy. However, women who use OCPs and who smoke are at an increased risk of adverse side effects such as stroke.

For several years, hormone replacement therapy (HRT) has been used to reduce the uncomfortable symptoms, such as hot flashes, that are seen with estrogen loss at menopause, and to reduce calcium loss from bones. However, research has now shown that HRT may lead to increased risk of stroke, heart attack, breast cancer, and perhaps dementia. Therefore, HRT is no longer recommended for long-term use in menopausal women.

SPECIAL CONSIDERATIONS IN PREGNANT AND BREASTFEEDING WOMEN

Pregnant and breastfeeding women may have both chronic diseases and acute problems, either of which may require drug treatment. Giving medicine to pregnant women poses a big challenge. In pregnancy, the drug is really going to two people, so you must consider how the drug may affect the growing fetus. The benefit of any drug to a pregnant patient must be carefully weighed against the possible (or potential) risk to the fetus. All mothers want to have perfect babies, so it is important for pregnant women to avoid as many drugs as possible, especially those drugs with **teratogenic** potential, or those likely to cause malformations or damage in the embryo or fetus. In addition, you must be aware of the changing body chemistry of the mother throughout the pregnancy, as well as that of the growing fetus, and how this will affect the action of the drug itself.

Since the reports in 1961 of severe fetal malformations caused by the drug thalidomide, which was given to control nausea and vomiting in pregnant women, greater precautions have been taken to consider the effect of medications on pregnant women. Medications that have been confirmed as teratogenic in humans include antithyroid compounds, aminoglycoside antibiotics, anticancer agents, androgenic hormones, tetracycline, thalidomide, warfarin (Coumadin) and other anticoagulants, lithium, diethylstilbestrol, penicillamine, vitamin A analogues, and many anticonvulsants, such as carbamazepine, primidone, valproic acid, and phenytoin. Alcohol, methadone, and cocaine also are known teratogens. The FDA has developed categories for classifying drugs according to their known level of risk to the fetus and to breastfed infants (Table 5-1; see also Appendixes A and B).

Factors such as what drug the mother takes, how much is taken, and the age of the fetus when the drug is taken are related to different types of malformations. Taking a drug during the first 2 weeks after conception (before implantation) results in an "all or nothing" effect. The ovum either dies from exposure to a lethal dose of a teratogen or recovers completely with no adverse effects. The critical period for morphologic, or structural, teratogenic effects in humans lasts from about 2 to 10 weeks after the last menstrual period (Figure 5-1). This embryonic period corresponds to the time of organ development (14 to 56 days), during which any teratogenic drug taken by the mother may produce major abnormalities in the embryo. Taking a teratogen later in the pregnancy during the fetal period (57 days to term) may result in minor structural changes, but abnormalities are more likely to involve problems with growth, mental development, and reproductive organ abnormalities. Clearly, it would be best if all women could stop taking any drugs before they got pregnant.

As the fetus grows, the placenta allows most drugs and nutritional products to cross from the mother to the baby. Thus you should assume that what the mother eats is also "eaten" by the fetus, with the exception of some drugs such as heparin and insulin. However, the reaction of a fetus to a medication is different from that

---

| Table 5-1 | *FDA Pregnancy Risk Categories* |

FDA CATEGORY	DEFINITION
A	Adequate, well-controlled studies in pregnant women have not shown an increased risk of fetal abnormalities.
B	Animal studies have revealed no evidence of harm to the fetus; however, there are no adequate and well-controlled studies in pregnant women. **OR** Animal studies have shown an adverse effect, but adequate and well-controlled studies in pregnant women have failed to demonstrate a risk to the fetus.
C	Animal studies have shown an adverse effect and there are no adequate and well-controlled studies in pregnant women. **OR** No animal studies have been conducted and there are no adequate and well-controlled studies in pregnant women.
D	Studies, adequate well-controlled or observational, in pregnant women have demonstrated a risk to the fetus. However, the benefits of therapy may outweigh the potential risk.
X	Studies, adequate well-controlled or observational, in animals or pregnant women have demonstrated positive evidence of fetal abnormalities. The use of the product is contraindicated in women who are or may become pregnant.

From Meadows M: Pregnancy and the drug dilemma, *FDA Consumer Magazine*, 2001. Available at www.fda.gov/fdac/features/2001/301_preg.html#categories, accessed June 2005.

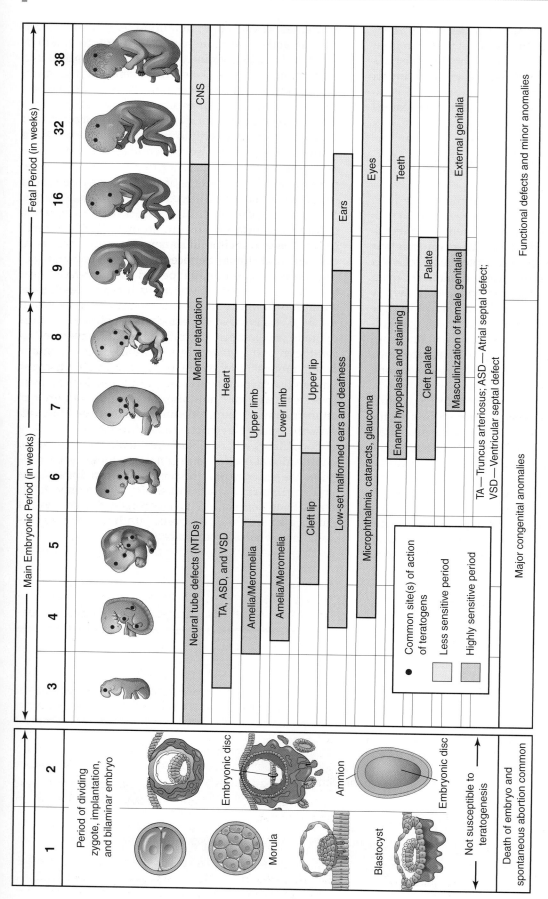

FIGURE 5-1 Critical periods in human development. The periods most susceptible to teratogenesis are indicated in *purple*; less sensitive stages are shown in *green*.

of the mother. Because of an immature blood-brain barrier, many medications are able to pass into the brain of the fetus, and because of the immaturity of the hepatic enzymes, the liver of the fetus is not developed enough to metabolize drugs.

Because pregnancy causes symptoms, many pregnant women require medications. The top 10 chemicals or drugs that pregnant women take are analgesics, antacids, antibiotics, antiemetics, antihistamines, diuretics, alcohol, iron supplements, sedatives, and vitamins. Health care workers should read the latest information to make sure that every drug given to a pregnant woman is safe.

Drugs can pass into human breast milk, and this is also a major concern for the baby. Most information about the amount of drug that goes into breast milk has come from measuring the chemical content of the drug in the milk itself. Sometimes it is possible to see the effect of the drug in the baby, but not always. Drugs that should not be taken by breastfeeding mothers include bromocriptine, cyclophosphamide, cyclosporine, doxorubicin, ergotamine, lithium, methotrexate, phenindione, amphetamines, nicotine, cocaine, heroin, marijuana, and phencyclidine.

If a mother is given a prescription while she is nursing, she can cut down the drug exposure by taking the medication just before the infant is due to have a lengthy sleep period or right after a feeding. A bottle can then be substituted for the next scheduled feeding. Nursing mothers should not take sustained-release formulations that slowly release the drug, or drugs with very long half-lives. If a feeding is skipped, the mother needs to express and discard her breast milk because the drug levels may build up in the milk. The infant should be watched for emotional changes, altered feeding habits, sleepiness, or restlessness. If short-term medication is required, the mother can consider stopping the breastfeeding for a short time, and pumping and discarding her milk.

SPECIFIC PRODUCTS USED THROUGHOUT THE LIFESPAN

Throughout the course of life, people may take many different types of medications. Some of these medications are used to help preserve health; others are given to help patients get well. Some of these common agents are discussed in this section.

IMMUNIZATIONS

The early immunization of children against diphtheria, pertussis, tetanus, chickenpox, measles, polio, and hepatitis is a national priority. Although many children are required to have their primary immunizations before beginning elementary school, the overall quality of the nation's health would be better if these immunizations were given much earlier. Immunizations are one of the main things that parents can do to protect the health of their children. (See Chapter 21 for information on primary immunizations.) However, many children fail to receive these protective injections because of two factors. First, health care providers may not give immunizations because of the mistaken belief that they should be withheld if the child has a mild illness when he is examined. Second, parents may refuse immunizations for their children because of concern about possible adverse effects. Statistically, there is a greater chance that getting a disease will harm the child more than getting the immunization for that disease. Failure to immunize children places the whole community at risk. To encourage everyone to get immunizations, the U.S. Department of Health and Human Services created the National Vaccine Injury Compensation Program. This "no-fault" system provides payment to individuals, or families of individuals, who have been injured by childhood vaccines.

People who travel outside the United States, are in the military, or work in handling food are required to have immunizations against many diseases. To maintain protection against many diseases, patients must return for additional "booster" immunizations so their immunity will continue. We are learning that greater attention should be paid to immunizing more adult and geriatric patients against common diseases.

People at high risk, such as health care workers, elderly people, and those who are immunocompromised, are encouraged to obtain yearly injections to help protect them against current strains of influenza. Children should also receive flu injections so that they avoid getting sick and bringing home infections to more vulnerable elderly or sick people at home.

ANTIDIABETIC AGENTS

For many years, it was not clear if it was important for diabetic patients to maintain strict blood glucose levels. But now, tight management of blood glucose levels has been proven to reduce organ damage in the diabetic.

ANTIHYPERTENSIVE AGENTS

The latest findings from research on hypertension demonstrate that lowering the blood pressure below 120/80 mm Hg reduces the patient's risk of myocardial infarction.

CHOLESTEROL-LOWERING DRUGS

It has been shown that lowering cholesterol levels helps reduce atherosclerosis and decreases the risk of heart attack and stroke.

STOP-SMOKING PRODUCTS

Smoking has been linked to lung cancer and many other health problems. Both the smoker and those who are exposed to secondhand smoke (passive smokers) suffer.

Fifty percent of cases of childhood asthma have been linked to the effects of passive smoking. It has been shown that the use of nicotine replacement products and drugs that reduce nicotine cravings, along with programs to change behavior, increase the chance that a person will be able to stop smoking. The risk of lung cancer and other adverse effects decreases in patients who are able to stop smoking.

WEIGHT LOSS DRUGS

Although they pose some risk, weight loss drugs, along with exercise and behavior change, may increase a person's ability to lose weight.

ANTIDEPRESSANT MEDICATIONS

Evidence exists that many people who have depression because of chemical imbalances or lack of various neurotransmitters in the brain may be helped through the use of antidepressant medications and counseling.

IMPOTENCE DRUGS

Prescriptions for drugs to treat erectile dysfunction have broken all records in terms of numbers of prescriptions written per day. These drugs are reported to increase blood circulation to the penis, thereby producing an erection. Men who have taken the drug report an amazing response that has given them potency with few side effects. It is clear that the increased physical activity associated with the return of elderly persons to sexual activity will place some individuals at risk for myocardial infarction. Patients with coronary heart disease should not use these drugs if they are not healthy enough to have sex. The possible long-term effects of these drugs will have to be determined through study of patients who use them repeatedly for a long time.

ASPIRIN

The benefits of aspirin in some patients who have had cardiovascular problems are clear. Research studies have shown these benefits in both men and women with a wide range of prior cardiovascular disease, ranging from a past heart attack or occlusive stroke to angina—including former coronary bypass surgery and angioplasty patients. Current guidelines for treating patients who may be having a heart attack call for them to chew and swallow a 325-mg aspirin tablet as soon as possible. This may place them at risk for bleeding, but the benefit is seen as greater than the risk.

CULTURAL INFLUENCES RELATED TO MEDICATIONS

Culture guides behavior in acceptable ways for the members of a specific group. The **culture** of a group represents the shared values, beliefs, customs, and behavior of the members. Each new generation learns the culture of the group through both formal teaching and informal life experiences. Factors such as the roles of men and women, the need for privacy or personal space, the meaning of food and nutrition, religious beliefs, the significance of transitions from one stage of life to another, and the amount of economic and personal freedom all influence the culture of the group. Changes in the group's social and physical environment often lead to the development of different cultural practices. Subcultures may develop within the larger group based on ethnicity, when the subgroup has a common heritage, or on race, when the subgroup members share specific physical characteristics. As subcultures continue to live within the majority group, their ideas and values change and they may grow to accept more of the practices of the dominant culture.

Over the years, cultural differences, or *diversity,* has increased among the citizens of the United States. There are many differences between the values and practices of the majority group of white, middle-class Americans and the minority subcultures that are growing in numbers. Some racial or ethnic group differences related to health care are obvious. People have different feelings, attitudes, and practices related to birth, death, and general health care; whether they might get specific diseases; how they respond to suffering, pain, and loss; standards of personal hygiene and need for privacy; acceptance of male and female children and tolerance of their behavior; rate of growth and development of children; and how they adjust to life changes. The words used to talk about their feelings and attitudes, and the ideas related to health care behavior and treatments for illness, are quite different in each cultural subgroup and arise from the accepted values of the group. Good nursing care, whatever the setting, depends on the nurse having the ability to assess these differences among cultures, and to adapt or change health care practices to better help the patient.

Cultural assessment involves talking with a patient about differences in values, religion, dietary practices, family lines of authority, family life patterns, and beliefs and practices related to health and illness. There are usually strong cultural beliefs about important transitions in life, such as birth, marriage, and death. Patients may also have strong beliefs about such things as toilet training, common medical problems, and the use of herbs and other forms of therapy. Many of these individuals have already talked with friends, family, and religious leaders, and may have incorrect notions about what is wrong with them and strong opinions about what should be done for them.

In the United States, health care workers are influenced by Western medical science and have been taught the values and beliefs of white, middle-class society. Many of the minority group patients that health care workers deal with do not always share these values and beliefs. Often today the health care workers themselves come from a minority culture. Thus there are many challenges to talking with each other, setting priorities, and agreeing on solutions. For example, many of the health care beliefs shared by different cultural groups are based on "folk medicine" passed down through the generations of a culture. Many cultures have their own "healers" in the form of a medicine man, shaman, or curandera, whose services may be a blend of both medicine and the religion. Members of the culture often seek the advice of such people before going to a Western or science-oriented health care provider. The various cures that these healers suggest may be difficult to accept and include in Western health care. The fact that Western medicine has not been able to explain why some practices work does not mean they are harmful or not effective. You must have respect for the person's cultural beliefs in all areas if you want the patient to listen to your advice and teaching.

You should attempt to accept and work with the cultural practices of patients as much as possible and should not force a patient to accept care that conflicts with her values. Forcing the patient to accept a particular type of care may even be harmful because feelings of guilt and of being separated from her religious or cultural group are likely to threaten the patient's well-being. Whether a patient will be willing to take the medication provided by a nurse depends on what meaning the medication has to the patient and the beliefs she has about its helpfulness or harm. So you must learn more about the patient's culture if you are to be effective.

A great deal of research is available about subcultures within the United States. If you work with minority groups on a regular basis, you will need to learn about these subcultures to provide good care to those patients. Usually, people are proud to tell someone about their background and beliefs. Because there is growing recognition of cultural diversity, many articles and texts are being published that also provide information helpful to health care workers. However, it is important not to assume that all African Americans, American Indians, or Hispanics are the same because they are members of a specific group. Within these larger groups are many subcultures with different histories, beliefs, languages, and values. What may be seen as acceptable behavior by one segment of the culture may be offensive to another. You should take care to ask minority group patients about what they prefer.

It is now recognized that there is also *health disparity*, or inequality in health care, for many minority group patients. Indeed, much has been written about the "culture of poverty" and its effects on health care. Many minority group patients are at risk for severe health problems but get less health care because of discrimination against them; lack of money, insurance, or knowledge; or other factors that make it difficult for them to get better care. For example, many minority group patients do not read English well enough to understand written instructions about their health problems, get prescriptions filled, or take drugs properly. The ability to read and understand this type of information is called *health literacy*. (See Chapter 2 for health literacy considerations in patient teaching.)

Finally, in addition to differences in health care beliefs, values, and attitudes, drug research has also shown important differences among racial and ethnic groups in their metabolic rates, clinical responses to drugs, and side effects. In particular, cardiovascular drugs and central nervous system drugs may produce varying clinical responses in various ethnic or racial groups, particularly the Chinese and other Asian groups.

GENETICS

The mapping of the human genome and the research on genes and DNA have shown that all individuals, no matter what race they belong to, are more similar than dissimilar. Research on individual races has concluded that African Americans are genetically the most heterogeneous (different) in their genetic profile. This may explain why this group as a whole has a greater rejection rate after organ transplantation, even with organs from living donors with similar tissue typing, and why they have particular unique responses to some types of medication. In people from some areas of the world, there is an unusually high number of cases of certain diseases, such as the thalassemia found in those of Eastern European and Mediterranean backgrounds. Research in genetics has shown that these diseases are passed down through families who carry certain genes. Hemophilia and sickle cell disease are other diseases that are the result of inherited traits in a family's DNA.

The area of genetics and the response of groups to medications is a topic of increasing interest to researchers. It has been suggested that, in the future, medications might be made specifically for different races and ages as we learn more about the role that heredity plays in both disease and treatment.

SPIRITUALITY AND RELIGION

Regardless of basic ethnicity or culture, many individuals have a strong belief in a "higher power" that watches over or guides their lives, or may be asked for assistance in dealing with problems. In times of illness, people often think about religion or become more spiritual, and they try to find answers to why they have become sick or why they fail to get well. The idea of religious belief has at times been both controversial and unpopular, and many health care professionals are not comfortable talking with patients about their religious beliefs. However, it does not seem wise for a good nurse to ignore one of the most basic aspects of a person—one that affects how they view life and death. Often, asking people about what they believe, and really listening to them, or helping them find a religious leader to meet their needs is all that is required.

Many research studies have been done about persons of faith. The results suggest that people who pray have better symptom relief. People who have a strong social support network through their religion also seem to do better than those without such support. How a person of faith interprets symptoms, disease, and death, and how these beliefs influence the actions of medications, is still under study.

EVALUATION OF FACTORS RELATED TO DRUG NONCOMPLIANCE

The goal of patient teaching for drug treatment plans is to work with patients to help them make informed decisions about taking their drugs (see Chapter 2). Many of the variables of age, culture, and belief affect a patient's willingness to take medications that are ordered. Patient difficulty with taking medications is a major unresolved problem. Drug **noncompliance** is the inappropriate self-administration of medications. Patients sometimes use medications in ways that vary from the health care provider's advice. The results of this self-administration often do not lead to behavior that is curative or helpful.

How does drug noncompliance begin? Often patients come to a health care provider almost as the last resort, after having already tried a number of remedies for their symptoms. The patient's age, sex, race, ethnic background, family, socioeconomic class, education, and past experience will have affected how the health problem is viewed and how the world in general is seen. Although today's patients are more likely to be better informed about medical care than patients were in the past, they are also more likely to be skeptical or distrusting of the medical profession. They may have read about medical mistakes and successful lawsuits, heard about bad experiences in medical care from friends, or had bad experiences themselves. They may come from a lower socioeconomic class, be less educated, or have value systems different from those of the health care provider. Patients do have underlying fears and concerns, and certain expectations for their care, but they are often reluctant to express these fears and expectations because they worry that others will think they are foolish.

Health care workers may often assume that a patient's value system is similar to their own and may not take the time to even determine the patient's beliefs

about and understanding of the illness. If this has happened, the patient may not have developed trust in the health care worker. So, many times a primary reason why patients are not compliant is because of their bad experiences with the health care system in the past.

Most studies of drug compliance have been done with hospital-based patients. These studies have usually found that patients are unfamiliar with their prescribed medications and how to take them, and that patients make errors in taking medications as much as 25% to 59% of the time. If the health care provider does not learn that the patient is not taking the medication as ordered, poor outcomes may be blamed on wrong dosage, failure of the drug plan itself, or incorrect diagnosis. Drug noncompliance often increases medical costs by leading to further hospitalization, by causing nursing home placement for elderly patients, and by increasing the use of outpatient services.

Reasons for drug noncompliance can be classified as errors of omission (a prescribed medication is not taken), errors of commission (a medication that has not been prescribed is taken), dosage errors (the wrong dose is taken), and scheduling errors (the medication is taken on the wrong schedule, for example, once daily instead of twice daily). There are six major reasons for patient noncompliance with drugs:

1. Noncompliance rates tend to be higher for care to prevent a problem than for treatment of an illness the patient already has. Also, compliance is better for "important" medications such as cardiac or anticonvulsant agents than for seemingly "less important" drugs like antacids or mild analgesics.
2. The extent of noncompliance increases with the length of therapy, as seen in chronic diseases such as diabetes, hypertension, epilepsy, and depression.
3. Noncompliance is highest for treatment regimens that require the patient to make significant changes in behavior, such as with plans to stop smoking or lose weight.
4. Poor understanding of instructions is a common cause of noncompliance.
5. People may not want to follow the treatment plan when it is very complex, for example, when many drugs are taken at different times or when drugs must be taken at frequent intervals or during the night.
6. People may not want to follow the treatment plan when there are unpleasant side effects.

Patients who have symptoms are more likely to take their medications than those who do not, especially if the symptoms are relieved by the medication. The patient's age, sex, race, education, occupation, income, and marital status usually do provide clues as to whether the patient will follow the instructions or not.

People who have a stable support system and stable family situation, however, are more likely to follow treatment plans. For example, a husband who has a wife who will help cook special foods for the diet and remind him to take his medicine will have better success than a person who lives alone.

Although many people believe that older adults are more likely not to cooperate with a treatment plan, most research indicates that aging does not affect compliance with prescribed medications. Elderly individuals may have fewer things to do every day, and this helps them focus on taking their medicines. For middle-aged and younger patients who have busy careers and families, the many activities they take part in each day may cause them to forget about their medications. Elderly patients, however, have been shown to have difficulty in opening some of the childproof drug bottles, and may have greater difficulty in reading or understanding new instructions.

If you establish a good relationship with the patient, this may help the patient do what he is instructed to do. A good relationship means that you can share information and talk easily with each other. Factors that have been identified as helpful in having a good relationship with the patient include the following:

- Being friendly
- Having a positive, confident approach
- Responding to patient complaints
- Encouraging patient questions
- Having a supportive, nonjudgmental method of getting information and talking to a patient who admits to noncompliance
- Encouraging patients to become actively involved in their own care
- Seeking active patient participation rather than physician- or nurse-dominated decision making
- Working together to create the treatment plan

- Identifying and resolving barriers to compliance
- Developing an agreement between patient and nurse in their understanding of a problem and its management
- Taking time to motivate the patient
- Working to help the patient be satisfied

Clearly, all these things take time, but you may often see the same patients over and over again in an office, clinic, or hospital. These positive activities can be included in the care plan as part of your regular work with the patient.

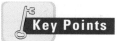
Key Points

- Efforts to individualize care by taking into account the patient's culture, beliefs, and age will make it more likely that the patient will participate actively in the plan to get well.
- The problems of disease and disability belong to the patient, not the provider.
- The goal of care throughout the life cycle should be to assist patients in taking charge of their own health and learning how to get well or stay well.
- You can help the patient follow the treatment plan through your own behavior.

Go to the free CD-ROM for an Audio Glossary, animations, video clips, and Review Questions for the NCLEX-PN® Examination.

evolve   Be sure to visit the companion Evolve website at http://evolve.elsevier.com/Edmunds/LPN/ for WebLinks, a link to the top 200 drugs by prescription, and sign-up pages for newsletter drug updates.

CRITICAL THINKING ?

1. Look up the drug digoxin. What doses are recommended for infants, children, adults, and elderly patients? What specific factors explain why these doses are different?

2. Among your classmates, discuss differences in beliefs about disease and death. What cultures produced these different beliefs? Whose beliefs are best?

3. Find resources that identify some of the different health care beliefs of various groups such as Chinese, Hispanics, and American Indians.

4. African Americans vary in their beliefs and values from other black people. Identify some of the differences in cultures of black people. If you treated everyone who is black in the same manner, what would be the likely results of your care?

5. Mrs. Green is 5 months pregnant. She has severe asthma but has not been taking her asthma medication because she is afraid it would hurt her baby. What are some of the factors that should be considered when you talk to Mrs. Green about this problem?

6. Ms. Kim, an elderly Korean woman, was brought in for surgery by her grandson, who speaks English perfectly. Now it is time for her first dose of presurgery medication, but her grandson is nowhere to be found. When you approach Ms. Kim with the medication, she smiles but shakes her head no. "No," she says, shaking her head emphatically. "No pill." What are some of the things you would want to explore with Ms. Kim regarding this medication?

7. You and your husband plan to begin a family. What medications are safe to take if you are pregnant and have a bad cold? Diabetes? Epilepsy? What products should you definitely avoid?

8. The last time you saw a health care provider for a minor primary care problem, did you get a prescription? Did you have it filled? Why or why not? Did you take all the medication as ordered? Why or why not?

9. When you are very busy giving care to patients, what things can you do to develop a good relationship? How will this help in teaching them about taking their medications?

10. Mrs. Jones tells you that she does not want her 6-month-old child to have immunizations. What would be the most therapeutic way to communicate with her?

6 Self-Care: Over-the-Counter Products, Herbal Therapies, and Drugs for Health Promotion

After reading and studying this chapter, you should be able to do the following:

1. List advantages and disadvantages of over-the-counter medications.
2. Describe some of the precautions to think about in taking herbals or other alternative or complementary therapies.
3. Identify common agents taken for health promotion.

Key Terms

Be sure to check out the bonus material on the free CD-ROM, including selected audio pronunciations.

alternative medicine (ăl-TĔR-nă-tĭv, p. 59)
complementary medicine (kŏm-plĕ-MĔN-tă-rē, p. 59)
health promotion (p. 64)
herbal (ĔR-băl, p. 60)
integrative practices (ĬN-tĕ-grā-tĭv, p. 59)

OVERVIEW

When we think of drugs used by patients, we often forget that many of the drugs patients take are those they buy in drugstores because they learned about them from their friends or they read about them in magazines or saw a television ad. More than ever before, people are learning about how to care for themselves and are more likely to purchase over-the-counter (OTC) products. Health care remedies that are not prescribed by health care providers also did a booming business in the United States in 1997; Americans spent $6 billion on nonprescription remedies. OTC drugs that patients buy and use are a majority of the drugs they take. What is safe for patients to take? What do they need to know about OTC products? What products should they be taking to keep them well? Can they believe all of the articles and stories about "wonder" drugs they can get without a prescription that promise such good results for chronic problems? How can you answer their questions?

DOCUMENTING PATIENT HEALTH CARE PRACTICES

It is important for you to be familiar with the many products that are now available to patients and that do not require prescriptions. First, many of these products contain chemicals that are useful in treating common health problems. If nurses are familiar with these products, they can help patients choose the safest product for their current problem or illness. Second, some of the active chemicals in these products may make existing medical problems worse or interact with a patient's prescribed medications.

You should always ask about OTC medications that patients may be taking when you ask about their drug history. Patients often neglect to tell their providers about these products. Many Americans consider herbal or OTC products to be safe because they are so easily available. But, they may not be safe for all patients. Through paying attention to information about OTC products, you should be able to ask about drugs a patient reports that she is taking and bring this to the attention of others caring for her.

It is also important to have the patients bring in all herbs or drug remedies they are using so that what they are taking may be accurately recorded. Seeing products in their original bottles or boxes gives more information that might be needed to tell if the drugs are safe. This action may be very helpful to prevent drug interactions or complications.

Patients who rely on complimentary and alternative medicine (CAM) may be taking alternative products (herbs, supplements, or other drugs) instead of prescription drugs, or they may use such products in addition to prescription drugs in a complementary way. When asking a patient about his use of CAM, you should not make judgments about these treatments. This approach is important if you wish to have the patient trust you enough to tell you the truth about what health regimens he is following or what herbal and OTC products he is taking. You should understand that patients who use these different treatments do so for many reasons:

1. They seek products that will keep their health good, prevent disease, or provide treatment for health problems they now have.
2. They have tried regular treatments without success.
3. The regular treatments had undesirable side effects.
4. There is no known therapy that will relieve their specific problem, but they keep searching for one.
5. Other people they trust in their family or community have told them about the product.
6. They are seeking a cheaper or nonprescription product to replace a drug that they want but cannot get or cannot afford.
7. Regular treatment violates the patient's religious or spiritual beliefs.

OVER-THE-COUNTER MEDICATIONS

The role of OTC agents in health care today is growing because there are now more people who are better educated and believe that they should take an active role in their own health care. The Nonprescription Drug Manufacturers Association (NDMA) estimates that more than 100,000 products are now available over the counter. These products contain 1 or more of about 700 active chemicals and come in a variety of dosage forms, sizes, and strengths. The sales of OTC products total more than $20 billion a year.

Nonprescription medications, or OTC products, are defined as drugs that are thought to be safe and effective for people to use without instructions from a health care provider about how to use them. OTC products differ from prescription medications in four ways:

1. The label information is more complete than with prescription medications and is often written in a style that is easier for consumers to understand.
2. With OTCs, there is a wider margin of safety because most of these drugs have undergone a lot of testing before advertising and many have been changed by the manufacturer based on information gathered after years of OTC usage by consumers.
3. OTCs are usually advertised directly to the consumer. (Many manufacturers of prescription drugs are now following this example by advertising directly to the public and asking people to talk with their health care provider about these drugs.)
4. OTCs are widely available.

The most common categories of OTCs are similar to those available by prescription. These include laxatives, peptic acid disorder products (antacids, H_2 receptor antagonists), analgesics, cough and cold products (antihistamines, decongestants, expectorants, antitussives), vaginal antifungals, stop-smoking products, and topical

steroids. Also, many drugs that were available only by prescription have now been given OTC status.

OTCs are sold in pharmacies, grocery stores, gas stations, and many other places. Less than one half of all OTC products are sold in pharmacies. Because there are so many different names and versions of these products, it is important to learn the drug name instead of just the product (trade) name. Many of these products have multiple ingredients. The cost of these combination products can be more than buying all of the ingredients singly, so it is important to check out commonly used products for price comparisons.

PRODUCT LABELING

The U.S. Food and Drug Administration (FDA) requires OTC product labels to contain important information in a manner that a typical person can read and understand. Drug companies are required to use a standard labeling format for all OTCs sold in the United States. Key information, beginning with active ingredients, followed by purpose(s), uses, warnings, and directions, is placed in the same order on all OTC packages, in an easy-to-read format. Surveys show that women are the family members most likely to buy OTC products, and they are also more likely to read labels before taking medications than men.

One of the most important things in reading labels for OTC products is to see if there are other chemicals in a product that might pose a risk. These "hidden" chemicals are used for different purposes: to help preserve the drug, to give color, and to help deliver the product or make it more stable. Consumers who have an allergy or intolerance to even small doses of any of these products may not be aware of the risk unless they read the label. Table 6-1 lists a number of common hidden chemicals in OTC products.

PATIENT TEACHING

There are some basic facts that health care providers should tell patients about OTC products. Sometimes this information is printed and given out to the patient because it is so important for patients to know about it. Whether they are given verbally or in writing, these are some of the key facts that patients should learn:

- Always read the instructions on the label.
- Do not take OTC medicines in higher dosages or for a longer time than the label says you should.
- If you do not get well, stop treating yourself and talk with a health care professional.
- Side effects from OTCs are relatively uncommon, but it is your job to know what side effects might happen from the medicines you are taking.
- Because every person is different, your response to the medicine may be different than someone else.
- OTC medicines often interact with other medicines, and with food or alcohol, or they might have an effect on other health problems you may have.

Table 6-1 | *Common "Hidden" Ingredients in Over-the-Counter Products*

HIDDEN DRUG	OVER-THE-COUNTER CLASS THAT MAY CONTAIN THE DRUG
Alcohol (ethanol)	Cough syrups and cold preparations, mouthwashes
Antihistamines	Analgesics, antiemetics, asthma products, cold and allergy products, dermatologic preparations, menstrual products, motion sickness products, sleep aids, topical decongestants
Antimuscarinic agents	Antidiarrheals, cold/cough/allergy preparations, hemorrhoidal products
Aspirin and other salicylates	Analgesics, antidiarrheals, cold and allergy preparations, menstrual products, sleep aids
Caffeine	Analgesics, cold and allergy products, diuretic and menstrual products, stimulants, weight control products
Estrogens	Hair creams
Local anesthetics (usually benzocaine)	Antitussives, cold sore products, dermatologic preparations, hemorrhoidal products, lozenges, teething/toothache products, weight loss products
Sodium	Analgesics, antacids, cough syrups, laxatives
Sympathomimetics	Analgesics, asthma products, cold/allergy preparations, cough syrups, hemorrhoidal products, lozenges, menstrual products, topical decongestants, weight control products

Modified from Katzung BG: *Basic and clinical pharmacology,* ed 9, New York, 2004, McGraw Medical.

- If you do not understand the label, check with the pharmacist.
- Do not take medicine if the package doesn't have a label on it.
- Throw away medicines older than the date on the package.
- Do not use medicine that belongs to a friend.
- Buy products that treat only the symptoms you have.
- Check the prices of OTC medicines, and buy generic products when you can.

Parents should know the following special information about using OTCs for children:

- Parents should never guess about the amount of medicine to give a child. Half an adult dose may be too much or not enough to be effective. This is very true of medicines such as acetaminophen (Tylenol) or ibuprofen (Advil), in which repeated overdoses may lead to poisoning of the child, liver destruction, or coma.
- If the label says to take 2 teaspoons and the dosing cup is marked with ounces only, get another measuring device. Don't try to guess how much should be given.
- Always follow the age limits listed. If the label says the product should not be given to a child younger than 2 years, do not do it.
- Always use the child-resistant cap and relock the cap after use.
- Throw away old, discolored, or expired medicine or medicine that has lost its label instructions.
- Do not give medicine containing alcohol to children.

COMPLEMENTARY AND ALTERNATIVE MEDICINE, INCLUDING HERBAL THERAPIES

The practices that are known as **alternative medicine** have often been somewhat mysterious, and the scientific basis for the action of alternative therapies has been uncertain. Because of the lack of research to explain therapeutic action, most medical and nursing schools do not teach their students about alternative medicine. Alternative therapies include herbal therapies, aromatherapy, chiropractic, acupuncture, massage, and homeotherapy. A similar type of treatment known as **complementary medicine** includes these same basic alternative therapies and is preferred by many because it uses these therapies together with standard medical care and not as an alternative. Another term to describe this type of treatment is **integrative practices.**

Recent studies have found that 40% to 50% of Americans are using some type of alternative therapy and even more are taking herbs and supplements. It is reported that, in 1994, 60 million people in the United States used alternative therapies at a cost of $13.7 billion. The estimated number of visits to providers of alternative medicine (425 million) exceeded those to all primary care physicians (325 million). More than 70% of patients who used alternative therapies did not tell their primary care providers. Patients often believe that they know more than their health care providers do, and that their providers do not listen to them or respect their choices.

There is more and more patient interest in herbs, supplements, and homeopathic remedies, but there is little scientific information in texts and reference books about these products. Most of the books and articles about herbal therapies are written to sell products. Responsible nurses, for their part, want good information about the choices that their patients are making. It is crucial that you have up-to-date, balanced, and scientific material to help you understand herbal therapies and to learn about strengths, weaknesses, clinical indications, proper dosages, toxicities, and interactions of different alternative drug therapies.

HERBAL THERAPIES AND SUPPLEMENTS

Use of **herbal** medicine (drugs made from plant sources) has always been a part of most cultures. China has used herbal products for centuries as a standard part of medical practice. People in the United States are now using herbal remedies in record numbers, believing that these products will prevent disease, treat illness, and improve health. Because herbal therapies have been used for a long time in different cultures, this has created the impression that they are safe and natural. This creates a false sense of safety and effectiveness for the consumer. The fact that something is "natural" does not mean it is safe or effective. There is growing belief in the medical community that if herbs are effective, then they should be used under the direction of a health care professional.

Product Labeling

Herbal preparations are not regulated anywhere in the world. Germany has done the most in terms of scientific research into the safety and efficacy of some of these herbs, but these studies have been small and do not begin to meet the scientific standard demanded by the FDA for prescription drugs. The FDA does not regulate herbal medicines, but it took action on April 24, 1998, to protect consumers from misleading health claims by the herbal industry. The goal of the FDA was to clarify for herbal drug makers what types of claims can and cannot be made for herbal products and dietary supplements so that consumers can make more informed and wiser choices.

The FDA actions were a result of the agency's attempts to conform with the Dietary Supplement Health and Education Act passed by Congress in 1994, which said health and disease claims are different than structure and function claims. The act says that labels cannot make claims that a product cures a disease or has a special benefit or health effect without special FDA approval. The act allows general statements about the product's function in the body. The new rules bar makers of supplements and herbal remedies from claiming to cure, prevent, or alleviate cancer, acquired immunodeficiency syndrome (AIDS), and other specific diseases. Companies are limited to making general claims about the product's ability to make the immune system stronger. Critics claim that most disease treatments can be described in terms of their effects on a structure or function of the body, so it will be difficult to tell the difference between structure and function claims, which are allowed, and disease claims, which are not.

Because of the wide use of alternative therapies, there has been growing interest in research on the action of various products. The scientific community has expressed concern about drugs that are not tested or regulated. Because some of these medications have "folk" acceptance, they may be cheaper than regular drugs, and there may be fewer barriers to purchasing them, so their use has increased. As more of these products are being used over longer periods of time, researchers are now starting to pay attention to them. Until there are more scientific studies, health care providers should urge caution in the use of these products.

Pros and Cons

Safety, purity, and effectiveness are the major issues in evaluation of herbal products. Important questions to consider in looking at herbal products include:
- How much of the herbal product does this product actually contain?
- What part of the plant was used to make the extract?
- What other chemicals does it contain?
- What are the active ingredients?
- What reliable information exists that this herb is useful and for what conditions?

Herbal products are made by grinding up parts of the plant and making them into pills, capsules, or liquids. One of the major criticisms of herbal products is that the plants vary so much in concentration or dosage because plants make different amounts of chemicals depending on the soil, water, and sun where they were grown. That is, the weight of one leaf may be the same as that of another, but the amount of biologically active chemical in each leaf may vary according to the amount of sunlight, the nutrition in the soil, and the extent of watering.

Hormone replacement therapy (HRT) has become a hot market for the use of "natural" products. Natural estrogens are really estrogen-like chemicals called *phytoestrogens*. Examples of plants containing natural estrogens or phytoestrogens are flaxseed, red clover sprouts, and soy flour. Herbs thought to contain chemicals that act as stimulants for hormones are licorice, ginseng, *Vitex*, and black cohosh. It generally takes 6 to 8 weeks to see an improvement in symptoms of menopause when taking these products. Again, these herbal preparations do not deliver the same amount of chemicals with each dose, and there is no way to know the purity of the product. There is also no way to know if the product will do what it is supposed to do. For example, many women in China have long used an herb called *dong kwai,* claiming it reduces or eliminates hot flashes. However, research thus far has failed to find estrogen, or estrogen-like chemicals, in dong kwai.

Many nonprescription products are advertised to have the same function as prescription drugs. For example, there are herbal preparations that are supposed to act like sildenafil (Viagra). Herbal antiobesity products were sold as alternatives to fenfluramine and dexfenfluramine when these products were taken off the market. Herbal products for depression, high cholesterol, and asthma are also for sale. However, products containing St. John's wort have not been completely tested for their effectiveness as antidepressants in the United States. They may also include 6-hydroxytryptophan (closely related to another chemical linked to a rare and potentially fatal blood disorder) and ephedra, an amphetamine-like compound that may cause high blood pressure, heart irregularities, strokes, and death. The claim that garlic reduces cholesterol to an acceptable level also has not been confirmed by scientific research. Patients who take these products in place of prescription drugs should consider that they are taking an experimental drug. Because of dangers such as these, the FDA took action to remove some of these products from the market and posts information about these products on their MedWatch home page (http://www.fda.gov/medwatch/).

There is a consortium of industry groups led by the Council for Responsible Nutrition that has developed voluntary guidelines that some herbal drug makers are using. Patients need to look for products that have been standardized by the manufacturer by measuring the amount of the key ingredient. However, the purity and potency of many products sold in the United States are unknown.

Some European countries have more extensive experience with selected herbal products than the United States. Many of the products now gaining attention in the United States have been used for years in other countries—either as OTC products or by prescription. A lot of information has been learned not only about the effects of these products, but also about how they interact with other foods and medications. For example, natural products that reduce blood glucose or blood pressure or have a sedating effect may be dangerous when taken along with prescription drugs with the same actions. Table 6-2 shows the herbs considered by non-U.S. regulatory authorities to be relatively safe and effective if used in recommended dosages and if they are made by companies that standardize their drug-making process. Table 6-3 lists herbs that are considered unsafe for use based on reports or observations.

Table 6-4 lists a few nonherbal natural remedies that are in common use and considered both safe and effective. Sometimes the products themselves, such as calcium, may be of proven use. However, if the calcium comes from oyster shells taken from polluted waters, the shells may be filled with lead, zinc, or arsenic. A similar problem occurs with melatonin, a hormone extracted from the pineal gland of the cow. If the drug maker does not make sure that the cow is disease free, the consumer may be at risk for diseases from the cow (for example, "mad cow" disease).

AROMATHERAPY

Essential oils extracted from the petals, leaves, bark, resins, rinds, roots, stalks, seeds, and stems of aromatic plants are used to promote health and well-being. It is also believed by some that these oils have medical properties that fight bacteria, viruses, bacterial toxins, and fungi. It is believed that the scents work by triggering hormones that govern bodily functions. Massage with oils or inhaling their vapors is effective, but these oils should never be swallowed or applied near the eyes. It is believed that when these oils are applied to the skin or the vapors are inhaled, their molecules attach to oxygen molecules in the lungs and circulate through the body, helping the body to heal itself. Although the practice of aromatherapy has many followers, there is very little research now available to support its use.

DRUGS FOR HEALTH PROMOTION: VITAMINS AND MINERALS

Another major category of drugs used for self-care is vitamins and minerals. People in the United States are using vitamins and minerals to prevent cancer, boost immunity, cope with stress, strengthen bones, and increase their overall sense of well-being. Sales of these products are now at record highs. Patients often decide on their own that they need such products. They may or may not seek advice from a health care provider or pharmacist about what to take. Many different products are for sale, and the price varies a lot for the same product. Costs for some products are high because of the claims made about their effectiveness, but not all such claims for vitamins and minerals have been proved. Does more expensive mean better? What is fact and what is fiction about the use of vitamins and minerals?

PROS AND CONS

What is known is that vitamin and mineral supplements are useful when the patient has a deficiency, as may be the case in women in their childbearing years and in the elderly population. The American Heart Association has suggested that people should eat more fruits, vegetables, and whole grains; implement an exercise program; replace saturated fats with oils from fish and nuts; and limit salt and alcohol intake. Most official sources suggest that, if a variety of healthy foods are eaten, the necessary vitamins can likely be obtained from diet alone. However, supplements may be required for some patients, mostly those who may be deficient. For supplementation, vitamins should have 50% to 150% of the Recommended Dietary Allowance

Table 6-2 | *Herbs Considered Safe and Effective*

COMMON NAME	USE FOR WHICH IT IS PROMOTED	SAFETY/EFFICACY/DOSAGE
Arnica	External remedy for healing bruises, muscle strains, and sprains; reduces inflammation	Toxic when taken orally
Black cohosh	Reduces menopause symptoms	Shown to be safe and effective
Chamomile	Antiinflammatory, antispasmodic, antiinfective	Safe and effective; 3 gm/250 mL hot water; drink 3–4 times daily or take in capsule form
Chaste tree	Female hormone regulation	Safe and effective; rare indigestion
Cholesten	Serum cholesterol reduction	Safe
Echinacea	Stimulates the immune system; used in treatment or prevention of colds and flu or urinary tract infections	6–9 doses (1 gm dried root) of *Echinacea* juice per day for 2 weeks; very safe, no side effects; probably effective
Fennel	Internal: increases milk flow in lactating women; external: oil eases muscle and joint pain	Safe and effective
Feverfew *(Tanacetum parthenium)*	Migraine headache prevention or reduces severity and frequency; inhibits platelet aggregation	Safe and effective; take 125 mg twice daily; do not use concurrently with aspirin or warfarin (Coumadin)
Garlic *(Allium sativum)*	May lower some blood lipids; inhibits platelet aggregation; lowers blood pressure	Safe and effective; destroyed by heat; take 2.5 gm/day raw or 0.4–1.2 gm/day dried; do not use concurrently with aspirin or warfarin
Ginger *(Zingiber officinale)*	Antiemetic, good for motion sickness; inhibits platelet aggregation	Safe and effective; take 1–2 gm/day; do not use concurrently with aspirin or warfarin
Ginkgo *(Ginkgo biloba)*	Improves blood flow to the brain and extremities; improves brain tissue tolerance to hypoxia; reduces capillary fragility; alleviates vertigo and ringing in the ears; may slow dementia	Safe and effective; take 60 mg twice daily of standard extract; avoid in patients taking aspirin or warfarin because it may cause serious bleeding; only useful to elderly or debilitated persons, of no use in persons with normal brain function
Ginseng	Taken for hot flashes but may make them worse	Safe, but questionable efficacy; not an aphrodisiac; no effect on fatigue or stress
Goldenseal	Prevention or resolution of upper respiratory infections	Safe and effective mullein expectorant, decreases bronchial spasms; reduces colds, bronchitis
Mullein	Expectorant, decreases bronchial spasms; reduces colds, bronchitis	Safe and effective
Rose hips	Fights infections by reducing capillary fragility; contains high concentration of vitamin C	Safe and effective
St. John's wort	Antidepressant	Safe and effective for mild depression; take 1–3 gm/day; do not use in addition to other antidepressants
Saw palmetto	Reduces benign prostatic hypertrophy	Safe and effective; take 0.5–1 gm/day
Valerian *(Valeriana officinalis)*	Mild tranquilizer and sleeping aid	Safe and effective; take 1–3 gm/day; enhances the effects of other drugs that sedate or tranquilize

Modified from Edmunds MW, Mayhew MS: *Pharmacology for the primary care provider,* ed 2, St Louis, 2004, Mosby.

Table 6-3 | *Herbs Considered Unsafe*

COMMON NAME	USE FOR WHICH IT IS PROMOTED	SAFETY/EFFICACY/DOSAGE
Blue cohosh	Labor induction; reduction of menopause symptoms	Birth defects in animals
Borage	Antidiarrheal, diuretic	Contains pyrrolidine alkaloids that are potentially carcinogenic and toxic to the liver
Broom (broom tops, drish broom)	Miscellaneous	Toxic
Calamus	Antipyretic, digestive aid	Has produced malignancy in rats
Chaparral	Natural antioxidant, blood purity, anti-cancer, acne treatment	Severe liver damage; two cases known in which liver transplants were required
Coltsfoot	Antitussive, demulcent	Contains carcinogenic alkaloids
Comfrey	Wound healing	Obstruction of blood flow from liver; has caused cirrhosis and death
Ephedra	Anorectic, bronchodilator	Ineffective as an anorectic; effective for bronchodilation; unsafe for those with hypertension, diabetes, or thyroid disease; unsafe with caffeine; may cause serious toxic reactions when taken concurrently with MAO inhibitors
Germander	Anorectic	Hepatotoxicity
Jin Bu Huan	Stomachache, insomnia, antitussive	Hepatitis, respiratory depression with bradycardia
Licorice	Expectorant, antiulcer	Effective, but safe only in small doses for short periods of time; may cause sodium retention and potassium loss
Lobelia	Bronchodilator	High doses can decrease respiration, raise heart rate, and lower blood pressure
Pennyroyal	Abortion agent	Severe hepatotoxicity, interference with clotting
Royal jelly	Insomnia, liver ailments	Serious to fatal allergic reactions
Sassafras	General tonic	Contains safrole, a carcinogen
Senna (Senna alexandrina)	Laxative	Electrolyte imbalance, particularly potassium loss
Stephania magnolia	Weight loss	Renal toxicity
Willow bark	Antipyretic	Gastritis, bleeding, and Reye's syndrome
Yohimbé	Aphrodisiac	Psychosis, loss of consciousness

Modified from Edmunds MW, Mayhew MS: *Pharmacology for the primary care provider,* ed 2, St Louis, 2004, Mosby.
MAO, Monoamine oxidase.

Table 6-4 | *Natural Remedies Other Than Herbs or Vitamins*

NAME	SOURCE	USES	SAFETY AND EFFICACY
Chondroitin	Cow cartilage	Eases aches and pains; protects and rebuilds cartilage	Safe and effective; 400 mg/day
Dehydroepiandrosterone (DHEA)	Androgen hormone synthesized from wild yams	Alleviates cancer, heart disease, and autoimmune disease; antiaging remedy	Believed to be safe but all side effects are not known; toxic to liver in sufficient quantities; efficacy not proven
Glucosamine	Oyster shells	Eases aches and pains; protects and rebuilds cartilage	Safe and effective if shells are not from polluted water; 500 mg q day
Melatonin	If produced from natural sources, it comes from the pineal glands of cows	Cure for jet lag; helps the body's clock; sleep aid; antiaging remedy	May inhibit sex drive in men; 1–3 mg at bedtime

Modified from Edmunds MW, Mayhew MS: *Pharmacology for the primary care provider,* ed 2, St Louis, 2004, Mosby.

(RDA), and daily treatment should not provide more than 2 to 10 times the RDA for a specific vitamin.

There are known dangers to vitamin use, especially high-dose use. When megadoses of most vitamins are taken, the excess amount is quickly excreted in the urine with no additional benefit to the patient. Occasionally, when large doses of vitamin A are taken, the amount not used rapidly by the body may be stored in the tissues, causing the skin to turn yellow. Most vitamin products can be toxic to children, and iron can be deadly to small children. Folic acid can react with anticancer treatment medications and mask signs of vitamin B_{12} deficiency. Sometimes, the body starts to rely on large doses of vitamin C when taken over a prolonged period of time, and the body may believe there is a deficiency when the patient returns to a normal dose. Patients with diarrhea may lose vitamin and mineral products unchanged in the stool. There is also some evidence that vitamin use may weaken the efficacy of immunizations for flu in the elderly population.

Overuse of minerals can also be dangerous. Large amounts of calcium can limit the absorption of iron and other trace elements. They can also cause constipation and reduce kidney function. Calcium is needed primarily in menopausal women and older men, particularly those who are at risk for bone loss.

Antioxidant vitamins have a prominent place in the current literature on nutritional supplements. The major antioxidant vitamins are vitamin E, or alpha-tocopherol; beta-carotene or provitamin A, which is a precursor to vitamin A; vitamin C, or ascorbic acid; and selenium. All of these vitamins are found in fruits and vegetables. Many research studies are being done to determine the mechanism of action of antioxidants. Current research suggests that, when low-density lipoprotein (LDL) cholesterol is oxidized, the oxidation is often incomplete. (The analogy has been made to wood that burns incompletely in a fireplace and "pops," sending sparks against the screen.) This incomplete oxidation produces free radicals that often lead to atherosclerotic plaques. It is believed that antioxidants slow or prevent LDL cholesterol oxidation because they are oxidized better than LDL cholesterol. This slows or eliminates atherosclerosis. It is also believed that antioxidants slow the process that may cause cells to become cancerous. This has caused a large increase in the sales of antioxidants in an attempt to decrease cardiovascular disease and cancer.

Although many major research studies have looked at antioxidants and have found they may have some benefits, no major clinical studies have found that antioxidants prevent cancer. There is evidence that those who eat fruits and vegetables regularly have less risk of cancer. However, there is no evidence that this is the result of antioxidants. Therefore taking antioxidant vitamins may be helpful to some extent. Research has also found that vitamins C, B_6, and B_{12} may be helpful to prevent coronary artery disease.

Advertisers suggest that natural products are better than synthetic vitamins. However, vitamins are probably the same whether they are natural or synthetic, costly or cheap. In fact, natural vitamins may contain other chemicals or impurities that may make them less effective than standardized synthetic products. The most important differences are that some preparations have been shown to dissolve better than others, or contain the product in amounts that increase the absorption of other vitamins and minerals taken at the same time.

National surveys have shown that those who least need extra vitamins and minerals are the most likely to take them, including people who eat right, exercise, and do not smoke. There is no evidence that people who take vitamins live longer or suffer less illness or disease. A benefit of vitamins and minerals to the average healthy individual who consumes a variety of foods has never been proven. The USDA's new My Pyramid tool reminds people to balance what they are eating so they get their essential nutrition every day.

Supplements cannot make up for a poor diet or unhealthy lifestyle practices such as smoking or lack of exercise. Patients who do not eat a well-balanced diet, and do eat lots of high-fat or "empty calorie" foods, may want to consider taking a multivitamin and mineral supplement. Most women in the United States 20 years of age or older eat about 1673 calories a day. Women who diet may eat fewer calories and may need to work harder to get the RDAs for essential vitamins and minerals. If patients cannot eat certain foods such as dairy foods, they may need to supplement their diet to make sure they are getting the nutrients they need.

An increasing amount of research suggests that taking specific nutrients may be helpful to protect against problems such as osteoporosis, birth defects, heart disease, stroke, infectious diseases, macular degeneration, and cataracts. These products are taken to maintain or improve a person's health and well-being, or for **health promotion.** Some of these products are discussed in the following sections. Chapter 24 provides a complete discussion of the types of vitamins and minerals, their actions, uses, adverse reactions, and drug interactions.

CALCIUM

In 1993, the FDA approved the use of a health claim on food and supplement labels about the role of calcium in reducing the risk of osteoporosis and the need for calcium supplements by people who do not get enough calcium from their diets. The current advice is for people over the age of 50 to consume at least 1200 mg of calcium daily. More than three glasses of low-fat milk per day would be required to provide this much calcium. Calcium-fortified (or enriched) products such as orange juice, sardines, salmon, tofu, and other dairy products help meet the daily requirements. The calcium citrate malate found in fortified orange juice is one of the best forms of calcium because it tends to be absorbed better than other types. The calcium carbonate found in Tums and other antacids is also acceptable. Vitamin D is important for calcium absorption. It is available as a supplement in multivitamins and fortified milk and naturally from exposure of the skin to the sun. Some calcium products also come with a small amount of magnesium, which also helps calcium absorption. Calcium supplements are absorbed the best when taken with food because food slows down their passage through the large intestine.

FOLIC ACID, VITAMIN B$_6$, AND VITAMIN B$_{12}$

There is now a significant amount of scientific data showing that eating foods containing folate (citrus fruits, cereals, leafy greens, and whole grains) or taking a multivitamin containing folic acid protects against birth defects such as neural tube defects, spina bifida, and anencephaly, and may also reduce the risk of heart disease and stroke. The neural tube of the fetus is formed within the first 28 days of pregnancy, before many women know they are pregnant. However, the evidence for folic acid in preventing neural tube defects is so strong that the U.S. Public Health Service issued an official recommendation that "all women of childbearing age in the United States who are capable of becoming pregnant should consume 0.4 mg of folic acid per day for the purpose of reducing their risk of having a pregnancy affected with spina bifida or other neural tube defects." This warning applies to women throughout their childbearing years. The dose of folic acid should be increased to 4 mg/day for at least 3 months before a woman plans to get pregnant.

Research has also shown that modestly elevated homocysteine levels in the blood are a risk factor for heart disease. Folic acid and vitamins B$_6$ and B$_{12}$ have been shown to reduce homocysteine levels. The intake of these three B complex vitamins, found primarily in vegetables and legumes, has been shown to be low in the United States, particularly in the elderly population. Vitamin B$_{12}$ is also found in meat and fish but is not absorbed as easily by people as they age. Some experts say that those at risk for heart disease should take a supplement that contains folic acid and vitamins B$_6$ and B$_{12}$. Folic acid may be more readily absorbed from supplements and enriched foods than from other sources.

IRON

Iron has long been known to be necessary for people who suffer from anemia caused by blood loss. Thus young women of childbearing age are often given iron supplements. Most menopausal women would probably benefit from a multivitamin containing 10 milligrams of iron or less. Iron supplements for people who do not have blood loss have not been shown to be needed or desired. High levels of iron in the blood can result in heart disease, cancer, and serious infection. However, it is hard to find a multivitamin without iron. People should take iron and calcium supplements at different times because these two minerals compete for absorption.

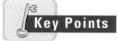

Key Points

- The nurse often serves, either formally or informally, as a teacher and adviser to the patient.
- It is important to be knowledgeable enough to answer questions about OTC medications, current trends in alternative therapies, and recent recommendations about vitamins and minerals.
- Keeping up on recent findings will help prepare you for this part of your nursing role.

Go to the free CD-ROM for an Audio Glossary, animations, video clips, and Review Questions for the NCLEX-PN® Examination.

evolve Be sure to visit the companion Evolve website at http://evolve.elsevier.com/Edmunds/LPN/ for WebLinks, a link to the top 200 drugs by prescription, and sign-up pages for newsletter drug updates.

CRITICAL THINKING ?

1. A patient you are caring for has hypertension. He tells you that he routinely takes Sudafed for colds and sinus infections. What would you tell him?

2. Mrs. Brown is recovering from a stroke. She has been given anticoagulant therapy and is about to go home. Although she is making good progress, she is quite depressed about her appearance and her ability to walk without assistance. Her family wants her to begin taking gingko. What will you tell them?

3. You develop a bad cold. When you go to the pharmacy, you see OTC medications labeled as decongestants and others labeled as antihistamines. Which will you buy and why?

4. Tylenol is a common product available in almost every home. Look at the dosages of Tylenol for infants, children, and adults. If you have a child under 2 years, a 6-year-old, and a 12-year-old, could you give them the same product? Look at the symptoms of overdosage. How easy do you think it would be to give an overdose of this medication to a child?

5. Make a list of the OTC medications in your bathroom. Would any of these products be dangerous if a child were to take them? Does this information make you reconsider how you store these products?

6. Your patient says that she plans to go to a health food store to buy some medication for menopausal hot flashes. What information would you give her about the products sold in these stores?

7. You discover that one of your Chinese patients makes a medicinal tea every morning. This patient has asthma and high blood pressure. What are some of the things you might want to talk about with this patient?

8. One of your very poor patients has been buying very expensive vitamins at a health food store. What information would you offer? What benefits exist for using these instead of less expensive vitamins available at the grocery store?

9. Which of the following individuals would you expect to need a daily multivitamin and mineral supplement: a 30-year-old woman who smokes; a thin, 5-year-old boy; a 20-year-old female who is a vegetarian; a 30-year-old man who drinks lots of coffee and eats erratically; a 40-year-old woman who has had six children; a 35-year-old homeless man with cirrhosis of liver; and a 60-year-old postal worker. Give a reason why or why not for each person.

10. Your new daughter-in-law tells you that she and your son plan to start a family. What vitamins and/or minerals will her health care provider most likely recommend that she take? Why?

CHAPTER 7

Review of Mathematical Principles

Objectives

After reading and studying this chapter, you should be able to do the following:

1. Work basic multiplication and division problems.
2. Interpret Roman numerals correctly.
3. Apply basic rules in calculations using fractions, decimal fractions, percentages, ratios, and proportions.

Key Terms

Be sure to check out the bonus material on the free CD-ROM, including selected audio pronunciations.

common denominator (dē-NŎM-ĭ-nā-tŏr, p. 70)
complex fraction (FRĂK-shŭn, p. 69)
denominator (p. 68)
fraction (p. 68)
improper fraction (p. 69)
mixed number (p. 69)
numerator (NŪ-měr-ā-tŏr, p. 68)
percent (p. 72)
proper fraction (p. 69)
proportion (p. 73)
ratio (RĀ-shē-ō, p. 72)
Roman numeral system (p. 68)

OVERVIEW

The ability to calculate basic mathematical problems accurately and quickly rests on the nurse having a good foundation of basic math. Although most nurses feel comfortable with addition and subtraction, many can profit from a review of basic concepts in multiplication and division, as well as fractions, percentages, and proportions, to increase their speed. These number relationships form important building blocks for tasks the nurse must master. By memorizing and drilling on these basic facts, you will have confidence and speed in calculating dosages and converting from one system of measures for drugs to another.

MULTIPLICATION AND DIVISION

Box 7-1 presents a basic grid for multiplication and division. To multiply two numbers, find one number in the top row and the other number in the left-hand column, and follow the row leading across and the column leading down from each number to where the row and the column intersect (cross each other) within the grid.

For example: What is 7×8? Find the number 7 on the left and follow across to the right; find the number 8 on the top and follow down from it. The two lines intersect at 56. Therefore $7 \times 8 = 56$. Another way to indicate that two numbers are to be multiplied is to place them in parentheses next to each other. Therefore, (30)(3) means 30×3.

To use this grid for division, find the number on the left-hand side of the chart that is the same as the divisor (the number you are dividing by). Follow the row to the right until you come to the exact number you are dividing, or the number closest to it. Follow the column up to the top to learn the number of times that larger number may be divided by the number on the left.

For example: How many times will 9 go into 81? Find 9 in the column on the left. Follow the row across until you come to 81. Follow the column up from 81 to the top, which is 9. Therefore $81 \div 9 = 9$. If you wanted to know how many times the whole number 9 would go into 84, you would still use the column containing the number 81, because it is the closest number in that row of the grid to 84. The answer would still be 9, but there would be a remainder of 3.

Memory Jogger

Multiplication Hint
Zero times any number is zero!

Box **7-1** | *Multiplication and Division Grid*

1	2	3	4	5	6	7	8	9	10	11	12
2	4	6	8	10	12	14	16	18	20	22	24
3	6	9	12	15	18	21	24	27	30	33	36
4	8	12	16	20	24	28	32	36	40	44	48
5	10	15	20	25	30	35	40	45	50	55	60
6	12	18	24	30	36	42	48	54	60	66	72
7	14	21	28	35	42	49	56	63	70	77	84
8	16	24	32	40	48	56	64	72	80	88	96
9	18	27	36	45	54	63	72	81	90	99	108
10	20	30	40	50	60	70	80	90	100	110	120
11	22	33	44	55	66	77	88	99	110	121	132
12	24	36	48	60	72	84	96	108	120	132	144

ROMAN NUMERALS

The numbers commonly used today in expressing quantity and value are called *Arabic numerals.* Examples of Arabic numerals are 1, 2, and 3. Another number system in common use is the **Roman numeral system.** Roman numerals from the values of 1 to 100 are commonly used as units of the apothecaries' system of weights and measures in writing prescriptions. They may also be used to express dates in copyrights and in formal manuscripts. Seven numerals make up the basic building blocks of the Roman numeral system (Box 7-2).

After memorizing the seven Roman numerals and their values, it is important to learn four rules in using roman numerals. These rules and some examples are presented in Box 7-3.

FRACTIONS

A good understanding of fractions is important to the nurse because all units of the apothecaries' system are written as common fractions for all amounts less than 1. Fractions also form the foundation in dosage calculations when medication is only available in a different dose form than the form that was ordered.

Box **7-2** | *Roman Numerals and Their Values*

I	= 1
V	= 5
X	= 10
L	= 50
C	= 100
D	= 500
M	= 1000

Box **7-3** | *Rules in Using Roman Numerals*

1. Whenever a Roman numeral is repeated, or when a smaller numeral *follows* a larger one, the values are added together. For example:

   II = 2 (1 + 1 = 2)
   LVII = 57 (50 + 5 + 1 + 1 = 57)
   CXIII = 113 (100 + 10 + 1 + 1 + 1 = 113)

2. Whenever a smaller Roman numeral *comes before* a larger Roman numeral, subtract the smaller value from the larger one. For example:

   IV = 4 (5 − 1 = 4)
   CD = 400 (500 − 100 = 400)

3. Numerals are never repeated more than three times in a sequence. For example:

   III = 3
   IV = 4

4. Whenever a smaller Roman numeral comes between two larger Roman numerals, subtract the smaller number from the numeral following it. For example:

   XIX = 19 (10 + [10 − 1] = 19)
   LIV = 54 (50 + [5 − 1] = 54)

In expressing dosages in the apothecaries' system, lowercase rather than capital Roman numerals are used. A dot is always placed over the Roman numeral i whenever lowercase numbers are used. For example, iii or vi is the proper form rather than III or VI.

BASIC PRINCIPLES

A **fraction** is one or more equal parts of a unit. It is written as two numbers separated by a line, such as ½ or ¾. The parts of the fraction are called the *terms.* The two terms of a fraction are the **numerator** and the **denominator.** The numerator is the top number (the number above the line). The denominator is the bottom number (the number below the line). In ½, 1 is the numerator and 2 is the denominator.

The denominator tells into how many equal parts the whole has been divided. The numerator tells how many of the parts are being used.

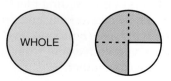

It is important not to confuse these two parts of the fraction. One way to remember which part belongs where is to think of the word NUDE. The N is on top; the D is on the bottom, like this:

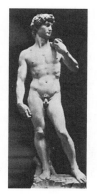

$$\begin{array}{c} \mathbf{N} \\ \mathbf{U} \\ \overline{} \\ \mathbf{D} \\ \mathbf{E} \end{array}$$

To use fractions in calculations, the numerator and the denominator must be of the same unit of measure. For example, if the numerator is in grains, the denominator must be in grains.

Fractions may be raised to higher terms by multiplying both terms of the fraction by the same number. For example, to raise ¾ to a higher term, multiply both the numerator and the denominator by 2, converting it to ⁶⁄₈. Thus ¾ and ⁶⁄₈ have the same value:

$$\frac{3}{4} \times \frac{2}{2} = \frac{6}{8}$$

Fractions are reduced to lower terms by dividing both the numerator and denominator by the same number. For example, to lower ³⁄₉ to a lower term, divide both the numerator and the denominator by 3, converting it to ⅓. Thus ³⁄₉ and ⅓ have the same value:

$$\frac{3}{9} \times \frac{3}{3} = \frac{1}{3}$$

A **proper fraction** has a numerator smaller than the denominator. The number ¾ is a proper fraction because it is less than 1; its numerator is less than its denominator.

An **improper fraction** has a numerator the same as or larger than the denominator. The number ⁶⁄₄ is an improper fraction because the numerator (6) is larger than the denominator (4).

A **mixed number** is a whole number and a proper fraction. Examples of mixed numbers are 4⅓, 3¾, and 5¹⁶⁄₃₅.

It is often necessary to change an improper fraction to a mixed number or to change a mixed number to an improper fraction when doing certain calculations. To change an improper fraction to a mixed number, divide the denominator into the numerator. The result is the whole number (quotient) and the remainder, which is placed over the denominator of the improper fraction.

For example, ¹⁷⁄₃ is an improper fraction. To convert it to a mixed number:

1. Divide the denominator (3) into the numerator (17):

$$\begin{array}{r} 5 \leftarrow \text{quotient} \\ 3\overline{)17} \\ -15 \\ \hline 2 \leftarrow \text{remainder} \end{array}$$

2. Move the remainder (2) over the denominator (3).
3. Put the quotient (5) in front of the fraction:

$$5\frac{2}{3}$$

To change the mixed number 5⅔ to an improper fraction, multiply the denominator of the fraction (3) by the whole number (5), add the numerator (2), and place the sum over the denominator. For example:

$$\begin{array}{r} 3 \times 5 = 15 \\ +2 \\ \hline 17 \leftarrow \text{sum} \end{array}$$

The sum (17) goes over the denominator of the fraction: ¹⁷⁄₃ is the improper fraction.

A **complex fraction** has a fraction in either its numerator, its denominator, or both. The following are examples of complex fractions:

$$\frac{\frac{1}{5}}{50} \qquad \frac{30}{\frac{2}{3}} \qquad 3\frac{\frac{1}{2}}{\frac{1}{8}}$$

Complex fractions may be changed to whole numbers or to proper or improper fractions by dividing the number or fraction above the line by the number or fraction below the line. For example, to change the following complex number to a proper fraction, divide the fraction above the line by the number below the line:

$$\frac{\frac{1}{2}}{100} = \frac{1}{2} \div 100$$

To divide by 100, or by ¹⁰⁰⁄₁, simply invert or reverse the numerator (100) and the denominator (1) and multiply by the result, or by ¹⁄₁₀₀. For example:

$$\frac{1}{2} \div 100 = \frac{1}{2} \div \frac{100}{1} = \frac{1}{2} \times \frac{1}{100}$$
$$= \frac{1}{2 \times 100} = \frac{1}{200}$$

Adding Fractions

If fractions have the same denominator, simply add the numerators, and put the sum above the common denominator. For example:

$$\frac{1}{11} + \frac{3}{11} = \frac{4}{11} \quad \frac{\text{(sum of } 1 + 3)}{\text{(same denominator)}}$$

Also:

$$\frac{2}{12} + \frac{3}{12} + \frac{6}{12} = \frac{11}{12} \quad \frac{\text{(sum of } 2 + 3 + 6)}{\text{(same denominator)}}$$

If the fractions have different denominators, they must be converted to a number that each denominator has in common, or a **common denominator.** One can always find a common denominator by multiplying the two denominators by one another. Sometimes, however, both numbers will go into a smaller number. For example, in the equation $\frac{1}{12} + \frac{3}{8} + \frac{3}{4} = ?$, what is the smallest common denominator?

1. The smallest whole number all these denominators (12, 8, and 4) have in common is 24; 24, then, is the lowest common denominator.
2. Divide the lowest common denominator (24) by the denominator of each fraction (12, 8, and 4) to determine the quotient, or the answer to be used to convert each fraction to a number with the common denominator:

$$\frac{12}{24} = ?$$
$$\frac{8}{24} = ?$$
$$\frac{4}{24} = ?$$

3. Next, multiply both the numerator and the denominator of each fraction by the quotient for each. This is often easier to see if the problem is written vertically:

$$\frac{1}{12} \times \frac{2}{2} = \frac{2}{24}$$
$$+ \frac{3}{8} \times \frac{3}{3} = \frac{9}{24}$$
$$+ \frac{3}{4} \times \frac{6}{6} = \frac{18}{24}$$

4. Then add the numerators and bring down the denominator:

$$\frac{2}{24} + \frac{9}{24} + \frac{18}{24} = \frac{29}{24}$$

5. Change the improper fraction to a mixed number:

$$\frac{29}{24} = 1\frac{5}{24}$$

When adding mixed numbers, first change them to improper fractions and proceed as indicated previously.

Subtracting Fractions

If fractions have the same denominator, subtract the smaller numerator from the larger numerator. Leave the denominator the same, and then reduce to the lowest terms, if necessary. For example:

$$\frac{5}{10} - \frac{1}{10} = \frac{4}{10} = \frac{2}{5}$$

If fractions do not have the same denominator, change the fractions so they have the smallest common denominator, subtract the numerators, and leave the denominator the same. For example:

$$\frac{15}{28} - \frac{3}{14} = ?$$

Because 28 is a multiple of 14 ($14 \times 2 = 28$), 28 is a common denominator of 28 and 14. Divide the lowest common denominator by the denominator of each fraction to determine the quotient, and multiply the numerator and denominator of the fraction by the quotient:

$$\frac{15}{28} \times \frac{1}{1} = \frac{15}{28} \text{ (no change necessary)}$$
$$\frac{3}{14} \times \frac{2}{2} = \frac{6}{28} \text{ (}28 \div 14 = 2\text{)}$$

Subtract the numerators and leave the denominators the same:

$$\frac{15}{28} - \frac{6}{28} = \frac{9}{28}$$

When subtracting mixed numbers, first change them to improper fractions and proceed as shown in the previous examples.

Multiplying Fractions

When multiplying fractions, reduce all terms to their smallest form to simplify the calculation. For example, $\frac{12}{24}$ is the same as $\frac{1}{2}$, but $\frac{12}{24}$ is more difficult to work with. To reduce to the lowest terms, divide the same number into both the numerator and the denominator. For example, in the fraction $\frac{2}{10}$, both 2 and 10 can be divided by 2; therefore, $\frac{2}{10} \div \frac{2}{2} = \frac{1}{5}$. Similarly, in the fraction $\frac{9}{36}$, both the numerator and the denominator can be divided by 9; therefore, $\frac{9}{36} \div \frac{9}{9} = \frac{1}{4}$.

When the fractions are in their simplest form, multiply the numerators together, and then multiply the denominators together. For example:

$$\frac{1}{20} \times \frac{5}{3} \times 3 =$$
$$\frac{1}{20} \times \frac{5}{3} \times \frac{3}{1} =$$
$$\frac{1 \times 5 \times 3}{20 \times 3 \times 1} = \frac{15}{60}$$

This can be simplified as follows:

$$\frac{15}{60} = \frac{1}{4}$$

If the number is a mixed number (a whole number and a fraction), change it to an improper fraction before solving. For example:

$$2\frac{1}{2} \times \frac{2}{3} \times 6 = \frac{5}{2} \times \frac{2}{3} \times \frac{6}{1}$$

Simplify:

$$= \frac{5}{\overset{}{\underset{1}{2}}} \times \frac{\overset{1}{\cancel{2}}}{\overset{}{\underset{1}{3}}} \times \frac{\overset{2}{\cancel{6}}}{1}$$

$$= \frac{10}{1} = 10$$

Memory Jogger

Multiplying Fractions

Because 3 is a whole number, it is the same as ³⁄₁; the 1 can be added as a denominator if it makes calculations easier to understand.

Dividing Fractions

To divide a fraction by a fraction, invert (or turn upside down) the fraction that is the divisor and then multiply. For example:

$$\frac{4}{6} \div \frac{2}{6} = ?$$

Invert the divisor:

$$\frac{4}{6} \times \frac{6}{2} = ?$$

Simplify, then multiply the numerators and then the denominators:

$$\frac{\overset{2}{\cancel{4}}}{\underset{1}{\cancel{6}}} \times \frac{\overset{1}{\cancel{6}}}{\underset{1}{\cancel{2}}} = \frac{2}{1} = 2$$

If the number is a mixed number, change it to an improper fraction before solving. For example:

$$\frac{2}{3} \div 1\frac{1}{3} = ?$$

Change the mixed number to an improper fraction:

$$\frac{2}{3} \div \frac{4}{3} = ?$$

Invert the divisor:

$$\frac{2}{3} \times \frac{3}{4} = ?$$

Simplify:

$$\frac{\overset{1}{\cancel{2}}}{\underset{1}{\cancel{3}}} \times \frac{\overset{1}{\cancel{3}}}{\underset{2}{\cancel{4}}} = \frac{1}{2}$$

$$\frac{1}{1} \times \frac{1}{2} = \frac{1}{2}$$

DECIMAL FRACTIONS

A decimal fraction has a denominator of 10 or a multiple of 10. Instead of writing the denominator, a decimal point is added to the numerator. For example:

$$\frac{1}{4} = \frac{25}{100} = 0.25$$

All numbers to the left of the decimal point represent whole numbers. Numbers to the right represent fractions. Zeros may be placed to the right of the decimal without changing the value of the whole number (for example, 45 is the same as 45.0 or 45.00).

Decimals increase in value from right to left; they decrease in value from left to right. Decimals increase in value in multiples of 10. Each column in a decimal has its own value, according to where it lies in relation to the decimal point (Box 7-4).

Adding and Subtracting Decimal Fractions

Place the numbers so that the decimal points are stacked in a straight line. Keep the columns straight. Add zeros to the right of the decimal points if necessary so that each number has an equal number of digits to the right of the decimal point. Then add or subtract as for whole numbers. The decimal point goes in the answer just below the decimal points in the problem.

For example, to add 0.0678 and 1.082:

```
  0.0678
+ 1.0820    (add one zero)
  1.1498
```

Note that the decimal point in the answer is in line with the other decimal points.

To subtract 3.053 from 6.046:

```
  6.046
− 3.053
  2.993
```

Multiplying and Dividing Decimal Fractions

To multiply decimal fractions, multiply the two numbers as for whole numbers. Then count the number of decimal places in the multiplicand (the number that is multiplied) and the number in the multiplier (the

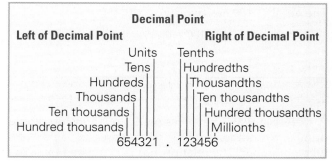

Box 7-4 | *Values Left and Right of the Decimal Point*

	Decimal Point	
Left of Decimal Point		**Right of Decimal Point**

```
                      Units  Tenths
                       Tens| Hundredths
                  Hundreds| |Thousandths
                 Thousands| ||Ten thousandths
             Ten thousands| ||Hundred thousandths
          Hundred thousands||||  ||Millionths
                   654321 . 123456
```

number you multiply by). Beginning at the right side of the product (answer), count off that total number of decimal places from right to left and insert a decimal point. For example:

44.61	Multiplicand (has two decimal places)
$\times$ 2.3	Multiplier (has one decimal place)
13383	
+ 89220	
102.603	Count off three places right to left and insert decimal point.

To divide by a decimal fraction, first move the decimal point in the divisor (the number you are dividing with) enough places right to make it a whole number. Then move the decimal point in the dividend (the number you are dividing) as many places as it was moved in the divisor. Place the decimal point in the quotient (answer) directly above that in the dividend. For example, to divide 32.80 by 8.2:

$$8.2\overline{)32.80} \quad \text{8.2 is the divisor; 32.80 is the dividend}$$

Move the decimal point in the divisor to the right to make it a whole number, then move it the same number of places in the dividend:

$$8.2\overline{)32.80}$$

Solve the problem:

$$\begin{array}{r} 4.0 \\ 82.\overline{)328.00} \\ -\underline{328.00} \\ 0 \end{array}$$

A shortcut may be taken when multiplying or dividing by 10, 100, or 1000. To multiply a decimal fraction by 10, 100, or 1000, move the decimal point as many places to the right as there are zeros in the multiplier. For example:

$$0.0006 \times 1000 = ?$$

In 1000 there are three zeros, so:

$$0.0006 \times 1000 =$$
$$0.0006 = 0000.6 = 0.6$$

To divide a decimal fraction by 10, 100, or 1000, move the decimal place as many places to the left as there are zeros in the divisor. For example:

$$0.5 \div 100 = ?$$

The number 100 has two zeros, so:

$$0.5 \div 100 = 000.5 = 0.005$$

RATIOS

A **ratio** is a way of expressing the relationship of one number to another number, or of expressing a part of a whole number. The relationship is expressed by sepa-

rating the numbers with a colon (:). The colon means division. The expression 1:2 means there is a ratio of one part to two parts. Ratios are commonly used to express concentrations of a drug in a solution.

For example, a ratio written as 1:20 means 1 part to 20 parts. The relationship may also be expressed as a fraction (e.g., 1:10 is the same as $\frac{1}{10}$).

PERCENTS

The term **percent** or the symbol % means parts per hundred. Thus a percentage may also be expressed as a fraction or as a decimal fraction. For example:

30% means 30 parts per hundred or $\frac{30}{100}$
70% means 70 parts per hundred or $\frac{70}{100}$

Percentages should also be reduced to their lowest common denominator, when appropriate. For example:

20% is $\frac{20}{100}$ or $\frac{1}{5}$
40% is $\frac{40}{100}$ or $\frac{2}{5}$

To change a fraction to a percentage, divide the numerator by the denominator, multiply the quotient (results) by 100, and add a percent sign (%). For example, to change $\frac{8}{10}$ to a percentage:

$$8 \div 10 = 0.8$$
$$0.8 \times 100 = 80\%$$

To change $\frac{2}{5}$ to a percentage:

$$2 \div 5 = 0.4$$
$$0.4 \times 100 = 40\%$$

To change a mixed number to a percentage, first change it to an improper fraction, then proceed as noted previously. For example, to change $1\frac{1}{4}$ to a percentage:

$$\frac{5}{4} = 5 \div 4 = 1.25$$
$$1.25 \times 100 = 125\%$$

To change a ratio to a percentage, the ratio is first expressed as a fraction. The first number, or term, of the ratio becomes the numerator, and the second number or term becomes the denominator (for example, 1:200 becomes $\frac{1}{200}$). The fraction is then changed to a percentage:

$$1{:}200 = \frac{1}{200}$$
$$1 \div 200 = 0.005$$
$$0.005 \times 100 = 0.5\%$$

To change a percentage to a ratio, the percentage becomes the numerator and is placed over the denominator of 100. For example, to change 20% and 50% to ratios:

20% is $\frac{20}{100} = \frac{1}{5}$ or 1:5
50% is $\frac{50}{100} = \frac{1}{2}$ or 1:2

Box 7-5 | *Rules for Changing Between Percentages, Decimals, Fractions, and Ratios*

CHANGING FRACTIONS

- To change a fraction to a ratio, write the two numbers with a colon between them instead of the dividing line.

  Example: $\frac{1}{5}$ = 1:5

- To change a fraction to a decimal fraction, divide the numerator by the denominator.

  Example: $\frac{1}{5}$ = 0.20

- To change a fraction to a percentage, divide the numerator by the denominator (use as many decimal places as needed); then move the decimal point two places to the right and add the percent sign.

  Example: $\frac{1}{5}$ = 0.20 = 20%

CHANGING PERCENTAGES

- To change a percentage to a decimal fraction, move the decimal point two places to the left and omit the percent sign.

  Example: 10% = 0.10

- To change a percentage to a fraction, drop the percent sign, write the number as the numerator, with 100 as the denominator, and reduce to the lowest terms.

  Example: 10% = $\frac{10}{100}$ = $\frac{1}{10}$

- To change a percentage to a ratio, drop the percent sign, use the number as the first term and 100 as the second term, and reduce to the lowest terms; *or* change to a fraction and then use a colon instead of the dividing line.

  Example: 10% = 10:100 = 1:10 *or* 10% = $\frac{1}{10}$ = 1:10

CHANGING DECIMALS

- To change a decimal fraction to a percentage, move the decimal point two places to the right (multiply by 100) and add the percent sign.

  Example: 0.20 = 20%

- To change a decimal fraction to a common fraction, omit the decimal point and place the number over the appropriate denominator of 10, 100, or 1000, and reduce to the lowest terms.

  Example: 0.20 = $\frac{20}{100}$ = $\frac{1}{5}$

- To change a decimal fraction to a ratio, write the number as the first term; then put 10, 100, or 1000 as the second term; finally, reduce to the lowest terms.

  Example: 0.20 = 20:100 or 1:5

CHANGING RATIOS

- To change a ratio to a fraction, write the numbers with a dividing line instead of a colon.

  Example: 1:20 = $\frac{1}{20}$

- To change a ratio to a decimal fraction, divide the first term by the second term.

  Example: 1:20 = 0.05

- To change a ratio to a percentage, divide the first term by the second term, move the decimal point two places to the right in the answer, and add a percent sign.

  Example: 1:20 = 0.05 = 5%

A percentage may easily be expressed as a decimal, a fraction, or a ratio. For example:

$$20\% = 0.20 = \frac{20}{100} = \frac{1}{5} = 1:5$$

It is very easy to change between fractions, percentages, decimals, and ratios. The rules that summarize these changes are presented in Box 7-5.

PROPORTIONS

A **proportion** is a way of expressing a relationship of equality between two ratios. In other words, the first ratio listed is equal to the second ratio listed. The two ratios are separated by a double colon (::), which means "as." The numbers at each end of the relationship are the extremes, and the two numbers in the middle are the means. In any proportion, *the product of the extremes equals the product of the means.* This means that, if one of the terms is not known, it may be calculated. The unknown term is defined by an *x*. For example:

5:500 :: 2:*x*

(where *x* is the unknown) can be read as "5 is to 500 as 2 is to *x*" or "The relationship of 5 to 500 is the same as the relationship of 2 to *x*." Then:

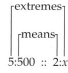

In this proportion, 5 and x are the extremes, and 500 and 2 are the means. Therefore:

$$5 \times x = 500 \times 2$$

To find x, express the proportion as a relationship of two fractions, cross multiply, and solve:

$$\frac{5}{500} = \frac{2}{x}$$
$$5x = 500 \times 2$$
$$5x = 1000$$
$$x = \frac{1000}{5}$$
$$x = 200$$

Because a proportion is a relationship of equality, both ratios in the proportion must also be written in the same system (for example, minims are to grains as minims are to grains; milliliters are to grams as milliliters are to grams). For example:

15 ⓜ : 60 ⓖⓡ :: 13 ⓜ : x ⓖⓡ   Correctly written

15 ⓜ : 60 ⓜ :: 13 ⓜ : x ⓖⓡ   Incorrectly written

The calculation of ratios and proportions provides one of the major foundations in drug dosage calculations.

Often you know the desired concentration of a drug and need to calculate how much to give of a medication on hand. You will be able to figure how much medication to give by using the principles of proportion.

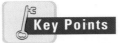
Key Points

- You must understand and be able to use basic math principles to administer drugs.
- These basic math principles include the use of multiplication, division, and Roman numerals, as well as the calculation of fractions, decimal fractions, percentages, ratios, and proportions.

Go to the free CD-ROM for an Audio Glossary, animations, video clips, and Review Questions for the NCLEX-PN® Examination.

evolve Be sure to visit the companion Evolve website at http://evolve.elsevier.com/Edmunds/LPN/ for WebLinks, a link to the top 200 drugs by prescription, and sign-up pages for newsletter drug updates.

CRITICAL THINKING ?

1. Match the following mathematical expressions or components (marked in bold) on the left with their appropriate labels in the right-hand column:
   a. $\frac{2}{3}$ _____ ratio
   b. $^{25}/_4$ _____ denominator
   c. $5\frac{1}{8}$ _____ improper fraction
   d. **1**   _____ mixed number
   e. **3**   _____ numerator
   f. **3:4**   _____ percent
   g. **75%**   _____ proper fraction
   h. $\frac{1}{4} + \frac{2}{5} = \frac{13}{20}$ _____ common denominator

2. Review multiplication and division by doing the following problems:

   $7 \times 11 =$ $9 \div 3 =$ $8 \times 7 =$

   $(252)(41) =$ $98 \times 7 =$ $360 \div 3 =$

3. Calculate the following division problems:

   $516 \div 7 =$ $637 \div 4 =$ $7849 \div 60 =$

4. Change the following Roman numerals into Arabic, and the Arabic numerals into Roman numerals:

   CDVIII =   93 =
   XXXIV =   562 =
   LXXVII =   1934 =
   MCMXIII =   2597 =

5. Find the common denominators and add or subtract (reduce, if necessary):
   a. $\frac{1}{4} + \frac{2}{5} =$ b. $\frac{4}{25} + \frac{3}{25} =$
   c. $\frac{1}{4} + \frac{2}{3} =$ d. $\frac{3}{4} - \frac{4}{7} =$

6. Subtract the following:
   a. $\frac{5}{6} - \frac{7}{9} =$ b. $\frac{4}{25} - \frac{3}{20} =$
   c. $5\frac{3}{8} - 2\frac{3}{4} =$ d. $7\frac{1}{3} - 4\frac{2}{5} =$

7. Multiply the following fractions and reduce to lowest terms:
   a. $\frac{2}{7} \times \frac{3}{5} =$ b. $\frac{4}{11} \times \frac{3}{8} =$
   c. $\frac{5}{12} \times \frac{2}{3} \times \frac{1}{2} =$ d. $\frac{3}{4} \times \frac{4}{5} \times \frac{2}{3} =$

8. Divide the following fractions:
   a. $\frac{5}{9} \div \frac{2}{3} =$ b. $\frac{3}{4} \div \frac{3}{5} =$
   c. $5\frac{1}{2} \div 2\frac{3}{4} =$ d. $7\frac{1}{5} \div 4\frac{2}{5} =$

9. Change the following decimals to fractions:
   a. $0.591 =$ b. $1.34 =$ c. $2.547 =$

10. Convert to common fractions or mixed numbers in lowest terms:
    a. $1.56 =$ b. $5.27 =$ c. $3.375 =$

11. Calculate the following:
    a. $11.019 + 52.70 + 7.141 =$ b. $97.30 - 9.071 =$
    c. $1.59 \times 2.301 \times 1.977 =$ d. $121.4 \div 8.12 =$

12. Change to a percentage:
    a. $0.65 =$ **b.** $5\frac{3}{7} =$ **c.** $\frac{4}{9} =$

13. Change to decimal fractions:
    a. $23\% =$ **b.** $116\% =$ **c.** $\frac{2}{7}\% =$

14. Express as decimals:
    a. $7\frac{3}{8} =$ **b.** $321\% =$ **c.** $52\% =$

15. Express as percentages:
    a. $2.47 =$ **b.** $1.55 =$ **c.** $2\frac{2}{3} =$

16. Express as ratios:
    a. $\frac{1}{6}$ to $\frac{1}{5}$
    b. 2 feet to 6 inches
    c. 100 mph

17. Calculate the following:
    a. $\frac{3.5}{6.7} = \frac{x}{8.9}$
    b. $\frac{2}{3} = \frac{x}{0.49}$
    c. $0.3 : 1 :: 0.5 : x$

8 Mathematical Equivalents Used in Pharmacology

Objectives

After reading and studying this chapter, you should be able to do the following:

1. Use the apothecaries' system to convert from one measure to another.
2. Use the metric system to convert from one measure to another.
3. State the values of common household measures and their equivalents.
4. Compare the units used in the apothecaries', metric, and household measures systems.
5. Use common abbreviations and symbols to interpret and solve medication problems.

Key Terms

Be sure to check out the bonus material on the free CD-ROM, including selected audio pronunciations.

apothecaries' system (ă-PŎTH-ĭ-kăr-ēz, p. 76)
Celsius (SĔL-sē-ĕs, p. 80)
Fahrenheit (FĂR-ĕn-HĪT, p. 80)
gram (p. 77)
liter (LĒ-tĕr, p. 77)
meter (MĒ-tĕr, p. 77)
metric system (MĔ-trĭk, p. 77)

OVERVIEW

Three established systems of weights and measures are used to compute and prepare medications. Perhaps the most commonly known system is that of general household measures. This system is adequate when more accurate measures are either not available or not needed, and is used primarily in the home. The English have used the apothecaries' system for many centuries. It relies on different units for solid and liquid measures. The metric system was developed in France and is based on the decimal system, with measures expressed in increments of tens, hundreds, and thousands. The metric and apothecaries' systems are commonly used by physicians and pharmacists as medication is ordered and prepared. The metric system is used the most often.

You may wonder why we include the older and less precise household and apothecaries' measurement systems in textbooks today. Although our world has grown smaller, there are still many parts of the world where technology is far behind that of Western civilizations. Nurses today often travel or work in different parts of the world and need to understand the basic principles of drug calculation. Even in the United States, there are many areas of the country where small rural hospitals, clinics, or offices do not have sophisticated medication delivery systems and packaging. In these settings, there may also be few registered nurses, and responsibility will fall on the licensed practical/vocational nurse to accurately calculate how much medicine should be given to a patient. You can never tell when mastering these different measurement systems will help you in the future.

You must be able to use all three systems of measures to calculate medication dosages accurately. You may feel somewhat nervous about learning these new systems because they seem unusual or difficult. However, once the basic words and values are memorized, you should be able to solve problems with confidence.

APOTHECARIES' SYSTEM

The **apothecaries' system** uses the basic units of grain (gr) for solids and minim (m) for liquids. Whole numbers and fractions are used in this system. The whole numbers are written as lowercase Roman numerals such as iv and x; decimals are not used. A few Arabic symbols are used to express dram (℥) and ounce (℥) and fractions. When ½ is desired, a special abbreviation from Latin, ss, may be used. In the apothecaries' system, the unit abbreviation comes before the quantity (for example, gr ½ [grains one half] or m xxx [minims 30]). If no abbreviation is used, the quantity comes before the unit (for example, ½ grain or 30 minims).

The apothecaries' system makes a clear distinction between solid and liquid measures. One minim (a liquid measure) equals 1 grain (a solid measure). Although there are many units of measure in the system, only a few are commonly used. These common measures are listed in Box 8-1.

| Box 8-1 | *The Apothecaries' System* |

LIQUID MEASURES

60 minims (m) = 1 fluid dram (ʒ)
8 fluid drams = 1 fluid ounce (fl oz or ℥)
16 fluid ounces = 1 pint (pt)
2 pints = 1 quart (qt)
4 quarts = 1 gallon (gal)
480 minims = 1 ounce (oz)

SOLID MEASURES

60 grains (gr) = 1 dram (ʒ)
8 drams = 1 ounce (oz or ℥)
480 grains = 1 ounce (oz)
12 ounces = 1 pound (lb)*

*Generally not used. Instead, 16 oz =1 lb is commonly used from the avoir-dupois table.

METRIC SYSTEM

The **metric system** relies on a decimal system; it is built on multiples of 10. The metric system uses **meter** (m) for the unit of length, **liter** (L) for the unit of volume, and **gram** (gm) for the unit of weight. The most common measures used in the metric system are listed in Box 8-2.

Memory Jogger

Common Metric Equivalents

Milliliters, cubic centimeters, and grams are approximately equivalent; 1 mL, or 1 cc, weighs approximately 1 gm.

| Box 8-2 | *The Metric System* |

MEASURES OF LENGTH (METER)

1 meter (m) = 100 centimeters (cm) = 1000 millimeters (mm)
1 centimeter (cm) = 0.01 meter (m)
1 millimeter (mm) = 0.001 meter (m)

MEASURES OF VOLUME (LITER)

1 decaliter (daL) = 10 liters (L)
1 liter (L) = 10 deciliters (dL) = 1000 milliliters (mL) or 1000 cubic centimeters (cc)

MEASURES OF WEIGHT (GRAM)

1 kilogram (kg) = 1000 grams (gm)
1 gram (gm) = 1000 milligrams (mg)
1 milligram (mg) = 1000 micrograms (mcg)

Converting within the various units of the metric system may be less complicated than converting from the metric system to other systems. For example:

1 mL or 1 cc weighs 1 gm, whereas 1 kg weighs 2.2 lb

Relying on what you know about the decimal system, it is simple to change measures within the metric system. To change milligrams to micrograms, move the decimal point three places to the right (multiply by 1000):

$$000.00007 = 000000.07$$

To change micrograms to milligrams, move the decimal point three places to the left (divide by 1000):

$$000000.07 = 000.00007$$

To change grams to milligrams, move the decimal point three places to the right (multiply by 1000):

$$1.000067 = 1000.067$$

To change milligrams to grams, move the decimal point three places to the left (divide by 1000):

$$1345.0789 = 1.3450789$$

Memory Jogger

Metric System Prefixes

Prefixes of the metric system indicate the multiples or fractions of the unit:
- milli = one thousandth
- centi = one hundredth
- deci = one tenth
- deca = ten
- hecto = hundred
- kilo = thousand

METRIC AND APOTHECARIES' EQUIVALENTS

Most problems are easier to solve when metric system numbers are involved. Most nurses find it helpful to change all the units in the apothecaries' system to the metric system in drug calculations.

Units in the apothecaries' and metric systems are not quite equivalent or equal, but they are close enough that they are commonly used. In calculating the changes from one system to another, fractions sometimes make a difference. There are actually 64 mg in 1 grain and 16 grains in 1 gm, but 60 and 15 are much

| Box 8-3 | *Approximate Equivalents in the Apothecaries' and Metric Systems** |

APOTHECARIES'		METRIC
1 gallon (gal)	=	4000 mL or 4000 cc or 4 L
1 qt or 32 oz	=	1000 mL or 1000 cc or 1 L
1 pt or 16 oz	=	500 mL or 500 cc or 500 gm
1 oz or 8 drams	=	30 to 32 mL or 30 to 32 cc or 30 to 32 gm
1 dram, 60 to 64 grains, or 60 to 64 minims	=	4 to 5 mL or 4 to 5 cc or 4 to 5 gm
15 to 16 grains or 15 to 16 minims	=	1 mL, 1 cc, or 1 gm
2.2 lb	=	1000 gm or 1 kg
1 grain	=	60 or 64 mg or 0.06 gm
1/60 grain	=	1 mg

*Fifteen rather than 16 grains is often used in calculations; 60 is often used in place of 64. These account for the variances seen in the table.

easier to work with and they are often employed in making calculations.

Rounding a number up or dropping to a lower number is often significant. When working with small portions such as minims, it is important to be precise. You should not give vague equivalents or round off calculations for dosages in milliliters, dosages for infants or children, dosages of cardiovascular or cancer drugs, or tablets, capsules, or medications for diagnostic tests. Additionally, dosages for heparin or other anticoagulants and insulin must be calculated precisely.

Rather than memorizing all the different units in the apothecaries' and metric systems, you should do the following:

1. Master the most familiar units system.
2. Learn equivalents in the two systems.
3. Know where information may rapidly be found to help in calculating less common unit dosages.

Most hospital units, clinics, and offices have some basic pharmacologic text with information on conversion from one system to another. This information should always be consulted when the nurse is unclear about a mathematical calculation.

There are a number of common equivalent values for the apothecaries' and metric systems of measurement. Basic rules for conversion are based on the assumption that you have mastered these basic relationships. You should study the information in Box 8-3 and memorize the equivalent values presented.

There are a few basic rules that may be followed to convert measurements from one system to another. These rules are presented in Box 8-4. In the apothecaries' system, 1 minim weighs 1 grain. This equivalency allows you to change the units of measure if you need to convert a liquid amount to a solid amount, or vice versa. If you are using measures from two different systems, always convert all of the numbers to one system, using whichever system is easiest to convert. For example, if a prescription calls for a certain number of grains of a drug, but the drug is only available in measurements of milligrams, you should

| Box 8-4 | *Rules for Converting Between Apothecaries' and Metric System* |

- To convert grains to grams, divide by 15 or 16. To convert grams to milligrams, move the decimal point three places to the right. To convert grams to grains, multiply by 15 or 16.
- To convert grains to milligrams, multiply by 60 or 64. To convert milligrams to grams, move the decimal point three places to the left. To convert milligrams to grains, divide by 60 or 64.
- To convert minims to milliliters, divide by 15 or 16. To convert milliliters to minims, multiply by 15 or 16.

convert the amount in grains to grams, and then to milligrams.

Sometimes when working with new number systems, it is difficult to keep things in proper perspective. The number you get after doing the calculation may appear abnormally small or tremendously large. As you gain experience, common sense will help you determine whether or not the answer is correct. When you must convert numbers from one system to another, you will soon learn shortcuts to help with mathematical calculations. For example, converting between grams and grains often produces large fractions that are difficult to reduce. It is often easier to change the grams to milligrams and then carry out the calculation.

HOUSEHOLD MEASURES

The final system of measures that nurses need to be able to use involves common household measures. These measures are often used when dosages do not need to be exact.

The basic units of liquid measure in the household system involve drops, teaspoons, tablespoons, and

Box 8-5   *Common Household Measures*

60 drops (gtt)	=	1 teaspoonful (t or tsp)
3 to 4 teaspoonsful	=	1 tablespoonful (T or Tbs)
2 tablespoonsful	=	1 ounce (oz)
6 to 8 teaspoonsful	=	1 ounce (oz)
6 ounces	=	1 teacupful
8 ounces	=	1 glass or cup

ounces. Their values are presented in Box 8-5. Although teaspoons and tablespoons found in the home come in varying sizes, these measures refer to the specialized measuring spoons one would use in baking or cooking. These measurements are not precise enough to substitute in hospital calculations.

Household measures may be converted either to the apothecaries' system or to the metric system. The drop (gtt) is the unit in the household system that is equivalent to the minim and the grain. However, household measures are very rough equivalents; for example, 1 tablespoonful equals 3 or 4 teaspoonsful. Thus it is possible to accept calculations converting household measures to the metric or apothecaries' system when the amounts are very small (for example, 60 gtt equals 1 teaspoonful). As the size of the dosage (or the volume) increases, there is less and less accuracy in the dosage calculated (for example, somewhere between 360 and 240 gtt equals 1 tablespoonful). Thus it would be foolish to try to calculate the number of drops in 1 tablespoonful. It is better to refer to a standard table of equivalents instead.

In comparing the metric, apothecaries', and household measurement systems, several obvious differences appear. These differences are summarized in Table 8-1. Examples of common conversions between household measures, apothecaries' system measures, and metric system measures are shown in Table 8-2.

When converting between these measurement systems, it may be difficult at times to keep the quantities in perspective because the calculations may involve unfamiliar units. Other common equivalents with more familiar units may help you to understand the relative sizes and weights involved in some of these measures. These are included in Box 8-6.

Table 8-1   *Comparison of Metric, Apothecaries', and Household Systems*

APOTHECARIES'	METRIC	HOUSEHOLD
UNITS OF MEASURE		
Grain, minim, dram, ounce	Milligram, gram, milliliter, cubic centimeter, liter	Drops, teaspoons, tablespoons, ounces, grams
STRUCTURE		
Ancient English system including familiar household measures; some measures in this system not commonly used	Built on decimal system (French) so logic of change from one unit to another is clear	Commonly used for small amounts when dosages need not be exact
FORMAT		
Roman numerals and common fractions are used; abbreviations or symbols are given before the amount number	Arabic numbers and decimal fractions are used; the amount number is given before the abbreviation	Arabic numbers are used; the amount number is given before the abbreviation

Modified from Edmunds MW, Mayhew MS: *Pharmacology for the primary care provider*, ed 2, St Louis, 2004, Mosby.
MAO, Monoamine oxidase.

Table 8-2   *Conversions Among Household, Apothecaries', and Metric Systems*

HOUSEHOLD		APOTHECARIES'		METRIC
1 teaspoonful	=	1 dram or 60 minims	=	4 or 5 mL
1 tablespoonful	=	3 or 4 drams	=	15 or 16 mL
2 tablespoonsful	=	8 drams or 1 ounce	=	30 or 32 mL
1 teacupful	=	6 ounces	=	180 mL
1 glassful	=	8 ounces	=	240 mL

Box 8-6 | *Common Equivalents for Metric Measures*

METRIC EQUIVALENTS

1 meter = 39.37 inches = 3.28 feet = 1.09 yards
1 centimeter = 0.39 inch
1 millimeter = 0.04 inch
1 kilometer = 0.62 mile
1 liter = 1.06 liquid quarts
1 gram = 0.04 ounce
1 kilogram = 2.2 pounds

COMMON MEASURE EQUIVALENTS

1 inch = 25.4 millimeters
1 foot = 0.3 meter
1 yard = 0.91 meter
1 mile = 1.61 kilometers
1 ounce = 28.35 grams
1 pound = 0.45 kilogram

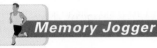

Memory Jogger

Converting Household Measures

The key relationship to understand in converting household measures to other systems is that 1 drop equals 1 minim and weighs 1 grain.

CONVERTING TEMPERATURE READINGS

For years nurses have used the Fahrenheit (F) scale to take temperatures. In the last 20 years, institutions have placed increasing emphasis on the centigrade, or Celsius (C), scale for hospital use. Although electronic thermometers with digital readouts are used in some hospitals, nurses may use either Fahrenheit or Celsius thermometers on occasion.

Thermometers used in many hospitals come in either Fahrenheit or Celsius scale. Oral thermometers come with either a long, flat tip or oblong or stubby tips. The oblong or stubby tips may also be used for rectal or axillary temperatures.

On the **Fahrenheit** scale, 212° is the boiling point and 32° is the freezing point. Outdoor temperature thermometers generally include these points. The Fahrenheit thermometer that is used for medical measurement ranges from 95° to 105°, with individual divisions representing 0.2°. Because body temperature generally does not vary more than a few degrees, this smaller range is sufficient to measure the normal body temperature range of 97.6° to 99.4° F and any common variations from normal.

The **Celsius** scale has a boiling point of 100° and a freezing point of 0°. The Celsius thermometer also has

a restricted range for medical use, with each division on the scale representing 0.1°. The normal body range as measured on the Celsius scale varies from 36.5° to 37.5° C.

Because both Fahrenheit and Celsius scales are commonly used in hospitals, the nurse must understand how to read each thermometer accurately, correctly note changes from normal, and convert from one scale to another. If you need to give an antipyretic medication to help lower an elevated temperature, you must clearly understand the variations from normal in either scale.

The formulas for converting from one scale to another are very simple. Because the normal range of temperatures varies so little in individuals, even a little experience in converting temperatures will aid you in rapidly understanding this process.

The formula for converting Fahrenheit to Celsius is as follows:

$$(^\circ F - 32) \times \frac{5}{9} = {^\circ}C$$

For example:

102° F is ?° C?
$$(102 - 32) \times \frac{5}{9} = 70 \times \frac{5}{9} = 38.9^\circ C$$

The formula for converting Celsius to Fahrenheit is as follows:

$$\left(^\circ C \times \frac{9}{5}\right) + 32 = {^\circ}F$$

For example:

40° C is ?° F?
$$\left(40 \times \frac{9}{5}\right) + 32 = 72 + 32 = 104^\circ F$$

For individuals who find nonfraction methods for changing temperature easier, they must master two other formulas:

Changing Celsius to Fahrenheit: multiply temperature by 1.8, then add 32

Changing Fahrenheit to Celsius: subtract 32 from the temperature, then divide by 1.8

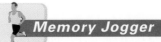

Memory Jogger

Converting Temperatures

The key relationships to understand in converting temperatures are as follows:

- One degree on the Fahrenheit scale equals 9/5 of one degree on the Celsius scale.
- One degree on the Celsius scale equals 5/9 of one degree on the Fahrenheit scale.

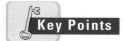

Key Points

- Many physicians' orders use a variety of the basic scales for weights and measures in the apothecaries', metric, and household systems.
- It is important to master the common equivalents in the three systems and the procedures for converting from one system to another.
- You must be able to use these different measurement systems accurately and appropriately. It is important for you to be able to complete these calculations with confidence.

Go to the free CD-ROM for an Audio Glossary, animations, video clips, and Review Questions for the NCLEX-PN® Examination.

evolve   Be sure to visit the companion Evolve website at http://evolve.elsevier.com/Edmunds/LPN/ for WebLinks, a link to the top 200 drugs by prescription, and sign-up pages for newsletter drug updates.

CRITICAL THINKING ?

1. Convert the following using the metric and apothecaries' systems where applicable:
   a. 0.065 gm = _____ gr
   b. m vi = _____ cc = _____ mL
   c. 4 gm = _____ mg
   d. 35 mg = _____ gm
   e. gr 3/4 = _____ mg = _____ gm
   f. 45 cc = _____ mL

2. Convert the following using the appropriate systems:
   a. 50 cc = ? dr = ? oz
   b. 160 cc = ? oz = ? dr = ? pt
   c. 7 cc = ? dr = ? tsp
   d. 1/150 gr = ? mg
   e. 7 kg = ? lb
   f. 8 L = ? liquid quarts
   g. 80 gm = ? oz
   h. 9 liquid quarts = ? L
   i. 36° C = ?° F
   j. 137 lb = ? kg

3. Your patient's drug order reads, "3600 mL PO q24h." How many glassfuls would the patient have to drink?

4. If a solution contains gr 1/40 of drug/mL, how many minims would you give for gr 1/160?

5. If 150 mL of solution contains 75 gm of alcohol, how many grams of alcohol are there in 25 mL of solution?

6. It takes 7 gm of a substance to make 35 mL of solution. How many milliliters of solution can be made with 42 gm of the substance?

7. A certain medication comes in an 18-fl-oz bottle with four bottles to a package. The same medication is also sold in a package containing two 1-liter bottles. Which contains more medicine, the four-pack or the two 1-liter bottles?

Calculating Drug Dosages

Objectives

After reading and studying this chapter, you should be able to do the following:

1. Use formulas to determine the dosages of tablets, capsules, or liquids.
2. Use formulas to determine the total number of tablets or capsules or the amount of liquid to be ordered for a specified time.
3. Use information about the apothecaries', metric, and household measurement systems to accurately calculate drug dosages.
4. Calculate dosages for parenteral injections, including those for special preparations such as insulin.
5. Calculate flow rates for infusions.
6. List three different rules used to calculate medication dosages for children.

Key Terms

Be sure to check out the bonus material on the free CD-ROM, including selected audio pronunciations.

body surface area (BSA) (p. 90)
Clark's rule (p. 89)
dimensional analysis (dĭ-MĔN-shŭn-ăl ă-NĂL-ĭ-sĭs, p. 90)
drop factor (p. 88)
flow rate (p. 88)
Fried's rule (frēdz, p. 90)
nomogram (NŌM-ō-grăm, p. 90)
Young's rule (p. 90)

OVERVIEW

How medications are ordered differs among physicians, drugs, and health care agencies. Some agencies require physicians to order generic products or only those drugs stocked by the pharmacy. Some drugs are traditionally ordered in units of a specific measurement system. (For example, atropine usually comes in metric units, such as 0.6 mg, whereas other drugs come in apothecary units, such as morphine sulfate, which comes as ¼ grain [gr].) Physicians' patterns in ordering drugs develop from their experiences in medical school and in the health care agencies where they have worked. Some physi-

cians are highly influenced by pharmaceutical salespeople. Thus there are many reasons why medication orders appear in a variety of forms, and the nurse must be prepared to understand them all.

CALCULATION METHODS

Calculating dosages involves the following three steps:
1. Determine whether the drug dosage desired (what is written in the physician's order) is in the same measurement system as the drug dosage available. If they are not in the same measurement system, convert between the two systems.
2. Simplify by reducing to the lowest terms whenever possible.
3. Calculate the dosage quantity to be administered. This may be done by using fractions, ratios, or proportions.

FRACTION METHOD

When using fractions to compute drug dosages, write an equation consisting of two fractions. First, set up a fraction showing the number of units to be given over x, the unknown number of tablets or milliliters. For example, if the physician's order states, "ibuprofen 600 mg," you would write $\frac{600 \text{ mg}}{x \text{ tablets}}$. On the other side of the equation, write a fraction showing the drug dosage as listed on the medication bottle over the number of tablets or milliliters. The ibuprofen bottle label states, "200 mg per tablet," so the second fraction would be $\frac{200 \text{ mg}}{1 \text{ tablet}}$. The equation then reads:

$$\frac{600 \text{ mg}}{x \text{ tablets}} = \frac{200 \text{ mg}}{1 \text{ tablet}}$$

Note that the same units of measure are in both numerators and the same units of measure are in both denominators. Now solve for x:

$$\frac{600 \text{ mg}}{x \text{ tablets}} = \frac{200 \text{ mg}}{1 \text{ tablet}}$$
$$\frac{600}{x} = \frac{200}{1}$$
$$200x = 600$$
$$x = 3 \text{ tablets}$$

RATIO OR PROPORTION METHOD

In using the ratio method, first write the amount of the drug to be given and the quantity of the dosage *(x)* as a ratio. Using the previous example, this would be 600 mg:*x* tablets. Next, complete the equation by forming a second ratio consisting of the number of units of the drug in the dosage form and the quantity of that dosage form, as taken from the bottle. Again, using the previous example, the second ratio would be 200 mg:1 tablet. Expressed as a proportion, this would be:

$$600 \text{ mg} : x \text{ tablets} :: 200 \text{ mg} : 1 \text{ tablet}$$

Solving for *x* determines the dosage:

$$600 \times 1 = 200 \times x$$
$$600 = 200x$$
$$x = \frac{600}{200}$$
$$x = 3$$

This method, again, gives a dosage of 3 tablets.

"DESIRED OVER AVAILABLE" METHOD

A third method for drug dosage calculation combines the conversion of ordered units into available units and the computation of drug dosage into one step. The general equation for doing this is:

Desired units ($\times$ Conversion factor) $\times$

$$\frac{\text{Quantity of drug form (caps, tabs, etc.)}}{\text{Quantity Available}}(\times \text{ Conversion factor}) = x \text{ (Quantity to give)}$$

If a physician orders 10 gr of a drug and the drug is available only in 300-mg tablets, the dose may be easily calculated with this formula. Substitute 10 gr **(Desired)** for the first element of the equation. Then use a conversion factor ($^{60 \text{ mg}}/_{1 \text{ gr}}$) so that the desired amount can be expressed in the same units as the dose available in the second portion of the formula. The second element of the equation shows the quantity of drug form (capsule or tablet) for the dose **Available** (1 tablet contains 300 mg). The completed equation then is:

$$10 \text{ gr} \times \left(\frac{60 \text{ mg}}{1 \text{ gr}}\right) \times \frac{1 \text{ tablet}}{300 \text{ mg}} = x \text{ tablets}$$

Once the conversion factor has been used, you can see the underlying relationship between dose **Desired** and dose **Available**:

$$\text{Dose } \mathbf{Desired} = 10 \text{ gr} \times \frac{60 \text{ mg}}{1 \text{ gr}}$$
$$= 600 \text{ mg}$$

Thus, the previous equation can be reduced to:

$$600 \text{ mg} \times \frac{1 \text{ tablet}}{300 \text{ mg}} = x, \text{ or}$$

$$\frac{(\text{Dose } \mathbf{Desired}) \ 600 \text{ mg}}{(\text{Dose } \mathbf{Available}) \ 300 \text{ mg}} \times 1 = x \text{ tablets}$$

$$\frac{600}{300} = 2 \text{ tablets}$$

By solving for *x*, you will find that the patient should receive two 300-mg tablets.

As you can see, all three methods of drug calculation (fraction, proportion, and desired over available methods) use the same information and much of the same format in solving the problems. With minor variations, they do the same thing. One or another of these methods will seem to make more sense to you or be easier to follow. Throughout the calculation sections, you should use the method for drug calculation that makes the most sense. Return here for review if you are having difficulty.

CALCULATING DOSAGES

ORAL MEDICATIONS

Although there are many forms of oral products, oral medications usually come in capsules, tablets, or liquids. Medications dispensed through the unit dose system are packaged by the pharmacist according to the dosage ordered. You usually do not have to calculate the medication dosage, but you should check the accuracy of the preparation.

When medication is ordered individually or through an open stock system, you usually will calculate the proper drug dosage. Drug calculations are required when any of the following conditions are true:

- The drug available is in a smaller dose than that ordered.
- The drug available is in a larger dose than that ordered.
- The drug available is in a different unit of measure than that ordered.

Memory Jogger

Parentheses in Math Problems

When parentheses are used in a math problem, it means to do all the calculations inside the parentheses first, then complete the rest of the problem.

Capsules and Tablets

Capsules cannot be broken or divided. This makes calculating the drug dosage more difficult. Additional capsules may be given to provide an accurate dosage; a part of one capsule cannot. Manufacturers of drugs provide capsules in different dosages to help in arriving at

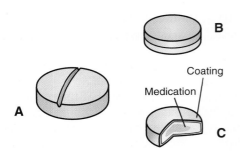

FIGURE **9-1** **A,** Scored tablet. **B** and **C,** Unscored tablets. The tablet in **B** is layered, and the tablet in **C** is coated.

the proper dosage. If the calculations specify that a fraction of a capsule should be given, give an additional capsule if the fraction is ½ or more; do not give an additional capsule if the fraction is less than ½. (For example, if the calculations work out to 2¾, give three capsules; if it is 2¼, give two.)

Some tablets may be easily divided if they are "scored" (Figure 9-1, *A*). Examples of unscored tablets are layered tablets (see Figure 9-1, *B*) and coated tablets (see Figure 9-1, *C*). If a tablet is not scored, it should *not* be broken or cut apart. Sometimes tablets may be cut to fill a smaller drug dosage order, or they may be combined to fill a larger drug dosage order.

The medication order usually states the dose of grams, grains, or milligrams to give. Therefore, you know the dose that is **Desired.** The order also specifies how often the medication is to be given, such as twice a day (bid) or four times a day (qid). It may or may not specify for how many days the medication is to be given. If the order does not indicate a specific length of time (for example, give for 5 days), the drug is given on a continuous basis, unless the institution has a specific policy limiting the length of time a drug may be given without reordering. (Antibiotics and narcotics usually have an automatic stop date after a certain period of time.) Therefore, you may also need to calculate how much medication to order, depending on the length of time the patient will receive the medication. You need to know how much medication is **needed.**

Memory Jogger

Dosage Formula Hint

To help you remember the usual formula, remember **Desired** over **Available,** D/A, or "DA." A District Attorney (DA) often helps solve a mystery. You are helping to solve the mystery of the dosage needed.

For example, the order reads: "diazepam (Valium) 10 mg PO stat and 2 mg bid × 10 days." The medication

Desired is diazepam 10 mg and diazepam 2 mg. You need to know the dosage **Available** for the medication. A check with the pharmacy reveals that diazepam comes in 2-, 5-, and 10-mg tablets.

You **need** one 10-mg diazepam tablet and enough 2-mg tablets for 10 days, or enough 2-mg tablets to fill the whole order. Thus you need to order:

One 10-mg tablet + One 2-mg tablet ×
2 times/day × 10 days = 1 × 2 × 10 =
Twenty 2-mg tablets + one 10-mg tablet

or, because five 2-mg tablets are the same as one 10-mg tablet, you may order:

Five 2-mg tablets + one 2-mg tablet ×
2 times/day × 10 days =
5 + (1 × 2 × 10) = 25 tablets

The formula to calculate the number of capsules or tablets to order is a basic ratio or proportion problem (review proportions in Chapter 7):

Dose **Desired** : Dose **Available** :: Tablets or capsules per dose : Drug form (tablets or capsules)

Written as an equation, this becomes:

Dose **Desired** × Drug form (tablets or capsules) =
Dose **Available** × Tablets or capsules per dose

In simple terms, this means:

$$\frac{\text{Dose }\textbf{Desired}}{\text{Dose }\textbf{Available}} \times \frac{\text{Drug form}}{\text{(tablets or capsules)}} = x \text{ (number of tablets or capsules per dose)}$$

For example, the order reads: "sulfadiazine 1.0 gm q6h × 3 days." Sulfadiazine comes in 300- or 500-mg tablets. Using the simplified equation and converting from milligrams to grams:

$$\frac{\text{(Dose Desired) 1.0 gm}}{\text{(Dose Available) 500 mg (= 0.5 gm)}} \times 1 \text{ tablet} = x \text{ (number of tablets per dose)}$$

$$\frac{1.0 \text{ gm}}{0.5 \text{ gm}} = 2 \text{ tablets}$$

Therefore, give two 500-mg tablets every 6 hours for 3 days. Two tablets given four times a day for 3 days equals 24 tablets total.

Memory Jogger

Steps to Complete Dosage Formula

1. First change dosages to the same unit of measurement.
2. Reduce to the simplest terms.
3. Calculate the dosage, using fractions, ratios, or proportions.
4. Use common sense to check the answer.

To illustrate, here are a few examples:

The order reads, "ASA gr x stat and prn for temperature elevation." Acetylsalicylic acid (ASA) is labeled as 0.3 gm/tablet.

$$\frac{\text{Dose \textbf{Desired}}}{\text{Dose \textbf{Available}}} = \frac{\text{gr x}}{0.3 \text{ gm}} \times 1 = x \text{ tablets}$$

$$\left(\text{Conversion factor: 16 gr = 1 gm, so } \frac{\text{gr x}}{16} = 0.6 \text{ gm} \right)$$

$$\frac{\textbf{D}}{\textbf{A}} = \frac{0.6 \text{ gm}}{0.3 \text{ gm}} \times 1 = 2 \text{ tablets}$$

The order reads: "Methocarbamol 1.5 gm daily." The medication comes in 750-mg tablets.

$$\frac{\text{Dose \textbf{Desired}}}{\text{Dose \textbf{Available}}} = \frac{1.5 \text{ gm}}{750 \text{ mg}} \times 1 = x \text{ tablets}$$

$$(\text{Conversion factor: 1.5 gm = 1500 mg})$$

$$\frac{\textbf{D}}{\textbf{A}} = \frac{1500 \text{ mg}}{750 \text{ mg}} \times 1 = 2 \text{ tablets}$$

Liquids

The process and formulas used to calculate dosages of liquids are the same as those used to compute dosages of capsules or tablets. Only the unit of measure is different. To review:

$$\frac{\text{Dose Desired}}{\text{Dose Available}} \times \frac{\text{Drug form}}{(\text{minims, milliliters, drams})} = x \text{ (amount of liquid per dose)}$$

For example, the order reads: "phenobarbital elixir 0.2 gm at bedtime." The drug is available in 20 mg/5 mL. Again, the formula is a basic proportion problem:

$$0.2 \text{ gm } (= 200 \text{ mg}) : x \text{ mL} :: 20 \text{ mg} : 5 \text{ mL}$$

Written as an equation, this is:

$$200 \text{ mg} \times 5 \text{ mL} = 20 \text{ mg} \times x \text{ mL}$$

Thus:

$$\frac{\text{(Dose \textbf{Desired}) 200 mg}}{\text{(Dose \textbf{Available}) 20 mg}} \times 5 \text{ mL} = x$$

$$\frac{200 \text{ mg}}{20 \text{ mg}} \times 5 \text{ mL} = 50 \text{ mL/dose}$$

Memory Jogger

Dosage Solution Formula

$$\frac{\text{Dose Desired}}{\text{Dose Available}} \times \frac{\text{Drug form}}{(\text{Dilution or amount of solution})} = \text{Amount of solution per dose}$$

PARENTERAL MEDICATIONS

When medication is to be injected, it comes in three different forms:

1. A prefilled syringe labeled with a certain dosage in a certain volume (for example, meperidine [Demerol] 100 mg in 1 mL).
2. A single- or multiple-dose ampule labeled with a certain dosage in a certain volume (for example, epinephrine [Adrenalin] 1:1000 in 0.1 mL).
3. A vial with a powder or crystals that must be mixed or reconstituted with sterile water or normal saline (NS) solution. The drug may be measured in grains, grams, milligrams, or units. The amount of solution to be added varies and must be calculated according to the instructions provided with the vial. Medications given intradermally or subcutaneously generally involve very small amounts of solution, whereas intravenous (IV) preparations may involve 50 mL of solution or more.

Again, proportion is the standard method for calculating this dosage:

$$\text{Dose \textbf{Available}} : \text{Dilution} :: \text{Dose \textbf{Desired}} : x$$

Written as an equation, this becomes:

$$\text{Dose Available} \times x = \text{Dose Desired} \times \text{Dilution}$$

or

$$\frac{\text{Dose \textbf{Desired}}}{\text{Dose \textbf{Available}}} \times \text{Dilution} = x$$

To illustrate, here are a few examples:

The order reads: "digoxin 0.2 mg IM." The drug is available as 0.5 mg/mL.

$$\frac{\text{(Dose \textbf{Desired}) 0.2 mg}}{\text{(Dose \textbf{Available}) 0.5 mg}} \times 1 \text{ mL} = x$$

$$\frac{2}{5} \times 1 \text{ mL} = 0.4 \text{ mL, or 6 minims}$$

Clinical Landmine

Accurate Calculations

Again! Do not forget your common sense! If the answer tells you to inject 20 mL, you know you have made a mistake!

The order reads: "Quinidine gluconate 200 mg IM q6h." The medication comes in a multiple-dose vial with 80 mg/mL.

$$\frac{\textbf{D}}{\textbf{A}} = \frac{200 \text{ mg}}{80 \text{ mg}} \times 1 \text{ mL} = 2.5 \text{ mL}$$

The order reads: "Demerol 35 mg IM daily." The drug is available in 50-mg/mL ampules.

$$\frac{D}{A} = \frac{35 \text{ mg}}{50 \text{ mg}} \times 1 \text{ mL} = 0.7 \text{ mL}$$

Many chemicals are very fragile. Heat, light, and time cause the medication to change or deteriorate. To avoid these problems, some medications are manufactured as powders or crystals, making them more stable. When the medication is ordered, liquid must be added to the drug to dissolve the medication in the solution (reconstitute the drug). The medication must then be given within a few hours or it will decay.

Some chemicals come in a single-dose vial. When the medication is ordered, usually 1 to 2 mL of liquid is added, the solution is gently shaken to dissolve it, and the whole amount is drawn into a syringe and injected. This is very common for some antibiotics.

At other times, an ampule will contain several doses of the powdered medication. The instructions for adding the liquid (diluent) must be followed carefully. Some multiple-dose vials for steroids contain the diluent in the top part of the bottle, separated from the powder in the bottom part of the container. Pushing on the top part forces the liquid down into the bottom part, dissolving the medication. The instructions are usually found on the package, on the vial label, or on the package insert in the box, and they must be followed exactly. Once powders have been dissolved in liquid or reconstituted, the bottle must be carefully labeled so that further doses may be accurately given from it. It is especially important to note the date and time the powder was dissolved, as well as the concentration of the reconstituted medication.

If instructions are not given for diluting the medication, it is common to dissolve the drug in enough diluent so that the dose ordered may be given in no more than 0.5 to 1 mL. A modification of the familiar proportion formula may be used to calculate the correct amount of diluent:

Dose **Desired** : 1 mL :: Total drug **Available** : x mL

In this formula, the relationship of the dose desired to the known amount of liquid is compared with the relationship of the total amount of the drug to an unknown amount of liquid. Expressed as an equation, this becomes:

Dose **Desired** $\times x$ = Total drug **Available** $\times$ 1 mL
Drug **Available**/Dose **Desired** $\times$ 1 mL = x

Note that, in this formula, the dose **Available** is on the top of the formula; the dose **Desired** is on the bottom. Think clearly when establishing the problems. Keep the logic of the proportions clear. **Desired** does not always go over **Available**!

To illustrate, here are a few examples:

The order reads: "cephalothin (Keflin) 500 mg q6h IM." The drug comes in a multiple-dose vial containing 3 gm of powder. Prepare it so that 500 mg equals 1 mL. First, convert 3 gm to 3000 mg. Then apply the proportion formula:

$$500 \text{ mg} : 1 \text{ mL} :: 3000 \text{ mg} : x$$
$$500 \text{ mg} \times x = 3000 \text{ mg} \times 1 \text{ mL}$$
$$\frac{3000 \text{ mg}}{500 \text{ mg}} = 6 \text{ mL}$$

Therefore, 6 mL of diluent must be added to obtain a concentration of 1 mL = 500 mg/mL. Expressed more simply:

$$\frac{\text{(Drug } \textbf{Available}) \ 3000 \text{ mg}}{\text{(Dose } \textbf{Desired}) \ 500 \text{ mg}} \times 1 \text{ mL} = 6 \text{ mL to be added}$$

The order reads: "Give 500,000 units penicillin IM." Dilute 1,000,000 units of penicillin so that 500,000 units equals 1 mL. Thus:

$$500,000 \text{ units} : 1 \text{ mL} :: 1,000,000 \text{ units} : x$$
$$\frac{1,000,000}{500,000} = 2 \text{ mL diluent}$$

or

$$\frac{A}{D} = \frac{1,000,000 \text{ units}}{500,000 \text{ units}} \times 1 \text{ mL} = 2 \text{ mL diluent to be added}$$

The order reads: "Give cephalosporin 200 mg in 1 mL IM." The drug is manufactured in 1-gm units of powder. What is the amount of diluent to add?

$$\frac{\text{(Drug } \textbf{Available}) \ 1 \text{ gm } (\ = 1000 \text{ mg})}{\text{(Dose } \textbf{Desired}) \ 200 \text{ mg}} =$$
$$\frac{1000 \text{ mg}}{200 \text{ mg}} \times 1 \text{ mL} = 5 \text{ mL diluent}$$

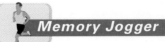

Memory Jogger

Dosage Formula

$$\frac{\text{Total drug available}}{\text{Dose desired}} \times 1 \text{ mL} =$$

Amount of diluent that must be added to vial powder so that dose order equals 1 mL

Hypodermic Tablets

Some narcotics come as sterile tablets. A tablet is put into a syringe, 1 to 2 mL of diluent is drawn into the syringe, and the medication is dissolved by gently turning the syringe. Rather than breaking the tablet, the proper amount is calculated and any extra solution is discarded before the medication is injected. The usual dilution is 1 mL. The standard formula is used:

Dose **Available** : 1 mL :: Dose **Desired** : x mL

For example, the order reads: "Give morphine gr ⅙." The available tablets are gr ¼.

$$\frac{\text{Dose \textbf{Desired}}}{\text{Dose \textbf{Available}}} = \frac{\text{gr } \frac{1}{6}}{\text{gr } \frac{1}{4}} \times 1 \text{ mL}$$

$$= \frac{1}{6} \times \frac{4}{1} \times 1 \text{ mL} = \frac{2}{3} \text{ mL or 11 minims}$$

Insulin

Insulin is a parenteral medication that replaces insulin not being produced by the patient. Great accuracy is important in preparing and administering insulin because the quantity given is very small and even minor variations in dosage may produce adverse symptoms in the patient.

Calculating and preparing insulin dosages is unique in the following three ways:

1. There are many kinds of insulin, but they all come in a standardized measure called a *unit*. Insulin is available in 10-mL vials and in two strengths (concentrations): U-100 (100 units per 1 mL of solution) (Figure 9-2) and U-500 (500 units per 1 mL of solution). U-500 is five times stronger (more concentrated) than U-100. This preparation is rarely used.

2. Insulin should be drawn up in a special insulin syringe that is calibrated in units (Figure 9-3). If an insulin syringe is not available, a tuberculin (TB) syringe that is calibrated in minims may be used (Figure 9-4).

3. The insulin order, the insulin bottle, and the insulin as drawn up should always be rechecked by another nurse for maximum accuracy. Small errors can cause big problems.

When the insulin order and the syringe are both U-100, all you have to do is draw up the number of units ordered. For example, the order reads: "48 units Lente insulin [insulin zinc suspension] U-100 1 hour before breakfast." Using a U-100 syringe, you would draw up 48 units of regular insulin.

When the order calls for two different types of insulin, both may be given at the same time in the same syringe. One will be short-acting (regular) insulin, and the other will be an intermediate or longer acting type

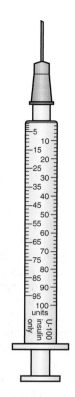

FIGURE **9-3** U-100 syringe.

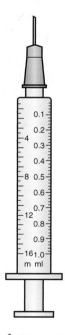

FIGURE **9-4** Tuberculin syringe.

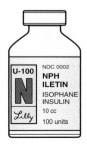

FIGURE **9-2** U-100 vial.

(neutral protamine Hagedorn [NPH] or zinc suspension). Draw up the regular insulin first, then the longer acting type. Give both in the same syringe. For example, the order reads: "20 units regular (Iletin) insulin U-100 and 30 units NPH [isophane insulin suspension] U-100 before breakfast." Using a U-100 syringe, draw up 20 units of regular insulin; then draw up 30 units of NPH insulin to equal 50 units in the syringe.

Sometimes U-100 syringes are not available and a TB syringe must be used. The number of minims that will equal the units ordered must be calculated. The formula for determining insulin dosage when a TB syringe is used is as follows:

$$\frac{\text{Insulin \textbf{Desired}}}{\text{Insulin \textbf{Available}}} \times 16 \text{ minims} =$$

Number of minims to administer

For example, the order reads: "80 units of regular (Iletin) U-100 insulin." When this insulin is to be given in a TB syringe, the dosage calculation is:

$$\frac{\text{Dose \textbf{Desired}}}{\text{Dose \textbf{Available}}} = \frac{80 \text{ units}}{100 \text{ units}} \times 16 = \frac{64}{5} = 12.8 \text{ minims}$$

Clinical Landmine

Accurate TB Syringe Calculations

NOTE: You *must* use 16—not 15—minims/mL for these very accurate calculations.

Intravenous Infusions

Flow Rates. Regulating the IV infusion rate is a common nursing task. Some institutions have automatic infusion pumps that make flow rate calculations easy. Each nurse will learn to use the equipment available. However, all nurses must learn to calculate infusion rates without relying on equipment in case of power or equipment failures, or when working in agencies where no automatic pumps are available. The completeness of physicians' orders for IV infusions varies widely. Some physicians are more specific in their instructions than others. A complete order specifies not only the type of solution and the volume to be infused (usually 500 or 1000 mL) but also the length of time that the medication should be given. More commonly, the nurse is left to calculate the flow rate, or how fast the medication will be infused.

There are three mathematical procedures that the nurse must be familiar with regarding IV infusions:
1. Calculating the flow rates for IV fluid administration
2. Making modifications in flow rates for infants
3. Calculating total administration time for IV fluid

To *calculate the flow rate for IV fluid administration,* two concepts must be understood: the flow rate and the drop factor. The rate at which IV fluids are given is the **flow rate,** and this is measured in drops per minute. The **drop factor** is the number of drops per milliliter of liquid and is determined by the size of the drops. The drop factor is different for different manufacturers of IV infusion equipment, and it must be checked by reading it on the infusion set itself. Regular infusion sets generally range between 10 and 15 drops/mL. Infusion sets have different drop factors for use with blood infusion sets (usually 10 to 12 drops/mL) because the drops are larger, whereas pediatric setups use very small drops called *microdrops* (often with 50 or 60 microdrops/mL).

Once the nurse has learned the drop factor for the equipment being used, the flow rate may be calculated by using the following formula:

Drop factor × Milliliters/minute =

Flow rate (drops/minute)

To illustrate, here are a few examples:
The order reads: "IV infusion to run at a slow rate to keep vein open." The rate to keep a vein open is 2 mL/min. The IV infusion set delivers 10 drops/mL. The goal is to determine the flow rate in drops/minute:

10 drops/mL (drop factor) × 2 mL/min = 20 drops/min

The order reads: "1000 mL NS to be administered in 5 hours." The drop factor is 15. To calculate the flow rate, use:

$$\frac{\text{Total of fluid to give}}{\text{Total time (minutes)}} \times \text{Drop factor (drops/milliliter)} =$$

Flow rate (drops/minute)

$$\frac{1000 \text{ mL}}{300 \text{ min}} \times 15 \text{ drops/mL} = \frac{15,000 \text{ drops}}{300 \text{ min}} = 50 \text{ drops/min}$$

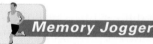

Memory Jogger

IV Fluid Administration

- The flow rate for infusions can be calculated.
- The drop factor for infusions depends on the type of equipment and must be read from the setup label.

Flow Rates for Infants and Children. Infants and small children are very sensitive to extra amounts or volumes of fluids. Smaller total amounts of IV fluids are often ordered, and the infusions are given in very small drops to avoid quickly overloading the infant's circulation. This is a built-in safety mechanism to try to prevent fluid overloading resulting from accidental delivery of too much fluid.

The drop factor must be determined from the infusion setup. Usually 60 microdrops/mL is the drop factor for infants. For calculating the flow rates in infants, the same formula is used, but the microdrop drop factor must be substituted into the formula for the adult drop factor:

$$\frac{\text{Total of fluid to give}}{\text{Total time (minutes)}} \times \frac{\text{Drop factor}}{\text{(microdrops/milliliter)}} =$$

$$\text{Flow rate (drops/minute)}$$

For example, the order reads: "Give 50 mL D_5W [5% dextrose in water] IV in 4 hours." The drop factor is 60 microdrops/mL. Thus:

$$\frac{50 \text{ mL}}{240 \text{ min}} \times 60 \text{ microdrops/mL} = \frac{300}{24} =$$

$$12.5 \text{ microdrops/min}$$

Total Infusion Time. Sometimes physicians' orders tell how fast they want infusions to run. To plan nursing care of the patient and to anticipate when new IV bottles may be needed, you need to calculate the total time the infusion will run.

Calculating the total administration time for IV fluid depends on calculating the total number of drops to be infused. Using this information, plus the drop factor, the total infusion time can be easily determined by using the following formula:

$$\frac{\text{Total drops to be infused}}{\text{Flow rate (drops/minute)}} \times 60 \text{ (drops/hour)} =$$

$$\text{Total infusion time (hours and minutes)}$$

To calculate the total infusion time:
1. *Determine the total number of drops ordered.* The total number of drops to be infused comes from the physician's order for the amount of fluid. This amount is multiplied by the drop factor (read from the infusion setup) to determine the total number of drops.
2. *Determine the number of minutes that the IV is to flow.* The number of drops per minute (50) is multiplied by 60 to give the number of drops infused in 1 hour (3000). This figure is then divided into the total number of drops. This will give the number of hours and minutes for the total infusion.

For example, the order reads: "1000 mL D_5W to be given at 50 drops/min with a drop factor of 10 drops/mL." Thus:

$$1000 \text{ mL} \times 10 \text{ drops/mL} = 10,000 \text{ drops}$$
$$\frac{10,000 \text{ drops}}{3000 \text{ drops/hr}} = 3.33 \text{ hr or 3 hr, 20 min}$$

Other Factors Influencing Flow Rates. There are many other factors that influence the flow rate of an infusion. The nurse has no control over many of them, such as the age, size, and condition of the patient; the size of the vein; the type of fluid; and the need for the fluid. Other factors such as the size of the needle, the needle's position in the vein, the height of the IV pole, the condition of the filter, the air in the air vent, and movement of the patient, may be changed or altered to assist in infusion of IV fluids. If the fluid does not infuse at the calculated rate, the IV setup should be carefully checked from the IV bottle to the site of the needle's insertion.

CALCULATING DOSAGES FOR INFANTS AND CHILDREN

Drug dosages are calculated to give the highest possible blood and tissue concentration of a medication without causing overdosage or adverse effects. Because infants are very sensitive to medications, and because infants and children are so much smaller than adults, almost all dosages given to infants and children are smaller than those given to adults. Most pharmaceutical companies list the recommended dosages for a child or infant for their drugs. If this information is not listed in the instructional material provided with the medication, the nurse should question whether the medication may safely be given to a child.

Although children's dosages were frequently calculated in the past, there remain only a few medications that require the nurse to calculate how much to give a child. Over the years, several general rules have developed to calculate these special reduced dosages for infants and children.

One of the most popular methods for determining the dosage for children is based on the child's body weight and is known as **Clark's rule.** Again, ratios and proportions may be used to calculate the pediatric value. If we assume that an average normal adult weighs 150 lb and we know the adult dosage, then if we know the child's weight, we can calculate the child's dosage:

Adult weight : Adult dosage :: Child's weight : x (Child's dosage)

For example, if the adult dose of Demerol is 100 mg, what is the dose for a 50-lb child?

$$\frac{\text{Weight of child}}{\text{Weight of adult}} \times \text{Adult dose} = \text{Child's dose}$$

so

$$\frac{50 \text{ lb}}{150 \text{ lb}} \times 100 \text{ mg} = \frac{100}{3} = 33 \text{ mg}$$

Other formulas substitute kilograms for pounds in calculating the weights. The formula remains the same. Clark's rule is by far the most popular method of assessing children's dosages. If no other formula is specified, you should use Clark's rule to determine a child's dosage.

Two other popular methods for calculating pediatric dosages involve the child's age. **Young's rule** is used for children ages 2 to 12; **Fried's rule** is used for infants and children younger than age 2. Obviously, all children of the same age are not the same size. When the pediatric patient is approximately the "normal" size for her age, these rules may be used. If the child is unusually large or small for her age, it is better to use a weight calculation.

Young's rule for children from 2 to 12 years of age states:

$$\frac{\text{Child's age}}{\text{Child's age} + 12} \times \text{Adult dose} = \text{Child's dose}$$

Fried's rule for children younger than 2 years states:

$$\frac{\text{Infant's age in months}}{150} \times \text{Adult dose} = \text{Infant's dose}$$

For example, using Young's rule, if the adult dose of aminophylline is 0.5 gm, what is the dose for a child who is 8 years old?

$$\frac{8\text{ yr}}{8\text{ yr} + 12\text{ yr}} \times 0.5\text{ gm} = \frac{8}{20} \times 0.5 = \frac{4}{20} = 0.20\text{ gm}$$

Using Fried's rule, if the adult dose of Staphcillin is 1 gm (1000 mg), what is the dose for a child who is 3 months old?

$$\frac{3\text{ months} \times 1000\text{ mg}}{150} = \frac{3000\text{ mg}}{150} = 20\text{ mg}$$

Medications that require very careful dosage use the **body surface area (BSA),** or total tissue area, of the child, which is the most accurate method for determining pediatric dosages. The reason for using the BSA is that children have a greater surface area than adults in relation to their weight. For drugs that require careful dosage, charts known as nomograms are used to calculate the BSA in square meters. A **nomogram** is a chart that displays the relationships between two different types of data so that complex calculations are not necessary. BSA charts are constructed from height and weight data. The surface area-to-weight ratio varies inversely (opposite) to length. Thus infants would have proportionally more surface area because they weigh less and are shorter than children. These charts may be used only if the child has normal height for weight. Even with the use of standardized charts, the calculated dosages are more accurate for children than for very young infants.

An example of a nomogram used to calculate BSA is shown in Figure 9-5. A straight edge is placed from the patient's height in the left column to his weight in the right column, and the intersection on the BSA column indicates the patient's BSA. The total BSA value is determined and is put into the following formula:

Surface area of the child (m^2) × Usual adult dose ÷
Surface area of an adult (1.73 m^2) = Child dose

Use the nomogram to solve these two sample problems, using the BSA to calculate pediatric dosages (use 1.73 m^2 as the accepted adult BSA):

1. If the adult dose of kanamycin is 0.5 gm, what is the pediatric dose for a 10-month-old child who weighs 22 lb and is 29 inches long?
2. If the adult dose of sulfisoxazole is 500 mg, what is the pediatric dose for an 8-year-old child who weighs 48 lb and is 47 inches tall?

DIMENSIONAL ANALYSIS CALCULATIONS

Anything that a nurse can do to eliminate medication errors is important. Some find that using dimensional analysis reduces frustration and confusion in dosage calculation. **Dimensional analysis** provides a single method to use for all kinds of drug problems, even those with two or three steps. This method provides a visual guide used by the nurse to construct a problem in an orderly, stepwise fashion. The numbers in the dosage calculation problem are placed on a grid along with their labels. The labels are then cross-canceled in order to assure that only one label is left—the one that is needed for the final answer. After cross-cancellation, numbers are multiplied across the top and bottom of the grid, which yields a fraction. This fraction is divided and the final label is applied for the answer. This method reduces the chance of incorrect placement or inversion of drug calculation factors and is especially suited for complex problems or those that call for unit conversions. An understanding of ratio and proportion provides a solid foundation for the use of dimensional analysis in dosage calculations. Following are the steps to construct a dimensional analysis problem. For example:

The physician orders vitamin C, 1500 mg PO to be given after breakfast. Tablets on hand are 500 mg per 1 tablet (tab).

1. **Identify the final answer label.** Look at the problem and ask, "What is the term that I will use to label the final answer to this dosage calculation? Is it milliliters, tablets, or liters?"

State, "The final answer to this dosage calculation will be labeled as 'tablets' (tabs)."

Ask, "How many tablets will need to be administered to this patient?"

Write this question as:

? tab =

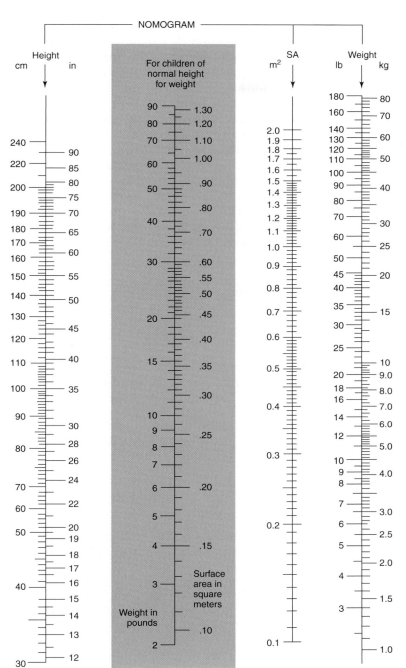

─── NOMOGRAM ───

FIGURE **9-5** Nomogram for body surface area of a child. *SA*, surface area.

2. **Draw a grid to the right of the label.**

$$? \text{ tab} = \underline{} \Big| \underline{} =$$

In this format, the horizontal bar means "divide" and the vertical bar means "multiply."

3. **Find a given factor in the dosage calculation problem that is labeled with the same name as the final answer label.**

The physician orders vitamin C (ascorbic acid) 1500 mg PO to be given after breakfast. Tablets on hand are 500 mg per 1 tablet (tab).

Insert that unit label directly to the right, and in the top or numerator position on the grid.

$$? \text{ tab} = \frac{1 \text{ tab}}{} \Big| \underline{} =$$

4. **Write the numbers in the problem in the correct form that shows a relationship or ratio.** In this case, it is given that 1 tablet contains 500 mg of vitamin C; in other words, 500 mg per 1 tab is available. So, with the label of 1 tab above the grid line, the corresponding term of "500 mg" is written below the line. This indicates the relationship or ratio of 1 tab to 500 mg.

$$? \text{ tab} = \frac{1 \text{ tab}}{500 \text{ mg}} \bigg| \quad =$$

5. **Check for the given number with the same label that appears in the first, lower space or denominator position on the grid. Place the number that belongs with this label in the next upper (numerator) space of the grid.**
   *The physician orders vitamin C (ascorbic acid) **1500 mg** PO to be given after breakfast. Tablets on hand are 500 mg per 1 tablet (tab).*
   In this problem, the given factor 1500 mg will be placed in the next grid space.

$$? \text{ tab} = \frac{1 \text{ tab}}{500 \text{ mg}} \bigg| \frac{1500 \text{ mg}}{} \quad =$$

6. **Cancel labels.** After all factors in the problem have been accounted for, proceed to *cancel out* the unit labels by making a single diagonal line through cross-matching labels as illustrated. This is called "cross-cancellation." If the dosage calculation problem has been properly set up, only the final answer label "tab" will remain uncanceled.

$$? \text{ tab} = \frac{1 \text{ tab}}{500 \text{ mg}} \bigg| \frac{1500 \text{ mg}}{} \quad =$$

7. **Calculate.** All numbers above the line are multiplied horizontally, left to right. All numbers below the line are multiplied horizontally, left to right. The final answer will appear as a fraction—which is actually a division problem. Divide the top number (numerator) by the bottom number (denominator) and then attach the final answer label left (tabs) to the answer.

$$? \text{ tab} = \frac{1 \text{ tab}}{500 \text{ mg}} \bigg| \frac{1500 \text{ mg}}{} = \frac{1500}{500} = 3 \text{ tabs}$$

It is wise to **reduce** numbers prior to the multiplication step. This helps to decrease large numbers that will be multiplied and simplifies the problem. This is helpful when problems become more complex and contain more factors. For example:

$$? \text{ tab} = \frac{1 \text{ tab}}{\underset{1}{500 \text{ mg}}} \bigg| \overset{3}{1500 \text{ mg}} = \frac{3}{1} = 3 \text{ tabs}$$

8. **Ask: "Does this answer make sense?"**
   Using dimensional analysis for dosage calculations is particularly valuable when the nurse must convert between systems of measurement. For example:
   The physician has ordered the thyroid hormone levothyroxine (Synthroid), 0.1 mg PO, for the patient. The pharmacist states that levothyroxine 50 mcg = 1 tablet is in stock.

1. **Identify the final answer label.**
   State, "The final answer to this dosage calculation will be labeled, 'tablets' (tabs)."
   Ask, "How many tablets will need to be administered to this patient?"
   Write this question in abbreviated form to the far left of the calculation paper.

$$? \text{ tab} =$$

2. **Draw a grid.**

$$? \text{ tab} = \frac{}{} \bigg| \quad =$$

3. **Find a given factor in the dosage calculation problem that is labeled with the same name as the final answer label.** Begin the process with the dosage relationships that are already known. In this example, the physician has ordered a total of **0.1 mg** of the drug and the pharmacy has **tablets** of **50 micrograms (mcg)** each.

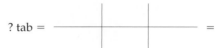

$$? \text{ tab} = \frac{1 \text{ tab}}{} \bigg| \quad =$$

4. **Write the numbers in the problem in the correct form that shows a relationship or ratio.** In this case, it is given that 1 tablet contains 50 mcg of levothyroxine; in other words, 50 mcg per 1 tab is available. So, with the label of 1 tab above the grid line, the corresponding term of "50 mcg" is written below the line. This indicates the relationship or ratio of 1 tab to 50 mcg.

$$? \text{ tab} = \frac{1 \text{ tab}}{50 \text{ mcg}} \bigg| \quad =$$

5. **Check for a given factor with the same label that appears in the first, lower space or denominator position on the grid. Place the number that belongs with this unit label in the next upper (numerator) space of the grid.** The answer to this drug calculation problem is the number of tablets that will equal the physician's ordered dose of 0.1 mg.
   There is a missing link in the problem because the drug available is labeled in micrograms (mcg) and the dosage desired is labeled in milligrams (mg). Placement of the unit labeled "mg" in the next upper

space would not allow for cancellation. A conversion from mcg to mg is necessary to fill in that missing link.

$$? \text{ tab} = \frac{1 \text{ tab}}{50 \text{ mcg}} \left| \frac{0.1 \cancel{\text{mg}}}{} \right| 0.1 \text{ mg} =$$

$$? \text{ tab} = \frac{1 \text{ tab}}{50 \text{ mcg}} \left| \frac{1000 \text{ mcg}}{1 \text{ mg}} \right| 0.1 \text{ mg} =$$

6. **Cancel labels.**

$$? \text{ tab} = \frac{1 \text{ tab}}{50 \cancel{\text{mcg}}} \left| \frac{1000 \cancel{\text{mcg}}}{1 \cancel{\text{mg}}} \right| 0.1 \cancel{\text{mg}} =$$

7. **Calculate.** Reduce numbers if needed. Do this where possible in order to reduce the large numbers that need to be multiplied and divided.

$$? \text{ tab} = \frac{1 \text{ tab}}{\underset{1}{\cancel{50}\cancel{\text{mcg}}}} \left| \frac{\overset{20}{\cancel{1000}\cancel{\text{mcg}}}}{1\cancel{\text{mg}}} \right| 0.1 \cancel{\text{mg}} = \frac{2}{1} = 2 \text{ tabs}$$

8. **Ask: "Does this answer make sense?"**

Memory Jogger

Dimensional Analysis
- Dimensional analysis does not diminish the importance of math accuracy.
- Hint: Memorize common unit equivalencies (for example, 1000 mg = 1 gm).
- Mastery of dimensional analysis requires a few weeks of focused effort.

How does dimensional analysis work if the answer needs to be labeled with more than one term, such as milliliters per hour (mL/hr) or drops per minute (gtt/min)? These are common answer labels when the nurse is calculating IV rates. For example:

A patient has sustained a life-threatening hemorrhage. The physician orders 1000 mL of lactated Ringer's IV solution to be infused at 80 gtt/min. The drop factor is 10 gtts = 1 mL. The nurse must set the IV pump to milliliters per hours. How many milliliters per hour will be infused?

1. **Identify the final answer label(s).**
   State, "The final answer to this dosage calculation will be labeled 'milliliters per hour (mL/hr)'."
   Ask, "How many mL/hr need to be administered to this patient?"

Write this question in abbreviated form to the far left of the calculation paper.

$$\frac{? \text{ mL}}{\text{hr}} =$$

2. **Draw a grid.**

$$\frac{? \text{ mL}}{\text{hr}} = \frac{}{} \left| \frac{}{} \right| =$$

3. **Find a given factor in the dosage calculation problem that is labeled with the same name as the top answer label.** It does not have to match the bottom label at this point.

$$\frac{? \text{ mL}}{\text{hr}} = \frac{1 \text{ mL}}{} \left| \frac{}{} \right| =$$

4. **Write the numbers in the problem in the correct form that shows a relationship or ratio.** First, place those factors that exist in a relationship or ratio in the grid. In this case, place the relationship **1 mL = 10 gtts** first.

$$\frac{? \text{ mL}}{\text{hr}} = \frac{1 \text{ mL}}{10 \text{ gtts}} \left| \frac{}{} \right| =$$

5. **Check for the given factor with the same unit label that appears in the first, lower space or denominator position on the grid. Place the number that belongs with this label in the next upper (numerator) space of the grid.** Place the corresponding number and label in the grid below.

$$\frac{? \text{ mL}}{\text{hr}} = \frac{1 \text{ mL}}{10 \text{ gtts}} \left| \frac{80 \text{ gtts}}{1 \text{ min}} \right| =$$

The answer needs to be in mL/hr and, if the calculation is performed at this point, the final answer will appear as mL/min. A conversion factor must be entered as follows:

$$\frac{? \text{ mL}}{\text{hr}} = \frac{1 \text{ mL}}{10 \text{ gtts}} \left| \frac{80 \text{ gtts}}{1 \text{ min}} \right| \frac{60 \text{ min}}{1 \text{ hr}} =$$

Examine the problem for the necessary numbers needed for calculation—ignore those that are not needed (extraneous) to arrive at the correct answer. There is one remaining factor in this calculation problem that has not been included in the grid. Through reasoning, you know that the 1000 mL factor is not necessary to calculate the mL/hr rate. Should there be some doubt as to whether or not to use this number in a calculation, the fact that there is no logical place for it on the dimensional analysis grid provides a tip that it is not needed in the calculation for the answer of mL/hr.

6. **Cancel labels.** In this problem, labels that remain after cancellation are mL and hr, indicating that the final answer will be labeled correctly.

$$\frac{? \text{ mL}}{\text{hr}} = \frac{1 \text{ mL}}{10 \text{ gtts}} \left| \frac{80 \text{ gtts}}{1 \text{ min}} \right| \frac{60 \text{ min}}{1 \text{ hr}} =$$

7. **Calculate.** Reduce numbers if needed.

$$\frac{? \text{ mL}}{\text{hr}} = \frac{1 \text{ mL}}{10 \text{ gtts}} \left| \frac{80 \text{ gtts}}{1 \text{ min}} \right| \frac{60 \text{ min}}{1 \text{ hr}} = \frac{480}{1} = \frac{480 \text{ mL}}{\text{hr}}$$

8. **Ask: "Does this answer make sense?"** In this case, 480 mL/hr is a large amount of fluid to infuse intravenously, and you would correctly question the answer. However, the problem indicated that replacement of a significant intravascular deficit was necessary, so the answer does make sense.

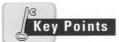

Key Points

- This chapter presented concepts and examples that illustrate common calculations that you will be required to perform in administering medications.
- Mastery of this information is important for accuracy and speed.
- The foundation of multiplication facts, fractions, decimals, ratios, and proportions, added to the principles of metric, household, and apothecaries' systems, comes together in the practical application of dosage calculations.
- This chapter should be reviewed if one has difficulty with dosage calculations or needs to review material that has not been worked with for some time.

Go to the free CD-ROM for an Audio Glossary, animations, video clips, and Review Questions for the NCLEX-PN® Examination.

evolve Be sure to visit the companion Evolve website at http://evolve.elsevier.com/Edmunds/LPN/ for WebLinks, a link to the top 200 drugs by prescription, and sign-up pages for newsletter drug updates.

DRUG CALCULATION REVIEW

1. The physician orders guaifenesin (Robitussin) syrup 1 tablespoon PO every 6 hours prn for a patient recovering from pneumonia who is being discharged from your unit. Pharmacy sends a 500-mL bottle of guaifenesin to send home with the patient. If the patient takes one dose (1 tablespoon) each night before bed, how long will a 500-mL bottle last?

2. A physician orders 30 units of isophane insulin suspension (NPH) subcutaneously. The vial contains 100 units per 1 mL. Only TB syringes are available for administration. How many milliliters of insulin must be administered?

3. A physician orders 500 mg of the antibiotic cefazolin sulfate (Ancef) IM. The vial of powder is labeled with the following instructions: "Add 2.5 mL of sterile water for injection. This will provide an approximate volume of 330 mg/mL." How many milliliters of solution should the nurse prepare?

4. A patient is to receive 2500 mL of normal saline to infuse IV over 24 hours. The drop factor is 10 gtt = 1 mL. What is the flow rate in gtt/min of this infusion?

5. A 50-kg patient has recently experienced a myocardial infarction and the physician orders a lidocaine infusion to suppress dysrhythmias. The order is:

   lidocaine 500 mg in 250 mL of D$_5$W at
   150 microdrops (mcgtt) per minute

   What will be the rate of this IV infusion in milligrams per kilogram per minute (mg/kg/min) when the nurse uses a microdrop setup of 60 mcgtt = 1 mL?

6. The physician has ordered 7500 units of heparin subcutaneously daily. The pharmacy has provided an ampule that contains 5000 units per 1 mL. How many milliliters will the nurse prepare for this injection?

7. As part of preoperative care, the physician has ordered atropine, gr $\frac{1}{300}$ IM. The multidose vial reads "1 mL = gr $\frac{1}{150}$." How many milliliters will be administered to this patient?

8. The physician orders metoprolol (Lopressor) 50 mg PO twice daily. The pharmacy has provided scored tablets of 0.1 gm each. How many tablets of

this antihypertensive medication should the nurse administer to the patient?

9. The physician has ordered digoxin (Lanoxin) elixir 0.25 mg PO. The nurse notes that the bottle is labeled 0.05 mg/mL. How many milliliters should be administered to the patient?

10. For an adult female patient, the physician has ordered erythromycin 1 gm PO at 1 PM, 2 PM, and 11 PM on the day before intestinal surgery. The nurse prepares to administer the first of the three doses and finds erythromycin 400-mg scored tablets available. How many tablets should be prepared for each dose of this intestinal antisepsis therapy?

CRITICAL THINKING ?

1. The drug order is for 0.6 gm PO. The drug of choice is available only in 240-mg capsules. How many capsules would you give?

2. An IV infusion of tetracycline 4 mg/mL is ordered; tetracycline 500 mg/100 mL is available. The drop factor is 10 drops/mL. What is the flow rate? How much medication is received per minute?

3. The drug order reads "Give 250 mL IV over 24 hours." The drop factor is 60 microdrops. What should the flow rate be? Would this IV administration rate be realistic? Why or why not?

4. The adult dose of a given drug is 0.8 mg. What would be the dose for a 40-lb child?

5. Penicillin 500,000 units q8h is ordered. The drug is available as penicillin 1,000,000 units per 5 mL. How many milliliters would be given?

6. The physician orders 0.0015 gm once daily of a drug. The drug is available in tablets labeled 2.5, 1.5, and 10 mg. Which would you order, and how many would you give for each dose?

10 Preparing and Administering Medications

Objectives

After reading and studying this chapter, you should be able to do the following:

1. Compare dosage forms for drugs given by the enteral route.
2. Outline procedures for giving medications enterally, parenterally, and percutaneously.
3. Identify anatomy landmarks used for giving parenteral medications.
4. List processes to prevent human immunodeficiency virus (HIV) transmission.

Key Terms

Be sure to check out the bonus material on the free CD-ROM, including selected audio pronunciations.

ampules (ĂM-pūls, p. 108)
asepsis (ā-SĔP-sĭs, p. 97)
barrel (p. 106)
buccal administration (BŬK-ŭl, p. 133)
capsules (CĂP-sūlz, p. 97)
elixirs (ĭ-LĬK-sĭrz, p. 97)
emulsions (ĭ-MŬL-shŭnz, p. 97)
intramuscular (IM) injections (ĭn-tră-MŬS-kū-lăr, p. 116)
intravenous (IV) route (ĭn-tră-VĒN-ĕs, p. 119)
lozenges (LŎZ-ĭn-jĕz, p. 97)

Mix-o-vial (p. 111)
nasogastric (NG) tube (nā-zō-GĂS-trĭk, p. 100)
needle (p. 106)
parenteral route (pĕ-RĔN-tĕr-ăl, p. 104)
percutaneous administration (pĕr-kū-TĀ-nē-ŭs, p. 130)
piggyback infusion (ĭn-FŪ-zhŭn, p. 124)
pill (p. 97)
plunger (p. 106)
subcutaneous injections (sŭb-kū-TĀ-nē-ĕs, p. 113)
sublingual administration (sŭb-LĬNG-wăl, p. 133)
suspensions (sŭs-PĔN-shŭnz, p. 97)
syringes (sĭ-RĬN-jĕz, p. 106)
syrups (SĬR-ŭps, p. 97)
tablets (p. 97)
tip (p. 106)
topical medications (TŎP-ĭ-kăl, p. 131)
vials (p. 108)

OVERVIEW

This chapter gives an overview of basic principles of medication administration. Section One discusses information about drugs taken by the enteral route: oral, nasogastric, or rectal. Section Two describes how to give drugs parenterally. Section Three describes the methods for giving medications percutaneously.

SECTION ONE
Enteral Medications

Enteral medications are given directly into the gastrointestinal (GI) tract through the oral, nasogastric, or rectal route.

ORAL ADMINISTRATION

The most common route of administration of medications is through the mouth, or orally. The order is often written, "give PO," meaning *per os* or "by mouth." Advantages of oral preparations are as follows:

- They are easy for the nurse to give and for the patient to swallow.

- Most medications come in this form.
- It is usually not very expensive to make oral preparations.
- If a patient takes too much of an oral medication, the drug can be removed by pumping the patient's stomach (gastric lavage) or by having the patient vomit.

The major disadvantages of oral preparations are as follows:

- They cannot be given to patients with a lot of nausea, who are vomiting, or who are unconscious.
- Some chemicals are not effective if mixed with gastric secretions.

- The onset of action may vary because the drug may be slowly absorbed in the GI tract.

There are many different forms of oral medications. Each form is desired for a specific reason (for example, to increase absorption, delay absorption, or reduce gastric irritation). The term **pill** is often used by patients to describe capsules or tablets. Tablets and capsules are very common and are made up of several different chemicals. Tablets may be covered with a special coating that resists the acidic pH of the stomach but will dissolve in the alkaline pH of the intestine.

Box 10-1 summarizes the various oral dosage forms and their characteristics.

PROCEDURE FOR ADMINISTERING ORAL MEDICATIONS

The basic procedure in administration of medication is the same, regardless of type or route of administration. The equipment available and the agency policies may vary because nurses work in many different settings. General principles that underlie all procedures include accuracy, taking responsibility, and **asepsis** (preventing of infection). The legal policies and rules, along with the nursing process and knowledge about the drug, are all part of giving medications. The steps in giving medications by the various routes should be followed exactly as outlined in the following sections. Procedure 10-1

Box 10-1 | *Oral Medication Forms*

Capsules are gelatin containers that hold powder or liquid medicine. Timed-release or sustained-release capsules contain granules that dissolve at different rates, providing slow and constant release of medications. Capsules are available in a variety of sizes and shapes. They provide an easy way to administer medications that have an unpleasant taste or odor. Capsules must not be opened, crushed, or chewed because irritation and excessive or lessened drug activity may be produced.

Elixirs are liquids made up of drugs dissolved in alcohol and water that may have coloring and flavoring agents added. The alcohol makes the drug more dissolvable than water alone.

Emulsions are solutions that have small droplets of water and medication dispersed in oil, or oil and medication dispersed in water. These preparations help disguise the bitter taste of a drug or increase its solubility.

Lozenges are medicine mixed with a hard sugar base to produce small, hard preparations of various sizes or shapes. Medication is released slowly when the lozenge is sucked.

Suspensions are liquids with solid, insoluble drug particles dispersed throughout. These solid particles tend to settle out in layers, so the medication must be shaken before pouring.

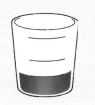

Syrups are liquids with a high sugar content designed to disguise the bitter taste of a drug. These are often used for pediatric patients.

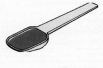

Tablets are dried, powdered drugs compressed into small shapes. These shapes are small enough so that they may be swallowed whole. Tablets usually contain trademarks, designs, or words for product identification and may have a line through the middle so the tablet may be divided (this is known as a scored tablet). Tablets may also contain coatings of various types to increase solubility or absorption.

PROCEDURE 10-1

Administering Oral Medications

STEP ONE: GETTING READY

1. Check the accuracy of the order as written and the time to be given. Clarify any information now known about the patient or the medication, such as allergies.
2. Wash your hands. This is essential to avoid contaminating the medication. Although it seems an obvious step, it is often neglected by busy nurses.
3. Assemble the medication equipment. Obtain the medication cups, glass, water or juice, and straw if needed (*A* through *F*). Unlock medication cart if necessary.

A

Soufflé cup

B

Nipple

C

Graduated medication cup

D

Medication spoon

E

Medication dropper

F

Syringe for administering oral medications

STEP TWO: PREPARING THE MEDICATION

1. Read the order on the medication form and obtain the correct medication from the cabinet or cart (*G*). Medications may come in a cardboard or plastic container, a bottle, or an individually wrapped package.
2. Compare medication order with label on container. First check for the right patient, drug, route, dosage, and time of administration.
3. Open the container and pour the correct number of tablets or capsules into the medication cup.
   - Do not touch the medication with your hands, but pour the medication directly into the bottle lid or the cup.
   - Return any extra medication to the container (*H*).

G

H

PROCEDURE 10-1—cont'd

- To avoid errors, hold the medication cup at eye level when pouring liquids *(I)*.
- If the unit dose system or nurse service is used, the medication will come in a labeled package. It is not removed from the wrapping until the nurse is at the patient's bedside *(J)*.

4. Compare the information on the medication card with the label on the container. This is the second check for accuracy.
5. Close the box or replace the lid on the container, and check the information on it for the third time with the medication card.
    - Medication lids are always replaced immediately after use. Medication that requires special storage (such as refrigeration) should be replaced immediately.
6. Put the medication container back on the shelf.
7. Place the cup containing the medication next to the medication card on the tray.
8. Repeat this process for each medication ordered for the patient. All of the tablets for one patient may be placed in the same medication cup.

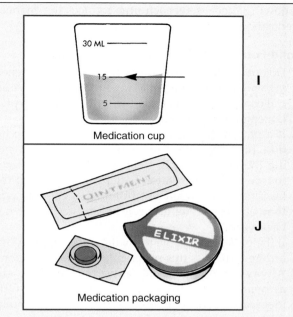

Medication cup

Medication packaging

STEP THREE: ADMINISTERING THE MEDICATION

1. Go to the patient's bedside. Help the patient into an upright position, if possible. Ask patient his name at the same time you are checking the patient's identification bracelet and bed tag. Never give medication without identifying the patient. Confused or critically ill patients may answer to any name.
2. Explain what you are giving and answer any of the patient's questions. Give any special instructions or teach the patient about the medication as needed. Make any special assessments required. If the patient makes any comment about the medication looking different from usual, having just taken the medication, or not having had that medication before, recheck the medication order.
3. Give the patient a glass of water or juice and have the patient place the medication in the back of his mouth, take a sip of water, and swallow. Most medication dissolves better and causes less stomach discomfort when it is taken with adequate liquid.
4. Remain at the beside until the medication is swallowed. Do not leave medication at the bedside for the patient to take later. You are responsible for making certain the medication is given when ordered.

STEP FOUR: CONCLUDING

1. Throw away the medication cup. Wash your hands.
2. Note on the chart the time that the medication was given and sign your name or initials. Record accurately that the medication was given as ordered. Also record if the drug was refused or omitted.
3. Later, check the patient again and note any responses or adverse effects that should be recorded on the chart and reported.

shows the procedure for administering oral medications. Following these steps each time reduces the chance of medication error.

Solid-Form Oral Medications

1. Do not crush tablets or break capsules without checking with the pharmacist. Many medications have special coatings that are essential for proper absorption.
2. Lozenges should be sucked, not swallowed.
3. If a patient has difficulty swallowing the medication, have her take a few sips of water before placing the medication in the back of her mouth, then follow with more water. Patients should keep their heads forward while swallowing, as they do when they eat. It is generally not helpful to tilt the head backward.
4. If the patient is unable to swallow the medication as ordered, discuss this problem with the physician.
5. Always give the most important tablets, such as heart medications and antibiotics, first. Other medications might even be withheld until you talk with the doctor if the patient has great difficulty taking them.

Liquid-Form Oral Medications

1. Liquids or solutions often must be shaken before they are poured. Although this is common sense, always check to make sure the lid is tightly closed before shaking the bottle.
2. Take the lid off the bottle and place the lid upside down (outer surface down) on a flat surface. This protects the inside of the lid from dirt or contamination.
3. When pouring liquids from a bottle into a medication cup, you should hold the bottle so the label is against your hand. This prevents medicine from running down onto the label so that it cannot be read.
4. Hold the medication cup at eye level to read the proper dose. Often the medication in the cup is not level but is higher on the sides than in the middle. Read the level at the lowest point in the medication cup.
5. Wipe any extra medication from the bottle top and replace the lid quickly to avoid contamination.
6. Do not dilute a liquid medication unless ordered to do so by the physician.
7. The medication could also be drawn up from the bottle or medication cup with a syringe or a medicine dropper. These methods are useful in helping you be accurate when a small dose is ordered and are often used when giving medications to infants or small children. The syringe or medicine dropper is placed halfway back in the baby's mouth, between the cheek and gums, and slowly emptied, giving the baby time to swallow it. The medication in the syringe or medicine dropper could also be emptied into a nipple on which the baby is sucking.

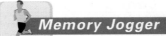
Memory Jogger

General Principles That Underlie All Procedures

- Accuracy
- Acceptance of responsibility
- Asepsis

NASOGASTRIC ADMINISTRATION

The **nasogastric (NG) tube** is another route for enteral medication. Patients who cannot swallow or who are weak or nauseated may be able to take medications through this tube, which leads directly through the nose and into the stomach. The tubing and the clamp allow you to easily give medications over a long period of time to patients who are unable to take food or medicine by mouth. Some patients find the NG tube so irritating to the nose that the medication must be given another way. In such cases, a percutaneous endoscopic gastrostomy (PEG) tube may be surgically placed directly through the abdomen and into the stomach.

PROCEDURE FOR ADMINISTERING NASOGASTRIC MEDICATIONS

The process for giving nasogastric medications is similar to that given for oral medications, but with the following precautions:

- Liquid medications may be ordered for patients who have disorders of the esophagus, are in a coma, or cannot swallow. Some tablets may be crushed, mixed with 30 mL of water, and given through the NG tube.
- Because many of the patients getting medications by NG tube are seriously ill or in a coma, it is especially important to be accurate in all phases of giving the medication. The patient may not be able to help by telling you if there are any problems in giving the medicine.
- Make certain that the NG tube is in the stomach. Aspirate (take out) stomach contents with a syringe, or inject (put in) 5 or 10 mL of air into the tube and listen for a gurgling sound in the abdominal area caused by the air. This may be heard by placing a stethoscope over the stomach. You might also listen for breath sounds, showing that the tubing might be in the lung, by holding the tubing to your ear. Of course, medication must not be given if there is any question about where the NG tube is located. Usually the NG tube is left in place once it is put into the patient.
- The procedure for giving nasogastric medications is very similar to steps 1, 2, and 4 of the procedure for giving oral medications. The major difference is that the medicine is put into the tube rather than

having the patient swallow it. If nasogastric suction is attached to the tubing, disconnect it and clamp the suction tube shut. Clamp the NG tube and attach a bulb syringe. Next, pour the medication into the syringe, unclamp the NG tube, and let the medication run in by gravity. Add water, usually at least 50 mL, to flush and clean out the tubing when the medicine has all passed through the tube. Reclamp the tube. The tube should remain clamped for at least 30 minutes

before the suction tube is reattached so that there is time for the medication to be absorbed. This procedure is shown in Figure 10-1.

• The process for giving medication through a PEG tube is very similar to that for the NG tube. In addition to the tubing, the PEG has a gastrostomy feeding button (a small, flexible silicone device that has a mushroom-shaped dome at one end and two small wings at the other end) that can be used to close the tube between uses. This button should

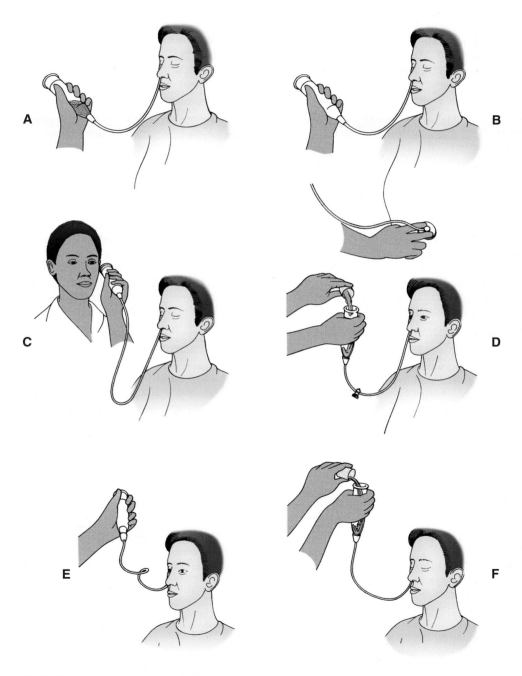

FIGURE **10-1** Administration of medication by nasogastric tube. Make certain the nasogastric tube is in place by **A,** aspirating stomach contents; **B,** listening for gurgling sound in stomach with stethoscope; or **C,** listening for breath sounds. **D,** Put the medication into tubing and **E,** let it run in by gravity. **F,** After the medication is almost out of the tubing, add water to flush the tubing.

be irrigated with 5 to 10 mL of tap water after food and medication have been given and wiped with a cotton-tipped applicator to help keep the tube open. The PEG tube itself should be cleaned with 25 to 50 mL of tap water after giving food to prevent it from getting clogged up.

RECTAL ADMINISTRATION

When a patient has severe nausea or vomiting, medication may need to be put into the rectum, thus avoiding the mouth and stomach. Unlike an enema, when medication is given rectally, the medication should be left to be absorbed and not expelled. Accurate dosage through rectal administration is somewhat more difficult and harder to predict than are the small, accurate doses used in oral medications. This is true for a variety of reasons:

- Some required medications do not come in suppository or enema form.
- Sometimes the patient has diarrhea and cannot hold the medication.
- Sometimes other rectal problems may make using this route a problem.
- If the patient has a lot of fecal material, the medication may not be well absorbed.
- Medications are not absorbed from the rectal mucosa at a standard or predictable rate.

The procedure for administering rectal medications is described in Procedure 10-2. You should note that steps 1, 2, and 4 again are similar to those for administering oral medications.

PROCEDURE 10-2

Administering Rectal Medications

STEP ONE: GETTING READY

1. Check the medication order on the Kardex. Check the accuracy of the order as written and the time to be given. Clarify any information known about the patient or the medication.
2. Wash hands. This is essential to avoid contaminating the medication.
3. Assemble all the necessary equipment. In addition to the medication order or card, get the medication tray, soufflé or medication cups, medication cart, lubricant, and rubber gloves.

STEP TWO: PREPARING THE MEDICATION

1. Read the order on the medication card and get the correct medication from the cabinet, refrigerator, or cart. Medication may come in a bottle, in a plastic container, or as a suppository wrapped in foil.
2. Compare the medication card with the label on the container. First check for the right patient, drug, route, dosage, and time of administration.
3. Obtain the proper amount of liquid, disposable medicated enema, or suppository. Suppositories should be firm or they cannot be properly inserted. If the suppository has melted, it may be hardened by being put in a small container of ice for a few minutes.
   - If the unit dose system or nurse service is used, the medication comes in a labeled package. It is not removed from the wrapping until the nurse is at the patient's bedside.
4. Compare the information on the medication card with the label on the container. This is the second check for accuracy.
5. Replace the medication container and check the information on it for the third time with the medication card.
   - Medication such as suppositories requiring special storage (refrigeration) should be replaced immediately.
6. Place the cup containing the medication next to the medication card on the tray. Suppositories should be given promptly to avoid melting.

STEP THREE: ADMINISTERING THE MEDICATION

1. Go to the patient's bedside. Help the patient turn over on her side with one leg bent over the other in a Sims' position. Protect the patient's modesty as much as possible by closing the drapes and draping the patient. Ask the patient her name at the same time you are checking the patient's identification bracelet and bed tag. Never give medication without identifying the patient.
2. Explain what you are giving and answer any of the patient's questions. Give any special instructions, such as holding the medicine inside and not letting it come out, and teach the patient about the medication as needed. Make any special assessments required.
3. Put on gloves. If you are giving a suppository, remove the suppository from the foil packet and place a small amount of water-soluble lubricant on the tip of the suppository and on the inserting finger. Tell the patient that you are ready to begin. Hold the suppository at the anal sphincter for a few seconds, and tell the patient to take a deep breath and to bear down slightly. This will relax the sphincter so you may push the suppository into the rectum about 1 inch (*A* through *D*). Use your fourth finger (which is smaller) for children. The patient should remain on her side for about 20 minutes. With children, you may have to hold their buttocks together to prevent them from releasing the suppository.

   If you are giving the patient medication by disposable enema, the procedure is the same except that the lubricated tip is inserted into the rectum and the 50 to 150 mL of medication is slowly squeezed from the disposable container (*E* through *G*).

STEP FOUR: CONCLUDING

1. Dispose of the foil packet or plastic containers and the gloves. Clean the medication tray or cart.
2. Leave patients with tissues to wipe themselves if needed and a way to wash their hands.
3. Wash your hands.

PROCEDURE 10-2—cont'd

4. Note on the chart the time that medication was given and sign your name or initials. Record accurately that the medication was given as ordered.

5. Check the patient again later and note any response or adverse effects that should be recorded on the chart and reported. Medicated enemas may be given for severe asthma, to relieve constipation, or to instill steroids used to treat bowel disorders. The nurse should always look for and report any response to the medicated enema.

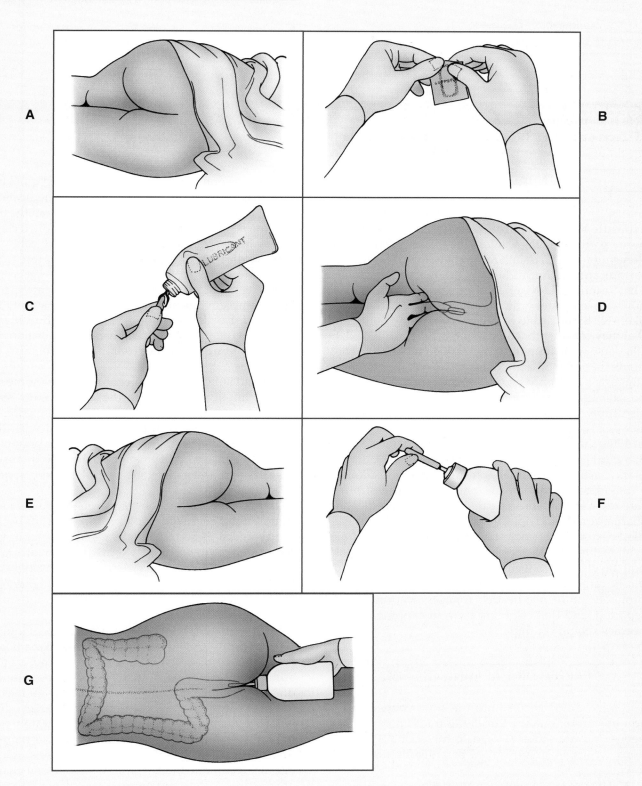

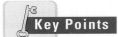

Memory Jogger

Safe Medication Administration Equation

Legal regulations
+ Nursing process
+ Knowledge about pharmacology
Safe medication administration

Key Points

- This section of the chapter has focused on the nursing procedure in the administration of enteral medications.
- Specific steps have been outlined for giving medications orally, by NG tube, and rectally.
- Specific precautions have also been presented for administering medications by the different routes.

SECTION TWO
Parenteral Medications

STANDARD PRECAUTIONS

In 1987, in an effort to protect health care workers from exposure to HIV, hepatitis B virus, and other blood-borne pathogens, the Centers for Disease Control and Prevention (CDC) issued recommendations for universal precautions for all health care workers to follow. They recommend that health care workers use gloves, gowns, masks, and protective eyewear when they were likely to be exposed to patient blood or body fluids, and that they consider that all patients might be infected. In 1988, an update from the CDC clarified the specific body fluids that may be a problem (Box 10-2). Evidence has suggested that only blood, semen, vaginal fluid, and possibly breast milk could carry HIV. These precautions also apply to a variety of other body fluids and tissues (see Box 10-2), although the risk from these is unknown. In 1996, the CDC published revised guidelines, called Standard Precautions, that are considered to be the primary ways to prevent the transmission of infections.

Standard Precautions recommend the use of puncture-resistant containers for disposing of all needles and sharps. You should not try to put the cap back on a needle, because most needlestick injuries occur at this time. Without breaking the needle off the syringe, they should both be placed in a well-marked "hazardous material" plastic canister directly after use. Research suggests that probably more needlestick injuries occur than are reported, and that efforts to prevent capping of used needles should continue.

PARENTERAL ADMINISTRATION

The **parenteral route** (into the skin) of medication administration may be through intradermal, subcutaneous, intramuscular (IM), or intravenous (IV) injections. Drugs are administered parenterally for the following reasons:

- The patient cannot take an oral medication.

- The action of the medicine is required quickly.
- Gastric enzymes might destroy the medication.
- The medication might be removed from the body on a "first pass" through the liver before it can get to the tissues in the body where it will act.
- Medication must be given at a steady rate to provide a constant blood level.
- The medication is not available in an enteral form.

For example, vomiting or unconscious patients may receive IM or IV antibiotics; IV medication may be given in a life-threatening emergency; or a patient may receive continuous IV medication to control heart dysrhythmias.

IM and subcutaneous injections require some time for the medication to reach the bloodstream, so the onset of action may be slower than if the medication were given IV. If an individual is filled with fluid (edema), has large quantities of fat, or has poor circulation (for example, if in shock), the rate of absorption may be unusually long for IM or subcutaneous injections.

IV injections or infusions may be needed when medication must go directly into the bloodstream because the action of these methods is rapid. IV medications may be effective for only a short time, requiring frequent doses. Overdosage errors of IV medications can be very serious. Also, the cost is generally higher for IV medication, even though the total dose may be smaller than if the medication were given orally.

Although all medication administration should be 100% accurate, the nurse giving parenteral medication has a special responsibility for careful and accurate administration because any errors in technique or dosage may have serious consequences. Once injected, the medication cannot be withdrawn. Precise administration of drug dosage is essential. Accurately locating the site of injection is required to avoid pain and damage to tissues, nerves, or blood vessels. Aseptic (sterile) technique must be followed to lessen chances of infection. A slow and gradual rate of injection of the

| Box 10-2 | *Summary of Standard Precautions: Prevention of Transmission of Human Immunodeficiency Virus, Hepatitis B Virus, and Other Blood-Borne Pathogens in Health Care Settings*

Under Standard Precautions, blood and certain body fluids of all patients are considered to possibly contain human immunodeficiency virus (HIV), hepatitis B virus (HBV), and other blood-borne pathogens. Blood is the single most important source of transmission of HIV, HBV, and other blood-borne pathogens in health care settings. Infection control efforts for HIV, HBV, and other blood-borne pathogens must focus on preventing exposure to blood, as well as on delivery of HBV immunization.

Research has shown that only blood, semen, vaginal secretions, and possibly breast milk may transmit HIV. Although the risk is unknown, universal precautions also apply to tissues and the following fluids: cerebrospinal fluid, synovial fluid, pleural fluid, peritoneal fluid, and amniotic fluid. Standard Precautions do not apply to feces, nasal secretions, sputum, saliva (except in situations in which contamination with blood is likely, such as dental settings), sweat, tears, urine, and vomitus unless they contain visible blood. The risk of transmission of HIV and HBV from these materials is extremely low to nonexistent.

Health care workers are at risk for exposure to blood from patients and must consider all patients as possibly infected with blood-borne pathogens. Therefore, health care workers must always follow infection control precautions for all patients.

PRECAUTIONS TO PREVENT TRANSMISSION OF HIV

General Precautions
- Consider all patients potentially infected.
- Wear gloves when touching blood, body fluids containing blood, and body fluids to which Standard Precautions apply; for handling items or surfaces soiled with blood or other fluids; and for doing venipuncture or other procedures involving blood. Change gloves after each contact with a patient.
- Use masks, protective eyewear or face shields, and gowns or aprons when doing procedures that may produce blood or body fluid droplets or splashes.
- Wash hands and skin surfaces immediately and thoroughly with warm soap and water if they get splashed with blood or body fluid to which universal precautions apply; wash between patients and after removal of gloves even when they are not torn or punctured.
- Take precautions to prevent injuries from needles, scalpels, and other sharp instruments during procedures, when cleaning instruments, during disposal, or when handling. To prevent needlestick injuries, needles should not be recapped, bent or broken by hand, or removed from disposable syringes. After they are used, disposable syringes and needles, scalpel blades, and other sharp items for disposal

should be placed in puncture-resistant containers located within the patient's room.
- Use mouthpieces, resuscitation bags, or other ventilation devices when mouth-to-mouth resuscitation is likely to be performed in emergency situations.

Special Considerations
- Health care workers who have sore, draining lesions or wet skin conditions should not be giving direct patient care and should not handle patient care equipment until the condition resolves.
- Pregnant health care workers are not known to be at greater risk of getting HIV infection than health care workers who are not pregnant; however, if a health care worker is infected with HIV during pregnancy, the infant is at risk of infection from perinatal transmission. Because of this risk, pregnant health care workers should be especially familiar with and strictly follow precautions to lower the risk of HIV transmission.

PRECAUTIONS FOR INVASIVE PROCEDURES
An invasive procedure is defined as any surgical entry into tissues, cavities, or organs, or repair of major traumatic injuries. General blood and body fluid precautions listed earlier, combined with the precautions listed below, should be the minimal precautions for all such invasive procedures.
- All health care workers who participate in invasive procedures must use appropriate barrier procedures to prevent skin and mucous membrane contact with all patients' blood and other body fluids to which universal precautions apply.
- Gloves and surgical masks must be worn for all invasive procedures.
- Protective eyewear or face shields should be worn for all procedures that commonly produce droplets or splashes of blood, body fluids containing blood, or other body fluids.
- Gowns or aprons made of materials providing a barrier should be worn during an invasive procedure in which there is likely to be splashing of blood or other body fluids.
- All health care workers who perform or assist in vaginal or cesarean delivery should wear gloves and gowns when handling the placenta or the infant until blood and amniotic fluid have been removed from the infant's skin. Gloves should be worn until postdelivery care of the umbilical cord.
- If a glove is torn or a needlestick or other injury occurs, the glove should be removed and a new glove put on as promptly as patient safety permits; the needle or instrument involved in the incident should also be removed from the sterile field.

Data from Centers for Disease Control: Recommendations for prevention of HIV transmission in health care settings, *MMWR* 36(suppl 25), 1987; Update universal precautions for prevention of transmission of human immunodeficiency virus, hepatitis B virus, and other bloodborne pathogens in health care settings, *MMWR* 37(24), 1988; and *MMWR* 38(suppl 6):9-18, 1989.

medication into the tissues is important for most drugs. This will reduce pain, prevent overdosage, and decrease adverse reactions such as respiratory collapse or heart dysrhythmias.

BASIC EQUIPMENT

SYRINGES

Syringes, or instruments for injecting liquids, come in 1-, 3-, 5-, 10-, 20-, and 50-mL sizes and in plastic or glass. Plastic syringes are the preferred equipment because

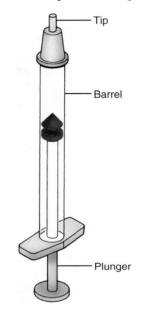

FIGURE **10-2** Parts of a syringe.

they may be used once and thrown away. This makes them convenient in terms of packaging and disposal, but they are more expensive than glass and cannot be used with some medications; also, dosage lines or calibration may be more difficult to read. Reusable glass syringes cost far less, but they may break, may become loose with constant use, and must be cleaned, repackaged, and sterilized each time they are used.

Syringes are made up of three main parts (Figure 10-2). The **tip** is the portion that holds the needle. The needle screws onto the tip or fits tightly so it does not fall off. The **barrel** is the container for the medication. The calibrations are printed numbers on the barrel, and they indicate the amount or volume of medication in either minims (m), milliliters (mL), units, or cubic centimeters (cc) (Figure 10-3). The **plunger** is the inner portion that fits into the barrel. The medication is forced out through the needle when the plunger is pushed into the barrel.

NEEDLES

The needle must be selected according to the needs of the medication. The **needle** is made up of the hub, or bottom part, which attaches to the syringe; the shaft, which is the hollow part through which the medication passes; and the pointed or beveled tip, which pierces the skin (Figure 10-4). The longer the pointed tip of the needle, the more easily the needle enters the skin. The diameter of the needle is called the *gauge*. The larger the number of the gauge, the smaller the hole. (For example, a 25-gauge needle is smaller than a 17-gauge needle.) Thick solutions require larger diameters for injection. The needle gauge is written on the needle hub and on the package. Needles also come in varying lengths, from ⅜ inch

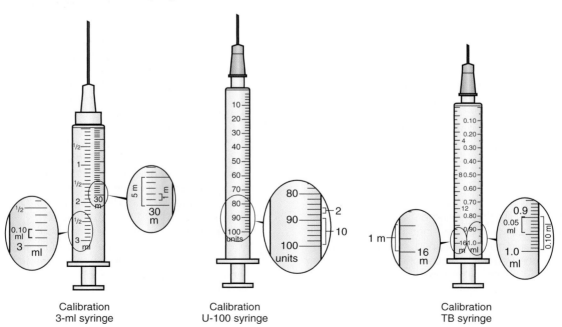

FIGURE **10-3** Comparison of different types of syringes.

to 3 inches. Generally, the smaller the needle (larger the gauge), the shorter the needle. The smallest needles are used for intradermal or subcutaneous injections because they do not need to go very far into the skin.

There are also several specialized IV needles that are used when a needle is to be left in place in the vein for a long period of time. Short, small needles with plastic "wings" are used in infants and children, in the smaller veins of the hands in elderly patients, or in adults who are able to move around. These needles are referred to as scalp vein, butterfly, or wing-tipped needles, and all have small pieces of plastic on either side of the needle that can be pinched together when the needle is going in and then flattened against the skin and held in place with tape. These needles have a small, capped plastic tube attached to the hub that can be used when withdrawing blood specimens or injecting drugs such as heparin. Other special needles include plastic needles, or intracatheters, that use a stainless steel needle for insertion and leave a plastic catheter tube in the vein after the metal needle is withdrawn. Because no metal tip is left inside the vein, there is less chance for the catheter to cut the tissue near it and less damage to the vein wall itself (Figure 10-5). Some needles have a filter to reduce the chance that crystals, medicine plugs (precipitates), or debris might go into the syringe. Needles with special tubing and dose control systems that allow patients to give themselves pain medicine (patient-controlled analgesia [PCA] and patient-controlled epidural analgesia [PCEA]) are also available. These systems have cut down on the need for nurses to give IM medications, thus lowering the chance of nurses sticking themselves with the needle.

The sizes of the needle and syringe are determined by how viscous (thick) the medication is and by the amount to be injected. For example, blood is very thick and requires a 15- to 19-gauge needle. Sometimes when the volume is very small and the dosage must be very accurate (as with heparin or insulin), a small-gauge needle (such as a 27-gauge) is used so no medicine is lost. If more than 3 mL of medication is to be given IM, the medication should be divided and given in two injections so that a large pool of medicine does not form in the tissue, which would irritate the tissue. The hub of the syringe should be ¼ to ½ inch above the skin surface when the drug is injected. This allows the needle to be easily grabbed and pulled out if the patient jerks or the needle breaks. (This rarely happens.) A general guide for choosing the best syringe and needle sizes is presented in Table 10-1.

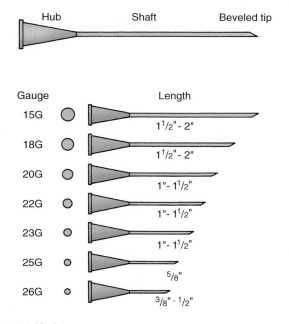

FIGURE **10-4** Parts of the needle and various needle gauges.

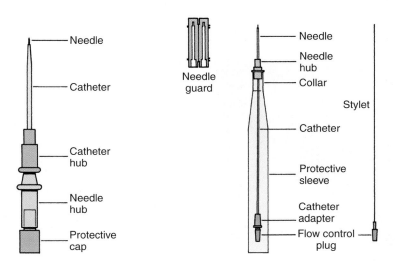

FIGURE **10-5** Over-the-needle catheters. Puncture the vein with a metal large-bore needle. Thread a 4- to 6-inch small-gauge plastic catheter inside and up into the vein before removing the metal needle. Use this type of needle when intravenous therapy must continue for several days.

Table 10-1	*Suggested Guide for Selecting Syringe and Needles*		
ROUTE	GAUGE (G)	LENGTH (in)	VOLUME TO BE INJECTED (mL)
Intradermal	25-27	⅜-½	0.01-0.1
Subcutaneous	25-27	½-1	0.5-2
Intramuscular	20-22	1-2	0.5-2
Intravenous	15-22	½-2	Unlimited

A "needleless" syringe (such as Vitajet, Medi-Jector, and Precijet 50) uses pressure to force small droplets of medication into tissue and is used for immunizations and sometimes insulin. Various needleless infusion lines are also used (Figure 10-6). This type of delivery system is growing in popularity because it removes the risks associated with reusing needles and needle disposal.

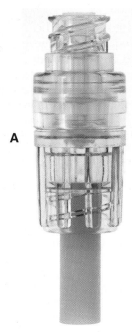

A

B

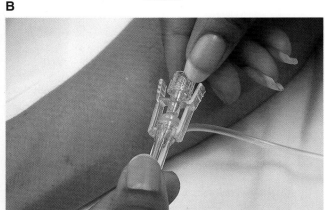

FIGURE **10-6** **A,** Clearlink® Luer Activated Valve. **B,** Needleless device using valvelike system. (**A,** Copyright Baxter Healthcare Corporation, Deerfield, IL.)

PROCEDURE FOR PREPARING AND ADMINISTERING PARENTERAL MEDICATIONS

The basic procedure for preparing and administering parenteral medications is similar to that for oral medications (Procedure 10-3). You will note in the following discussion that there is greater emphasis on sterile technique in giving parenteral medications, because the risk for infection is high. There is also a need to correctly determine the proper site for the injection. The type of parenteral injection and the medication itself often require special equipment or injection techniques. Accurate selection of the syringe and needle and the packaging of the medication help determine the specific steps to follow in drawing up the medication.

All equipment and medication used in parenteral injections should be clearly labeled. All packages should be closely inspected to make certain the contents are sterile. Any equipment that appears old or has crumpled or torn packaging should be thrown away. Dates should be checked to make certain the sterilization date has not expired. Any medication with a questionable seal or with changes in color or appearance should be returned to the pharmacy.

FORMS OF PARENTERAL MEDICATIONS

Parenteral medications are supplied in a variety of different containers. Ampules, vials, Mix-o-vials, and prefilled tubes are the most common dosage forms.

Small single- or multiple-dose glass containers of medication are called **vials.** The top of the glass container is covered first with a rubber diaphragm and then with a small aluminum lid. A tightly fitting metal band holds the rubber diaphragm in place. First the metal lid is removed, then the rubber diaphragm is cleansed with an alcohol wipe, and the needle is inserted through the rubber diaphragm into the medication. An amount of air equal to the amount of solution to be withdrawn is injected into the vial to assist the withdrawal of the medication (Figure 10-7). The vial may contain a solution, or it may contain a powder to which a liquid must be added just before administration to make a solution. You should read the label carefully to determine the amount of diluent that is required and what the diluent should be (for example, normal saline, sterile water, or glucose solution).

Needles should always be inserted into the vial with the bevel up so the nurse may inspect the needle as it goes into the rubber stopper. The needle is always changed before administering the medication to the patient because forcing the needle through the rubber stopper may make it dull or create sharp, irregular edges called "burrs" that would produce pain when inserted into the patient.

Ampules contain one dose of medicine in a small, breakable glass container. The narrow neck of the

PROCEDURE 10-3

Preparing and Administering Parenteral Medications

STEP ONE: GETTING READY

1. Check the medication order on the Kardex. Check the accuracy of the order as written and the time to be given. Clarify any information now known about the patient or the medication.
2. Wash your hands. This is essential to avoid contaminating the medication and equipment. Although it seems an obvious step, it is often neglected by busy nurses.
3. Assemble all the necessary equipment. In addition to the medication order or card, obtain the medication tray, the proper size needles and syringes, alcohol swabs, tubes, and medication cart. Make certain the equipment is sterile. The expiration date on the plastic or paper wrapping should indicate when the equipment must be thrown away or sterilized again.

STEP TWO: PREPARING THE MEDICATION

1. Read the order on the medication card and obtain the correct medication from the cabinet or cart. The medication may come in an ampule, a vial, a Mix-o-vial, or an infusion set.
2. Compare the medication card with the label on the container. First check for the right patient, drug, route, dosage, and time of administration.
3. Attach the needle to the syringe, keeping the needle covered with a cap.
4. Ready the medication for withdrawal by opening the ampule, if necessary.
5. Compare the information on the medication card with the label on the container. This is the second check for accuracy.
6. Insert the needle into the medication container and fill the syringe with the proper amount of medication. (See the following discussion regarding drawing up medications from different dosage forms.) If any air bubbles are present, tap barrel of syringe so air moves into needle and can be removed. Check the information on the container for the third time with the medication card.
   * Do not mix more than one medication in a syringe without checking to see if the medications can be mixed together.
7. Put the unused medication containers away.
8. Change the needle for a new sterile needle if medication has been withdrawn through a rubber stopper or from a multidose vial.
9. Place the syringe and alcohol swabs next to the medication card on the tray.

STEP THREE: ADMINISTERING THE MEDICATION

1. Go to the patient's bedside. Help the patient get into the proper position for the injection. The patient may need to turn over, roll onto his side, or remove his gown. Ask the patient his name at the same time you are checking the patient's identification bracelet and bed tag. Never give medication without positively identifying the patient. Confused or very ill patients may answer to any name.
2. Explain what you are giving and answer any of the patient's questions. Give any special instructions or teach the patient about the medication as indicated. Make any special assessments required. Examine previous injection sites for signs of necrosis, infection, or swelling. Examine the site to be injected. If the patient makes any comments about the medication being different from usual, having just taken the medication, or not having had that medication before, recheck the medication order.
3. Put on gloves. Using an alcohol wipe, carefully rub the skin for several seconds to cleanse it. Following the specific procedure for intradermal, subcutaneous, or intramuscular injection (described in detail in the chapter text), insert the needle firmly, pull back slightly on the plunger to aspirate for blood, and inject the medication. (To aspirate is to look for blood, indicating that the needle has been accidentally placed in a blood vessel, artery, or vein.) If blood comes into the syringe when the plunger is pulled back, remove the needle and set the syringe aside for disposal, prepare new medication for administration, and select another site for injection.
4. Assist the patient to a comfortable position.

STEP FOUR: CONCLUDING

1. Dispose of the alcohol wipe. Return to the nursing station and dispose of the syringe and needle according to hospital procedure. Do not attempt to put the cap back on the needle, because you may accidentally stick yourself. All hospitals have the policy that any accidental scratch or prick from a used needle should be reported because of the risk of AIDS or hepatitis. Clean the medication tray or cart. Wash your hands.
2. Note on the chart the time the medication was given, and sign your name or initials. Record that the medication was given as ordered or was refused.
3. Check the patient again later and note any particular response or adverse effects that should be recorded and reported. Particularly note any complaints of pain, numbness, or tingling at the injection site.

ampule may have to be cut with a small ampule file, or may have a line (score) or ring around it, indicating a weakened area where the top can be broken off. All the medicine can be shifted to the bottom of the ampule by flicking the top lightly with a finger. Grasp the top above the scored or ringed area with an alcohol wipe or gauze pad and pull down sharply on the glass top. The top should easily fall off, allowing insertion of the needle into the ampule to draw up the medicine (Figure 10-8). A filter needle should be used to prevent glass shards from being drawn up into the syringe with the medication. Ampules were very common forms of medication storage in the 1960s and 1970s, after which their popularity decreased because of the availability of less

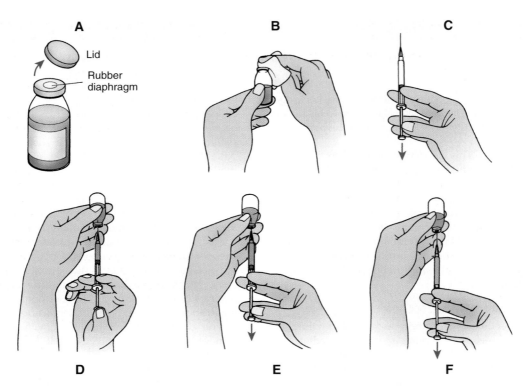

FIGURE **10-7 A,** Example of a vial. **B,** Remove the metal lid and cleanse the diaphragm with an alcohol wipe. **C,** Pull into the syringe an amount of air equal to the amount of solution to be withdrawn. **D,** Insert the needle with the bevel up, and inject the air into the space above the solution. **E,** Withdraw the medication. **F,** Move the needle downward to allow needle to continue to fill.

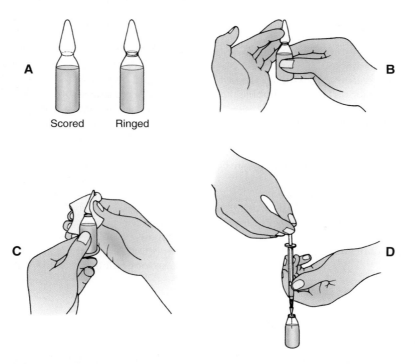

FIGURE **10-8 A,** Examples of scored and ringed ampules. **B,** Shift medication from the top to the bottom portion of the ampule by flicking the top lightly with a finger. **C,** Wrap a gauze pad around the neck of the ampule and use a snapping motion to break off top of ampule along prescored line at neck. Always break away from the body by bending the top toward you. **D,** Insert the filter needle into the ampule and draw up the medication.

expensive vials. There is interest in using ampules again as a way to reduce allergic reactions to the latex stoppers in the vials. Therefore, the American Society of Health Systems Pharmacists has recommended the use of ampules whenever possible.

Occasionally two medications may be ordered that may be given in the same syringe. Two compatible medications are often ordered to be given together as a preoperative medication before surgery (for example, meperidine [Demerol] and promethazine HCl [Phenergan]). Another example is the common practice of ordering two types of insulin (for example, regular and neutral protamine Hagedorn [NPH]) to be given together. In contrast, many antibiotics must be given in separate syringes because chemically they harden, separate into layers, or become inactive if mixed together. It is important when mixing medications in one syringe to remember the following:

- The compatibility of the two medications must be known.
- Air must be injected into both bottles before any medication is withdrawn (to avoid sucking medication already in the syringe down into another bottle).
- The medication with the shorter action or weaker dosage must be withdrawn first. (This idea can be understood if insulin is used as an example. Regular insulin acts more quickly than NPH insulin. If regular insulin is put into the syringe first and a small amount accidentally drops into the NPH insulin bottle when this insulin is being added to the syringe, the patient will not be affected. However, if the longer acting NPH insulin accidentally contaminates the regular insulin bottle, it could change the time at which the patient experiences the onset of the action of the insulin.)

- New guidelines for drawing up nonanimal insulins state that insulin may now be shaken before being drawn up. This reverses previous precautions.
- When regular and Lente mixtures of insulin are mixed in one syringe, they should be injected within 5 minutes of drawing. If this is not possible, the effect of the regular insulin is diminished. The excess zinc from the Lente insulin binds with the regular insulin and forms a Lente-type insulin. NPH-regular insulin mixtures are stable and are absorbed as if injected separately.

Medications that come as a powder must have a solution added immediately before use. The diluent for the powder and the amount to be used should be specified on the label. Frequently, normal saline solution or sterile water is used. The diluent may be drawn into a 1- or 2-mL syringe and added to the powder. The vial should be carefully rolled to make certain all the powder is dissolved in the liquid. If the powder does not completely dissolve, the medication should not be administered. Some of these medications come in a two-compartment vial called a **Mix-o-vial.** The top compartment contains a sterile solution; the bottom compartment contains the medication powder. A rubber stopper separates the two areas. Pressure on the rubber plunger of the top compartment forces the rubber stopper below to fall into the bottom compartment, letting in the solution to dissolve the powder. The vial is gently rolled to help dissolve the powder, and then a needle may be inserted to withdraw the solution (Figure 10-9).

Any multiple-dose vial or newly mixed (reconstituted) powder solution must be clearly labeled when it is first opened. The date, time, and concentration should be included, as well as the expiration time of the medication. The nurse who opened or mixed the medication should also initial the label.

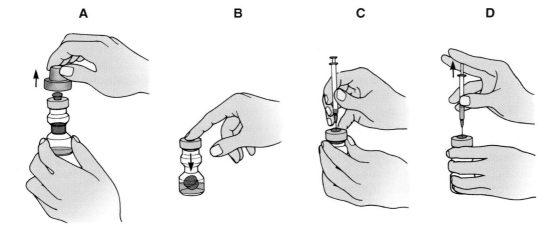

FIGURE **10-9** **A,** Remove the protective sterile cap from the Mix-o-vial. **B,** Push the rubber plunger on the top compartment; this will force the rubber stopper into the bottom compartment and let the solution dissolve the powder. The solution is mixed by gently rolling the container. **C,** The needle is inserted through the top rubber diaphragm into the solution. **D,** The required dose is withdrawn into the syringe.

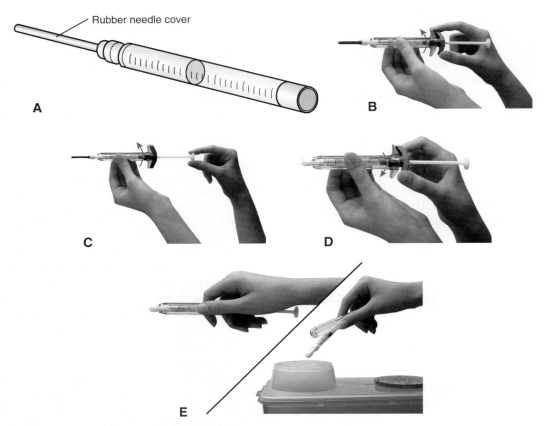

FIGURE **10-10** **A,** Example of a disposable prefilled medication cartridge. **B,** To load, place cartridge, Luer tip first, into open end of holder. Twist blue lock to close. **C,** To engage, turn plunger rod clockwise. Proceed with injection in normal manner, leaving tip guard on until just before use. **D,** To disengage, turn plunger rod counterclockwise. Pull plunger back fully. Twist blue lock open to release. **E,** Place thumb on cartridge and slide back. Invert holder and release used cartridge unit into disposal bin.

Many narcotics and emergency drugs (such as adrenalin) come in prefilled syringes and cartridges. These medication cartridges may be quickly slipped into a plastic holder and screwed into place; after the needle is added, the medication is administered (Figure 10-10). Prefilled syringes are particularly helpful when time is important (such as during a cardiac arrest) or when the dosage of medication rarely varies.

Medications or solutions to be given intravenously come in large plastic or glass containers that hold from 50 to 1000 mL. The opening to the glass container is plugged with a hard rubber stopper, a thin rubber diaphragm, and a metal cover. The metal cover and diaphragm are removed just before inserting the infusion tube that connects the bottle to the tube through a small hole in the hard rubber stopper. In many products, there is also a second small hole in the rubber stopper that allows air to enter the container to replace the amount of medication being infused. The plastic container comes sealed in another plastic bag, which is not opened until the infusion is to begin. Air may enter the plastic bag either at the bag opening or farther down on the infusion tubing (Figure 10-11).

Some medications, such as antibiotics, are ordered to be given every few hours. This medication would come from the pharmacy already mixed or as a solution to be injected into a smaller bottle, usually containing 50 to 250 mL of fluid, and hung with new tubing that is "piggybacked" or "secondary" to an infusion that is already running. The existing solution is clamped off while the piggyback medication is administered, usually over 20 to 60 minutes, and then the original solution is restarted.

After studying these general procedures for administering parenteral medications, you should examine specific techniques necessary for administration of intradermal, subcutaneous, IM, and IV medications. The equipment, sites of injection, and technique must be completely understood.

ADMINISTERING INTRADERMAL INJECTIONS

Intradermal injections are used to determine if someone has an allergy (allergy sensitivity testing), for vaccination, and for allergy desensitization shots. They are also used for injection of local anesthetics before wart

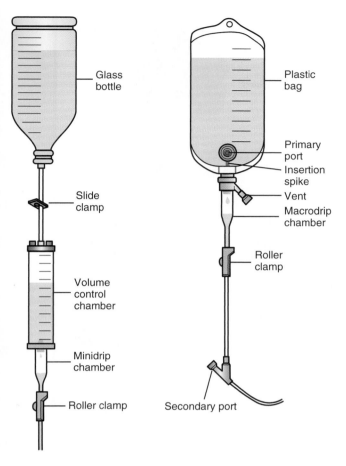

FIGURE **10-11** Intravenous bottle or bag and tubing.

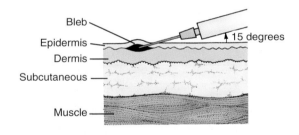

FIGURE **10-12** Anatomy of skin showing placement for intradermal injections.

removal, during suturing of the skin for minor cuts, and for minor procedures. The medication is injected into the intradermal space between the upper two layers of the skin, the epidermis and the dermis (Figure 10-12). Injections are made into the inner aspect of the forearm, the scapular area of the back, and the upper chest if these areas are reasonably hairless. Usually, just a small volume is injected, producing a small bump like a mosquito bite, called a *bleb*. The blood supply to this area of the skin is less than in other areas, so there is very slow absorption from the intradermal layer. Once the medication has been injected, the patient should not wear tight clothing over the area.

Equipment and Technique

Usually 0.01 to 0.1 mL is injected, so a needle that is both small (25 gauge) and short (⅜ inch) is used. The needle should be inserted firmly at a 15-degree angle. The bevel or slanted tip of the needle should be pointing upward. The medication is injected, and the needle is swiftly removed. The small bleb should be seen on the skin at the point where the medication was injected into the intradermal space.

If the injection was given for allergy or sensitivity testing, it is important to record the concentration of the medication used and the site of the injection (Figure 10-13). Many reactions to intradermal injections are not apparent for several hours or even days after injection. It is sometimes helpful to draw a circle around the injection site with a pen to help identify the site accurately at a later date when it is inspected for any reaction. The patient has an allergic reaction, or a clinically significant reaction to testing, if there is a wheal (elevated area) at the site where the diluted dose of medication was injected. The amount of swelling should be measured at 5, 10, and 15 mm.

If the patient has an allergy, the injection site may also become red, swollen, and very itchy (pruritic). The patient should not scratch this area and should use cool, wet compresses to reduce the irritation. The patient should call the physician or go to an emergency room if he has any symptoms in any other body systems, particularly trouble breathing, shortness of breath, puffiness of the face, or hives.

Skin reactions to intradermal allergy injections or to testing for tuberculosis (purified protein derivative [PPD] test) must be checked at a predetermined time after the injection. Each agency has a policy on how the patient reaction should be evaluated and recorded. When testing is done on an outpatient basis, a reliable patient is often told to look at injection site and mail in a postcard showing a picture that is most similar to the reaction. Table 10-2 shows common reactions to intradermal injections and how they are described.

ADMINISTERING SUBCUTANEOUS MEDICATIONS

Subcutaneous injections involve placing no more than 2 mL of fluid into the loose connective tissue between the dermis of the skin and the muscle layer (Figure 10-14). (This is a little deeper than the intradermal injections we have been discussing.) Because less blood is normally supplied to this area than to muscle, any medication injected here will be slowly, but completely, absorbed. This means there will be a slow onset of medication action but a long duration of drug action. Medications injected into the subcutaneous tissue are usually very strong, but concentrated into small doses. For example, insulin and heparin are the most frequently given subcutaneous injections. Because these medications are often given every daily for a long time

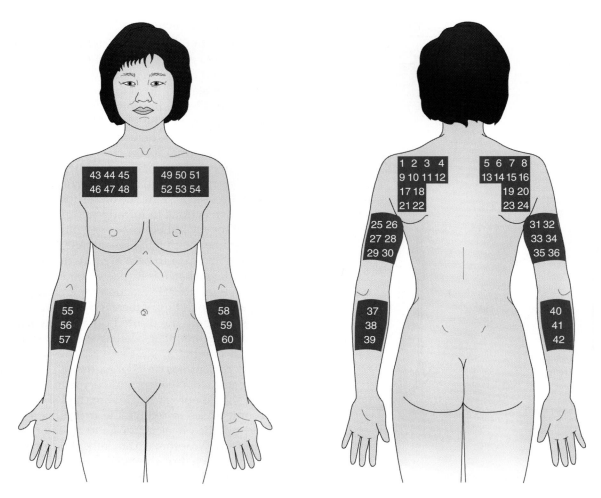

FIGURE **10-13** Sites used in intradermal skin testing for allergy.

Table 10-2 | *Description of Intradermal Skin Reactions*

OBSERVATION OF SKIN	RECORDING SYMBOLS		REACTION
	−	(0)	No reaction
	+	(1+)	Redness or erythema of skin
	++	(2+)	Redness and elevated lesions or papules up to 5 mm in diameter
	+++	(3+)	Redness, papules, and vesicles (fluid-filled elevated lesions) up to 5 mm
	++++	(4+)	Generalized blister larger than 5 mm

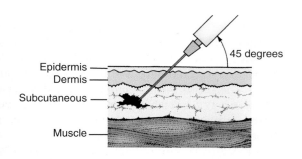

FIGURE **10-14** Anatomy of skin showing placement for subcutaneous injections.

in patients with chronic illnesses, special care must be taken not to irritate the tissue with repeated injections in the same area.

Equipment and Sites for Injection

In preparing the subcutaneous injection, only a small syringe and needle are needed. Usually a 25- or 27-gauge needle is used, and one that is no longer than ⅝ inch in length.

The sites used for subcutaneous injection depend on whether the nurse or the patient is giving the injection.

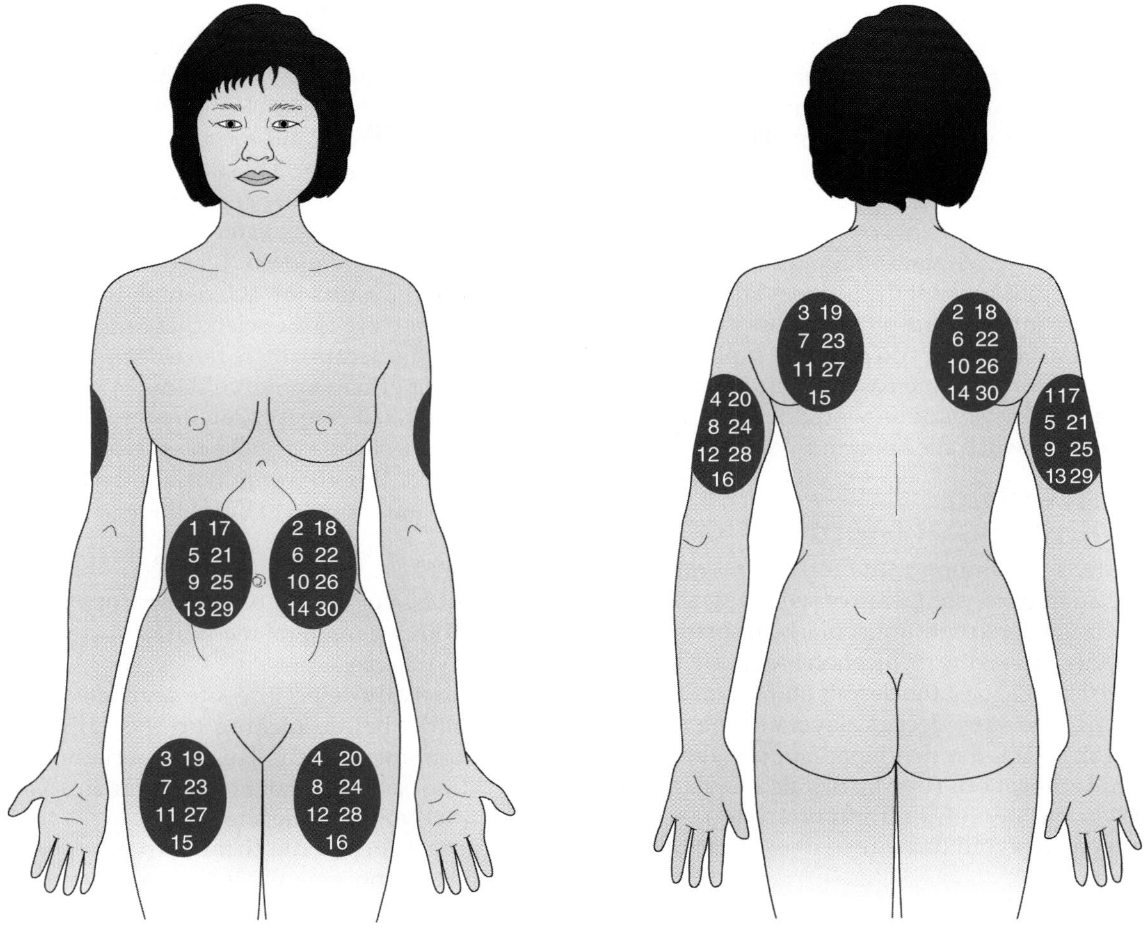

FIGURE 10-15 Body rotation sites for subcutaneous injections.

Commonly, the nurse gives subcutaneous injections in the upper arms, upper back, or scapular region. The nurse in the hospital will often need to teach the patient how to give herself the subcutaneous injection while she is in the hospital and can practice under the nurse's supervision. The patient is able to inject herself most easily in the upper arms, anterior thighs, and abdomen. The patient should agree on a rotation plan for injection sites, and this should be posted with the patient's medications or by the patient's bedside. The front view in Figure 10-15 shows areas usually used for self-injection. The back view shows less commonly used areas that may be used by the nurse. The site used should be part of the information recorded about the injection.

Insulin injections are absorbed 50% faster from the abdomen than from other areas. Other sites for injection include arms, thighs, and buttocks. Because it may be difficult for patients to remember where they last injected the insulin, a "tape-dot" method has been developed. Using the face of a clock, patients inject themselves in the abdomen at 3, 6, 9, and then 12 o'clock. After each injection they put a small dot of tape over the injection site. When they get around to the

3 o'clock position again, they move to the extremities and then back to the abdomen, 1 inch to the side of their previous injection, and start their new series of dots. Thus the sites are rotated in an organized manner. Diabetic patients should avoid injecting within 1 inch of a previous injection site for 1 month in order to avoid tissue damage.

Technique

The technique for subcutaneous injection is identical to that for other parenteral medications with the following three exceptions:

1. Because the dosages are so small and so potent, it is important to draw up the prescribed dose of medication and then add 1 to 2 minims of air. This forces all of the medicine into the tissue when it is injected so no drops are left in the needle. It is especially important that the exact dose is given, especially in children, in whom small variations in dose might have a large effect.
2. In injecting the medication, grasp the skin and hold it flat with one hand, and insert the needle firmly at a 45-degree angle with the other hand.

When you are giving an injection in the scapula or abdomen, it is often easier to grasp the skin with one hand, pull it up into a small roll, and insert the needle quickly at a 90-degree angle. Slowly inject the agent while watching for a small wheal or blister to appear.

3. The policy when giving an IM injection is to always make sure that the needle is in the muscle and that you have not accidentally entered a vein or artery. To do this, pull back on the plunger and check the syringe for any blood (aspirate) before injecting the medication. However, you must not aspirate when giving heparin. The increased vacuum on the tissues caused by aspiration would lead to damage and bruising when the heparin is injected.

ADMINISTERING INTRAMUSCULAR MEDICATIONS

The IM route is a common route for parenteral injections. Many antibiotics, preoperative sedatives, and narcotics are administered intramuscularly. In **intramuscular (IM) injections,** the medication is deposited deep into the muscle mass, past the dermis and subcutaneous tissue and into the very deepest layers of the muscle (Figure 10-16), where the rich blood supply allows for rapid and full absorption. The muscles also contain large blood vessels and nerves, so it important to place the needle correctly to avoid damage to these structures.

Equipment

The syringe chosen has to be large enough to hold the amount of medicine to be injected. Generally, 0.5 to 2 mL is injected IM, although infants and children rarely receive more than 1 mL. On the rare occasions when more than 3 mL of medicine is ordered, it should be given in two doses rather than in one syringe. The needle length should also be chosen to allow deeper placement of the needle. Usually 1- or 1½-inch needles are used. Very obese patients may require an even longer needle; very thin or emaciated patients may require a shorter needle. The gauge of the needle should be determined by the type of medication and how free-flowing it is. Usually 20- to 22-gauge needles are used.

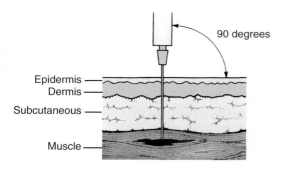

FIGURE **10-16** Anatomy of skin showing placement for intramuscular injections.

Sites for Injection

Five muscles are commonly used for IM injections: the deltoid, dorsogluteal, rectus femoris, vastus lateralis, and ventrogluteal muscles. Each site has advantages and disadvantages, and must be correctly identified for safe administration. These sites have been selected because they are usually away from major blood vessels and nerves, and so are safer to use. Some of these sites are not used for children. Use of the dorsogluteal site most often results in accidental injury to patients because it is close to the sciatic nerve. It is rarely used for IM injections because there have been so many lawsuits related to permanent nerve damage caused by a needle. However, if care is taken to properly identify landmarks, it is a site that may be used when other sites cannot be used. Box 10-3 summarizes the five sites for IM injections and how to identify them.

Technique

The process for giving of IM injections is the same as that for other parenteral medications, except for several additional items:

1. Carefully select the site and identify the landmarks before picking up the syringe. Have all equipment ready. This is especially true for children, who will not hold still for a prolonged time after you find the site.

2. Insert the needle firmly, usually at a 90-degree angle, and give the injection. After withdrawing the needle, apply gentle pressure to the site with a dry cotton pad. (Use of an alcohol swab may cause burning.) Massaging the area may increase pain if a large amount of medication has been injected. Because bleeding often occurs after IM injections, a small bandage may be necessary. Rotate the site of injection when repeated injections are needed.

3. Some medications are irritating or may stain the skin (for example, iron). Use the "Z-track technique" of injection (Figure 10-17) for these medications. The Z-track technique uses the skin itself as a "door" to seal in the drug and prevent it from leaking back out. Medications of the type that require the Z-track technique should be injected into the ventrogluteal site. Use a long needle and add 0.5 mL of air to the syringe after drawing up the medication to ensure that all of the medication is injected from the needle. Stretch or pull the skin approximately 1 inch to one side. Insert the needle, aspirate, inject the medication slowly, and wait approximately 5 seconds. Remove the needle and let the skin slide back to its normal position. Do not massage the injection site. The patient should avoid putting pressure on the area from clothing, although walking helps increase absorption.

Box 10-3 | *Sites for Intramuscular Injections*

DELTOID MUSCLE

The deltoid muscle is easily reached but used infrequently because the muscle is small and can accommodate only small doses of medications. The deltoid is also near the radial nerve. No more than 2 mL may be injected here (less in children), and the medication should not be irritating and should be quickly absorbed. For this site, seat the patient upright or have the patient lie flat with the arms apart. Two imaginary lines should be drawn across the armpit at the level of the axilla and the lower edge of the acromion, the sharp point of the shoulder. Two more imaginary lines should be drawn down on either side, one third and two thirds of the way around the outer lateral aspect of the arm. This creates a small rectangle in which medication can be safely given.

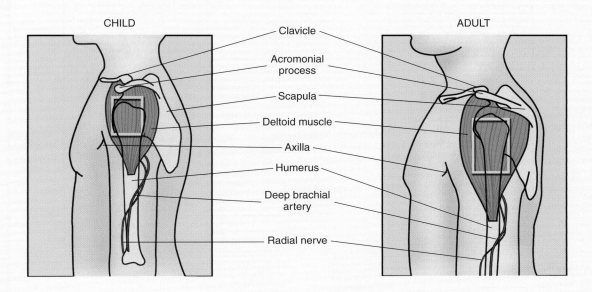

CHILD | ADULT

Clavicle
Acromonial process
Scapula
Deltoid muscle
Axilla
Humerus
Deep brachial artery
Radial nerve

DORSOGLUTEAL MUSCLE

The dorsogluteal muscle is a common injection site for adults because it is relatively free from nerves and major blood vessels. However, the muscles are not developed enough for this site to be used for children younger than 3 years of age. The patient must lie prone (on stomach) on a flat surface and point the toes inward to relax the muscles. An imaginary cross should be drawn from the anus laterally, and from the posterior superior iliac spine down the leg. The injection should be given in the upper, outer quadrant of the cross. Hold the syringe perpendicular to the flat surface and inject the medication. Many nurses are afraid to use this site because the sciatic nerve may be injured when nurses fail to properly identify the landmarks.

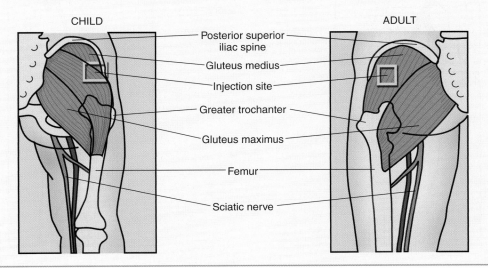

CHILD | ADULT

Posterior superior iliac spine
Gluteus medius
Injection site
Greater trochanter
Gluteus maximus
Femur
Sciatic nerve

Continued

Box 10-3 | *Sites for Intramuscular Injections*—cont'd

RECTUS FEMORIS MUSCLE

The rectus femoris muscle lies medial to (toward the middle of the body from) the vastus lateralis muscle, but does not cross the midline of the anterior thigh. It is used in both children and adults, especially for self-injection. Injections here may be painful if the muscle is not well developed. For this site, position the patient in bed either sitting up or lying flat.

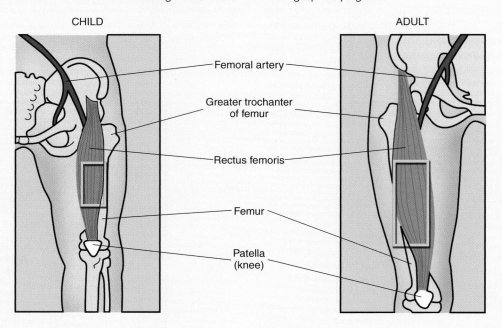

CHILD   ADULT

Femoral artery

Greater trochanter of femur

Rectus femoris

Femur

Patella (knee)

VASTUS LATERALIS MUSCLE

The vastus lateralis muscle is located on the anterior lateral thigh away from blood vessels and nerves. It can absorb a large volume of medication. This is the preferred site for IM injections in infants; it is also a good site for healthy, ambulatory adults because there are few near major blood vessels and nerves. The muscle mass here tends to shrink or become smaller in elderly or very ill patients and may be inadequate. The muscle extends from one handbreadth below the greater trochanter to one handbreadth above the knee.

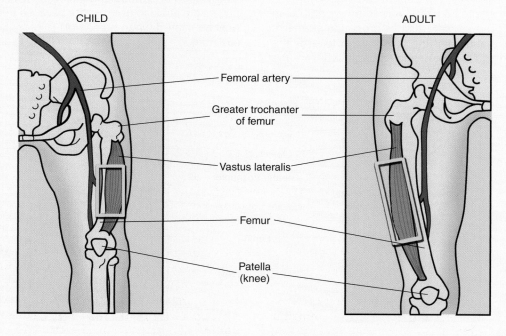

CHILD   ADULT

Femoral artery

Greater trochanter of femur

Vastus lateralis

Femur

Patella (knee)

Box 10-3 | *Sites for Intramuscular Injections*—cont'd

VENTROGLUTEAL MUSCLE

The ventrogluteal muscle is a large muscle mass that is free of major nerves and adipose tissue, and is also remote from the rectum (minimizing the risk of contamination). Whether the site may be used for children depends on the extent of muscle development. The patient should lie on the side with the upper leg flexed, or the patient should lie prone (on stomach) and point the toes inward to relax the muscles. The palm of the nurse's hand should be placed on the lateral portion of the greater trochanter, the index finger on the anterior superior iliac spine, and the middle finger extended to the iliac crest. The injection should be made into the center of the V formed between the index and middle fingers, with the needle directed slightly upward toward the crest of the ilium.

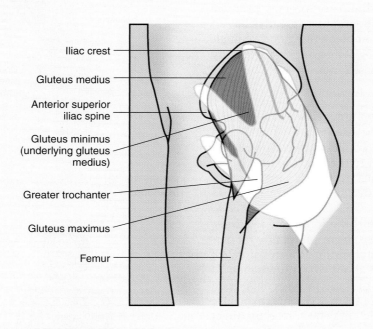

Iliac crest

Gluteus medius

Anterior superior iliac spine

Gluteus minimus (underlying gluteus medius)

Greater trochanter

Gluteus maximus

Femur

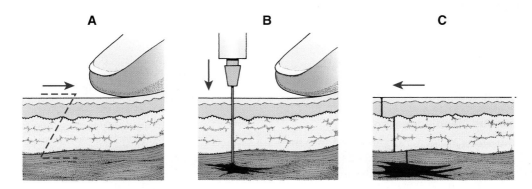

FIGURE **10-17** Z-track injection technique. **A,** Pull the tissue laterally. **B,** Insert the needle straight down into the muscle and inject the medication. **C,** Release the tissue as the needle is withdrawn; this allows the skin to slide over the injection track and seal the medication inside.

ADMINISTERING INTRAVENOUS MEDICATIONS

The **intravenous (IV) route** is used when it is necessary for medication to enter the bloodstream directly. Sometimes large doses of medication must be given, either every few hours or over a long period of time. Because IV medication has not been exposed to other enzymes or tissues before reaching the bloodstream, the rate of absorption and the onset of action are faster. In addition, some medications cannot be given orally, and may be very painful or irritating if given IM. In emergencies, medication may be injected directly into a vein, but usually the IV medication is given on a scheduled basis or infused slowly through IV tubing or an infusion line that is already in the vein.

If a patient must have numerous medications injected daily, both the patient and the nurse generally prefer IV administration. Some patients do not like to be "tied down" by the tubing and feel general discomfort and irritation from the needle and the medication. Nurses must use greater skill to administer medication intravenously than with other routes, and must be especially careful to prevent infection at the needle site. In addition, because the effect of the medication is immediate, drug overdosages, errors in dosage calculation, or failure to control the rate of administration may produce serious problems for the patient. Thus the nurse has an increased responsibility for implementing and evaluating the medication given. Registered nurses are usually the nurses who will give these types of medicines.

Equipment

IV solutions come in large-volume, plastic or glass containers, ranging from 250 to 1000 mL. Medications in vials, ampules, or prefilled syringes marked specifically "for IV use" may be added to these containers. Many hospitals receive IV solutions from the pharmacy with the medications already added.

Some hospitals have "IV teams" who can be called to insert the IV needle and start the initial medications. More frequently, the nurse has the responsibility for performing the venipuncture and starting the infusion. All hospitals have clear policies about what nurses may do in starting infusions. Most of these policies have been updated to protect the nurse from accidental exposure to HIV and hepatitis B, which may be spread by direct contact with blood and other body fluids and may lead to the development of acquired immunodeficiency syndrome (AIDS) and hepatitis, respectively. It is mandatory that nurses review these policies before attempting to start an IV, for their own protection and the protection of others. Policies clearly state that gloves should be worn and state how to dispose of the equipment that is contaminated with the patient's blood.

Sites for Intravenous Needle Insertion

Needles for IV infusions are generally inserted into the smallest veins and as close to the hands as possible. Arteries are not used. As more infusion sites are needed, the needle is inserted farther and farther up the vein, closer to the patient's heart. This principle allows one vein to be used multiple times. The metacarpal, dorsal, basilic, and cephalic veins are commonly used in adults (Figure 10-18). Veins in the lower extremities, veins over sharp, bony areas or joints, and veins in areas of recent injury or surgery should be avoided. Veins commonly used in infants and children include the scalp vein in the temporal area, veins in the dorsum of the foot, and those in the back of the hand (Figure 10-19). Elderly or emaciated patients generally have such fragile skin that needles will not stay in the veins of the hand.

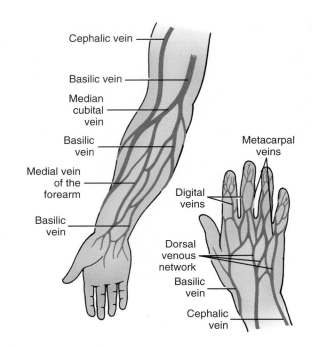

FIGURE **10-18** Intravenous sites used in the hand and forearm of adults.

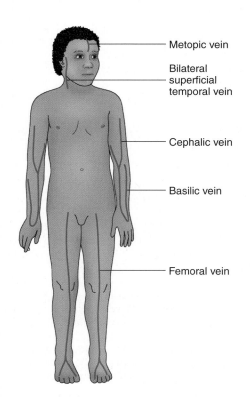

FIGURE **10-19** Intravenous sites used in children.

Venipuncture and Intravenous Infusion

The procedures for venipuncture and starting an IV infusion are somewhat different from those with other routes of administration. Procedure 10-4 summarizes the steps involved in venipuncture and IV infusion.

PROCEDURE 10-4

Preparing and Administering Intravenous Medications

STEP ONE: GETTING READY

1. Check the medication order on the Kardex. Check the accuracy of the order as written and the time to be given. Clarify any information known about the patient or the medication. Complete any calculations needed for dosage, flow rate, and length of infusion.
2. Wash your hands. This is essential to avoid contaminating the medication and equipment. Although it seems an obvious step, it is often neglected by busy nurses.
3. Assemble all the medication equipment. In addition to the medication order or card, obtain the medication tray, proper size needles, tubing, tape, IV infusion poles, alcohol swabs, and medication cart. Make certain that the equipment is sterile. The expiration date on the plastic or paper wrapping should indicate when the equipment must be thrown away or sterilized again.

STEP TWO: PREPARING THE MEDICATION

1. Read the order on the medication card, and obtain the correct medication from the cabinet or cart. Medications may come in an ampule, a vial, a Mix-o-vial, or an infusion set.
2. Compare the medication card with the label on the container. First check for the right patient, drug, route, dosage, and time of administration.
3. Attach the needle to the syringe, keeping the needle covered with a cap.
4. Ready the medication for withdrawal by opening the ampule, if necessary.
5. Compare the information on the medication card with the label on the container. This is the second check for accuracy.
6. Insert the needle into the medication container and fill the syringe with the proper amount of medication. (See the text for a discussion of drawing up medications from different dosage forms.) Check the information on the container for the third time with the medication card. Dilute the medication in the proper volume and type of solution. Always follow the manufacturer's recommendations.
   - Do not mix medications with blood or albumin. Do not administer any solution that is hazy or cloudy or that has a precipitate or any particles in it.
   - Once mixed, label the container with the medication, date, time, and your initials. IV infusions are generally usable for 24 hours. Any solution not used during that time should be returned to the pharmacy.
   - Some medications require special precautions such as shading from sunshine or infusion over a certain time period.
   - Make certain that the infusion is completely infused and that the tubing is cleared before other medication is added.

7. Put the unused medication containers away.
8. If using an IV bottle, remove the metal covering over the IV bottle top. Cleanse the top of the rubber diaphragm on top of the IV bottle or plastic IV bag with an alcohol wipe. Insert the needle with an unused syringe through the rubber diaphragm or medication port into the IV container and withdraw air, creating a vacuum inside the IV container. Now insert the needle with the syringe containing the medication and inject the contents into the IV container through one of the medication ports.
9. Place the syringe and alcohol preps next to the medication card on the tray. Bring other needed equipment to the bedside.

STEP THREE: INSERTING THE NEEDLE INTO THE VEIN

1. Go to the patient's bedside. Help the patient get into the proper position to receive the infusion. The patient may need to turn over, roll onto one side, or remove her gown. Ask the patient her name at the same time you are checking the patient's identification bracelet and bed tag. Never give medication without positively identifying the patient.
2. Explain what you are giving and answer any of the patient's questions. Give any special instructions or teach the patient about the medication as indicated. Make any special assessments required. Assess previous sites of injections for signs of necrosis, infection, or swelling. Examine the site to be injected. If the patient makes any comments about the medication being different from usual, having just taken the medication, or not having had that medication before, recheck the medication order.
3. Before performing the venipuncture, tear strips of adhesive tape for anchoring the needle. Open up the infusion set, insert the tubing into the IV container, allow the solution to run into the tubing, and then clamp it shut. Hang the container on the IV pole.
4. Put on gloves. Use correct barrier procedures, as determined by hospital policy, to protect yourself from HIV infection.
5. Apply a tourniquet 2 to 3 inches above the proposed insertion site. Use a slip knot to allow quick release of the tourniquet.
6. Identify the vein to be used and palpate it with the fingers.
7. Using an alcohol wipe, carefully rub the skin for a few seconds to cleanse. Wipe firmly in a circular pattern, moving inside to outside. Let the skin air dry.
8. Grasp the needle in your dominant hand, stretch the skin with the other hand, and stabilize the vein. With the needle bevel up at an angle less than 45 degrees, insert the needle into the skin about ½ inch below the point of entry into the vein. Then decrease the angle to

Continued

PROCEDURE 10-4—cont'd

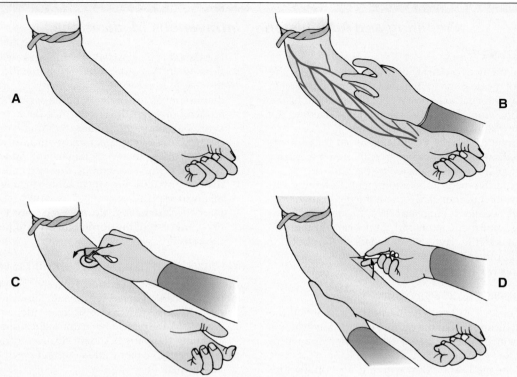

Insertion of needle for venipuncture. **A,** Select site and apply a tourniquet. **B,** Palpate vein to be used for infusion. **C,** Wipe skin with an alcohol swab, moving in a circular pattern. **D,** With the bevel up and the syringe at a 45-degree angle, the needle is inserted through the skin and into the vein. Slowly reduce the angle and thread the needle up into the vein once blood is seen in the syringe. Remove tourniquet and apply adhesive dressing.

15 degrees and slowly push the needle into and along the vein. Blood will flow down into the tubing when the needle is in the vein.
9. Connect the tubing to the needle, release the tourniquet, and cleanse the area to remove any blood that may have gotten on the skin or tubing. Remove the gloves.

10. Anchor the tubing with adhesive tape. Mark on the tape the time that the needle was inserted and your initials.
11. Immobilize the arm or hand by taping it to an infusion board.
12. Adjust the rate of infusion. An infusion pump may be used to monitor the flow rate and to alert you with an

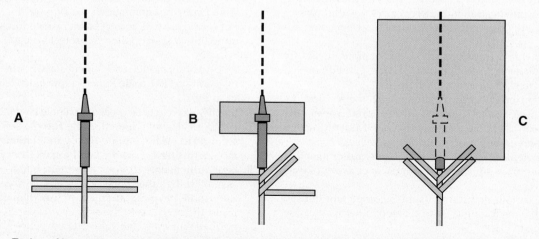

Taping of intravenous tubing after insertion. **A,** Place two small adhesive tape strips under the needle or the catheter with the adhesive side up. **B,** Cross adhesive tapes and fasten them securely to the skin on both sides. **C,** Place a large piece of tape over the tubing and skin to stabilize the needle. Mark the date and time of insertion and your initials or name.

PROCEDURE 10-4—cont'd

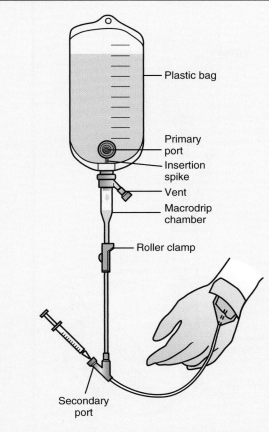

- Plastic bag
- Primary port
- Insertion spike
- Vent
- Macrodrip chamber
- Roller clamp
- Secondary port

Adding IV push medication to an IV line. Close the IV tubing with a roller clamp. Insert the syringe with the medication into the secondary port. Inject the medication slowly. Release the IV tubing at the roller clamp and allow the infusion to resume.

alarm if a problem develops. There are many types of pumps to control infusion rate. The nurse is responsible for checking the equipment's functioning and accuracy.

13. Assist the patient to a comfortable position.

STEP FOUR: CONCLUDING

1. Dispose of the alcohol wipes and gloves according to the hospital procedure. Clean the medication tray or cart and put away the equipment.
2. Note on the chart the time the medication was given and sign your name or initials.
3. Check the patient again later and note any particular responses or adverse effects that should be recorded and reported. Particularly note any complaints of pain, burning, or stinging at the needle insertion site. Note the infusion rate.

Modifications in Technique for Specific Situations

Adding Medication by Syringe to an Infusion. IV medications are commonly added by syringe to an IV infusion that is already running. This is done by using the medication portal available on the IV tubing. You should wear gloves while carrying out this procedure. The tubing should be clamped above the self-sealing IV portal of the infusion tubing. The portal should be cleaned with an alcohol swab, and a syringe containing the medication should be inserted through the portal. A short needle should be used to avoid accidentally pushing the needle all the way through the tubing. The plunger on the syringe should be drawn back until blood is seen in the tubing above the needle at the skin insertion site. This confirms that the needle is in the vein. The medication should then be slowly injected into the IV line, according to the prescribed rate of infusion for that medication. Once all the medication is injected, the needle is withdrawn and the tubing is unclamped. Any blood or fluid is cleaned up, and the

rate of infusion is readjusted. You should then remove your gloves and wash your hands.

All gloves, needles, swabs, and equipment must be taken to the nurses' station or to the dirty utility room for disposal according to hospital policy. You should then wash your hands again.

Adding Medication to a Plastic Bag or an IV Bottle. The top of the plastic bag or the IV glass bottle has an air portal, a tubing portal, and an injection portal (Figure 10-20). Identify the proper portal and cleanse it with an alcohol wipe. Allow the portal top to air dry. Fill the syringe with medication and inject the medication slowly with a small needle through the medication portal into the IV container. Slow administration will allow air to escape from the container while the medication is being injected. The nurse should label the bottle or bag with the date, time, dosage, and medications added and sign her initials.

Adding Medication to a Volume Control. Draw up the medication in a syringe. Fill the volume chamber with

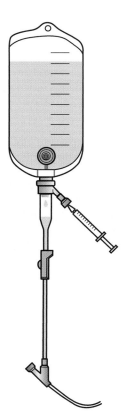

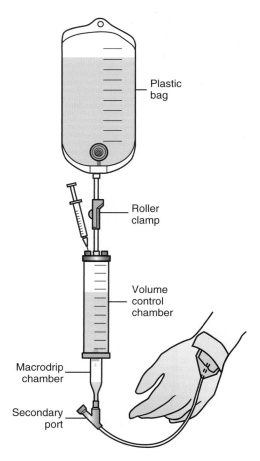

FIGURE **10-20** Adding medication to an IV plastic bag or glass bottle. Close the IV tubing with a roller clamp. Clean medication port with alcohol swab. Add the medication to the primary port of the bottle or the medication vent on the rubber stopper of the IV bag. Air must be let out of the container to equal that of the medication being injected or the medication will leak back out. Gently rotate container to mix the medication in the solution. Release the roller clamp and start the infusion.

FIGURE **10-21** Adding medication to a volume control chamber. Remove the IV container from the pole and squeeze all the liquid from the volume control chamber back into the container. Close the IV tubing with the roller clamp. Rehang the IV container on the pole. Add the medication in the syringe to the volume control chamber through the medication portal. Reopen the roller clamp and slowly infuse the medication.

the specified amount of IV solution and clamp the tubing between the IV bottle or bag and the volume control chamber. Cleanse the medication portal on the volume control chamber with an alcohol wipe and slowly inject the medication into the chamber. Adjust the rate of flow, allowing for infusion of the fluid in the tubing and the volume control chamber within the specified time limit (Figure 10-21). The nurse should label the container with the date, time, dosage, and medication added and sign his initials.

Adding a Medication by Piggyback Infusion. While an infusion is running to keep a vein open, it may be clamped off and a second IV infusion added to allow administration of medication. In this case, rather than injecting medication directly into the medication portal, the medication is added to a second, small IV bottle or bag, which is connected to the medication portal with a small needle. If this second IV container, or **piggyback infusion,** is hung slightly higher than the

first IV container and the tubing to the first container is clamped off, the medication from the smaller container will be infused (Figure 10-22). Usually antibiotics are given in this manner. The smaller IV container should be labeled with the time, date, medication, and dosage, and the nurse's initials. The order will specify the time in which the piggyback infusion should be completed. Once the smaller volume is infused, the setup is removed and the clamp on the original bottle is reopened.

Administration of Medication When There Is Only an Intermittent Infusion Device. When a butterfly or scalp vein needle is inserted and left in place, it also may become a portal for intermittent infusion. These units were formerly called heparin locks or saline locks, depending on what solution was used to flush them. They are now more often referred to as *intermittent infusion devices.* You should wear disposable gloves and use an alcohol wipe to cleanse the top of the rubber

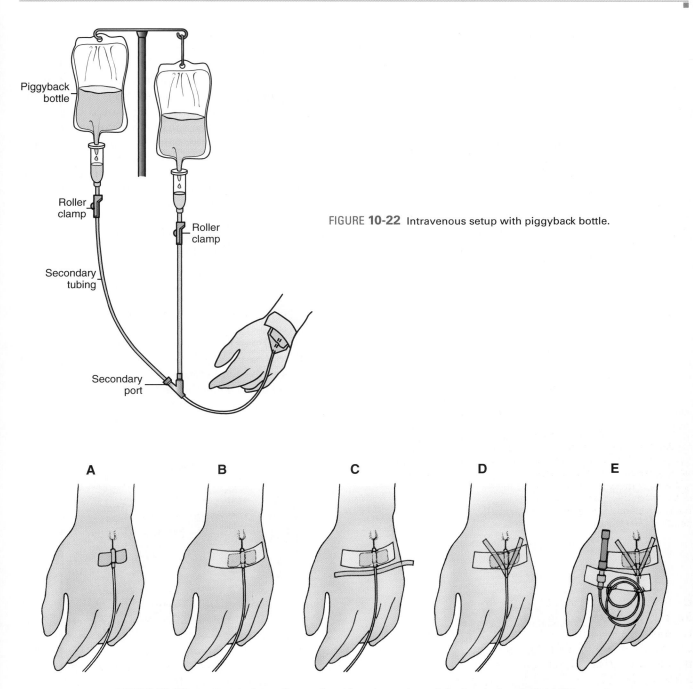

FIGURE **10-22** Intravenous setup with piggyback bottle.

FIGURE **10-23** Taping of a butterfly needle with an intermittent infusion device. **A,** Hold the two plastic wings together and insert the butterfly needle into the vein. **B,** Flatten the plastic wings out and place a strip of adhesive tape over them. **C,** Place another strip of tape just below the wings and under the IV tubing, adhesive side up. **D,** Cross the tape over the wing-tips to anchor the tubing into place. **E,** Coil IV tubing and tape it into place.

diaphragm at the end of the tubing. Pull back the plunger to aspirate blood into the tubing and then slowly inject the medication into the tubing. Follow this by inserting another syringe with 1 to 2 mL of normal saline to flush the medication out of the tubing. Some institutions also use 1 mL of heparin to help keep the tubing open. The nurse must carefully follow the hospital's policy. Clean up any spilled blood or fluid, remove the gloves, and dispose of the equipment properly. Figures 10-23 and 10-24 illustrate the taping of an intermittent infusion device and the addition of medication.

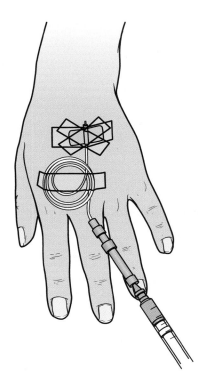

FIGURE **10-24** Adding medications through intermittent infusion device. Cleanse the main adapter plug on the end of the tubing with an alcohol wipe and allow it to air dry. Slowly inject the medication with a syringe. Withdraw the syringe and cleanse the diaphragm again with an alcohol wipe. Using another syringe containing saline, flush the reservoir with 1 to 2 mL of sterile saline. Remove syringe and cleanse diaphragm a final time with an alcohol wipe.

Intravenous Infusion Rates

Because so many factors influence the gravity flow, a solution may not necessarily continue to flow at the rate originally set. Therefore, IV infusions must be monitored frequently to verify that the fluid is flowing at the intended rate. The IV flask or bag should be marked with tape to indicate the rate so that you can tell at a glance whether the correct amount has been infused. The flow should be calculated when the solution is originally hung, and then rechecked at least hourly. To calculate the flow rate, the number of drops delivered per milliliter must be determined. This number varies depending on the equipment used and is usually printed on the solution set packaging. A formula that can be used to calculate the drop rate is as follows:

gtt/mL of given set/60 (min in 1 hr) ×

total hourly volume = gtt/min

A variety of infusion pumps are available to assist in IV fluid delivery. These devices allow more accurate administration of fluids and medications than is possible with routine gravity-flow setups. Some pumps have flow rates calibrated in terms of milliliters per hour and are referred to as *volumetric pumps* (Figures 10-25, 10-26, and 10-27). Others are calibrated in drops per minute

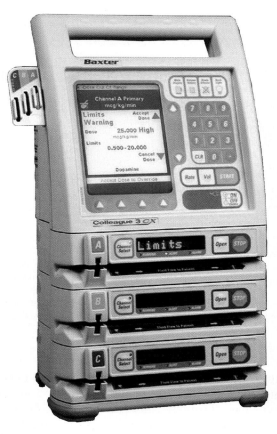

FIGURE **10-26** Colleague® 3CX Volumetric Infusion Pump with Guardian® Feature. (Copyright Baxter Healthcare Corporation, Deerfield, IL.)

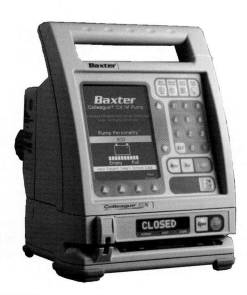

FIGURE **10-25** Colleague® CX Volumetric Infusion Pump. (Copyright Baxter Healthcare Corporation, Deerfield, IL.)

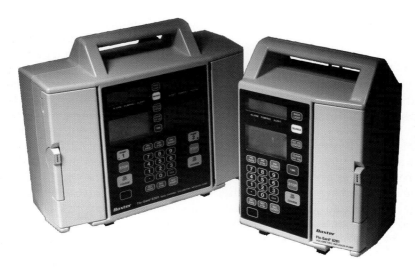

FIGURE **10-27** Flo-Gard® 6201 and Flo-Gard® 6301 Volumetric Infusion Pumps. (Copyright Baxter Healthcare Corporation, Deerfield, IL.)

and are referred to as *infusion controllers*. It is important to read the manufacturer's directions carefully before using any infusion pump or controller because there are many variations in available models. Use of these devices does not eliminate the need for frequent monitoring of the infusion and the patient.

Small pumps weighing about half a pound are now available as portable infusion systems for continuous drug treatment of certain patients with type 1 diabetes or cancer. The systems currently in use generally consist of a battery, a programmable electronic "brain," an electric motor and a pump, and a syringe. All of these parts can be removed as a unit from the small needle kept in place in either subcutaneous abdominal or thigh tissue in the diabetic patient or by a Silastic catheter inserted into an artery supplying the malignant tumor in a cancer patient. Some systems are designed to be worn externally over clothing, stored in a pocket, or suspended from a belt or a neck chain (Figure 10-28). Others are implanted within a subcutaneous pocket in the lower abdomen or elsewhere. The starting dosage levels and six other parameters of therapy are programmed initially by the physician. With this open-loop system, the patient measures the blood glucose levels throughout the day and calculates any necessary adjustments in the baseline infusion rate. The patient places the day's supply of insulin in a syringe and inserts the syringe into the pump. A length of special tubing is connected to the hub of the syringe, and a subcutaneous needle is attached to the distal end. The patient inserts the needle into the abdomen in the same manner used for a subcutaneous injection. The needle is then taped in place, and the infusion begins. The patient can also push a button that releases a bolus dose to cover each meal consumed. The infusion site is changed every 2 days and kept dry to prevent bacterial contamination.

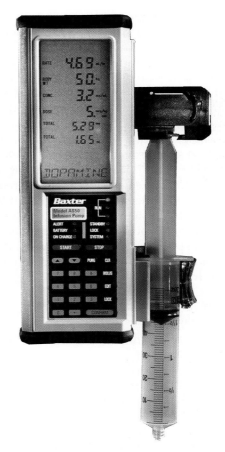

FIGURE **10-28** Auto Syringe® AS50 Infusion Pump. (Copyright Baxter Healthcare Corporation, Deerfield, IL.)

A second type of pump is a closed-loop system, sometimes called an *artificial pancreas*. This unit consists of a device that constantly measures blood glucose levels and sends information to a small computer, which calculates the needed dose of insulin and triggers the batter-powered delivery system. The insulin is then delivered through a subcutaneous needle that is usually implanted in the abdomen.

Additional Delivery Systems

Several other sites may be used for long-term administration of fluids and medication following special placement of catheters by a physician.

The *Hickman catheter* has been used for years as a venous access device. This device is commonly used for obtaining blood samples and to administer medications or hyperalimentation. This catheter and other similar venous access devices are implanted in a large vein such as the cephalic or internal jugular vein. The tip extends into the right atrium, and the end of the catheter exits the vessel through the chest wall. The end of the catheter has an intermittent infusion port attached. The flushing and special care of this tubing are required to keep it patent (open and unblocked).

Using the *epidural route*, a catheter is placed into the spinal column through a lumbar puncture. Anesthesia and narcotic analgesics are often administered by this route during surgery and postoperatively. The procedure for injecting or infusing medication through the epidural catheter follows that used for the IV route. The epidural route requires much lower doses of medication than the IV route; in addition, the effects of the medication last longer.

PCA and PCEA systems are often used in both venous and epidural sites for continuous pain control. These systems control the medication dose but allow the patient to control when analgesia is delivered. There is a lockout period if the patient has exceeded the authorized dose. These systems are left in place for extended periods of time. The almost routine placement of a PCA system in hospitalized patients provides a method for nurses to administer medication repeatedly to patients and avoid frequent IM injections.

General Nursing Actions for a Patient with an Intravenous Infusion

A patient receiving an IV infusion should be checked hourly, and the rate of infusion should be closely monitored. When an infusion runs behind schedule, the infusion rate should never be increased to "catch up." Too much fluid could overwhelm infants and patients with congestive heart failure, arrhythmias, pulmonary edema, or kidney failure. Intake and output records should be closely monitored. The patient should maintain an hourly output of 30 mL of urine or more. Any decrease in this level should be reported to the physician.

When one IV infusion has been completed and another is started, the rate should be turned down very low to keep the vein open but not stopped. Using aseptic technique, the old infusion container is clamped off, the old container is exchanged for a new container, and the drip chamber is filled halfway before the tubing is unclamped and the rate is recalculated.

If the completed infusion is to be discontinued, you should explain to the patient what is to happen, then clamp the tubing, loosen the adhesive tape, and put on gloves. Holding a gauze pad in your nondominant hand, you should apply gentle pressure on the venipuncture site with the pad as you carefully withdraw the needle with your dominant hand. The needle should be inspected to make sure it is intact. The area should be cleaned with an alcohol wipe and elevated if possible, and direct pressure should be applied to stop any bleeding at the site. Check for bleeding after 1 to 2 minutes. Follow institutional procedure in applying an antibiotic ointment, povidone-iodine (Betadine), or just a clean pressure dressing to the area. Dispose of all contaminated equipment in the authorized way.

In evaluating the patient receiving an infusion, there are six primary areas of concern.

Failure to Infuse Properly. Occasionally, the tubing may become bent or the patient may be lying on the tubing, preventing proper infusion. At other times, the needle may become lodged against the wall of the vein; pulling back slightly on the needle and reanchoring it will start the flow again. Sometimes the rate of infusion is so slow that a small clot may form at the end of the needle, blocking the flow. The IV container might have to be elevated to keep adequate pressure for infusion, or blood pressure cuffs or tight gowns that are restricting fluid flow might have to be removed. Starting at the bottle and moving downward, check every part of the infusion setup for problems. If the IV container is placed below the needle site and the needle is in place and not obstructed, gravity should cause blood to run back into the tubing. If blood fails to return to the tubing, you should suspect that the needle is out of place or blocked.

Infiltration. Another common complication occurs when the needle becomes dislodged from the vein, allowing infusion of medication and fluid into the tissues (infiltration). This produces pain, swelling of the area, and redness. When some kinds of medication accidentally leak into tissue, they can irritate and damage the tissue. Whenever IV infiltration is discovered, the infusion site must be carefully inspected for signs of injury. The infusion should be discontinued and the physician contacted, especially if necrosis, sloughing, blistering, or unusual swelling is seen. Warm, moist compresses should be applied to the area. Sometimes other drugs are injected to counteract the medication that accidentally infused into the tissue.

Air in the Tubing. Air that is infused into a patient is potentially dangerous, producing a bubble in the bloodstream. If air is seen in the tubing, the tubing should immediately be clamped below the air bubble and, using aseptic technique, the air should be withdrawn through a syringe and a needle should be inserted at the piggyback portal, or at the hub of the needle. All air, fluid, and blood in the syringe should then be discarded. Small amounts of air probably will not harm the patient. Should a larger amount of air actually enter the patient through the tubing, he should be placed with the head down and turned on the left side, and the physician notified. The patient should be given oxygen if he complains of shortness of breath.

Signs of Infection. Redness, swelling, warmth, and burning along the course of the vein are signs of infection or inflammation of the vein (phlebitis) and are often produced or aggravated by irritating medication. They are commonly seen with medications such as potassium, antibiotics, or anticancer drugs but may occur with any infusion. The IV should be stopped, the physician should be notified, and warm, moist compresses should be applied to the area.

A contaminated infusion that causes a systemic infection is rare. If the patient suddenly develops chills, fever, nausea, vomiting, and headache, the infusion should be immediately stopped, the patient closely monitored, and the physician contacted. The solution should be saved so that cultures may be taken.

Allergic Reactions. Some products create an allergic response in the patient. Antibiotics often cause shortness of breath, temperature elevation, or rash. Reactions to blood or blood products are also common, producing shaking chills, hematuria, and temperature elevations. The medication infusion should be stopped and the physician notified.

Circulatory Problems. Problems in the systemic circulation are produced primarily in two forms: circulating particles (which can cause pulmonary embolism) or excess fluid volume (which can cause pulmonary edema).
1. *Pulmonary embolism.* When particles of medication or pieces of a blood clot break loose and travel in the patient's bloodstream, they may become trapped in the lungs, causing shortness of breath as blood flow is blocked. Poor color, chest pain, restlessness, and coughing up blood may also be signs of pulmonary emboli. Infusion containers and IV lines should be kept clean, medications should be adequately dissolved, and filters should be used routinely in the IV lines. Embolism is an emergency, and the physician should always be notified promptly.
2. *Pulmonary edema.* Elderly patients, emaciated patients, infants, and children are particularly sensitive to the amount of fluid infused. These individuals may have heart, lung, or kidney problems that decrease their ability to handle extra fluid. Circulatory overload may develop when fluids are infused too rapidly, or when the volume is too great. Signs of circulatory overload include dyspnea; weakness; lethargy; reduced urine output; edema; swelling of the extremities; dependent edema; weak, rapid pulse; and shallow, rapid respirations.

In some individuals, the excess fluid accumulates primarily in the lungs, producing coughing, difficulty breathing, crackles in the lung sounds, and frothy sputum. The infusion should be slowed and the physician notified if these symptoms develop.

Table 10-3 summarizes the problems that may occur with an IV infusion and the appropriate nursing actions to take.

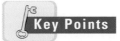

Key Points

- This section has stressed the procedures involved in administering parenteral medications, including the equipment, anatomic sites, and aseptic technique involved.
- The nurse should follow the standard agency procedure to ensure safe administration of parenteral medications and to protect staff from personal risk of infection.

Table 10-3 *Common Problems with Intravenous Infusions*

PROBLEM	NURSING ACTION TO TAKE
Failure to infuse properly	Check for bent tubing, needle against vein wall, or small clot at needle end; the IV pole may be too low, or the needle may be out of the vein. Check for damage done from tissue infusion. Stop infusion and restart it if required.
IV infiltration	Check to see if any tissue was damaged. Notify physician of any necrosis or sloughing. Apply wet compresses to the area to reduce pain. Stop infusion and restart it if required.
Air in tubing	Clamp tubing and remove the air with a syringe. If air was infused into the patient, put the patient in the head-down position, lying on the left side, and notify the physician.
Signs of infection	Check for local and systemic symptoms. Stop infusion, restart with a fresh setup, and notify physician. Treat symptomatically. Save the solution for testing.
Allergic reactions	Stop infusion and notify the physician.
Circulatory problems	Watch for symptoms of pulmonary edema: shortness of breath, poor color, weight gain, restlessness, edema. Notify the physician.
	Watch for symptoms of pulmonary embolus: poor color, shortness of breath, chest pain, coughing up blood. Notify the physician.

Percutaneous Medications

PERCUTANEOUS ADMINISTRATION

The topical application of medication for absorption through the mucous membranes or skin is called **percutaneous administration.** The medication acts locally to clean, soften, disinfect, or lubricate the skin. Many products are now given through transdermal systems to provide effects throughout the body (systemic effects).

It is difficult to predict how topical medications will be absorbed. They often have a short duration of action and require frequent applications. Some medications must be properly inhaled, spread, or shampooed to be effective. In addition, many of these medications are greasy or messy to apply and leave stains on clothing and bedding.

The amount of medication absorbed through the skin or mucous membranes depends on several factors:
- The size of the area covered by medication
- The concentration or strength of the drug
- The length of time the medication stays in contact with the skin

The general condition of the skin itself also makes a difference. Important factors include:
- The amount of skin irritation and breakdown
- The thickness of the skin involved
- The general hydration, nutrition, and tone of the skin

Methods of percutaneous administration include the following:
- Putting solutions onto the mucous membranes of the ear, eye, nose, mouth, or vagina

---

PROCEDURE 10-5

Preparing and Administering Percutaneous Medications

STEP ONE: GETTING READY

1. Check the medication order on the Kardex. Check the accuracy of the order as written and the time to be given. Clarify any information now known about the patient or the medication.
2. Wash your hands. This is essential to avoid contaminating the medication. Although it seems an obvious step, it is often neglected by busy nurses.
3. Assemble all the medication equipment. In addition to the medication order or card, obtain the medication tray; medication jars, tubes, or boxes; medication cart; gloves; plastic wrap; and tongue blades.

STEP TWO: PREPARING THE MEDICATION

1. Read the order on the medication card, and obtain the correct medication from the cabinet or cart. Medications may come in bottles, disks, patches, tubes, drops, sprays, and jars. Medication containers are commonly taken to the bedside for administration.
2. Compare the medication card with the label on the container. First check for the right patient, drug, route, dosage, and time of administration.
3. Place the medication next to the medication card on the tray.

STEP THREE: ADMINISTERING THE MEDICATION

1. Go the patient's bedside. Help the patient get into a position appropriate for the medication being given. Ask the patient his name at the same time you are checking the patient's identification bracelet and bed tag. Never give medication without positively identifying the patient. Confused or very ill patients may answer to any name.

2. Explain what you are giving and answer any of the patient's questions. Give any special instructions or teach the patient about the medication as indicated. Make any special assessments required. If the patient makes any comments about the medication looking different from usual, having just taken the medication, or not having had that medication before, recheck the medication order.
3. Cleanse the site of previous medication if necessary. Examine for signs of irritation, infection, or swelling.
4. Compare the information on the medication card with the label on the container. This is the second check for accuracy.
5. Put on gloves.
6. Before beginning administration, check the information on the container for the third time with the medication card.
7. Follow the specific procedure for applying the solution, powder, ointment, or shampoo. Cover the area with a plastic wrap or a dressing as ordered to increase absorption.

STEP FOUR: CONCLUDING

1. Discard all used dressings and gloves in the dirty utility room.
2. Note on the chart the time the medication was given and sign your name or initials. Record accurately that the medication was given as ordered.
3. Check the patient again later and note any particular responses or adverse effects that should be recorded and reported.

- Applying topical creams, powders, ointments, or lotions
- Inhaling aerosolized liquids or gases to carry medication to the nasal passages, sinuses, and lungs

PROCEDURE FOR ADMINISTERING PERCUTANEOUS MEDICATIONS

You should follow the same general procedures outlined for other routes of administration when applying medications to the skin or mucous membranes. You must also strictly follow the rules of safety. The general method for giving percutaneous medications is outlined in Procedure 10-5. However, the site of administration and the form of medication may require minor adjustments in the technique you will use for different types of medication.

ADMINISTERING TOPICAL MEDICATIONS

Topical medications are applied directly to the area of skin requiring treatment. The most common forms of topical medications include creams, lotions, and ointments, although there are many others. Each form of topical application has specific advantages and characteristics. Several forms are discussed in Box 10-4.

Technique

1. Always clean the skin before applying medication. This practice not only reduces the chance of infection but also removes any remaining medication from the previous application and prevents the buildup of medication in that area. Water-based and alcohol-based products may be removed with soap and water. Oil-based products may be removed with cottonseed oil and gauze. Coal tar products may be removed with corn oil and gauze.

Box 10-4 | *Common Forms of Topical Medications*

ASTRINGENTS
Astringents are alcohol-based medications used for cleaning oily skin, and for cooling and soothing skin. They have a drying effect.

CREAMS
Creams are semisolid emulsions (mixture of two liquids) that contain medication and a water-soluble base. They are rubbed into the skin.

DISKS OR PATCHES
A disk or a transdermal patch is a semipermeable membrane pad containing medication that is attached to the skin by its adhesive edges. The placement of the pad and length of time it is left in place are ordered by the physician. Medications may be left in place for 24 hours, providing gradual release of medication into the skin. Some estrogen products may be left on for several days. Nitroglycerin patches are often removed during the night to reduce the amount of tolerance the patient develops to the medication. The dosage the patient gets depends on the concentration of the medication and the area of skin covered.

LOTIONS
Lotions are aqueous (watery) preparations that contain suspended materials. They cleanse or soothe the skin, or act as a drawing agent or astringent. Lotions should be shaken thoroughly and applied sparingly by patting on the skin, not rubbing.

OINTMENTS
Ointments are semisolid preparations of medicines in an oily base, such as petrolatum or lanolin. Ointments provide good skin contact and are not easily removed. They are used sparingly, sometimes according to an application guide, and are often covered with dressings.

POWDERS
Powders are finely ground medication particles in a talc base. They are used for their drying, cooling, or protective effects.

SHAMPOOS
Shampoos are medications in an aqueous or alcohol base that are poured onto the hair, allowed to stand, and then rubbed into the hair and scalp before being rinsed off. They are designed to treat problems of the hair and scalp.

SOAPS
Medicated soaps may be used to cleanse the skin and to moisten dry skin. Some soaps also leave a residue that helps reduce bacteria and oil.

SOLUTIONS
Medicated solutions of chemicals mixed with water or normal saline are used as washes or baths, or are applied to wet dressings for wrapping the skin. Chemicals commonly used include boric acid, Burrow's solution, potassium permanganate, and silver nitrate. The mixing directions must be closely followed. Many of these solutions stain the skin and clothing.

2. You should wear gloves for protection. Many skin lesions (sores) contain infectious material that could be spread to you during the treatment process. Also, many medications may be absorbed through your skin as you apply them unless gloves are worn.

3. Lotions are shaken until they are a uniform color and are applied by dabbing the medication onto the skin with a cotton ball or gauze. Lotions are not rubbed into the skin.

4. Ointments and creams should be applied with a tongue depressor or a cotton-tipped applicator. Medication is scooped out or squeezed onto the applicator and then applied to the patient's skin with a firm stroke. If the area is to be covered with a dressing, the ointment may be applied directly to the gauze with the tongue depressor and then the gauze is applied to the skin. Creams are generally rubbed into the area, whereas ointments are just spread thinly and evenly over the skin. More is not better; this is an error that both patients and nurses commonly make with ointments.

5. Squeeze extra medication from wet dressings so they are not dripping. Follow directions closely. Dressings may be anchored with hypoallergenic tape, or the physician may request wraps, Ace bandages, gauze pads, plastic wrap, or gloves to cover the area. These coverings increase the sticking and absorption of the medication. They may also reduce staining and grease on clothes and bedding but may limit the patient's ability to move.

6. Many patients with skin lesions worry about their appearance. The treatment process and dressings also may draw attention to areas about which the patient feels embarrassed. These patients need to be cared for in private and given a chance to talk about their feelings about the problem and treatment. Take every chance to help the patient develop good self-esteem.

7. Many treatments for skin problems are continued after the patient leaves the hospital. Teach the patient how to apply the medication and the dressings. If possible, have the patient apply the medication and any dressings while you watch.

Technique for Nitroglycerin Ointment

Medicated ointment is an increasingly common method of giving nitroglycerin to patients with chest pain from angina. When properly applied, nitroglycerin ointment (Nitrol or Nitro-Bid) can provide constant medication to help prevent anginal attacks.

To apply nitroglycerin ointment, select a site on the chest, upper arm, or flank areas. An area without hair should be used. Adhesive tape applied to the skin and removed quickly should help remove small hairs. Do not shave the skin because this may cause skin irritation when medication is applied. Clean the skin gently with an alcohol wipe. The physician or health care provider will order the patient to apply a certain number of inches of nitroglycerin ointment. A measuring applicator paper that looks like a ruler is provided with the medication (Figure 10-29). The correct number of inches of medication is squeezed onto the applicator paper as a small ribbon. The applicator paper is then laid on top of the skin where the medication is to be applied. There are several ways to proceed:

1. The applicator paper is laid on the skin, ointment side down, and left in place. The area is not rubbed.

2. The applicator paper may be covered with plastic wrap that is taped in place to prevent stains on clothing. It must be changed every 3 to 6 hours, depending upon the prescriber's order.

3. The applicator paper is removed, and the area is covered with plastic wrap, spreading the nitroglycerin over a larger area.

Transdermal Delivery Systems

Disks or transdermal patches are another method of giving constant medication through the skin. Some medications using a transdermal delivery system include nitroglycerin, birth control pills, scopolamine, and clonidine. Various antismoking programs also use nicotine patches. The principles for administration are similar to those for applying nitroglycerin ointment.

The medication comes packed over a semipermeable membrane and an adhesive patch. A site is chosen for application according to a standard rotation pattern. The patch is carefully picked up, and the clear plastic backing is removed from the patch, showing the medication (Figure 10-30). The medicated side is then pressed firmly onto the skin. The outer edge of the patch is adhesive and will hold the patch tightly to the skin. Patches are changed daily, unless they become loose or come off and require replacement. Transderm-Nitro and Nitro-Dur and oral birth control patches may be worn while showering; all other medicated patches should be applied after bathing.

ADMINISTERING MEDICATIONS TO MUCOUS MEMBRANES

The mucous membranes are the other major route of percutaneous medication administration. In general, medication is easily absorbed across mucous membranes and it is easy to reach therapeutic dosages. However, all mucous membranes do not have the same sensitivity to medication or the same ability to absorb chemicals. The blood supply under the mucous membranes also varies. These differences may be used to good advantage. For example, putting medication in an oily base will slow its absorption and might help when administering antibiotics, whereas a water-based medication would be quickly absorbed and its action would stop rapidly.

There are seven places where medications are commonly applied to mucous membranes: under the

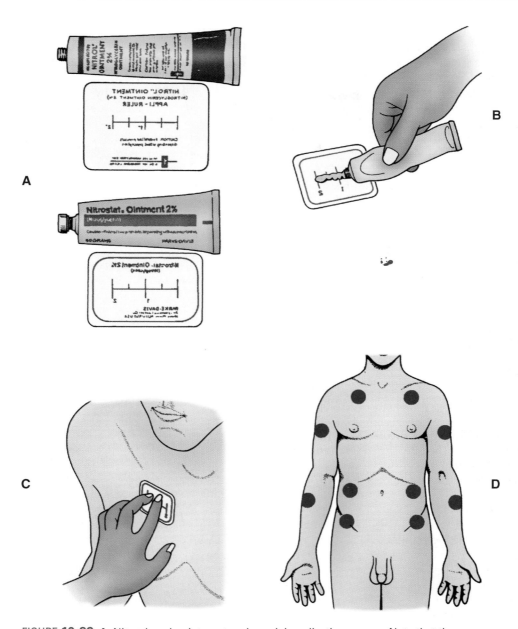

FIGURE **10-29 A,** Nitroglycerin ointment and special application papers. Note that the papers are printed backward. **B,** The correct amount of ointment is squeezed onto the paper. **C,** The paper is applied to the patient's skin in one of the sites shown in **D.** Clear plastic wrap may be applied over the paper to increase absorption and protect clothing from staining.

tongue (**sublingual administration**); against the cheek (**buccal administration**); in the eye, nose, or ear; or inhaled into the lung through an aerosol. Vaginal suppositories, creams, or douches also represent treatment through mucosal membranes. The medications for mucous membranes might come as tablets, drops, ointments, creams, suppositories, or metered-dose inhalers.

The procedure for applying medications to mucous membranes follows the general format already discussed. Different mucous membranes require minor changes in technique, which are listed in Procedure 10-6.

Additional Guidelines

1. All medications applied to mucous membranes must be administered aseptically or by clean technique. You must wash your hands before preparing medications. Gloves should be used to protect you from infections. Standard Precautions recommended by the CDC should be followed each time a medication is administered. Eye drops and eardrops must be instilled carefully to prevent contamination of the droppers or the spread of the infection from one eye or ear to the other. Equipment and dressings used during medication administration must be disposed of properly.

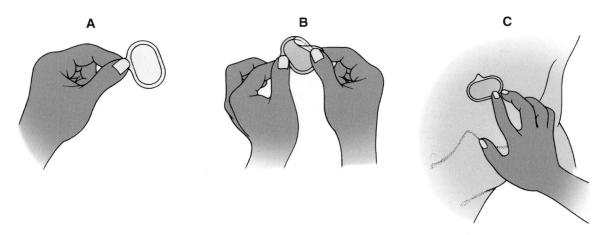

FIGURE **10-30** **A,** Nitroglycerin patch. **B,** Remove the plastic backing, being careful not to touch the medication inside. **C,** Place the side with the medication on the patient's skin and press the adhesive edges into place.

PROCEDURE 10-6

Administering Medications to Mucous Membranes

BUCCAL AREA OF CHEEK

The patient holds the medication between the cheek and molar teeth (*A*), where it is rapidly absorbed into the bloodstream and reaches the systemic circulation without being metabolized by the liver. This site is used for nitroglycerin tablets to relieve chest pain.

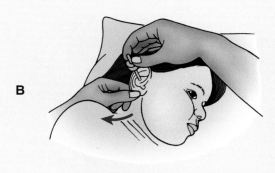

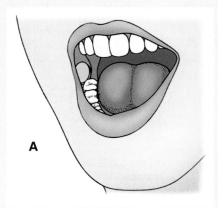

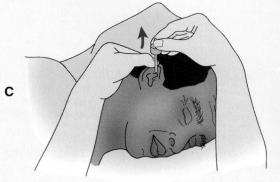

EAR

Localized infection or inflammation of the ear is treated by dropping a small amount of a sterile medicated solution into the ear. Very low dosages of medication are required, and the medication label must indicate that it is for otic (ear) usage. The medication should be at room temperature. The patient should lie on the side with the affected ear up. Shake the medication well and draw the medication up into the dropper. In children younger than 3 years, gently pull the earlobe down and back (*B*); in adults, gently pull the earlobe up and out (*C*). This will straighten the external canal so that the medication may be dropped into the canal. Do not touch the dropper to the ear. The patient is to remain in the same posi-

tion for 5 minutes to allow the medication to coat the surface of the inner canal. A cotton ball may also be inserted if ordered. Repeat in the other ear if indicated.

EYE

Sterile drops or ointments in very low dosage and specifically labeled for ophthalmic (eye) use may be applied to the eye. Gloves are used during the procedure. The eye may be

PROCEDURE 10-6—cont'd

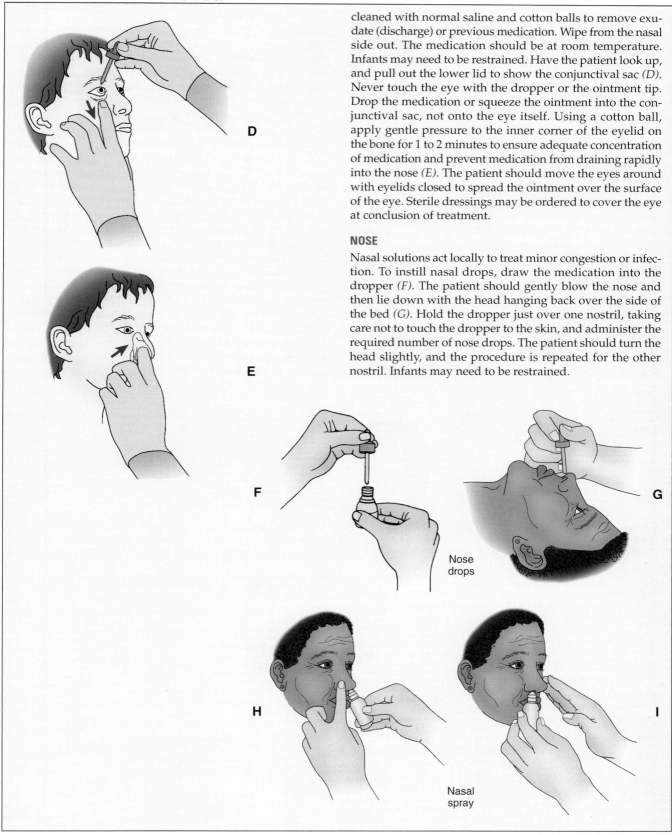

D

E

F

Nose
drops

G

H

Nasal
spray

I

cleaned with normal saline and cotton balls to remove exudate (discharge) or previous medication. Wipe from the nasal side out. The medication should be at room temperature. Infants may need to be restrained. Have the patient look up, and pull out the lower lid to show the conjunctival sac *(D)*. Never touch the eye with the dropper or the ointment tip. Drop the medication or squeeze the ointment into the conjunctival sac, not onto the eye itself. Using a cotton ball, apply gentle pressure to the inner corner of the eyelid on the bone for 1 to 2 minutes to ensure adequate concentration of medication and prevent medication from draining rapidly into the nose *(E)*. The patient should move the eyes around with eyelids closed to spread the ointment over the surface of the eye. Sterile dressings may be ordered to cover the eye at conclusion of treatment.

NOSE

Nasal solutions act locally to treat minor congestion or infection. To instill nasal drops, draw the medication into the dropper *(F)*. The patient should gently blow the nose and then lie down with the head hanging back over the side of the bed *(G)*. Hold the dropper just over one nostril, taking care not to touch the dropper to the skin, and administer the required number of nose drops. The patient should turn the head slightly, and the procedure is repeated for the other nostril. Infants may need to be restrained.

Continued

PROCEDURE 10-6—cont'd

If a nasal spray is used, the solution is shaken, the patient sits upright, one nostril is blocked, and the tip of the nasal spray is inserted into the nostril *(H)*. As the patient takes a deep breath, squeeze a puff of spray into the nostril *(I)*. Wipe tip of spray bottle if medication is to be sprayed into both nostrils. Less medication is required with the spray, and the medication is rapidly absorbed into the vascular areas of the nose for prompt action.

RESPIRATORY MUCOSA

Medication may be carried through the mouth or nose and down into the respiratory tract through use of aerosol neb-ulizers, Spinhalers, or metered-dose inhalers. These tech-niques require special equipment that must be kept very clean, and that breaks the medication up into very small par-ticles, which can be carried with air down into the lungs where the desired action takes place.

Aerosols

Aerosols use a special nebulizer mouthpiece, and medica-tions are diluted according to a special concentration. Oxy-gen is used to deliver the medication. The patient sits upright, places the nebulizer mouthpiece loosely in the mouth, and breathes in and out slowly and deeply while the oxygen is directed through the nebulizer until the medica-tion is gone. The equipment must be cleaned after it is used.

Metered-Dose Inhalers

Metered-dose inhalers are used to deliver specific amounts of corticosteroids or bronchodilators to nasal or lung tissue. These small canisters are pressurized with gas, which pro-pels the medication out and breaks it up into small particles that can be carried deep down into the lungs as the patient takes a deep breath. The medication is carried directly to the site of action with very little systemic effect. The onset of action is rapid. Some medications are designed to be administered through the mouth, and others through the nose. It is important to read the directions completely. The medication should be shaken before use. Instruct the patient to sit upright, and hold the nebulizer in the hand 1 to 2 inches in front of the mouth or at the opening of the nose *(J)*. If the patient cannot cooperate, she may place her lips around the mouthpiece. The patient should exhale, then squeeze the canister in its holder as the next inspiration begins. This will carry medication down into the lungs. The patient should hold her breath as long as possible before exhaling to allow the medication to settle before adminis-tering in the other nostril or taking another puff. It is impor-tant to time the squeezing of the nebulizer to ensure that medication travels in with the next breath and is not just squirted on the back of the throat or nose. The nebulizer must be cleaned with water after each use. It is important that the patient keep an adequate supply of medication on

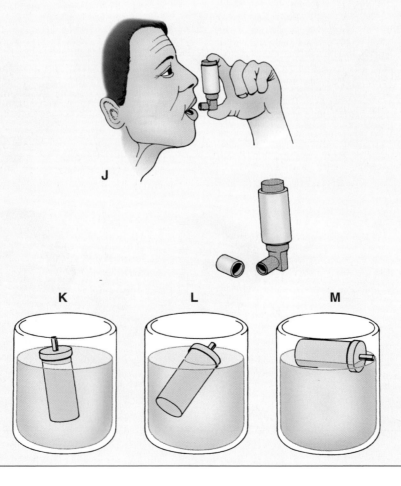

PROCEDURE 10-6—cont'd

hand. Check a metered-dose canister for medication by placing it in a glass of water. *K*, Canister is full. *L*, Canister is partially filled. *M*, Canister is nearly empty.

SUBLINGUAL MUCOSA

The patient places the tablet under the tongue (*N*), where it dissolves, is rapidly absorbed through the blood vessels, and enters the systemic circulation. This site is used for nitroglycerin tablets to relieve chest pain.

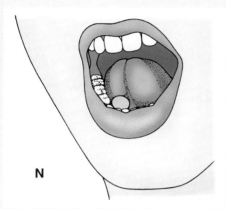

N

VAGINA

Medication to treat local infections or irritation may be applied vaginally through creams, jellies, tablets, foams, suppositories, or irrigations (douches). Room-temperature suppositories are inserted into the vagina with a gloved hand, much like a rectal suppository is inserted. Creams, jellies, tablets, and foams are inserted with a special applicator that comes with the medication. With the patient lying down, the filled vaginal applicator is inserted as far into the vaginal canal as possible and the plunger is pushed, depositing the medication (*O*). The patient is instructed to remain lying down for 10 to 15 minutes so all the medication can melt and coat the vaginal walls. The patient may need a perineal pad to catch any drainage or prevent staining. Gloves must be carefully discarded according to hospital regulations.

Some medicated solutions are used to wash the internal vaginal area when infection and irritation are present. These solutions are administered as douches. The patient may be on a bedpan or reclining in a bathtub. A douche bag containing a medicated solution is hung from an IV pole or shower head so that it is placed about 12 inches above the patient's hips. The tubing is clamped shut. The vulva is gently washed by slowly unclamping the tubing, and then the douche nozzle is inserted into the vaginal canal 3 to 4 inches and pointed downward toward the patient's tail bone (coccyx). The labia are held shut while the solution is gently introduced. As much solution as possible is allowed to fill the vaginal canal before the labia are opened and the solution flows out. The nozzle should be rotated gently to allow the solution to reach and wash all areas. When all the solution has been used, the nozzle is withdrawn, all the equipment is cleaned and put away, and the gloves are discarded.

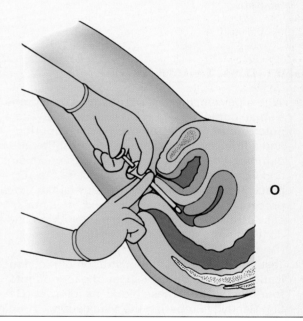

O

2. Accurate recording of medication administration should be made as soon as the medication is given. Medications involving site rotation should be carefully recorded. When medications are given for angina, you must return within a few minutes to assess the patient's response to the medication. Additional medication may be required, or the physician may need to be called.

3. Giving medications is an excellent teaching opportunity. You should take advantage of it each time medication is given and teach the patient about the medication's actions, the important points to follow in giving the medication, and problems to report. When the medication is to be taken at home, the patient should start giving herself the medicine under your supervision as soon as possible. This will provide additional chances for you to assess the patient's learning needs and to answer questions.

Key Points

- Percutaneous medication requires putting medication on the skin or the mucous membranes through a variety of procedures and preparations.
- The basic techniques in percutaneous administration do not usually require the accuracy and precision of parenteral or oral medications.
- The nurse's responsibility in medication administration remains significant.

Go to the free CD-ROM for an Audio Glossary, animations, video clips, and Review Questions for the NCLEX-PN® Examination.

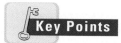 Be sure to visit the companion Evolve website at http://evolve.elsevier.com/Edmunds/LPN/ for WebLinks, a link to the top 200 drugs by prescription, and sign-up pages for newsletter drug updates.

CRITICAL THINKING ?

1. With a partner, use a jar of vitamins or aspirins or a small bottle of juice, a small paper cup, and a note card (for the Kardex) to practice pouring and administering tablets and liquids. Prepare to demonstrate each step as your partner explains, and vice versa, to the rest of the class. As you practice, keep in mind all the steps laid out in the procedure descriptions in the text—it is not as easy as it sounds to remember everything and to do it all in the right order as well!

2. Test yourself on the administration of rectal medications by sectioning a sheet of paper off into four blocks. Label these blocks as follows: "Getting Ready," "Preparing the Medication," "Administering the Medication," and "Concluding the Process." Now fill in as many steps within each phase of administration as you can remember. Without checking your work against the book, exchange lists with a partner and fill in steps you know of that she has left out. Now answer these two questions:
   a. Did your partner's list include anything that you left out of yours? What?
   b. Did your partner add anything to your list that you had not thought of?
   Now check your own work against the text. How many steps in this apparently "simple" procedure did you leave out altogether?

3. Write these three headings across the top of a sheet of paper: "Dose Form," "Description," and "Indications." Now put the oral dose forms listed below in column 1, skipping at least three spaces between each.

buccal forms	elixirs	emulsions
capsules	lozenges	pills
suspensions	syrups	tablets

Now distinguish these forms from one another by completing your table. How are they distinct not only in form but also in indications?

4. Describe techniques and considerations unique to PEG medication administration.

5. You have just entered the medication room where Lisa, another nurse, has just finished pouring capsules for Mr. Johnson, when she is called away in an emergency. As she rushes past you, she calls back, asking you to please give Mr. Johnson his medication. She points to the cup as she slips out the door. What should you do?

6. You have been responsible for Mrs. Davis's care for 2 days now, counting today. When you enter her room with her medication, she seems groggy and confused; she probably just woke up, you think. You greet her, set down the medication, but then discover that she no longer has on her identification band. However, it is time for her medication, you know her well, she answers to her name, and you do not want to delay her medication. Under these circumstances, can you administer her medication and then find out what happened to her identification band?

7. Describe Standard Precautions for preventing the transmission of HIV.

8. What is the purpose of the Z-track injection technique? Describe how it is given. Can this method be used for any intramuscular injection?

9. Point out the differences in site, absorption, and technique between each of the following parenteral routes: intradermal, subcutaneous, IM, and IV.

10. How do you get rid of bubbles in a filled syringe? Why should you bother?

11. List as many forms of percutaneous medications as you can. Now check your work in the text; add whatever you left out. Identify unique steps in the administration of each.

12. Your patient is due to receive an oral antiemetic around the clock to control his nausea and vomiting. As you enter his room to administer his next dose, you observe him beginning to vomit. You know his medication is available as a rectal suppository. Should you administer the medication as a suppository?

11 Allergy and Respiratory Medications

Objectives

After reading and studying this chapter, you should be able to do the following:

1. Identify major antihistamines used to treat breathing problems.
2. Describe the action of antitussive medications.
3. List medications used to treat and prevent asthma attacks.
4. Describe the major actions and the adverse reactions of the two main categories of bronchodilators.
5. Identify at least six medications commonly used as decongestants.
6. Describe the mechanism of action for expectorants.
7. List the major contraindications to the use of nasal steroids.

Key Terms

Be sure to check out the bonus material on the free CD-ROM, including selected audio pronunciations.

antihistamines (ăn-tĭ-HĬS-tă-mēnz, p. 142)
antitussives (ăn-tĭ-TŬS-ĭvz, p. 146)
bronchodilators (brŏn-kō-DĪ-lā-tŏrz, p. 150)
bronchospasm (BRŎN-kō-spăzm, p. 148)
contraindications (p. 143)
expectorants (ĕk-SPĔK-tŏr-ănts, p. 160)
histamine (HĬS-tă-mēn, p. 142)
leukotriene receptor inhibitors (lū-kō-TRĪ-ēn, p. 156)
ototoxic (ō-tō-TŎK-sĭk, p. 143)
perennial allergic rhinitis (PAR) (ă-LĔR-jĭk rī-NĪ-tĭs, p. 142)
perennial nonallergic rhinitis (PNAR) (NŎN-ă-lĕr-jĭk, p. 142)
precautions (p. 143)
prophylaxis (prō-fĭl-ĂK-sĭs, p. 148)
rebound effect (p. 143)
rebound vasodilation (vā-sō-dī-LĀ-shŭn, p. 157),
refractoriness (rē-FRĂK-tō-rĭ-nĕs, p. 151)
seasonal allergic rhinitis (SAR) (p. 142)
sympathomimetics (SĬM-păth-ō-mĭ-MĔT-ĭks, p. 150)
wheezing (p. 148)
xanthines (ZĂN-thēnz, p. 150)

OVERVIEW

This chapter looks at medications that affect the respiratory system. Section One, Antihistamines, describes medications used to treat breathing problems caused by allergies. Section Two discusses antitussives, or medications used to control coughing. Section Three describes the several different categories of medications used for the prophylaxis (prevention) and treatment of asthma and chronic obstructive pulmonary disease (COPD). Sections Four and Five cover decongestants and expectorants. The final section discusses nasal steroids used to treat respiratory problems.

RESPIRATORY SYSTEM

The respiratory system is made up of the lungs and the respiratory passages (Figure 11-1). The upper respiratory system—the oral and nasal cavity, sinuses, pharynx, larynx, and trachea—provide the passages for air to move into the bronchi and lungs (the lower respiratory system). The lungs are divided into lobes. The respiratory system acts to exchange gases (oxygen and carbon dioxide) between the blood and the air and regulates blood pH.

When you take a deep breath (inspiration), the diaphragm drops down; at the same time the intercostal muscles contract, which raises the ribs, increases the size of the chest, and creates a negative pressure. The negative pressure causes air to rush into the lungs through the respiratory passages. When you breathe out (exhalation), the muscles relax, the pressure increases in the chest, and air is passively forced out of the lungs. Thus, the chest works when breathing in, but rests when breathing out.

Any part of the respiratory passages or structures and the lungs themselves may be abnormal. Strictures (narrowed openings) or obstructions (blockage) caused by infection or mucus, collapse of the bronchioles caused by asthma, or infectious masses or tumors are common problems requiring medication. The upper airways are often the site of allergic reactions and bacterial and viral infections.

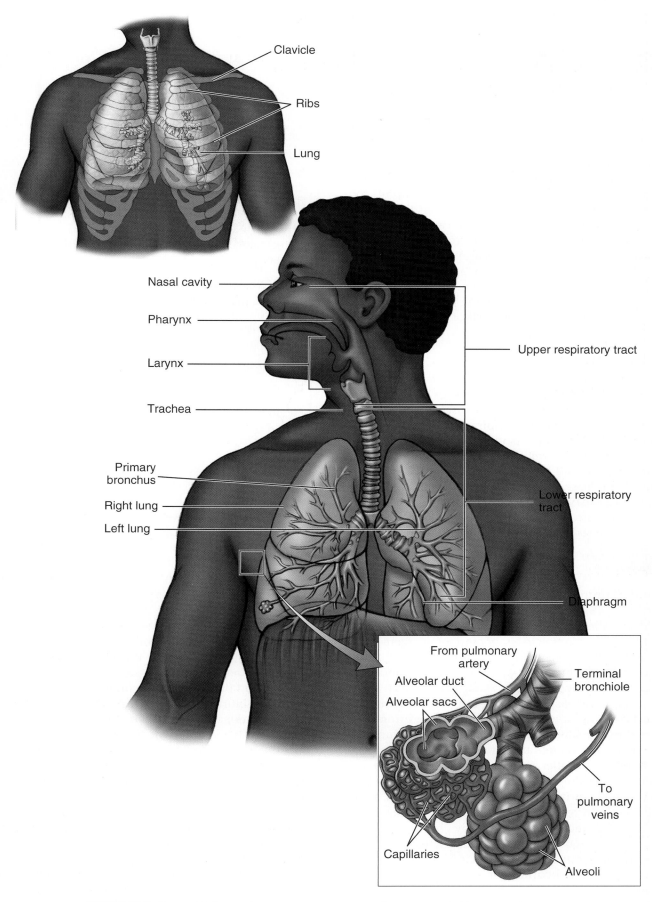

Clavicle

Ribs

Lung

Nasal cavity

Pharynx

Larynx

Trachea

Upper respiratory tract

Primary bronchus

Right lung

Left lung

Lower respiratory tract

Diaphragm

From pulmonary artery

Alveolar duct

Alveolar sacs

Terminal bronchiole

To pulmonary veins

Capillaries

Alveoli

FIGURE **11-1** Organs of the respiratory system: upper respiratory tract and lower respiratory tract.

Antihistamines

OVERVIEW

Histamine is a chemical produced by the body that causes the inflammatory response. The mast cells found near capillaries and the white blood cell basophils contain large amounts of histamine. When the body is injured, histamine is released and it causes the smooth muscle and vascular system to increase blood flow by opening up the capillaries. This also makes the skin turn red. Fluid then escapes from the capillaries into the tissues, causing swelling. The amount of histamine that is released after an injury or an allergic reaction varies. **Antihistamines** relieve the effects of histamine on body organs and structures.

ACTION

Antihistamines block the action of histamine by competing with it for the H_1 receptor sites on the effector structures (e.g., vascular and nonvascular smooth muscles, salivary glands, and respiratory mucosal glands). This acts to limit the vasodilation (opening) and increased capillary permeability and to reduce the edema (swelling) caused by histamine. Antihistamines also limit the release of acetylcholine, producing an anticholinergic (drying) effect, particularly in the bronchioles and gastrointestinal (GI) system. Antihistamines also have a sedative effect on the central nervous system (CNS).

USES

Antihistamines are used to treat **seasonal allergic rhinitis (SAR)** and **perennial allergic rhinitis (PAR).** Allergic rhinitis is a condition in which the patient has a reaction to either outdoor allergens (SAR) or indoor allergens (PAR). Histamine plays a central role in producing most of the typical eye and nasal signs and symptoms such as sneezing, nasal stuffiness, and postnasal drip. These signs and symptoms are also found in patients with **perennial nonallergic rhinitis (PNAR),** which involves inflammation of the mucous membranes of the nose caused by problems other than allergies. Antihistamines are also used to relieve symptoms of other allergic disorders (particularly urticaria [hives], angioneurotic edema, serum sickness, and reactions to blood or plasma) and as an adjunctive (additional) therapy in anaphylactic (shock) reactions. Antihistamines are used in combination cold remedy capsules to decrease mucous secretion and at bedtime for sedation so people can sleep.

There are six main groups of antihistamines, with various characteristics and actions. These groups and some specific drugs within each group are listed in Box 11-1.

| Box 11-1 | *Major Antihistamine Groups* |

ALKYLAMINES
brompheniramine
chlorpheniramine
dexchlorpheniramine

ETHANOLAMINES
clemastine
diphenhydramine

ETHYLENEDIAMINE
tripelennamine

PHENOTHIAZINE
promethazine

PIPERAZINE
hydroxyzine

PIPERIDINES
azatadine
cetirizine
cyproheptadine
fexofenadine
loratadine
phenindamine

ADVERSE REACTIONS

Some of the adverse reactions that may develop and that you should watch for in the patient receiving antihistamines include hypertension (high blood pressure), hypotension (low blood pressure), tachycardia (rapid heartbeat), blurred vision, confusion, dizziness, drowsiness, excitation, insomnia (inability to sleep), paradoxic excitation (when a patient shows stimulation rather than the usual sedation), restlessness, sedation, tinnitus (ringing in the ears), anorexia (lack of appetite), constipation, diarrhea, dry mouth, nausea, vomiting, difficult or painful urination, impotence, urinary retention or frequency, photosensitivity (abnormal response to exposure to sunlight), rash, urticaria (itching), nasal congestion, and thickening of bronchial secretions because of direct mucosal drying.

Antihistamine overdosage is potentially fatal, particularly in children. The symptoms of overdosage occur when the CNS is being stimulated and depressed at the same time.

DRUG INTERACTIONS

The sedative effect commonly seen with antihistamines is increased when other CNS depressants (such as hypnotics, sedatives, tranquilizers, depressant analgesics, and alcohol) are used along with the antihistamine. Antihistamines also add to the effect of anticholinergic drugs, and they can strengthen the anticholinergic side effects of monoamine oxidase (MAO) inhibitors, as well as tricyclic antidepressants. When antihistamines are used along with **ototoxic** drugs (drugs that may damage hearing, such as large doses of aspirin or other salicylates, or streptomycin), the ototoxic effects may be masked. Antihistamines can decrease the effect of corticosteroids and many hormones. They may also interfere with the effects of anticholinesterase drugs.

Nursing Implications and Patient Teaching

Assessment

You should learn as much as possible about the health history of the patient, including the presence of drug allergy, other drug use, and the presence of asthma, glaucoma, peptic ulcer, prostatic hypertrophy, bladder neck obstruction, or respiratory or cardiac disease, and the possibility of pregnancy. A patient with thyroid disease or migraine headaches may be unable to take antihistamines because of the tachycardia (rapid heartbeat) produced. These conditions are either **contraindications** (factors that rule out the use of a drug) or **precautions** (factors that indicate that a drug should be used with great care) for the use of antihistamines.

As you listen to the patient describe her symptoms, think about whether her problem is SAR, PAR, or PNAR. The patient may have a history of allergic reactions with allergic nasal congestion (usually seasonal in onset), runny nose, or cough related to a cold or allergy. You may observe symptoms of rhinitis: sneezing, nasal discharge, and inflamed nasal mucosa. The patient may also have edema, skin lesions, dermatographism (wheals, or a raised surface of the skin where it has been scratched), conjunctivitis (inflammation of the inner eyelid and eye), eczema (irritation of the skin), insect bites, or contact dermatitis. The nasal mucosa may be swollen, boggy (soft), and pale, and there may be nasal plugging or a clear watery discharge. Increased sinus pressure may be found when pushing on or palpating the frontal or maxillary sinuses.

The use of antihistamines in young children may cause hallucinations, convulsions, and even death. Elderly patients are also extremely sensitive to these drugs. Some products may cause teratogenic effects (deformities) in a fetus. Antihistamines should be used with caution in children with a family history of sleep apnea or sudden infant death syndrome (SIDS), or in children with symptoms of Reye's syndrome.

Diagnosis

Through reading the patient's history, you should learn both the type of allergic reaction—SAR, PAR, or PNAR—and whether the medication is being given for some other type of allergic reaction. The severity of the symptoms will help in making the diagnosis and in deciding about additional nursing actions you should take (for example, hydration of the patient [giving him lots of fluid] or looking for an infection).

Planning

The sedative effect is common to most antihistamines, except for products such as loratadine. The drowsiness caused by antihistamines makes it dangerous for the person taking them to operate heavy machinery or drive.

Some antihistamines may be given parenterally to treat hypersensitivity to blood products, as adjunctive therapy to analgesia, or in treating motion sickness. Most antihistamines are administered orally. Many are available in over-the-counter (OTC) preparations, although the forms with the highest dosage are available only by prescription. Most drug companies have at least one preparation that is available by prescription, so that people with Medicare/Medicaid benefits are able to get these drugs with their cards.

Implementation

Antihistamines should be taken only when needed. The type and dosage should be chosen for the desired effect and the person being treated. For example, ethanolamine derivatives make people very sleepy, and people who do tasks that require alertness probably should not use them. Some drugs cause less drowsiness but may not be as effective in getting rid of the symptoms for some people.

If tolerance (increased resistance to a drug caused by repeated use) to one type of antihistamine develops, switch to another type to see if it is helpful. Medications can be changed or rotated to keep the symptoms under control. You should remind the patient to not chew sustained-release tablets or capsules.

Giving oral doses with meals or milk can limit GI side effects. Antihistamines given orally are usually well absorbed; parenteral administration is rarely needed. When an intramuscular (IM) preparation such as diphenhydramine is used, it should be injected deep into the muscle to prevent tissue irritation. Antihistamines should not be given subcutaneously. Intravenous (IV) injection of these agents should be done slowly, with the patient lying down. Long-term use of topical nasal antihistamines increases the risk of sensitization, often causing a **rebound effect,** or an increase in the symptoms you are trying to stop.

Table 11-1 presents additional information on the antihistamines.

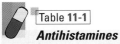

Table 11-1

Antihistamines

GENERIC NAME	TRADE NAME	COMMENTS AND DOSAGE
ALKYLAMINES		Alkylamines are effective at low dosages and are practical for daytime use. They may cause both CNS stimulation (excitation) and depression (drowsiness); the individual response is variable.
brompheniramine	Bromfed Dimetapp	Dimetapp tablets are available OTC. *Adults and children older than 12 yr:* 4 mg PO q4-6h. Do not exceed 24 mg in 24 hr.
chlorpheniramine	Chlor-Trimeton	Sustained-release forms are not for use in children younger than the age of 6; there is a low incidence of side effects. Available OTC. *Adults:* 2-4 mg PO 3 or 4 times daily; sustained-release tablets: 8-12 mg PO q8-12h during the day or at bedtime. *Children:* 1-2 mg PO 3 or 4 times daily.
dexchlorpheniramine	Polaramine 🍁	Same as for chlorpheniramine.
ETHANOLAMINES		Ethanolamines have the highest incidence of drowsiness, but GI side effects are infrequent.
clemastine	Tavist	*Adults:* 1.34 mg twice daily. *Children 6-12 yr:* 0.67 mg twice daily.
diphenhydramine	Benadryl Genahist Diphenhist Banophen	Drug has anticholinergic, antitussive, antiemetic, and sedative properties, with high incidence of CNS depressant effects; drowsiness increases with use. *Adults:* 25-50 mg PO 3 or 4 times daily. *Children weighing more than 20 lb:* 12.5-25 mg PO 3 or 4 times daily, or 5 mg/kg/day PO.
ETHYLENEDIAMINE		
tripelennamine	PBZ PBZ-SR	There is a low incidence of side effects; the elixir is very palatable. *Adults:* 25-50 mg PO q4-6h, maximum 600 mg PO in 24 hr; sustained-release tablet: 100 mg in the morning and evening. *Children older than 5 yr:* 50 mg PO in the morning and evening; maximum 300 mg in 24 hr.
PHENOTHIAZINE		Phenothiazines have a strong CNS depressant effect (drowsiness). Phenothiazines may suppress the cough reflex or mask signs of intestinal obstruction, brain tumor, or overdosage from toxic drugs. See additional information on phenothiazines in Section Three.
promethazine	Phenergan Promethazine	High incidence of side effects, including severe drowsiness; potent drug with prolonged action; use cautiously in ambulatory patients. *Adults:* 25 mg PO or IM at bedtime; may also give 12.5 mg PO before meals and at bedtime if needed. *Children younger than 12 yr:* 6.25 or 12.5 mg PO 3 times daily; may also give 12.5 mg IV or IM.
PIPERIDINES		
azatadine	Optimine	For SAR and PNAR. *Adults and children older than 12 yr:* 1 or 2 mg twice daily.
cetirizine	Zyrtec	For SAR and PAR. Can give to patients with hypersensitivity to hydroxyzine. *Adults and children older than 6 yr:* 5 or 10 PO daily, with or without food. Give 5 mg/day in patients with renal or hepatic dysfunction.
cyproheptadine	Periactin	For SAR and PAR, and hypersensitivity reactions. *Adults:* 4-20 mg daily. May start with 4 mg and reduce. *Children:* Calculate total daily dosage as ~0.25 mg/kg.
fexofenadine	Allegra	For SAR. Analogue of terfenadine (Seldane) but has none of the cardiac dysrhythmias that the other product had before removal from the market. *Adults and children older than 12 yr:* 60 mg twice daily. 60 mg daily in patients with renal dysfunction.

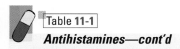

Table 11-1

Antihistamines—cont'd

GENERIC NAME	TRADE NAME	COMMENTS AND DOSAGE
PIPERIDINES—CONT'D		
loratadine	Claritin	Place rapidly disintegrating tablets under the tongue. *Adults and children older than 12 yr:* 10 mg PO daily. *Children 6-11 yr:* 10 mL syrup PO daily. Give same dose every other day if patient has renal or hepatic dysfunction.
phenindamine	Nolahist	*Adults and children older than 12 yr:* 25 mg q4-6h, not to exceed 150 mg in 24 hr. *Children 6-11 yr:* 12.5 mg, not to exceed 75 mg in 24 hr.
PIPERAZINE		
hydroxyzine	Atarax Vistaril	For pruritus, sedation, adjunct to analgesia, antiemetic. *Adults:* 25 mg 2 or 3 times daily. *Children 6 yr and older:* 50-100 mg daily in divided doses. *Children younger than 6 yr:* 50 mg daily in divided doses. *Parenteral:* Adults only—25-100 mg IM as a single dose, then q4-6h prn.
MISCELLANEOUS		
azelastine	Astelin Nasal Spray	For SAR. Prime delivery system with 4 sprays or until a fine mist appears. Reprime with 2 sprays if unused for 3 days. *Adults and children older than 12 yr:* 2 sprays per nostril twice daily. Avoid spraying in eyes.

Evaluation

The therapeutic effect of antihistamines should stop the allergy symptoms. You should watch for any adverse reactions, which are common but mild. Antihistamine use in children and infants is discussed in the Pediatric Considerations box.

Elderly patients are more likely to develop side effects such as dizziness, syncope (light-headedness and fainting), confusion, dyskinesia (difficulty in movements of the body), and tremor. These are called *extrapyramidal reactions*. Considerations for antihistamine use in the elderly are discussed in the Geriatric Considerations box.

The respiratory tract may become dry and the mucus may thicken when using an antihistamine. The patient must drink large amounts of water to thin the secretions and keep the tissues moist.

If any skin reactions occur, the patient should stop taking the drug at once. The CNS depressant effects of antihistamines may be increased if the patient takes more than the recommended dosage or drinks alcohol while using the product. This could be dangerous.

Patient and Family Teaching

You should tell the patient and family the following:
1. The patient should take the medications as ordered and not take more than the recommended dosage.

 Pediatric Considerations

Antihistamines

- Infants and young children often have anticholinergic side/adverse effects.
- Closely watch pediatric patients with spastic paralysis or brain damage, because they often have an increased reaction to these agents, requiring a dosage reduction.
- Anticholinergics, especially in high doses, may cause a paradoxical reaction of increased nervousness, confusion, or hyperexcitability.
- Where hot weather prevails or environmental temperatures are high, children receiving these agents have an increased risk of developing a rapid body temperature increase because the anticholinergic drugs suppress sweat gland activity.
- Start with low doses and increase gradually as needed and tolerated.

Modified from McKenry LM, Salerno E: *Mosby's pharmacology in nursing*, ed 20, St. Louis, 1998, Mosby.

Geriatric Considerations

Antihistamines

The elderly often have anticholinergic side effects, especially constipation, dry mouth, and urinary retention (usually in males).

- Memory impairment has been reported with continuous use of these agents, especially in older patients.
- When usual adult doses are given, some elderly people may have sedation or a paradoxical reaction: hyperexcitability, agitation, or confusion.
- Anticholinergic dosing in the elderly population should begin at the lowest dose with gradual increases, until maximum improvement is noted or intolerable side effects occur.

From McKenry LM, Salerno E: *Mosby's pharmacology in nursing,* ed 21, St. Louis, 2003, Mosby.

2. Most antihistamines cause drowsiness, and the patient must avoid tasks such as driving, for which she needs to be alert.
3. These drugs may cause dizziness, thickening of secretions, and upset stomach, which may require the attention of a nurse, physician, or other health care provider if they continue.
4. If the medication causes stomach upset, taking it with meals or milk can decrease this problem.
5. Although a patient may experience many side effects from one agent, another antihistamine may produce few side effects.
6. Tolerance may develop after use of an antihistamine. If one product seems to stop working over time, the patient can try another antihistamine for better control of symptoms.
7. The patient should stop using antihistamines for 48 hours before having skin tests for allergies.
8. Many antihistamines can be purchased over the counter; some need a prescription. Make certain the patient has a prescription if it is needed.
9. The patient should not take any other medications without the knowledge of the nurse, physician, or other health care provider; it is especially important for the patient to not take alcohol or other sedative drugs while taking an antihistamine.
10. This medication must be kept out of the reach of children and others for whom it is not prescribed; overdosages may be very serious.

SECTION TWO

Antitussives

OVERVIEW

Drugs used to relieve coughing are called **antitussives.** These drugs may either (1) act centrally on the cough center in the brain, (2) act peripherally by anesthetizing stretch receptors in the respiratory tract, or (3) act locally, primarily by soothing irritated areas in the throat. Products vary in their effectiveness. Antitussives are commonly combined with other drugs and are usually sold as OTC drugs. Medications containing narcotics are controlled substances and most require a prescription, although some states may allow codeine combination products to be sold over the counter if the patient signs for them.

ACTION

The main action of an antitussive depends on whether a narcotic is included or not. Narcotic antitussives suppress the cough reflex by acting directly on the cough center in the medulla of the brain. Nonnarcotic antitussives reduce the cough reflex at its source by anesthetizing stretch receptors in respiratory passages, lungs, and pleura, and by decreasing their activity.

USES

Antitussives are used for the relief of overactive or nonproductive coughs.

ADVERSE REACTIONS

Adverse reactions to antitussives include constipation, drowsiness, dry mouth, nausea, and postural hypotension (low blood pressure when a person suddenly stands up).

DRUG INTERACTIONS

Narcotic antitussives have an additive effect with other CNS depressants, and so the dosage should be reduced. Antitussives increase the analgesic effect of aspirin, which may be helpful.

Nursing Implications and Patient Teaching

Assessment

You should learn as much as possible about the health history of the patient, including allergy to antitussives, presence of COPD, possibility of pregnancy, and other drugs or alcohol that the patient takes that may cause drug interactions. These conditions may be contraindications or precautions to the use of antitussives.

The patient may have a history of a nonproductive cough or an overactive cough, which may keep the patient awake at night or cause muscular pain.

Diagnosis

Care should be taken to confirm the cause of a productive cough. Signs of infection, allergy, or other problem should be considered in determining the source of the cough.

Planning

Do not give antitussives to patients with hypersensitivity (allergy) to these drugs or to patients with COPD. Narcotic antitussives may cause drug dependence. Some of the antitussives are Schedule II controlled substances.

These preparations may cause drowsiness, so the patient should be cautioned to avoid tasks requiring alertness after taking the medication.

Implementation

Antitussives come only in oral forms. They should be used only for short periods of time because they can be addictive.

Table 11-2 provides additional information on antitussives.

Evaluation

You should watch for therapeutic effects: the cough stops or there is a decrease in frequency and duration of coughing spells, and the patient is able to sleep better at night. You should watch the patient for adverse reactions and drug tolerance.

Patient and Family Teaching

You should tell the patient and family the following:
1. The patient should take the medication as ordered and not alter the dosage or frequency.
2. Narcotics may cause drowsiness, and the patient must use caution when doing tasks that require alertness.
3. Overuse of the codeine-containing antitussives may cause severe constipation and may also lead to addiction.
4. These drugs increase the effects of alcohol and other drugs that slow the nervous system; the patient should not take any other medications while taking an antitussive.
5. The patient may become nauseated during the first few minutes after taking the medication; this problem goes away if the patient lies down.
6. These drugs occasionally cause lightheadedness, dizziness, or fainting when the patient gets up from a lying or sitting position; tell the patient to change positions slowly.
7. The patient should take the drug with food or milk to decrease stomach upset.
8. This medication must be kept out of the reach of children and others for whom it is not prescribed.

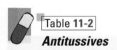

| Table 11-2 |
| **Antitussives** |

GENERIC NAME	TRADE NAME	COMMENTS AND DOSAGE
NARCOTIC ANTITUSSIVES		

codeine
  codeine phosphate
  codeine sulfate
		The average antitussive dose ranges from 10 to 20 mg q4-6h and is effective at this level. Protect codeine from light; do not use in children younger than 12 years of age.
		Adults: 10-20 mg q4-6h.
		Children: 5-10 mg PO 3 to 4 times daily.

hydrocodone	Hycodan	*Adults:* 1 tablet q4-6h.
NONNARCOTIC ANTITUSSIVES		
benzonatate	Tessalon Perles	Anesthetizes stretch receptors. Do not chew drug, because local anesthesia of the mouth will develop. *Adults and children over 10 yr:* 100 mg PO 3 times daily as needed; maximum of 600 mg in 24 hr.
dextromethorphan	Benylin DM Robitussin Vicks Formula 44	Centrally depresses the cough center. *Adults:* 10-20 mg PO q4h or 30 mg PO q6-8h; maximum of 120 mg daily. *Children 2-12 yr:* 2.5-10 mg PO q4h or 15 mg PO q6-8h; maximum of 60 mg daily.
diphenhydramine	Tusstat	Potent antihistamine; safe and effective antitussive. *Adults:* 25 mg PO q4h; maximum of 150 mg daily. *Children:* 6.25-12.5 mg PO q4h; maximum of 75 mg daily.

OVERVIEW

Asthma is a condition in which there is increased inflammation and mucus production, leading to bronchiolar collapse. The patient has no trouble breathing air into the lungs, but the lumens (spaces inside the bronchial tubes) become smaller as the patient attempts to breathe out. This traps air inside the lungs. The patient feels a lack of oxygen, and acts by breathing faster, trapping even more air inside the lungs. As some air is forced out through the small, mucus-lined passages during respiratory expiration, a musical respiratory sound called **wheezing** is heard.

Asthma is caused by a variety of factors, such as deficiencies of some respiratory enzymes, reaction to an allergy, reflex response to cold dry air, or hard exercise. Some individuals have a genetic tendency to develop asthma, and asthma often starts in childhood. For some individuals, it becomes a chronic condition. For others, it may be seen only with acute illnesses or exercise.

The National Heart, Lung, and Blood Institute of the National Institutes of Health has published *Guidelines for the Diagnosis and Management of Asthma.* These guidelines recommend a stepwise plan for using asthma drugs that puts a heavy emphasis on the early use of inhaled antiinflammatory drugs. Asthma is grouped into classes of asthma severity. These classes are (1) mild intermittent, (2) mild persistent, (3) moderate persistent, and (4) severe persistent. In each category, the severity and frequency of daytime symptoms, nighttime symptoms, and lung function are evaluated. The health care provider should work with the patient on prevention, identification of allergens, patient education regarding self-care, and effects of cultural and ethnic influences on asthma management. Because asthma is primarily a disease of inflammation, corticosteroids (both oral and inhaled) are also used in treatment. Some of the steroids used in treating respiratory problems are discussed briefly here, and in greater detail in Chapter 20.

COPD is a slowly worsening, disabling disorder that is identified by abnormal tests of expiratory flow (air that is breathed out) that do not change very much over several months. The damage to the body results from gradual destruction of the alveolar walls, creating unequal areas of ventilation and perfusion. Thus, circulating blood and inhaled air may not come together so that oxygen can be transferred to the blood and waste products in the blood can be removed. COPD attacks or exacerbations are seen with increases in inflammation from pulmonary infections and in response to allergic or nonallergic triggers. Unlike asthmatics, patients with COPD are seldom symptom free, and the disease keeps getting worse. Medications that dilate or open the bronchioles and help thin secretions are helpful in reducing symptoms of dyspnea (uncomfortable breathing).

ASTHMA PROPHYLAXIS (PREVENTION) MEDICATION

ACTION
Cromolyn sodium helps in treating asthma by slowing down the destruction of sensitized mast cells. As mast cells are destroyed, they release histamine and the slow-reacting substance of anaphylaxis (SRS-A) that are created by breathing in specific antigens. By slowing the destruction of mast cells, the symptoms of asthma can be prevented. Cromolyn may also provide hyposensitization (decrease in allergic response) after long-term use by preventing the release of phospholipase. This enzyme assists in the release of chemical mediators from nonsensitized mast cells.

USES
Cromolyn and nedocromil sodium, a drug with actions similar to those of cromolyn, are used to manage bronchial asthma in some patients. How these drugs should be used is clearly described in the national guidelines. These drugs have no antihistaminic, antiinflammatory, or bronchodilator activity. Thus they are effective only for **prophylaxis** (prevention of or protection against disease) and should not be used in an acute attack of asthma. They are also used in some patients with food allergies to prevent GI and systemic reactions; in patients with allergic rhinitis, eczema, and other forms of dermatitis; for patients with chronic urticaria; and for those with postexercise **bronchospasm** (narrowing or collapse of bronchial airways).

ADVERSE REACTIONS
Adverse reactions to cromolyn or nedocromil include dizziness, headache, vertigo (feeling of dizziness or spinning), rash, nausea, bad taste in the mouth, throat irritation, damage to teeth, dysuria (painful urination), urinary frequency, bronchospasm, cough, nasal congestion, wheezing, anaphylaxis, tearing of eyes, and swollen parotid glands. Because these drugs are rapidly eliminated from the body, they are nontoxic except to those who have a hypersensitivity to the drug.

DRUG INTERACTIONS

No drug interactions with cromolyn or nedocromil have been reported.

Nursing Implications and Patient Teaching

Assessment

You should learn as much as possible about the health history of the patient, including specific respiratory signs and symptoms, other medications, allergy, possibility of pregnancy, and presence of infection.

The patient may have a history of allergies, asthma, bronchitis, emphysema, recurrent acute or chronic attacks of wheezing, cough with or without mucoid sputum, dyspnea, fatigue, intolerance to exercise, and, in severe cases, cyanosis (bluish color to the skin). Acute upper or lower respiratory tract infections may precede the onset of acute symptoms.

Diagnosis

Confirm that the patient's condition is stable. These products are not effective in an acute asthma attack. The patient should have no signs or symptoms of illness.

Planning

The patient should begin taking these drugs when an acute attack of asthma is over, the airways are clear, and the patient can breathe easily. Cromolyn is reported to be more effective in children than in adults.

The amount of drug that the lungs are able to use depends on the proper use of the inhaler, the degree of bronchospasm present, and the amount of secretion in the tracheobronchial tree. Only about 5% to 10% of the inhaled drug reaches the lungs.

Implementation

Cromolyn and nedocromil are not absorbed through the GI tract, so they are ineffective when taken orally. Cromolyn is available under the name Intal as an inhaler in 20-mg capsules for inhalation using an oral inhaler called a Spinhaler. A capsule is inserted into the Spinhaler, and the patient sucks in hard on the inhaler, which then spins the medication into small particles that move down into the lungs with each deep breath. The Spinhaler is washed after each use. Adults and children 5 years and older should begin with 20-mg doses inhaled at four equal intervals daily. The dosage can be decreased slowly to the minimum effective level, usually 20 mg three times daily. Nedocromil is a similar product taken by standard inhaler. Two inhalations four times daily at regular intervals is the standard regimen.

Occasionally, cough and bronchospasm may follow administration of cromolyn or nedocromil. Thus some patients may not be able to continue using these drugs even when taking bronchodilators at the same time.

Because of the bad taste, throat irritation, and potential damage to teeth, good oral hygiene is important. Patients should brush their teeth and rinse their mouth after using the Spinhaler.

Be careful when decreasing the dosage or stopping the use of cromolyn or nedocromil; this decrease in dosage can cause asthmatic symptoms to start up again.

You should teach the patient about the proper use and care of the Spinhaler, and have the patient return a demonstration of the procedure.

The cromolyn capsules should be protected from light, moisture, and heat.

Evaluation

Symptoms of asthma should improve within 4 weeks of using cromolyn or nedocromil. The therapeutic effect is shown when asthma attacks stop. Because the drug should be given when a patient's condition is stable, a visit should be scheduled 2 weeks after the first dose, and at least once more within the first 4 weeks to see how effective the medication has been.

Watch the patient carefully when the dose is being reduced or stopped. The drug regimen must be checked if there is no effect within 4 weeks.

Patient and Family Teaching

Cromolyn. You should tell the patient and the family the following:

1. The patient should not swallow the capsules.
2. The capsules should be protected from light, heat, and moisture.
3. The airway should be cleared of as much mucus as possible before taking the drug.
4. The patient should avoid using these drugs if he cannot take a deep breath and hold it, or if he feels he is having an asthma attack.
5. These drugs must be taken every day at regular intervals.
6. If the patient is using a bronchodilator at the same time, it should be used first; then after several minutes the cromolyn or nedocromil may be taken.
7. Throat irritation, dryness of the mouth, and hoarseness may be prevented by rinsing and gargling after each dose.
8. To deliver the appropriate dosage of cromolyn, the patient must use the Spinhaler correctly and keep it clean.
9. Stopping the medication quickly can make the patient have an acute attack of asthma.
10. The nurse, physician, or other health care provider should be called if symptoms do not improve or if they get worse.
11. The patient should avoid breathing moisture into the inhaler. Because the drug is a powder, moisture may cause the powder to clump and may prevent the correct dosage.

Nedocromil. You should tell the patient and the family the following:

1. The inhalation canister must be primed by pressing three times before the first use. Repeat this if the canister remains unused for 7 days.
2. The patient should take the medication at regular intervals and at the same time every day.
3. In a patient whose asthma symptoms are under control, other asthma medication may be decreased as the patient is stabilized.

BRONCHODILATORS

Several types of **bronchodilators** may be given to open the bronchi and allow air to pass out of the lungs more freely; these include the sympathomimetics and the xanthine derivatives. The **sympathomimetics** are beta-adrenergic agents, and they dilate the bronchi through their action on beta-adrenergic receptors. They are also known as adrenergic stimulants. The **xanthines** act directly to relax the smooth muscle cells of the bronchi, thereby dilating or opening up the bronchi.

SYMPATHOMIMETICS

Action

The main action of sympathomimetic bronchodilators in asthma and other respiratory diseases is to relax the smooth muscle cells of the bronchi by stimulating $beta_2$-adrenergic receptors. They also stimulate alpha-adrenergic receptors, which produces a vasoconstriction (narrowing of the blood vessels) response all through the body (systemically), especially a narrowing or contraction in the blood vessels of the bronchial mucosa. This results in less mucosal and submucosal edema. Sympathomimetic bronchodilators also stimulate $beta_1$ receptors, which results in an increased rate and force of the heart's contractions. The sympathomimetic drugs vary in their actions on beta receptors. Some act solely on $beta_2$ receptors, and others have $beta_1$ and $beta_2$ effects. If the drug action is specific to $beta_2$ receptors, there are fewer side effects.

Uses

Sympathomimetic bronchodilators are used for relief of symptoms of bronchospasm occurring in acute and chronic asthma, bronchitis, and emphysema (COPD).

Adverse Reactions

Adverse reactions to sympathomimetic bronchodilators include symptoms related to stimulation of other alpha and beta receptors throughout the body: dysrhythmias (irregular heartbeats), hypotension, tachycardia, anorexia, anxiety, headache, insomnia, nausea, pallor, perspiration, polyuria (excretion of a large amount of urine), restlessness, vomiting, weakness, and urinary hesitancy and retention. These symptoms get worse if there is an overdosage.

Drug Interactions

Thyroid drugs, some antidepressants (tricyclics, MAO inhibitors), some antihistamines, and amphetamines increase the effects of sympathomimetic drugs. Two or more sympathomimetic drugs taken together may cause the symptoms of adverse reactions to become worse. Patients on digitalis or diuretics may experience dysrhythmias if they are given sympathomimetic drugs. Many general anesthetics also cause dysrhythmias when they are used with these drugs. Nonselective beta blockers and beta-adrenergic blocking agents such as propranolol may block the bronchodilating effects of these beta receptor–stimulating drugs. Sympathomimetics can block the action of some antihypertensive medications.

Nursing Implications and Patient Teaching

Assessment

You should learn as much as you can about the health history of the patient, including whether the patient is pregnant or breastfeeding; has a history of hyperthyroidism, heart disease, hypertension, diabetes, glaucoma, seizures, or psychoneurotic disease; is taking other drugs that may interact with the bronchodilators; or has a history of allergy. These conditions may present contraindications or precautions to the use of sympathomimetic bronchodilators.

The patient may have a history of allergies, asthma, bronchitis, emphysema, recurrent acute or chronic attacks of wheezing, and cough. The patient may have had an acute upper or lower respiratory tract infection before the onset of acute symptoms.

Diagnosis

As you work with the patient, you will confirm that the patient is having an asthma attack or has respiratory difficulty from COPD. The asthma pattern shows the severity of asthma. The severity of asthma determines the treatment. In addition, you may determine that the patient has a need for hydration, strategies to reduce anxiety, and education about her condition.

Planning

To relieve bronchial spasm, $beta_2$ receptors in bronchial smooth muscle cells must be stimulated. One of the drawbacks of adrenergic bronchodilators is that their effects are not limited to $beta_2$ receptors. Some agents also stimulate $beta_1$ receptors, which increase the rate and force of cardiac contraction, and alpha receptors, which control vasoconstriction. Thus these bronchodilator drugs should be given with extreme caution to individuals who already have cardiovascular, endocrine, or convulsive disorders.

Implementation

The routes of administration of bronchodilators vary according to how sick the patient is and the preparation to be used. Drugs may be given parenterally, orally, or by oral inhalation (nebulizers, or metered-dose inhalers [MDIs]). The medications selected depend on whether short-term treatment or long-term management is required. A patient who is using an inhaler for the first time should be shown how to use the inhaler, as well as given written instructions that he can refer to later. Every time the patient comes in for health care, he should show how he is using the MDI, because research shows that many patients do not use this device correctly.

Use of more than one sympathomimetic agent at a time is contraindicated.

Refractoriness, or lack of response to a drug that a patient has used before with good effectiveness, may occur if the drug is given too frequently. Patients also may get less relief from aerosols if they are used too often. Irritation of the bronchial tree and oropharynx may occur with use of powdered drug forms.

Table 11-3 provides a list of sympathomimetics and other medications used for the treatment of asthma and COPD.

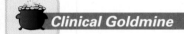

Clinical Goldmine

Monitoring the Dosage

The dosage of a sympathomimetic must be carefully monitored to prevent tachycardia, decreased or increased blood pressure, nausea, headache, and other CNS symptoms.

Evaluation

You should check the patient's pulse and blood pressure to see if the heart is affected by the drug. Response to therapy varies among patients. The patient should be watched carefully to see if the breathing problems have improved.

Patients should be watched for increasing tolerance, which will result in less response to the drug.

Patient and Family Teaching

You should tell the patient and family the following:
1. The patient should take the medication as directed by the nurse, physician, or other health care provider; the dosage should not be changed.
2. Overuse of these drugs may result in severe side effects.
3. The nurse, physician, or other health care provider should be contacted if the drug is not helping the patient.
4. The patient should contact the nurse, physician, or other health care provider if she has bronchial irritation, dizziness, chest pain, insomnia, or any change in symptoms.
5. Drinking lots of fluid, especially water, makes the mucus thinner and helps the medication work better.
6. The patient must not take any other medications without checking first with the nurse, physician, or other health care provider.
7. The patient should take the last dose a few hours before bedtime so that the drug does not produce insomnia.
8. The drug should be protected from light; colored solutions should be thrown away.

XANTHINE DERIVATIVES

Action

The main action of xanthine-derivative bronchodilators is to relax the smooth muscle cells in the bronchi and the blood vessels in the lungs. These drugs also act directly on the kidneys to produce diuresis (increased production and excretion of urine). These drugs cause CNS effects. Other actions are myocardial stimulation, increased rate of breathing, effects on metabolism, and release of epinephrine from the adrenal medulla.

Uses

Xanthine derivatives are used as adjunctive therapy to treat the symptoms of bronchospasm in acute and chronic bronchial asthma, bronchitis, and emphysema and in treating neonatal apnea. They may also be used to treat acute pulmonary edema by promoting bronchodilation and diuresis. The correct way to use them is carefully described in the National Institutes of Health *Guidelines for the Diagnosis and Management of Asthma*.

Adverse Reactions

Adverse reactions to xanthine derivatives include dysrhythmias, flushing, marked hypotension, tachycardia, headache, insomnia, restlessness, diarrhea, epigastric pain, nausea, vomiting, and rash.

Overdosage causes serious adverse reactions that increase in severity, including confusion, respiratory failure, shock, bizarre behavior, extreme thirst, delirium (extreme confusion, often with delusions or disorientation), and hyperthermia (abnormally high body temperature). Excessive overdosage may lead to seizures and death without warning. Children are particularly at risk for this problem.

Drug Interactions

Xanthines may increase the CNS stimulation caused by ephedrine, sympathomimetics, and amphetamines.

Table **11-3**

Medications for Asthma and Chronic Obstructive Pulmonary Disease

GENERIC NAME	TRADE NAME	COMMENTS AND DOSAGE
SYMPATHOMIMETIC BRONCHODILATORS		
albuterol	Proventil Ventolin	Selective for beta$_2$ receptors and thus has fewer cardiac side effects than other adrenergic drugs and a long duration of bronchodilation; comes as an inhaler with about 200 doses, or in tablet form. *Adults and children:* 1-2 inhalations q4-6h or 2-4 mg PO 3 or 4 times daily.
bitolterol ephedrine sulfate	Tornalate	2 inhalations in 1-3 minutes, followed by third inhalation if needed. Has a long duration; it is used to treat milder forms of COPD. *Adults:* 25-50 mg PO q3-4h or 25-50 mg subcutaneously or IM q3-4h. *Children 6-12 yr:* 6.25-12.5 mg PO q4-6h. *Children 2-6 yr:* 0.3-0.5 mg/kg PO q4-6h.
epinephrine	Adrenalin Chloride Sus-Phrine Primatene-Mist	Reserved for acute attacks of bronchospasm. It has a rapid onset of action (3-10 min) when given subcutaneously or by inhalation. Light, air, and heat can change the color. 1-2 min should be allowed between inhalations if successive dosage is needed. <ul><li>*For Adrenalin and epinephrine* *Adults:* 0.2-1.0 mg subcutaneously or IM. *Children:* 0.01 mg/kg or 0.3 mg/m^2 to a maximum of 0.5 mg.</li><li>*For Sus-Phrine* *Adults:* 0.1-0.3 mL subcutaneously. *Children:* 0.005 mL/kg subcutaneously.</li></ul>
isoetharine	Isotharine	Hand nebulizer: 3-7 inhalations undiluted.
isoproterenol	Isuprel Medihaler-Iso	Selective for beta receptors; helpful for those no longer benefiting from use of epinephrine; may decrease blood pressure; may make saliva pink. *Adults:* 10-20 mg sublingually (SL), not to exceed 60 mg/day. *Children:* 5-10 mg SL, not to exceed 30 mg/day. *Inhalation:* 1-5 treatments as needed daily.
metaproterenol	Alupent	More selectivity for beta$_2$ receptors of the bronchi and less effect on beta$_1$ receptors of the heart than isoproterenol; well absorbed from the GI tract. *Adults:* 20 mg PO 3 or 4 times daily. *Children over 9 yr or over 60 lb:* 20 mg PO 3 or 4 times daily. *Children 6-9 yr or less than 60 lb:* 10 mg PO 3 or 4 times daily.
pirbuterol	Maxair	2 inhalations q4-6h.
salmeterol	Serevent	Long-acting inhaled beta$_2$-receptor agonist used to prevent attacks but not in acute conditions. *Adults and children 4 yr and older:* Usual dosage is 1 inhalation (50 mcg) twice daily (morning and evening, approximately 12 hr apart)
terbutaline	Brethine Bricanyl	Has a negligible effect on beta$_1$ receptors; has an affinity for beta$_2$ receptors of the bronchial tree, peripheral vascular beds, and the uterus. Often effective when other drugs are not. *Adults:* 5 mg PO 3 times daily at 6-hr intervals. *Children 12-15 yr:* 2.5 mg PO 3 times daily; or 2.5 mg subcutaneously 3 times daily, not to exceed 7.5 mg subcutaneously in 24 hr.

Table 11-3

Medications for Asthma and Chronic Obstructive Pulmonary Disease—cont'd

GENERIC NAME	TRADE NAME	COMMENTS AND DOSAGE
XANTHINE BRONCHODILATORS		
aminophylline		A synthetic preparation that is a prototype for many of the theophylline compounds. It plays a significant role in management of conditions with bronchial constriction and spasm. It is especially useful when differentiation cannot be made between bronchospasm and pulmonary edema. This agent is commonly prescribed by its generic name and contains 78% theophylline and 12% ethylenediamine. IM injection is painful.
		• *Asthma attacks*
		Adults: 500 mg PO stat; 200-315 mg PO q6-8h maintenance. For rectal suppositories, usual dose is 500 mg daily or twice daily, not to exceed 1 gm/day, or 500 mg IM as necessary. With rectal solutions, use 300 mg daily to 3 times daily or 450 mg twice daily. Timed-release tablets can be given at 300-600 mg q8-12h.
		Children: 7.5 mg/kg PO stat; 5-6 mg/kg PO q6-8h maintenance; or give 7 mg/kg rectal suppository, or use rectal solutions at 5 mg/kg.
dyphylline	Dilor	Few side effects.
	Lufyllin	*Adults:* Give up to 15 mg/kg PO q6h; individualize dosage. For IM dosage, give 250-500 mg injected slowly.
		Children 40-100 lb: 80-240 mg for acute attacks; 27-80 mg for maintenance in 3-4 hr.
		Children under 40 lb: 40-80 mg for acute attacks; 13-17 mg in 3-4 hr for maintenance. For IM dosage, give 2-3 mg/lb daily in divided doses.
oxtriphylline	Choledyl SA ❦	Less irritating to gastric mucosa, is readily absorbed from GI tract, and more stable and soluble than aminophylline. Useful for long-term therapy of bronchospasm.
		Adults: 200 mg PO 4 times daily.
		Children 2-12 yr: 100 mg/60 lb 4 times daily.
theophylline	Bronkodyl	Popular and effective drug in management of bronchial constriction and spasm. Timed-release capsules slowly provide medication for 8-12 or 12-24 hr.
	Elixophyllin	*Adults:* 200-250 mg PO q6h.
	Quibron T	*Children:* 3-6 mg/kg q6h.
	Slo-Phyllin	• *For timed-release capsules:*
		Adults: 300 mg PO q12h.
		Children 12-16 yr: 200 mg PO q12h.
		Children 9-12 yr: 150 mg PO q12h.
		Children under 9 yr: 100 mg PO q12h.
LEUKOTRIENE RECEPTOR INHIBITORS		
montelukast Na	Singulair	Well-tolerated product used for chronic asthma.
		Adults and children older than 15 yr: One 10-mg tablet daily, taken in the evening.
		Children 6-14 yr: One 5-mg chewable tablet daily, taken in the evening.
zafirlukast	Accolate	Nursing women should not take this medication. Store medication at 68°-77° F and protect from light and moisture.
		Adults and children older than 12 yr: Take 20 mg twice daily 1 hr before or 2 hr after eating.
zileuton	Zyflo	*Adults:* 600 mg PO 4 times daily. May be taken with meals and at bedtime.

Continued

Table 11-3

Medications for Asthma and Chronic Obstructive Pulmonary Disease—cont'd

GENERIC NAME	TRADE NAME	COMMENTS AND DOSAGE
CORTICOSTEROIDS: SYSTEMIC		
methylprednisolone		*Adults:* 7.5-70 mg daily in single dose or 4 times daily as needed for control. *Children:* 0.25-2 mg/kg daily in single dose or 4 times daily as needed for control. • *For short-course "burst":* *Adults:* 40-60 mg/day as single or 2 divided doses for 3-10 days. *Children:* 1-2 mg/kg/day, maximum 60 mg/day, for 3-10 days.
prednisolone		*Adults:* 7.5-70 mg daily in single dose or 4 times daily as needed for control. *Children:* 0.25-2 mg/kg daily in single dose or 4 times daily as needed for control. • *For short-course "burst":* *Adults:* 40-60 mg/day as single or 2 divided doses for 3-10 days. *Children:* 1-2 mg/kg/day, maximum 60 mg/day, for 3-10 days.
prednisone		*Adults:* 7.5-70 mg daily in single dose or 4 times daily as needed for control. *Children:* 0.25-2 mg/kg daily in single dose or 4 times daily as needed for control. • *For short course "burst":* *Adults:* 40-60 mg/day as single or 2 divided doses for 3-10 days. *Children:* 1-2 mg/kg/day, maximum 60 mg/day, for 3-10 days.
CORTICOSTEROIDS: INHALED		
beclomethasone dipropionate	QVAR Vanceril	*Adults:* 2 inhalations 3 or 4 times daily. *Children 6-12 yr:* 1 or 2 inhalations 3 or 4 times daily.
budesonide	Pulmicort Turbuhaler	*Adults:* 200 mcg 1-3 times daily. *Children older than 6 yr:* 200 mcg 1-2 times daily.
flunisolide	AeroBid	*Adults:* 2 inhalations twice daily. *Children 6-16 yr:* 2 inhalations twice daily.
fluticasone propionate	Flovent	*Adults:* Prophylactic or maintenance dose is 100-500 mcg twice daily. *Children 4-11 yr:* 50-100 mcg twice daily.
triamcinolone acetonide	Azmacort	*Adults:* 2 inhalations 3 or 4 times daily. *Children 6-12 yr:* 1 or 2 inhalations 3 or 4 times daily.

Cytochrome P-450 interactions between xanthines and erythromycin, lincomycin, and clindamycin may increase blood levels of theophylline. Beta-blocking agents may interfere with (antagonize) the effect of xanthines. Xanthines also increase the action of some types of diuretics. Xanthines may increase the risk of toxicity when taken with digitalis glycosides. Large doses of these agents may reverse the effect of oral anticoagulants. Lithium carbonate is excreted more rapidly in the presence of xanthines. The use of furosemide with theophylline increases the serum levels of theophylline and may cause toxicity. Xanthine derivatives shorten prothrombin and clotting times.

Clinical Landmine

Factors Affecting Blood Levels

The efficacy of theophylline is directly related to the blood levels achieved from its administration. The desired therapeutic range is considered to be 10 to 20 mcg per milliliter of serum. The factors affecting blood levels include the following:
1. Differing levels of theophylline in each product
2. Variance in rates of absorption
3. Metabolism and elimination of each drug
4. Age of the patient receiving the medication

Nursing Implications and Patient Teaching

Assessment

You should learn as much as possible about the health history of the patient, including whether the patient is pregnant or has a history of smoking, allergy, renal or liver dysfunction, heart disease, cardiac dysrhythmias, peptic ulcer, severe hypertension, or glaucoma. These conditions are contraindications or precautions to the use of xanthines.

Diagnosis

The severity of the asthma or COPD is determined by history and is linked to the treatment. Look for any other problems that may require your help: need for increased hydration, insomnia, or feelings of anxiety.

Planning

The half-life of xanthine bronchodilators is shorter in smokers than in nonsmokers, which may make it necessary to use a higher dosage for smokers.

It is not necessary to use drug formulations that contain alcohol; they may be harmful.

Implementation

Xanthine products are available in a number of forms: capsules, coated tablets, sustained-release tablets and capsules, aqueous solutions and suspensions, hydroalcoholic elixirs, suppositories, rectal solutions, and IV and IM injections.

The amount of the theophylline base varies in xanthine products, and the preparations are not therapeutically equal. This inequality may cause difficulty when the patient is switched from one product to another. The critical factor is to measure the theophylline blood levels to get the desired therapeutic effect.

The rate of absorption of oral theophylline depends on the dosage form used. Oral liquids have the fastest absorption rate, followed by uncoated tablets. Enteric-coated or sustained-release tablets and capsules produce inconsistent blood levels and should usually be used only at night. Food does not influence the absorption of theophylline. Absorption of rectal suppositories is slow and sometimes unpredictable. The rate of absorption for rectal solutions and IM injections is usually equivalent to that of an oral solution.

The rates of metabolism and excretion of theophylline are also variable. Xanthines are metabolized in the liver and excreted by the kidneys. The serum half-life of the drugs can range from 3 to 12 hours in adults and 1¼ to 9 hours in children. Heart failure, liver dysfunction, and pulmonary edema can slow excretion, and smoking can increase excretion. Children under 9 years of age require larger doses of theophylline than adults to maintain the same therapeutic blood levels of the drug. Thus the dosage must be prescribed on an individualized basis and be carefully monitored. It is common for an initial loading dose to be indicated.

Because of the need to increase or decrease the amount of medication based on the symptoms, the use of fixed-combination bronchodilator products (that is, a sympathomimetic, a xanthine, and an expectorant combined in one product) is not recommended. Fixed-combination products do not make it possible to change the doses of each individual drug, and a fixed-combination drug may lead to toxicity from some of the drugs. Use of selected sympathomimetic and xanthine bronchodilators administered at the same time, however, may have a synergistic effect.

For more information about the xanthine derivatives, see Table 11-3.

Evaluation

The patient's breathing status and symptoms should be watched for any change. You should be alert for signs of toxicity, such as tachycardia or dysrhythmias, vomiting, dizziness, and irritability.

The drug dosage may be changed based on the therapeutic blood levels of theophylline, the amount of theophylline base in each preparation, and the clinical response of the patient.

Children and elderly patients should be carefully watched for CNS stimulation because they are highly sensitive to these drugs.

To minimize GI symptoms, administer the drug with food and water. Rectal irritation may develop from use of suppository forms.

Patient and Family Teaching

You should tell the patient and family the following:

1. The patient should take the medications as ordered; this often means every 6 hours if taking a sustained-release medication.
2. Any unusual symptoms should be reported to the nurse, physician, or other health care provider, especially seizures, rapid heartbeat, irregular heartbeat, vomiting, dizziness, and irritability.
3. The patient should avoid drinking large amounts of caffeine-containing drinks such as tea, coffee, cocoa, and cola drinks.
4. Some other medications interfere with the drug action if taken at the same time. The patient should avoid taking any other drugs without first checking with the nurse, physician, or other health care provider. This includes drugs the patient may buy over the counter, because they may also have an effect on the respiratory system (for example, cough syrups and hay fever and allergy medicine).
5. The patient should take the medicine with a glass of water or with meals to avoid an upset stomach.
6. If a dose is missed and this is noticed within an hour, the patient should take the prescribed dose

as soon as possible. If more than an hour has passed, the dose should be skipped and the patient should stay on the original dosing schedule.

7. Some suppositories must be refrigerated, whereas others may not need refrigeration. The patient should check with the pharmacist about this.

8. The nurse, physician, or other health care provider should be called if use of suppositories causes burning or irritation of the rectal area.

LEUKOTRIENE RECEPTOR INHIBITORS

ACTION

The **leukotriene receptor inhibitors** belong to the newest category of drugs used in treating asthma. These drugs are not bronchodilators but act to block receptors for the cysteinyl leukotrienes C_4, D_4, and E_4. Cysteinyl leukotrienes (leukotrienes bound to the amino acid cysteine) are potent bronchoconstrictors. By blocking receptors that control bronchoconstriction, vascular permeability, and mucous secretion, the leukotriene receptor inhibitors can reduce the symptoms of asthma.

USES

These products are substitutes for inhaled glucocorticoid therapy in patients with mild, persistent asthma who cannot take the inhaled medications. These drugs may also be added to regular therapy because they have a different type of action. They provide medication options for patients with aspirin sensitivity. They are used for chronic asthma therapy and can also be used during acute attacks, although they will not reverse bronchospasm.

These drugs are rapidly absorbed orally. Food interferes with their absorption, so they should be taken on an empty stomach. The safety of these drugs has not been established in pregnancy and breastfeeding, or in children under the age of 10.

ADVERSE REACTIONS

These drugs are generally safe and well tolerated. Headache is the most common side effect. A few individuals may have infection, nausea, and diarrhea.

DRUG INTERACTIONS

These drugs interact with warfarin, erythromycin, theophylline, and aspirin.

Nursing Implications and Patient Teaching

Assessment

You should learn as much as possible about the health history of the patient in order to determine the status of the patient's asthma and what other medications the patient might be taking. Ask about the possibility of pregnancy, breastfeeding, or liver disease.

Diagnosis

You should carefully evaluate the patient to determine the possibility of infection, the presence of anxiety, a lack of knowledge, or anything else that may complicate his asthma treatment regimen.

Planning

These drugs are not started if the patient is having an acute asthma attack. They are adjunctive drugs given as part of an asthma treatment regimen. Watch to see if there might be adverse drug interactions with other medications the patient is taking. Some of these medications involve special storage requirements.

Implementation

Most of these medications are given twice daily. They are usually well tolerated, and no significant problems are associated with them.

See Table 11-3 for specific information on the drugs in this category.

Evaluation

Therapeutic effect is seen with a reduction in number and severity of asthma attacks. Patients should report to their health care provider if they have an increase in asthma attacks.

Patient and Family Teaching

You should tell the patient and family the following:

1. Taking food with these medications reduces the drug absorption, except for zileuton.

2. Women should not take these drugs if they are pregnant or breastfeeding.

3. These medications should be kept out of the reach of children or others for whom they are not ordered.

4. These medications are used together with other types of asthma medication. They should be continued if the patient has an acute asthma attack. The patient should not suddenly stop the medication or decrease doses.

5. Zafirlukast must be kept protected from extremes of temperature, light, and humidity. It should be stored in the airtight container in which it is supplied.

CORTICOSTEROIDS

ACTION

Corticosteroids are the most powerful (potent) and consistently effective medications for the long-term control of asthma. Their action on the inflammatory process may account for their effectiveness. They block the reaction to allergens and reduce airway hyperresponsiveness. They inhibit cytokine production, protein activation, and inflammatory cell migration and activation.

USES

Inhaled corticosteroids are used in the long-term control of asthma. They are often used to reduce the need for oral corticosteroids. Systemic corticosteroids are often used to get quick control of the disease when beginning long-term therapy. They are also used to speed recovery from moderate to severe episodes, and to prevent more of these episodes.

ADVERSE REACTIONS

Inhaled steroids may produce cough, dysphonia (hoarseness), and oral thrush. In high doses, systemic effects such as slowing of growth in children and osteoporosis in adults may occur. Systemic steroids used for a short time may cause many problems such as brief abnormalities in glucose metabolism, increased appetite, fluid retention, weight gain, mood alteration, hypertension, and peptic ulcer. Long-term use suppresses the adrenal axis and may produce serious and systemic symptoms.

DRUG INTERACTIONS

The inhaled products have a local effect and do not interact to a great extent with other drugs. However, systemic products interact with many drugs (see Chapter 20).

Nursing Implications and Patient Teaching

Assessment

You should learn everything you can about the severity of the patient's asthma. Look for symptoms of other respiratory infection, allergens, or stress that might have triggered an asthma attack. Ask questions about whether the patient takes her asthma medication correctly. Does patient have other conditions that could be made worse by systemic corticosteroids?

Diagnosis

Classify symptoms of asthma by severity and identify asthma triggers. Diagnose needs for patient teaching. Does the patient need to take in more fluids? Does the patient need more education?

Planning

Develop a teaching plan to meet the educational needs that have been discovered. Oral products should be used at the lowest effective dose for the shortest time possible. Develop a plan to look for adverse effects that may develop from the medication.

Implementation

Stay with the patient and help him with breathing exercises if he is having an acute asthmatic attack. Also begin giving the patient a lot of water to reduce the thickness of secretions, and help the patient cough them up and spit them out. Show the patient the proper way to hold the medication canister, take a breath, and compress the canister so that the medication is released into the lungs and not into the mouth. Begin teaching the patient about the disease process, the medication regimen, equipment, and procedures. Using a spacer/holder chamber device and washing out the mouth after inhalation will decrease local side effects and improve systemic absorption.

For more information about these products, see Table 11-3.

Evaluation

Have the patient show you how to use the inhaler. Watch for improvement in the patient's breathing.

Patient and Family Teaching

Education should focus on the disease process, triggers to asthma attacks, and appropriate therapy.

The patient and family should learn about taking the medicine and knowing when it is not effective. Make sure the patient understands when to contact the health care provider.

Explain how corticosteroid medications are used together with other products. This information should be put in writing so the patient can refer to it later.

Children need to be taught as much as possible and given the responsibility of helping to determine when they need medication, what type of medication they need, and whether it is effective.

Decongestants

OVERVIEW

ACTION

Decongestants directly affect the alpha receptors of blood vessels in the nasal mucosa, causing vasocon-striction. This action reduces blood flow, fluid movement, and mucosal edema. Many agents also act on beta receptors, which may cause **rebound vasodilation,** or an increase in blood flow leading to further congestion. This problem is commonly seen with prolonged use of the medication.

USES

Decongestants are used to relieve nasal congestion found with allergies and upper respiratory tract infections (URTIs). These drugs may also be used as additional therapy for middle ear infections and to decrease congestion around the eustachian tubes. Ear blockage and the pressure and pain caused by air travel may respond to nasal decongestants.

ADVERSE REACTIONS

Stinging and burning as a result of mucosal dryness sometimes follow topical administration of decongestants. Rebound congestion may occur after prolonged use of topical agents. When the drugs are absorbed from the GI tract, systemic effects such as nervousness, nausea, dizziness, tachycardia, dysrhythmia, and a transient increase in blood pressure may occur. Rarely, a severe shocklike syndrome with hypotension and coma has been reported in children. Psychologic dependence and toxic psychoses have been reported with long-term, high-dose therapy. The severity of overdosage varies, resulting in a variety of symptoms.

DRUG INTERACTIONS

The systemic effects of decongestants may be made stronger if they are given with other sympathomimetics, MAO inhibitors, tricyclic antidepressants, antihistamines, and thyroxine. Decongestants should be used with caution in stable hypertensive patients on guanethidine, bethanidine, or debrisoquine sulfate. Use of decongestants at the same time as high doses of digitalis or use of other drugs that may sensitize the heart to dysrhythmias should be avoided because anginal pain may result when there is coronary insufficiency.

Nursing Implications and Patient Teaching

Assessment

Learn as much as possible about the patient's health history. The patient may have a history of nasal congestion, postnasal drip, nasal discharge, sneezing, sore throat, headache, itchy eyes, lacrimation (excess tear production), nasal polyps, earache, decreased hearing, URTI, or allergies.

Ask about allergy to adrenergic agents, narrow-angle glaucoma, concurrent MAO inhibitor or tricyclic antidepressant therapy, and loss of sensation in the fingers and toes. These are contraindications to the use of decongestants. Use decongestants cautiously in patients with hypertension, dysrhythmias, heart disease, angina, hyperthyroidism, diabetes, advanced arteriosclerotic conditions, glaucoma, prostatic hypertrophy, or chronic cough because of the possibility of systemic vasoconstriction and tachycardia. Also use with caution in patients with a long history of asthma and emphysema

who also have degenerative heart disease. Excessive use of topical decongestants may result in GI absorption that causes systemic effects. The safe use of decongestants in pregnancy has not been established.

Diagnosis

The exact cause of the patient's problem must be found to make certain the treatment is appropriate. Determine if rhinitis is related to allergy or infection.

Planning

Frequent and continual use of the topical decongestants or use at dosages greater than recommended may result in a rebound effect. Topical decongestants should be used only in acute states, for no longer than 3 to 5 days, and should be used very carefully at low doses in children and the elderly.

Implementation

Oral decongestants are considered to be more effective and more prolonged than nasal preparations because they can reach all parts of the mucous membrane in the nasal passages. The disadvantage of the systemic agents is that their effects may not be limited to the nasal mucosa; they may also affect other parts of the body.

Topical forms may be supplied as drops, sprays, jellies, and oral inhalation agents. The advantage of topical administration is the rapid onset of action and direct stimulation of the nasal mucosa. Drops have a tendency to pass into the hypopharynx and then be swallowed, thus passing into the GI tract. Sprays deliver a fine mist that is easily trapped in the upper respiratory tract, so they are less likely to reach the GI tract. Topical preparations should not be used for more than 3 to 5 days because of the risk of a rebound effect. Oral preparations are more appropriate for long-term use.

The patient's head should be tipped back when giving drops to prevent swallowing of the drug. Use care not to touch the skin while administering solutions. Solutions can become contaminated with use and result in growth of bacteria and fungi.

Table 11-4 lists various nasal decongestant products.

Evaluation

You should watch to see that symptoms disappear and to see if rebound congestion develops with an increase in symptoms. If headache and nervousness develop, stop the treatment.

Patient and Family Teaching

There are many decongestants on the market that are available over the counter. Many of these OTC products contain combinations of medications to make them attractive to the patient with several symptoms. These

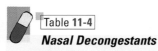

Table 11-4

Nasal Decongestants

GENERIC NAME	TRADE NAME	COMMENTS AND DOSAGE
SYMPATHOMIMETIC BRONCHODILATORS		
ephedrine	Pretz-D Kondon's Nasal	May produce burning, stinging, dryness of nasal mucosa, and sneezing. *Adults and children 6 yr and older:* 2 or 3 drops, or application of a small amount of jelly in each nostril q3-4h.
epinephrine	Adrenalin	Stimulates both alpha and beta receptors. Give 1-2 drops in each nostril q4-6h.
INHALERS		
naphazoline	Privine	Has rapid and prolonged effect; produces CNS depression when swallowed. *Adults and children 6 yr and older:* 2 drops in each nostril q3h.
oxymetazoline	Afrin Dristan 12 Hr Duration	Prolonged decongestant effect. Often overused by patients, leading to rebound congestion when used longer than 3 days in succession. *Adults and children 6 yr and older:* 2 squeezes each nostril twice daily, or 2-4 drops in each nostril twice daily.
phenylephrine	Neo-Synephrine Sinex	Drug ineffective if exposed to air, strong light, or heat. Very effective topical preparation, but it may cause marked local irritation. *Adults:* 0.25%-1.0% strength, 3-4 drops or 1-2 sprays q4h. *Children 6-12 yr:* Use 0.25%, 2-3 drops q3-4h. *Children 2-6 yr:* Use 0.167%, 2-3 drops q4h. *Infants:* Use 0.125%, 2-3 drops q3-4h.
pseudoephedrine sulfate	Sinex Sudafed	*Adults and children 12 yr and older:* 60 mg PO 3 to 4 times daily; or 120-mg timed-release capsule can be given PO q12h. *Children 2-12 yr:* 15-30 mg PO 3 or 4 times daily.
tetrahydrozoline	Tyzine	*Adults and children 6 yr and older:* 2 drops of 0.1% solution in each nostril as needed, but no more than q3h. *Children 2-6 yr:* 2-3 drops of 0.05% solution in each nostril no more than q3h.
xylometazoline	Otrivin	Action lasts 8-10 hr. Overdose can cause extreme CNS depression in children. *Adults:* 2-3 sprays or 2-3 drops in each nostril. *Children younger than 12 yr:* 2-3 drops of 0.05% q8-10h.

products may contain a decongestant and one or more antihistamine, analgesic, antitussive, expectorant, or anticholinergic products. Each additional medication increases the precautions for use of the product and the adverse effects that may occur. For example, drugs that contain anticholinergics cause drying of mucous secretions. They should be avoided in patients with asthma or COPD. The patient should consider whether there is a need for all of the drugs listed on the label of these combination products. Also, the types of drugs that make up even well-known products change frequently. Pharmacists are excellent sources of information about OTC medications, and patients should be encouraged to seek their professional advice.

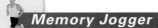

Memory Jogger

Administering Decongestants

You should provide the patient and family with the following instructions:
1. To administer drops:
   a. Blow the nose gently.
   b. Lie down with the head tipped back over the edge of the bed.
   c. Put 1 to 2 drops of solution on the lower nasal mucosa.
   d. Breathe through the mouth.
   e. Remain in this position for 5 minutes while turning the head from side to side; this will help the drops run back into the nose instead of down the throat.

Continued

Memory Jogger—cont'd

2. The patient should always rinse the dropper after putting drops into the nose. This will help prevent growth of bacteria and fungi.
3. To administer a spray:
   a. Keep the container upright to obtain a fine mist.
   b. Gently blow the nose.
   c. Squeeze the bottle firmly in each nostril.
   d. After 3 to 5 minutes, blow the nose again.
   e. Repeat the application if congestion remains.
4. Each person in the family should use a separate bottle of nasal spray. Topical decongestants should not be shared.
5. To administer jellies:
   a. Put a small amount on the finger.

b. Apply it to the nasal mucosa.
c. Snuff deeply through the nose.
6. To administer inhalers:
   a. Insert the open end of the plastic tube in each nostril.
   b. Inhale two times.
7. The patient should avoid excessive use of these medications or they will cause the symptoms that the patient is trying to reduce.
8. Missed doses may be taken within an hour of the scheduled time, and then the regular schedule may be resumed. If more than 1 hour has passed, the patient should skip that dose and return to the regular schedule.

SECTION FIVE

Expectorants

OVERVIEW

ACTION

Expectorants are agents that decrease the thickness of respiratory secretions and aid in their removal. It is believed that they work by increasing the amount of fluid in the respiratory tract. These increased liquid secretions promote ciliary action and decrease the amount of coughing while increasing the amount of sputum produced. There is considerable disagreement about whether they really work or not.

USES

Expectorants are used to treat symptoms of productive cough. These products may be useful in chronic respiratory disease when thick mucus is a complication.

ADVERSE REACTIONS

GI upset is a common adverse reaction to expectorants.

DRUG INTERACTIONS

Expectorants with guaifenesin may increase bleeding tendency. Patients taking anticoagulants must be closely monitored if they are given expectorants.

Nursing Implications and Patient Teaching

Assessment

You should learn as much as possible about the health history of the patient, including the history of cough,

presence of other respiratory disease, allergy, and other medications that may cause drug interactions.

Diagnosis

Are there needs for hydration? Diagnose any lack of knowledge.

Planning

Expectorants are not to be used for persistent cough without the advice of a physician or other health care provider.

Clinical Landmine

Chronic or Persistent Cough

Chronic or persistent cough may be the result of a serious condition and should not be ignored.

Implementation

The patient should take an increased amount of fluid each day and breathe humidified air. This will help liquefy secretions. Medication should be taken with at least one full glass of water.

Table 11-5 gives a summary of expectorants.

Evaluation

You should monitor for the expected effect.

If the patient uses more than the recommended dosage, adverse reactions may occur.

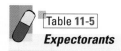

Table 11-5
Expectorants

GENERIC NAME	TRADE NAME	COMMENTS AND DOSAGE
guaifenesin	Anti-tuss Robitussin Organidin NR	Although there is a lack of convincing evidence to document clinical efficacy, this is a widely publicized product. *Adults:* 100-400 mg PO q4-6h; maximum dose 2.4 gm/day. *Children 6-12 yr:* 50-100 mg PO q4-6h; maximum dose 600 mg/day. *Children 2-6 yr:* 50 mg PO q4h; maximum dose 300 mg/day.
iodinated glycerol	Iophen R-Gen	Patients may develop dose-related dermatitis, gastrointestinal upset, or rash. Hypersensitivity, thyroid enlargement, and acute parotitis are rare. One drop is approximately equal to 3 mg. *Adults:* 60 mg PO 4 times daily with water; 1 teaspoonful (5 mL) elixir 4 times daily; or 20 drops of solution 4 times daily with water. May also be taken with juice or milk if diet allows. *Children:* Up to half of the adult dose, based on weight.
iodine products	Potassium Iodide SSKI	Do not use continuously, because prolonged use may lead to hypothyroidism. • *Potassium Iodide* *Adults:* 300 mg in liquid q4-6h. *Children:* 250-1000 mg daily in 2-4 divided doses. • *SSKI* *Adults:* 0.3-0.6 mL 4-12 times daily, diluted in a glass of water, juice, or milk.

Patient and Family Teaching

You should tell the patient and family the following:

1. The patient should be aware that these drugs will help make the sputum more liquid. This will make it easier to bring sputum up when the patient coughs.
2. The patient should use a humidifier and drink at least 2 quarts of water daily while taking an expectorant. These actions will help get the mucus out.
3. The nurse, physician, or other health care provider should be notified if the cough is present with a high fever, rash, or persistent headaches, or if the cough returns once the patient thinks it has been under control.
4. The patient should use the medication only in the dosage recommended to decrease chances of side effects.

SECTION SIX
Topical Intranasal Steroids

OVERVIEW

ACTION
The main action of topical intranasal steroids is an anti-inflammatory effect, which decreases local congestion.

USES
Topical intranasal steroids are used to treat allergic, mechanical, or chemically induced local nasal inflammation or nasal polyps only when the more usual treatment has been tried and found to not work. Some patients get good allergy relief from these products and require no other medications. These medications are gen-erally safe and have been used continuously for a decade by some patients without adverse or systemic effects.

ADVERSE REACTIONS
Adverse reactions to topical intranasal steroids include asthma, headache, light-headedness, loss of sense of smell, nasal irritation and dryness, nausea, nosebleeds, perforation of the nasal septum, bad taste and smell, rebound congestion, and skin rash.

DRUG INTERACTIONS
Intranasal steroids may interact with many products. Consult the earlier section on corticosteroids for more information.

Nursing Implications and Patient Teaching

Assessment

You should learn as much as possible about the health history of the patient, including allergy, fungal infections, tuberculosis, ocular herpes simplex, local infections (especially of the nose, sinus, or throat), and the possibility of pregnancy. These conditions are contraindications or precautions to the use of topical nasal steroids. You should ask about the patient's past experience with and response to nasal sprays.

Diagnosis

You should learn why the patient requires intranasal medication. Identify any other problem secondary to medication use or misuse, such as presence of adverse effects or patient education deficits.

Planning

The patient receiving topical intranasal steroids should not be given smallpox vaccination or immunizations because the immunologic response may be decreased. In the patient with latent tuberculosis or reactivated tuberculosis, close observation and possible chemoprophylaxis may be indicated. The effects of these drug are increased in patients with hypothyroidism and cirrhosis.

Implementation

The recommended dosage must not be exceeded. The dosage should be decreased when the patient begins to improve.

Table 11-6 provides a list of intranasal steroids.

Evaluation

You should watch for a reduction in nasal stuffiness, obstruction, and discharge, and for relief of sinus headaches. You should also monitor how often the medication is used and what dosage is used. Watch for cracked or bleeding nasal mucosa. You should be alert for adverse reactions such as signs of systemic absorption and fluid retention, increased blood pressure, weight gain, ankle edema, or evidence of local infection.

Nasal dryness and irritation are side effects and do not usually require stopping the drug. The dosage of these drugs should be gradually reduced to avoid adrenocortical insufficiency.

These drugs may decrease resistance to infection, as well as mask some common signs of infection. Elevation of blood pressure, retention of salt and fluid, and increased potassium and calcium loss may occur if the patient takes large doses. This may be treated with dietary salt restriction and potassium supplementation. Loss of the ability to smell, shortness of breath,

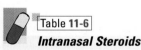

Table 11-6

Intranasal Steroids

GENERIC NAME	TRADE NAME	COMMENTS AND DOSAGE
beclomethasone dipropionate	Beconase	Use after other conventional therapy has been found to be ineffective. Symptomatic relief is not immediate, and therapy should be continued even with initial minimal response. Maximal response should be seen within 3 wk or medication should be discontinued. *Adults and children over 12 yr:* 1 inhalation in each nostril 2 to 4 times daily. Taper off gradually as relief is obtained.
budesonide	Rhinocort Aqua	*Adults and children over 6 yr:* 1 spray in each nostril 2-4 times daily (64 mcg/day). *Adults and children over 12 yr:* Dosage may be increased up to 4 sprays in each nostril once daily (256 mcg/day).
flunisolide	Nasalide Nasarel	*Adults:* 2 sprays in each nostril twice daily; may increase to 3 times daily if warranted. Do not use more than 8 sprays/day per nostril. Maintenance dose may be 1 spray/day per nostril. *Children 6-14 yr:* 1 spray in each nostril 3 times daily; may give 2 sprays in each nostril twice daily. Maximum dose is 4 sprays/day per nostril. Taper to 1 spray/day per nostril.
fluticasone propionate	Flonase	Diskhaler and diskus are effective new delivery forms. *Adults:* 2 sprays per nostril daily or 1 spray per nostril twice daily. *Children over 12 yr:* 1 spray per nostril daily.
mometasone furoate monohydrate	Nasonex	*Adults and children over 12 yr:* 2 sprays in each nostril daily.
triamcinolone acetonide	Nasacort AQ	*Adults and children over 12 yr:* 2 sprays in each nostril once daily (220 mcg/day). *Children 6-11 yr:* 1-2 sprays in each nostril once daily (110 mcg/day).

unrelieved stuffy nose, chest tightness, or wheezing indicates a need for intervention by a health care provider.

The patient should be watched for signs of systemic absorption because fluid retention and temporary inhibition of pituitary-adrenal function may develop.

Patient and Family Teaching

You should tell the patient and family the following:

1. The patient should not use these drugs if she has an infection. The patients should notify the nurse, physician, or other health care provider if she develops an infection while taking this drug.
2. The patient should not exceed the prescribed dosage and frequency; using the drug in the smallest effective dose for the shortest period of time will prevent general absorption.
3. There may be temporary dryness and irritation of the nose.

4. When stopping this drug, the dosage must be tapered slowly and not stopped suddenly, especially if the medicine has been used for long periods of time.
5. The nurse, physician, or other health care provider should be notified if symptoms do not improve or if they get worse.

COMPLEMENTARY AND ALTERNATIVE THERAPIES

Allergies, asthma, and coughs and colds are some of the conditions frequently treated with alternative products. See the Complementary and Alternative Therapies box for some of the most common preparations and their use.

Complementary and Alternative Therapies

SYMPTOMS	HERBAL PRODUCTS OR VITAMINS/MINERALS	COMMENTS
Allergy	Grape seed, stinging nettle, coleus, vitamin C	*Grape seed:* Contraindicated in active bleeding, hemostatic disorders; potential interaction with anticoagulants, aspirin, NSAIDs, antiplatelet agents.
		Coleus: Potential interaction with anticoagulants, aspirin, NSAIDs, antiplatelet agents, methotrexate.
		Vitamin C: High doses for diabetic patients may produce falsely high blood glucose readings.
Asthma	Cordyceps, tylophora, grape seed, coleus, vitamin C	*Cordyceps:* May interact with MAO inhibitors, anticoagulants, NSAIDs, antiplatelet agents.
		Tylophora: May interact with MAO inhibitors, anticoagulants, aspirin, NSAIDs, antiplatelet agents.
		Grape seed, coleus, vitamin C: See above.
Cold	Arabinoxylane, *Echinacea,* elderberry, astragalus, goldenseal, grapefruit seed extract, zinc, vitamin C	*Arabinoxylane:* High phosphorus content indicates caution in patients with renal failure.
		Echinacea: Do not use longer than 10 days; potential interaction with therapeutic immunosuppressants and corticosteroids.
		Astragalus: May interact with immunosuppressants.
		Grapefruit seed extract: Avoid taking with astemizole, cisapride, terfenadine, or other medications metabolized by cytochrome P-450 3A4 system.
		Vitamin C: See above.
Cough	Ground ivy, thyme, licorice, marshmallow	*Ground ivy:* Contraindicated in epilepsy.
		Thyme: Use with caution in patients with allergy to oregano.
		Licorice: Potential interactions with laxatives, corticosteroids, cardiac glycosides.
		Marshmallow: Potential interactions with insulin, oral hypoglycemic agents.

Modified from Krinsky DL, Lavella JB, Hawkins EB, et al: *Natural therapeutics pocket guide,* ed 2, Hudson, Ohio, 2003, Lexi-Comp, Inc.
NSAIDs, Nonsteroidal antiinflammatory drugs; *MAO,* monoamine oxidase.

CASE STUDY

Lisa Fines, 28 years old, comes to the clinic with a clear nasal discharge, red itchy eyes, and a cough of 3 days' duration.

1. What other important information would you like to obtain from her history?
2. What information would you like to obtain from the physical examination?
3. What pattern of subjective and objective findings would make you believe she had seasonal allergic rhinitis? Asthma? A URTI?
4. What would be the difference in treatment for seasonal allergic rhinitis, asthma, or a URTI?
5. Would there be any modifications in the recommended treatment if Lisa were pregnant? A child or only 2 years of age? An elderly patient with congestive heart failure?

CASE STUDY

Mrs. Plains is a 43-year-old African American woman who reports wheezing and tightness in her chest since early this morning. She went shopping today and has been outside during an unseasonable cold spell, which she believes is the cause of the wheezing. She has had one other episode of wheezing that occurred 3 days ago while she was outside in the cold. She has a slight cough that is productive of a small amount of clear sputum. For the last 3 or 4 days she has awakened at night, particularly early in the morning, with dyspnea and a cough. She has no other symptoms.

Physical examination: Afebrile and in no acute distress.
Cardiovascular: Heart rate 84 beats/min, blood pressure 114/84 mm Hg.
Respiratory: Breath sounds equal throughout both sides; scattered monophonic expiratory wheezes throughout lung fields.

1. The physician decides that Mrs. Plains has a moderately persistent, reversible airway obstruction that is responsive to bronchodilators and corticosteroids. She is started on an oral inhaler. What might the doctor order? Give the name, dosage, frequency, and patient instructions for each medication you select.

NAME	DOSAGE	FREQUENCY	PATIENT INSTRUCTIONS
a.			
b.			
c.			

2. Mrs. Plains comes back in 1 month. Two weeks ago she had a cold with nasal congestion, sneezing, and a sore throat. Since then, the cough has worsened and she is now producing large amounts of purulent sputum. What do you think has happened?
3. The physician orders erythromycin EES one tablet PO three times daily. Why?
4. Mrs. Plains returns 1 month later. Her cough and sputum production have resolved. She continues to have wheezing when she goes out in the cold. What self-management plans would you discuss with her?

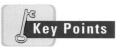

- The following respiratory medications are used to treat allergies or respiratory system disorders: antihistamines, or allergy medications; antitussives, or medications to control cough; asthma medications (bronchodilators, leukotriene receptor inhibitors, corticosteroids); decongestants; expectorants; and nasal steroids.
- Respiratory medications are available in many forms, as both prescription and OTC medications.
- Monitoring adverse reactions and teaching the patient about adverse reactions, administration, and dosage considerations are important responsibilities of the nurse in administering respiratory medications.

Go to the free CD-ROM for an Audio Glossary, animations, video clips, and Review Questions for the NCLEX-PN® Examination.

evolve Be sure to visit the companion Evolve website at http://evolve.elsevier.com/Edmunds/LPN/ for WebLinks, a link to the top 200 drugs by prescription, and sign-up pages for newsletter drug updates.

DRUG CALCULATION REVIEW

1. Order: Theophylline 300 mg by mouth twice a day
   Supply: Theophylline 100-mg tablets
   Question: How many tablets of theophylline are needed with each dose?

2. Order: Albuterol 4 mg by mouth three times daily
   Supply: Albuterol 2-mg tablets
   Question: How many tablets of albuterol are needed with each dose?

3. A 20-year-old woman presents to the emergency department with itching and red wheals present on her extremities. The physician orders diphenhydramine (Benadryl) 25 mg IM stat. You note that the multiple-dose vial read 50 mg/1 mL. Using dimensional analysis, how many milliliters should you prepare for this injection?

CRITICAL THINKING ?

1. Ms. Allbright comes into your clinic stating that her antihistamine dosage requires adjustment. You ask her to describe her symptoms, and she gives you the classic symptoms indicating a need for antihistamine. What are the signs and symptoms that would require an antihistamine?

2. The physician listens to your report of Ms. Allbright's complaints and then shakes his head. He tells you that Ms. Allbright has been taking an antihistamine for an extended period of time. The physician suspects that she has built up a possible psychologic dependence, leading to overuse and rebound reactions. What symptoms would lead you to suspect that Ms. Allbright is undergoing rebound phenomenon? How *might* you determine that the medication is not working . . . ?

3. Mr. Tracy enters the clinic with a severe cough. He demands loudly that he be given "cough drops right away!" What questions will you ask Mr. Tracy about his cough? In what situations would you not want to suppress a cough?

4. The physician agrees that Mr. Tracy should be given something to relieve his coughing. What class of drugs is commonly used to relieve coughing? What is "symptomatic relief"? Why are these medications used in nonproductive coughs?

5. Mr. Tracy has been prescribed an antitussive. Develop a patient teaching plan that includes a discussion of possible adverse reactions and drug interactions. What will you tell Mr. Tracy?

6. Ms. Henry has just been told she has asthma. She tells you that she has "suspected it for quite some time, but it is a surprise anyway." She asks you to tell her what causes asthma. Then she asks you to explain why she has to take medication right now, when she has not had an "attack" for several weeks. Explain the differences between treatment and prophylaxis and why she needs prophylactic therapy.

7. Ms. Henry has never used a Spinhaler before. Draw up a teaching plan for Ms. Henry, showing her how to place the capsules properly in the Spinhaler and how to inhale. Include strategies for reducing the coughing reaction and care of the Spinhaler itself.

8. Ms. Rochester has had several nasal polyps removed and has been placed on intranasal steroids. She is worried about taking any kind of steroid. "I wouldn't mind as much, I guess, if I just knew what to watch out for," she says. Identify the most common adverse reactions to nasal steroids; compare them with adverse reactions to systemic steroids.

9. Why are antitussives generally not recommended for patients with COPD?

10. Why would a patient be asked to discontinue his or her seasonal allergy antihistamines before receiving a purified protein derivative (PPD) for tuberculosis screening or before skin testing for other allergies?

11. You are working in a community clinic. As she is leaving after her appointment, Ms. Harris tells you she "is going straight to the drugstore because the doctor says she has a bad head cold and she needs something to drain her sinuses." When you review her medical history, you see that she is taking medication to control hypertension. What information does she need before choosing an OTC decongestant?

12 Antiinfective Medications

Objectives

After reading and studying this chapter, you should be able to do the following:

1. Identify the major antiinfective drug categories and the organisms against which they are effective.
2. Define "spectrum" and explain what this word means in antiinfective therapy.
3. List some of the most common adverse reactions to medications used to treat infections.
4. Outline the most important things to teach the patient who is taking antiinfective medications.

Key Terms

Be sure to check out the bonus material on the free CD-ROM, including selected audio pronunciations.

antibiotics (ăn-tĭ-bī-ŎT-ĭks, p. 166)
antimicrobials (ăn-tĭ-mī-KRŌ-bē-ălz, p. 166)
bactericidal (băk-tēr-ĭ-SĪD-ăl, p. 167)
bacteriostatic (băk-tēr-ē-ō-STĂT-ĭk, p. 167)
broad-spectrum drugs (p. 167)
generation (p. 166)
helminthiasis (hĕl-mĭn-THĪ-ă-sĭs, p. 188)
narrow-spectrum drugs (p. 167)
pathogen (PĂTH-ō-jĕn, p. 166)
spectrum (p. 167)
superinfection (SŪ-pĕr-ĭn-fĕk-shŭn, p. 167)

OVERVIEW

This chapter discusses medications used to treat various types of infections. Because of the many different types of infections and the numerous drugs that have been developed to treat them, antiinfective drugs are some of the most commonly given drugs. Thus, you will need to learn as much as possible about these drugs and how to teach patients who are taking them.

Organisms of many different types are always on the skin and inside the body of healthy individuals. These organisms do not make a person ill unless there is some change in the effectiveness of the skin as a barrier or a change that makes the person more vulnerable, such as being pregnant or developing acquired immunodeficiency syndrome (AIDS). Infants and young children and elderly people have the greatest risk of infection, as do people with poor circulation, poor nutritional status, or multiple diseases, and those who often come in contact with people who have infections. An organism that produces infection is a **pathogen.**

Pathogenic organisms come in a variety of forms. The term *bacteria* has been used to refer to unicellular, plantlike microorganisms lacking chlorophyll. This term is a generic term that is now often replaced by more specific names. *Fungi* are plantlike organisms growing in irregular masses, without roots, stems, or leaves, and without chlorophyll or other pigments involved in photosynthesis; they reproduce sexually or asexually. *Virus* is the term for a group of microbes that, with few exceptions, are capable of passing through fine filters that trap most bacteria; they cannot grow or reproduce apart from living cells. How a virus is classified depends on the features of its virion (the complete virus particle). A *parasite* is an organism that lives on or in another organism and draws its food from the other organism.

Each infection in a patient must be carefully evaluated to identify the specific organism causing the infection and the drug that will be most effective against it. Although some parasites may be seen with the naked eye, most infectious organisms are visible only under a microscope. The organisms must be carefully cultured and tested to see which medications are effective against them (medication sensitivity). Organisms can be identified by their shape, and many can be classed as gram positive or gram negative, depending on whether they are stained by Gram stain or not. Learning what organism is present allows the health care provider to use the medication that will best treat that particular organism.

Antiinfective agents, or **antimicrobials,** are chemicals that kill or damage the pathogenic organisms. Some of these chemicals are made from other living microorganisms (such as the penicillins), and are classified as **antibiotics.** Other chemicals are synthetics (such as sulfonamides) or are combinations of synthetic and naturally occurring microorganisms. Some drugs have become more refined, purified, and sensitive as a result of long-term testing. Each new group of these drugs that is developed from other similar drugs is called a **generation;** the original group of drugs are referred to as first-generation drugs, and later groups are called second-generation drugs, third-generation drugs, and so on.

Antiinfective medications work in many different ways. Usually they interfere with some important life process of a pathogen, thereby making it weaker, or incapable of reproducing; in some cases they actually kill the organism. Agents that are **bactericidal** kill the bacteria; those that are **bacteriostatic** limit or slow the growth of the bacteria, which weakens or eventually leads to the death of the bacteria. (The "cidal" or "static" part of the word gives a clue about the activity, whether it refers to bacteria or to fungi [fungicidal or fungistatic].) The number of organisms the medication is effective against is described in terms of its **spectrum.** Some antiinfective medications are effective against only a few organisms. These are called **narrow-spectrum drugs.** Other drugs are effective against a wide variety of organisms. These are known as **broad-spectrum drugs.**

Antibiotics often cause adverse reactions. These include allergy (penicillin and sulfa products cause the most allergies); ototoxicity, nephrotoxicity, and hepatotoxicity (damage to the ears, kidneys, and liver that may or may not be reversible if medication is stopped); and gastrointestinal (GI) distress so severe that it may require stopping the drug. Antibiotics can also result in **superinfection,** when other organisms that are not sensitive to a prescribed antibiotic (for example, yeast) are able to overgrow because the antibiotic also killed the organisms that would have kept them under control.

Overuse of antibiotics, especially when it was not known if the drug could kill the organism, has led to problems over the years: (1) patients now expect to get a prescription every time they feel ill; (2) the organisms that were weak may all have been killed over the years, leaving only the very virulent or strong pathogens; and (3) exposing organisms to antibiotics that did not kill them has led to the development of "super germs" that have built up a tolerance or resistance to common antibiotics. The result of these factors is that many common organisms infecting patients are now resistant to available drugs, and new antiinfectives have not yet been developed to fight them. Because many organisms have developed resistance to multiple drugs, vancomycin may be a drug of last resort in many patients. Vancomycin is effective against some gram-positive bacteria that are resistant to multiple drugs and is used in cases of severe infection. It may take several years before researchers are able to find new antiinfective drugs, and many patients may be left without effective drugs when they really do need them.

This chapter describes the main information about many types of antiinfective medications and is divided into three sections. Section One discusses antibiotics: penicillins, sulfonamides, and the broad-spectrum antibiotics. Section Two describes the drugs used in the treatment of tuberculosis. Section Three discusses drugs used to treat parasitic infections, including amebicides, anthelmintics, and antimalarial preparations. Antifungal medications are included in Chapter 13, along with other antiviral and antiretroviral drugs used in the treatment of AIDS.

SECTION ONE
Antibiotics

PENICILLINS

ACTION

Penicillin interferes with creation of the mucopeptide cell wall.

USES

Penicillins were the main antibiotics for many years. They were used for almost every type of infection, including those for which they were not effective. Over the years, overuse and inappropriate use of penicillin has led to the development of penicillin-resistant strains of disease. Allergy to penicillin has also become a problem. Although penicillin continues to be an important antibiotic, research on penicillin has led to the identification of many other types of antibiotics that may now be used to control infection. Penicillin is the broad-spectrum drug of choice for susceptible gram-positive and gram-negative organisms.

The choice of drug to give a patient depends on the infectious organism (as identified by cultures or smears) or on the basis of the clinical picture. Penicillin is effective in the treatment of the following susceptible organisms: alpha-hemolytic streptococci; group A beta-hemolytic streptococci; streptococci belonging to groups C, G, H, L, and M; and *Spirillum minus* (rat-bite fever), *Neisseria gonorrhoeae, Treponema pallidum* (syphilis), *Neisseria meningitidis, Clostridium perfringens, Clostridium tetani, Corynebacterium diphtheriae, Staphylococcus, Pasteurella meningitidis,* and other less common organisms. Penicillin is also used for prophylactic treatment against bacterial endocarditis in patients with rheumatic or congenital heart disease before they have dental procedures or surgery of the upper respiratory tract, genitourinary tract, or GI tract. Some penicillins may be useful against organisms used by terrorists as bioweapons.

ADVERSE REACTIONS

Adverse reactions to penicillin include neuropathy (with high parenteral dosages), fixed drug eruptions (usually a single spot that itches), nausea, vomiting, epigastric distress, anemia, blood dyscrasias, rash, erythema (redness or inflammation), urticaria (hives), angioedema (swelling of the skin and mucous membranes), laryngeal edema (swelling of the larynx), and anaphylaxis (shock).

DRUG INTERACTIONS

Bacteriostatic antibiotics such as tetracycline and erythromycin may decrease the bactericidal effect of penicillin. Probenecid prolongs blood levels of penicillin by blocking its renal clearance. Use of ampicillin and oral contraceptives together has produced menstrual irregularities and unplanned pregnancies. Indomethacin, phenylbutazone, or aspirin may increase serum penicillin levels. Antacids may decrease the absorption of penicillin. Penicillin may change the results of some laboratory tests.

Clinical Landmine

Drug Interactions and Women

Women who are taking oral birth control pills should use a backup method of protection if they begin taking an antibiotic. Many antibiotics interfere with the action of birth control pills, leaving the woman at risk of pregnancy.

Nursing Implications and Patient Teaching

Assessment

The patient in need of antibiotic therapy may vary from being asymptomatic (showing no symptoms) to being severely ill. You should look for common clues to infection, such as fever, redness, swelling, or pain.

You should learn as much as possible about the health history of the patient, including any other drugs she takes that may interact with penicillin; whether there is a prior history of penicillin allergy, asthma, or hypersensitivity (allergy) to procaine or tartrazine; and if the patient is pregnant or breastfeeding. These conditions may be contraindications or precautions to the use of penicillin.

Anaphylactic (shock) reactions have occurred with both oral and parenteral penicillin therapy. Penicillin should be used with caution in patients who have many other drug allergies.

Diagnosis

The type of infection will dictate the antibiotic to be used and whether treatment guidelines apply. Diagnosis of previous drug or food allergies, dementia, and dehydration may all influence the drug to be ordered, the dosage, and the rate of administration.

Planning

Prolonged use of penicillin may lead to liver, kidney, or blood disorders.

A minimum of 10 days of therapy is indicated to treat group A beta-hemolytic streptococci to reduce the risk of rheumatic fever, endocarditis, or glomerulonephritis. Resistant strains of pathogens have developed when penicillin is not given in effective doses and for the length of time required to kill organisms.

Clinical Goldmine

Antibiotic Therapy

Whenever possible, cultures should be drawn before starting antibiotic therapy. You may need to culture sputum, urine, blood, wound, or nonhealing sites on the skin.

Implementation

With intramuscular (IM) injections, the nurse should always aspirate (pull back on the plunger of the syringe to check for blood) to prevent medicine from accidentally being injected into a blood vessel.

The sexual partners of patients infected with syphilis or gonorrhea must be treated also.

While the patient is on penicillin therapy, the results of laboratory culture and sensitivity tests, as well as many other laboratory findings, may be incorrect because penicillin changes the results of many tests.

The dosage of penicillin ordered depends on the type and severity of the infection. Penicillins come in different forms and may be classified as natural (penicillins G and V), penicillinase resistant, broad spectrum (aminopenicillins), and extended spectrum. Table 12-1 presents a summary of penicillins.

Evaluation

You should take the patient's blood pressure and pulse before IM penicillin injections to have baseline information. The patient should be advised to wait 30 minutes after PO (by mouth) or IM administration before leaving an office or clinic. This allows time for you to watch for signs of adverse reactions. You should also watch the patient for signs of allergic reaction, although some allergic responses may not develop for days after taking the medication.

Table 12-1

Penicillins

GENERIC NAME	TRADE NAME	COMMENTS AND DOSAGE
NATURAL PENICILLINS		
penicillin G (benzathine)	Bicillin Permapen	Long-acting IM penicillin. In children, administer parenterally in midlateral aspect of thigh. In adults, give IM in gluteal muscle. Oral dosage exhibits poor absorption and is not recommended for routine use. *Oral dosages:* 400,000-600,000 units PO q6h. *Parenteral dosages:* • *Prophylaxis for rheumatic fever:* 1.2 million units IM twice a month on a continuous basis. • *Streptococcal upper respiratory infection, skin and soft tissue infection, scarlet fever, erysipelas:* *Adults:* 2.4 million units IM. *Children 30-60 lbs:* 900,000-1.2 million units IM. *Children under 30 lbs:* 600,000 units IM. • *Syphilis* *Early:* 2.4 million units IM. *Latent:* 2.4 million units IM once a week for 3 weeks.
penicillin G (potassium)	Pfizerpen	Given primarily to infants and children IV as 15-30 min infusions. *Infants up to 7 days:* 50,000 units/kg/day in divided doses every 12 hr; for group B *Streptococcus* or meningitis, give 100,000-150,000 units/kg/day. *Infants over 7 days and children:* 75,000 units/kg/day in divided doses every 8 hr. In meningitis, this may be increased from 200,000-300,000 units/kg/day every 6 hr.
penicillin G (procaine, aqueous) (APPG)	Wycillin	Contains procaine to decrease injection pain; determine if patient is allergic to procaine. Give deep IM injection in gluteal muscle; aspirate before injection. Rotate injection sites. This is the drug of choice for gonorrhea. • *Pneumonia* (pneumococcal): 600,000-1,200,000 units/day IM. • *Bacterial endocarditis* (group A beta-hemolytic streptococci): 600,000-1,200,000 units/day. • *Prophylaxis against bacterial endocarditis:* 1,000,000 units penicillin G with 600,000 units APPG IM 30-60 minutes before surgical or dental procedures, then 500 mg penicillin V q6h for 8 doses. • *Sexually transmitted diseases* (may vary, depending on disease): 4.8 million units IM (in 2 sites), with 1 gm probenecid, followed by 100 mg oral doxycycline twice daily for 10-14 days.
penicillin V		Stable in gastric juices; however, blood levels are higher when administered on an empty stomach. • *Streptococcal infection, scarlet fever, erysipelas:* 200,000-400,000 units PO q6-8h for 10 days. • *Pneumococcal infection:* 400,000-600,000 units q6h until afebrile for 2 days. • *Staphylococcal infection, fusospirochetosis:* 400,000-800,000 units PO q6-8h. • *Prophylaxis for rheumatic fever/chorea:* 200,000-250,000 units PO twice daily continuously.
penicillin V (potassium)	Beepen-VK Pen-Vee K	Used in the treatment of mild to moderately severe infections when patient can take oral medication. *Adults:* 250-500 mg PO 3 to 4 times daily. *Children:* 15-50 mg/kg/day in 3-6 divided doses.

Continued

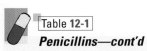

Table **12-1**

Penicillins—cont'd

GENERIC NAME	TRADE NAME	COMMENTS AND DOSAGE
PENICILLINASE RESISTANT		
cloxacillin	Cloxapen	Effective in the treatment of pneumococci. Also effective in the treatment of group A beta-hemolytic streptococci. *Adults and children over 20 kg:* 250-500 mg PO q6h. *Children under 20 kg:* 50-100 mg/kg/day PO in divided doses q6h.
dicloxacillin	Dycill Dynapen	Effective in the treatment of penicillinase-producing staphylococci. *Adults and children over 40 kg:* 125-250 mg PO q6h. *Children under 40 kg:* 12.5-25 mg/kg/day PO q6h.
nafcillin	Nallpen Unipen	*Adults:* 250 mg to 1 gm PO q4-6h; or 500 mg IM q4-6h. *Children:* 250 mg PO 3 times daily or 25-50 mg/kg/day in 4 divided doses; or 25 mg/kg/day IM in 2 doses. *IV dosage:* 500 mg q4h in 15-30 mL of sodium chloride, injected for 5-10 min or as slow drip to prevent thrombophlebitis.
oxacillin	Bactocill	Rare, reversible hepatocellular dysfunction has been reported. *Adults:* 500-1000 mg PO q4-6h for 5 days, or 250 mg to 1 gm IM q4-6h. *Children:* 50-100 mg/kg/day PO in divided doses q6h for 5 days; or 50-100 mg/kg/day parenterally in 4 divided doses.
AMINOPENICILLINS: BROAD-SPECTRUM PENICILLINS		
amoxicillin	Amoxil Trimox Wymox	*Adults and children over 20 kg:* 250-500 mg PO q8h. *Children under 20 kg:* 20-40 mg/kg/day PO in divided doses q8h. • *Uncomplicated gonorrhea:* 3 gm PO single dose with 1 gm probenecid; follow with tetracycline 500 mg PO 4 times daily for 7 days.
amoxicillin and clavulanate potassium	Augmentin	*Adults:* One 250-mg tablet q8h. *Children:* 20 mg/kg/day in divided doses q8h.
ampicillin	Omnipen Totacillin	Give with 1 gm probenecid for treatment of gonorrhea. *Adults:* 250-500 mg PO qid. *Children under 20 kg:* 50-100 mg/kg/day PO in divided doses q6h. *Children over 20 kg:* 250-500 mg PO 4 times daily. • *Uncomplicated gonorrhea:* 3.5 g PO with 1 gm probenecid.
ampicillin sodium (parenteral)	Omnipen	Used in treatment of a variety of serious infections and often used concomitantly with a sodium aminoglycoside or a cephalosporin. *Adults:* 250-500 mg IM or IV q6h. *Children:* 25-50 mg/kg/day IM or IV in divided doses q6-8h. • *Lower respiratory tract infections, skin infections, bone and joint infections:* 225-300 mg/kg/day. Give IV in divided doses of 3-4 gm q4-6h. • *Urinary tract infections:* 100-200 mg/kg/day. Give IV in divided doses of 2-3 gm q6h.
ampicillin sodium and sulbactam sodium	Unasyn	Give either IV or IM. *Adults:* 1.5-3 gm q6h.
bacampicillin	Spectrobid ✤	*Adults:* 400 mg q12h; dose may be doubled in severe infections. *Children under 25 kg:* 25 mg/kg/day in 2 equally divided doses q12h; dose may be doubled in severe infections. • *Gonorrhea:* Usual adult dosage for men and women is 1.6 gm bacampicillin plus 1 gm probenecid as a single oral dose.

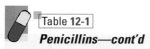

GENERIC NAME	TRADE NAME	COMMENTS AND DOSAGE
EXTENDED SPECTRUM		

carbenicillin	Geocillin	Products vary in amount of sodium per gram.
		• *Urinary tract infection*
		Adults: Uncomplicated: 1-2 gm IM q6h. Serious: 200 mg/kg/day IV drip.
		Children: 50-200 mg/kg/day IM in divided doses q4-6h.
		• *Septicemia, severe systemic respiratory, or soft tissue infections*
		Adults
		   Pseudomonas and anaerobes: 400-500 mg/kg/day IV in divided doses or continuous drip.
		   Proteus and *Escherichia coli*: 300-400 mg/kg/day.
		Children: 400-500 mg/kg/day IV in divided doses or continuous drip.

mezlocillin	Mezlin	Administered IM or IV. This product is reserved for use in severe or complicated infections. • *Urinary tract infections:* 1.5-3 gm q6h IV or IM. • *Lower respiratory tract infections, intraabdominal infections, skin and gynecologic infections:* 3-4 gm q4-6h IV or IM.
piperacillin	Pipracil	Effective against a wide number of gram-positive and gram-negative aerobic and anaerobic bacteria. • *Urinary tract infections, pneumonia:* 6-16 gm/day IV divided into 4-6 doses. • *Uncomplicated gonorrhea infections:* 2 gm IM single dose. • *Complicated or serious infections:* 12-18 gm/day IV into 4-6 doses.
piperacillin sodium and tazobactam sodium	Zosyn	Administer by IV infusion over 30 minutes. Usual dose is 3.375 gm q6h.
ticarcillin	Ticar	• *Uncomplicated urinary tract infection* *Adults:* 1 gm IM or IV q6h. *Children:* 50-100 mg/kg/day IM or IV in divided doses q6-8h. • *Complicated urinary tract infections:* 150-200 mg/kg/day in divided doses q4-6h. • *Systemic septicemia, respiratory tract infection, soft tissue infection:* 200-300 mg/kg/day in 3, 4, or 6 divided doses.
ticarcillin and clavulanate sodium	Timentin	Administer 3.1 gm q4-6h by IV infusion. Reduce dosage in renal impairment.

Patient and Family Teaching

You should tell the patient and family the following:

1. The patient should take the medication exactly as prescribed and not stop taking medication just because he feels better. Every dose should be taken.
2. The patient should use care when bathing and brushing the teeth while using this medication, and watch for any signs of itching, irritation, or infection.
3. The patient should notify the nurse, physician, or other health care provider if rash, hives, decreased urination, diarrhea, or other unusual symptoms develop. Penicillin allergies can develop at any time after the patient had started the treatment.
4. If medication is given on an outpatient basis, the patient should go to an emergency room quickly if he becomes short of breath or has difficulty breathing.
5. If treatment is for a sexually transmitted disease, the patient should not engage in sexual activity during treatment. All sexual partners should also be tested and treated.

SULFONAMIDES

ACTION

Sulfonamides have a bacteriostatic effect against a wide range of gram-positive and gram-negative microorganisms by inhibiting folic acid synthesis.

USES

Sulfonamides are usually used to treat acute and chronic urinary tract infections, particularly cystitis, pyelitis, and pyelonephritis, when these infections are caused by *Escherichia coli* or *Nocardia asteroides*. Other indications include trachoma (inclusion conjunctivitis), chancroid, lymphogranuloma venereum, toxoplasmosis, acute otitis media caused by *Haemophilus influenzae*, and prophylactic therapy in cases of recurrent rheumatic fever. Susceptible organisms include *Streptococcus pyogenes*, *Streptococcus pneumoniae*, some strains of *Bacillus anthracis*, *Corynebacterium diphtheriae*, *Haemophilus ducreyi*, and *Chlamydia trachomatis*, and other less common organisms. Several sulfonamides are useful only in the treatment of ulcerative colitis, as preoperative and postoperative therapy for bowel surgery, or in the treatment of dermatitis herpetiformis.

ADVERSE REACTIONS

Adverse reactions to sulfonamides include headache, drowsiness, fatigue, dizziness, vertigo (feeling of dizziness or spinning), tinnitus (ringing in the ears), hearing loss, insomnia (inability to sleep), peripheral neuropathy, hypothyroidism, hypoglycemia (low blood sugar level), anorexia (lack of appetite), nausea, vomiting, stomatitis (inflammation of the mouth), abdominal pain, drug fever, blood dyscrasias, generalized maculopapular or urticarial rash, fever, malaise (weakness), pruritus (itching), dermatitis, local irritation, periorbital edema (swelling around the eyes), anaphylactic shock, crystalluria (formation of crystals in the urine), hematuria (blood in the urine), and proteinuria (large amounts of protein in the urine). Other serious adverse effects, including toxemia (bacterial poisons in the bloodstream) and fever, may develop with overdosage and indicate that the patient may have a severe hypersensitivity to sulfonamides.

Clinical Goldmine

Superinfection

You must watch for superinfections, or overgrowth of normal bacteria, that may show up in the oral, vaginal, or rectal areas.

DRUG INTERACTIONS

Sulfonamides may potentiate or increase the effect of oral anticoagulants, methotrexate, sulfonylureas, thiazide diuretics, phenytoin, and uricosuric agents. Sulfonamides may be displaced from plasma albumin by probenecid, salicylates, phenylbutazone, promethazine, sulfinpyrazone, and indomethacin; this will cause the effects of sulfonamides to be increased. Penicillins may be less effective when used together with a sulfonamide. The sulfonamide's effect may be antagonized by drugs such as local anesthetics. Antacids may result in decreased absorption of the sulfonamide when they are taken together. Sulfonamides may change the results of various laboratory tests.

Nursing Implications and Patient Teaching

Assessment

You should learn as much as possible about the complete health history of the patient, including any allergy to sulfa drugs, aspirin, thiazides, or sulfonylureas; whether the patient is taking any other drugs that may interact with sulfonamides; whether the patient is pregnant or breastfeeding; and whether the patient has kidney or liver problems. These conditions are contraindications or precautions to the use of sulfonamides.

The patient in need of antibiotic therapy may vary from being asymptomatic to being severely ill. You should watch for symptoms of infection, such as fever, redness, swelling, or pain.

Diagnosis

Does the patient have allergy, dehydration, or other medical problems that would interfere with the administration of this drug?

Planning

The drug should be discontinued if the patient's urinary output is reduced or if a rash develops.

Warn the patient to stay out of the sun because severe photosensitivity (abnormal response to exposure to sunlight) can occur if the patient's skin is exposed to excessive amounts of sunlight or ultraviolet light.

The patient should drink adequate fluids to avoid crystalluria or urinary stone formation.

Implementation

Although most sulfonamides are given by mouth, several can be given parenterally, primarily intravenously (IV). Other parenteral routes are avoided because they can cause irritation of the skin. Some sulfonamides are given vaginally as creams or suppositories, or in eye or ear preparations.

Sulfonamide dosage depends on the severity of the infection being treated, the drug used, and the patient's response to and tolerance of the drug. Generally, the short-acting sulfonamides are given at more frequent intervals than are the intermediate- or long-acting sulfonamides. Also, short-acting sulfonamides usually require a special first dose that is larger than the dose that will be regularly taken (initial loading dose).

If sulfonamides are taken with food, their absorption tends to be delayed but not reduced. Table 12-2 provides a summary of sulfonamides.

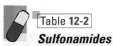

Table 12-2
Sulfonamides

GENERIC NAME	TRADE NAME	COMMENTS AND DOSAGE
sulfadiazine	Sulfadiazine	Requires a daily urinary output of at least 1500 mL plus alkalization to prevent crystalluria. Subcutaneous and IM routes are contraindicated. • *Urinary tract infection, rheumatic fever prophylaxis:* 500 mg daily for patients who weigh less than 30 kg; 1 gm daily for those over 30 kg. • *Intraocular infection:* 4 gm initially, then 1 gm q4h. • *Intravenous* *Adults:* 100 mg/kg up to total of 5 gm initially, then 30-50 mg/kg q6-8h. *Children and infants over 2 months:* 50 mg/kg initially, then 100 mg/kg daily in 4 divided doses.
sulfamethizole	Thiosulfil	A short-acting, readily soluble sulfonamide effective in the treatment of urinary tract infections. *Adults:* 2-4 gm initially, then 2-4 gm daily in 3-6 divided doses. *Children and infants over 2 months:* 75 mg/kg initially, then 150 mg/kg daily in 4-6 divided doses, total daily dose not to exceed 6 gm.
sulfamethoxazole	Gantanol	An intermediate-acting sulfonamide highly effective in urinary tract infections when used for 7-10 days. *Adults:* 2 gm initially, then 1 gm 2 to 3 times daily. *Children and infants over 2 months:* 50-60 mg/kg initially, then 25-30 mg/kg q12h.
sulfasalazine	Azulfidine SAS Enteric-500 🍁	• *Ulcerative colitis* *Adults:* 1-4 gm daily in 4-8 divided doses, then 2-3 gm daily in 4 divided doses as maintenance. *Children and infants over 2 months:* 40-60 mg/kg daily in 4-8 divided doses, then 30 mg/kg daily in 4 divided doses as maintenance.
sulfonamide combination vaginal product	Triple Sulfa	Contains equal amounts of sulfadiazine, sulfamerazine, and sulfamethazine, thereby reducing the possibility of crystalluria because the solubility of each sulfonamide exists independently in solution. • *Vaginal infection:* Insert 2.5-5.0 mL (one-half to one applicator full) cream intravaginally twice daily for 14 days. Used primarily for urinary tract infections. *Adults:* 2-4 gm initially, then 2-4 gm daily in 3-6 divided doses. *Children and infants over 2 months:* 75 mg/kg initially, then 150 mg/kg daily in 4-6 divided doses, with total daily dose not to exceed 6 gm.
SULFONAMIDE MIXTURES		
sulfamethoxazole and trimethoprim	Bactrim 🍁 Septra	Used for acute infections and as prophylaxis. May be used in patients with impaired renal function and for those unable to tolerate sulfonamides alone. • *Urinary tract infection* *Adults:* 2 tablets or 20 mL suspension q12h for 10-14 days. *Children and infants over 2 months:* 40 mg/kg sulfamethoxazole and 8 mg/kg trimethoprim daily in 2 divided doses q12h for 10 days. • *Acute otitis media:* Follow pediatric dosage given for urinary tract infection.

Evaluation

A complete blood cell count (CBC), urinalysis, and liver and kidney function tests should be done before the patient begins sulfonamide therapy and about once every month if the patient is on prolonged therapy.

You should watch the patient for signs and symptoms of blood dyscrasias, including sore throat, fever, pallor (paleness), purpura (bruising), and jaundice (yellow color of skin, eyes, and mucous membranes), and for renal or hepatic failure in high-risk patients.

Patient and Family Teaching

You should tell the patient and family the following:

1. Sulfonamides are more fully absorbed when they are taken on an empty stomach. Therefore, they should be taken either 1 hour before or 2 hours after meals, along with a full glass of water.
2. To prevent formation of crystals in the urine, the patient must drink large amounts of water while taking this medication.
3. The patient should avoid excessive exposure to sunlight or ultraviolet light to prevent possible redness and irritation of the skin.
4. The patient should take all the medication prescribed and should not stop taking medication when she feels better and the symptoms disappear.
5. The patient should contact the nurse, physician, or other health care provider if there is no improvement of symptoms within 2 to 3 days after beginning therapy.
6. The nurse, physician, or other health care provider should be notified quickly if a skin rash, blood in the urine, bruises, nausea, or other adverse effects of therapy develop.

BROAD-SPECTRUM ANTIBIOTICS

ACTION

Broad-spectrum antibiotics act in different ways to affect pathogenic bacteria. They may attack a bacterium's internal cell processes, which are vital to its existence, or may destroy the external cell wall. Thus the antibiotics may be either bactericidal or bacteriostatic.

USES

Broad-spectrum antibiotics represent a very large grouping of unrelated drugs used to treat infections caused by certain susceptible organisms. For the medication to be effective, the organism responsible for the infection should be identified by a culture. The medication that is most effective against that particular organism is then determined through sensitivity testing. Organisms are often classified as gram positive or gram negative, depending on whether they are stained by Gram stain.

Antibiotics are not effective against viral, parasitic, or fungal infections. However, it is common for a patient with a viral or fungal infection to also develop a bacterial infection because the body's defenses are weakened. A *secondary infection* occurs when one infection follows another. In a *mixed infection*, both infections are present at the same time. Table 12-3 summarizes the organisms against which specific antibiotics are effective or the primary problems for which the medication might be used.

ADVERSE REACTIONS

Several types of adverse reactions are seen with most broad-spectrum antibiotics. Superinfections may develop, particularly after long-term use. These reactions, such as diarrhea, oral thrush (*Candida* infection of the mouth), or vaginal itching, are usually irritating but mild. At other times, the superinfection may become life-threatening. Overgrowth of organisms is commonly seen in AIDS patients, whose immune systems may be totally overwhelmed by a mild superinfection. Oral antibiotics commonly produce mild episodes of nausea, vomiting, and diarrhea but rarely require stopping the drug. These effects are often dose related, and they result from GI irritation, changes in the normal bacteria in the bowel, and overgrowth of yeast.

All drugs have the potential to damage the tissue of certain organs. The usual organs that are affected are the ear (the auditory nerves), the kidney, and the liver (producing ototoxicity, nephrotoxicity, and hepatotoxicity). Certain antibiotics are much more likely to produce tissue damage than others. It is important to carefully identify patients who may already have damage to these organs before medication is started.

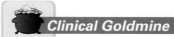
Clinical Goldmine

Antiinfectives

Aminoglycosides may cause significant damage to the kidney (nephrotoxicity) or ears (ototoxicity). Bacitracin may cause renal failure as a result of tubular and glomerular necrosis; therefore, the patient's renal status must be closely monitored.

Many individuals have allergic reactions to antibiotics. Allergic reactions may develop within minutes of taking the drug, or may appear days after stopping the medication. Hypersensitivity may also develop after repeated use of the medication. Allergy may range from a mild skin rash or fever to severe and possibly fatal anaphylaxis, characterized by shortness of breath, paralysis of the diaphragm, laryngeal edema, and shock. Patients must be closely questioned each time antibiotic therapy is ordered to determine sensitivity reactions. A

Table **12-3**
Sensitivity of Specific Organisms to Some Broad-Spectrum Antibiotics

ANTIBIOTIC	SUSCEPTIBLE ORGANISMS AND CLINICAL DISEASESE
aminoglycosides	Effective in the treatment of gram-negative infections when penicillin is contraindicated
bacitracin	Restricted to use in severe illness
	Effective in the treatment of staphylococcal pneumonia or empyema in infants
clindamycin	Used to treat severe infections caused by streptococci, pneumococci, staphylococci, or anaerobic bacteria when penicillin and erythromycin are contraindicated
erythromycin	Alternative treatment for patients hypersensitive to the penicillins
lincomycin	Used to treat severe infections caused by susceptible strains of streptococci, pneumococci, and staphylococci when penicillin and erythromycin are contraindicated
polymyxin B	Effective against all the gram-negative organisms, with the exception of *Proteus*
	Effective in the treatment of acute infections caused by susceptible strains of *Pseudomonas aeruginosa, Haemophilus influenzae, Escherichia coli, Enterobacter aerogenes,* and *Klebsiella pneumoniae*
spectinomycin	Drug of choice to treat gonorrhea in patients who are hypersensitive to the penicillins and to treat penicillinase-producing gonorrhea
telithromycin	New product for mild to moderate respiratory infections
	Used for *Streptococcus pneumoniae, H. influenzae,* in acute bacterial exacerbation, chronic bronchitis, acute sinusitis, community-acquired pneumonia
tetracyclines	Used to treat granuloma inguinale, rickettsial diseases, mycoplasmal infections, spirochetal relapsing fever, and *Chlamydia trachomatis*
	Indicated in patients sensitive to penicillin, especially to treat gonorrhea or syphilis
vancomycin	Used to treat severe infections in patients who are hypersensitive to the penicillins or cephalosporins
	Effective in the treatment of staphylococcal endocarditis, osteomyelitis, pneumonia, soft tissue infections, and methicillin-resistant staphylococcal infections
	Oral dosage effective in the treatment of staphylococcal enterocolitis

Clinical Landmine

Allergy
A patient may develop an allergic reaction to a drug at any time. This may include reactions to drugs that the patient has taken before without any symptoms.

patient who is sensitive to one type of antibiotic will often be sensitive to other types (cross-sensitivity).

In addition to these general reactions, some broad-spectrum antibiotics have specific adverse reactions associated with their use, and you should always watch for them. These reactions are summarized in Table 12-4.

Clinical Landmine

Antibiotic Cross-Sensitivity
Cross-sensitivity exists with many antibiotics. Any person who has several drug allergies should be carefully watched when taking any type of antibiotic.

DRUG INTERACTIONS

Antibiotics have many common drug interactions. These interactions often make the antibiotic ineffective or alter the effectiveness of the other drugs. Each patient taking an antibiotic must be watched carefully if he is taking other drugs. You should read the manufacturer's product information about specific drug interactions for each drug you administer. Use of some antacids with antibiotics may limit the absorption of tetracycline. Food, milk, dairy products, or iron preparations may also limit the absorption of some antibiotics. Some antibiotics interfere with the absorption of oral birth control pills, so the patient should use an additional form of birth control to avoid getting pregnant while she is taking the antibiotic.

Nursing Implications and Patient Teaching

Assessment
A patient in need of antibiotic therapy may vary from being asymptomatic to being severely ill. You should watch for common indicators of infection, such as fever, redness, swelling, or pain.

Table **12-4**

Significant Adverse Reactions Produced by Specific Broad-Spectrum Antibiotics

ANTIBIOTIC	ADVERSE REACTION
aminoglycosides	Significant renal toxicity, which is usually reversible; risk of toxicity increases in patients with renal impairment. Significant auditory and vestibular ototoxicity may occur in patients on prolonged therapy or those taking higher than recommended dosages.
bacitracin	Renal toxicity leading to tubular and glomerular necrosis has been reported. Also, increased serum drug levels without an increase in drug dosage and severe pain and rash with IM injection are seen.
cephalosporins	Painful IM injections; thrombophlebitis with IV therapy. May produce hemolytic anemia and other blood dyscrasias.
clindamycin	Severe and fatal colitis characterized by abdominal cramps, diarrhea, and rectal passage of blood and mucus (these symptoms may not appear until after treatment is completed).
colistin	Renal toxicity. Transient neurologic disturbances have been reported with colistimethate, as well as nephrotoxicity manifested by decreased urinary output and increased serum creatinine.
erythromycin	GI distress, sensorineural hearing loss, and hepatotoxicity.
lincomycin	Severe and fatal colitis characterized by abdominal cramps, diarrhea, or rectal passage of blood and mucus (these symptoms may not develop until treatment is completed). Hypotension and cardiac arrest may occur after rapid IV administration.
polymyxin B	Nephrotoxicity may develop, evidenced by proteinuria, cellular urinary casts, azotemia, decreased output, or elevated BUN. Neurotoxicity may be evidenced by irritability, weakness, drowsiness, ataxia, numbness of extremities, blurring of vision, or respiratory paralysis.
tetracycline	Black, hairy tongue.
vancomycin	Nephrotoxicity with toxic effect increased at high serum levels or with prolonged therapy; ototoxicity may also occur.

You should find out as much as you can about the patient's health history, including prior renal damage, hepatic problems, systemic lupus erythematosus, or alcoholism; drugs that may interact with an antibiotic; pregnancy or breastfeeding; age; and occupation. These factors may be contraindications or precautions to antibiotic drug therapy.

Drugs such as cephalosporins may be classed as first-, second-, or third-generation agents, based on their chemical development from other drugs. In general, second- and third-generation drugs are more effective than first-generation agents against a broad group of gram-negative organisms; however, they are also less effective against gram-positive organisms. Third-generation agents are also more effective against resistant organisms and have increased resistance to inactivation by beta-lactamase (an enzyme that some organisms make to protect them against the action of some antibiotics). However, these agents cost more and may have more side effects. Differences among drugs within categories are primarily based on the drug's activity.

Diagnosis

Are there other factors that may pose a problem to the patient requiring broad-spectrum antibiotics? For example, patients reporting any previous allergy to the penicillins may also be allergic to some cephalosporins. Cephalosporins should be used with extreme caution in these individuals because of a high incidence of cross-sensitivity. Nephrotoxicity has been reported with some cephalosporins, and the incidence is greater in elderly patients and in patients with poor renal function.

Planning

Many broad-spectrum antibiotics cross the placental barrier and are secreted in breast milk. The use of tetracycline in pregnancy and in children under 8 years of age may produce tooth discoloration or inadequate bone or tooth development.

Photosensitivity may occur with tetracycline treatment, so the patient should avoid exposure to the sun or ultraviolet rays.

Many of the parenteral antibiotics should be used with caution because of their toxic effects. Many antibiotics should be given with extreme caution to patients with poor renal function. The risk of toxicity is low in patients with normal renal function if they take no more than the recommended dosage.

Implementation

The nurse should make certain that the drugs are taken at the proper time and for the full course of the therapy. The dosage depends on the type and the severity of the infection. All chewable forms of erythromycin must be fully chewed to obtain the complete therapeutic effect.

The strength for erythromycin is expressed as the erythromycin base equivalence. Because of differences in absorption, 400 mg of ethylsuccinate is required to provide the same free erythromycin serum levels as 250 mg of erythromycin base, stearate, or estolate.

Many antibiotics may be administered orally or parenterally. Topical application should be avoided to prevent sensitization. The patient should be kept well hydrated (supplied with fluids). Drinking extra fluids to ensure a minimum urine output of 1500 mL decreases the chances of renal toxicity.

The nurse should always aspirate before an IM injection to prevent medication from accidentally entering a blood vessel.

Doxycycline (Vibramycin) is a particularly good drug, especially for the elderly population. It may be taken twice daily and is usually tolerated even by some individuals who have reduced renal function.

Lincomycin and tetracycline are best absorbed on an empty stomach, 1 hour before or 2 hours after meals, and should be taken with a full glass of water. The patient should particularly avoid taking milk products with tetracycline.

Ciprofloxacin (Cipro) has been approved for the treatment and prophylaxis of anthrax.

In the treatment of syphilis, gonorrhea, or chlamydial infections, the sexual partners of the infected patient also must be treated.

Tetracycline that is out of date (older than the expiration date on the label) should not be used because it may lead to damage of the proximal renal tubules. Tetracycline should be used with caution in patients with poor liver function because the drug may cause hepatotoxicity.

Table 12-5 presents a summary of the broad-spectrum antibiotics.

Evaluation

Allergic reactions ranging from mild erythema to anaphylaxis have been reported with use of broad-spectrum antibiotics. Vertigo may develop with the use of any of the tetracyclines; however, vertigo is more common with the use of minocycline.

Superinfection may occur in the patient who is taking extended antibiotic therapy. You should monitor for infections in the mouth and the rectal or vaginal areas.

Because of the possibility of ototoxicity in patients taking vancomycin, you should watch for tinnitus, which may be a sign that the patient is at risk for deafness.

Aminoglycosides have a narrow therapeutic range, so you must closely monitor blood levels of these drugs to avoid toxic levels. Dosage is calculated on the basis of the patient's weight and is increased or decreased based on blood levels so an effective level is maintained. The narrow therapeutic range (when the lowest and highest levels are not far apart) requires that the sample for the antibiotic blood level be drawn just before the next scheduled dose is given. This sample will show the lowest blood level of the antibiotic (found at the "trough"), rather than a blood level at a higher range (at or near the "peak"). Knowing the lowest blood level allows you to increase or lower the dosage without dropping below the effective level or going above the toxic level. Because of the nephrotoxicity of these agents, blood urea nitrogen (BUN) and creatinine levels should also be monitored during the course of therapy.

Erythromycin products cause severe GI distress in almost all patients. They are also very irritating when given IV. Thus careful monitoring of a patient's reaction to these products is essential because there may be a need to discontinue the drug.

With some broad-spectrum antibiotics, you should monitor for liver toxicity by checking for abdominal pain, jaundice, dark urine, pale-colored stools, or weakness. Blood or mucus in the stools may indicate colitis. If large doses of antibiotics are given, the patient should be monitored closely for sensorineural hearing loss. You should observe the patient for therapeutic effects, allergy, and superinfection.

Patient and Family Teaching

You should tell the patient and family the following:

1. The patient should take tetracycline and lincomycin on an empty stomach, 1 hour before or 2 hours after eating, and follow it with a full glass of water. Most other antibiotics should be taken with meals or food to decrease GI upset.
2. If GI upset occurs, the patient should eat a few plain crackers with the medicine.
3. The patient should take the drug exactly as prescribed, even after the symptoms disappear. The medication should not be saved, because taking out-of-date medication may cause rather severe anal irritation.
4. The patient taking tetracycline should avoid the sun or ultraviolet light.
5. The patient should use care when bathing and brushing the teeth while taking this medication, and watch for signs of infection in the mouth and the anal or vaginal areas.

Table **12-5**

Broad-Spectrum Antibiotics

GENERIC NAME	TRADE NAME	COMMENTS AND DOSAGE
amikacin	Amikin	May be used to treat unidentified infections before results of sensitivity tests are known. Do not mix with other drugs. *Adults and children:* 15 mg/kg/day IM or IV in 2-3 divided doses; do not exceed 1.5 gm/day. *Neonates:* 10 mg/kg loading dose, followed by 7.5 mg/kg q12h.
gentamicin	Gentamycin	Used to treat unidentified infections. Do not mix with carbenicillin or other drugs. *Adults:* 1 mg/kg q8h; may use up to 5 mg/kg/day in 3-4 divided doses parenterally. *Children:* 2-2.5 mg/kg q8h.
kanamycin	Kamycine ♦ Kantrex	*Adults:* 3-12 gm/day PO in divided doses; 250 mg 2-4 times/day by inhalation. *Children:* 12.5 mg/kg/day PO in 4 divided doses. *Suppression of intestinal bacteria:* 1 gm PO qh for 4 hr, followed with 1 gm PO q6h for the next 36-72 hr. *Hepatic coma:* 8-12 gm/day PO in divided doses.
neomycin	Mycifradin Neo-Fradin Neo-Tabs	Used in preoperative preparation for surgery. *Suppression of intestinal bacteria:* Give 1 gm at 19 hours, 18 hours, and 9 hours before surgery.
netilmicin	Netromycin	*Adults:* 1.5-2 mg/kg q12h.
paromomycin	Humatin	• *Intestinal amebiasis:* 25-35 mg/kg/day PO in 3 divided doses for 5-10 days with meals. • *Hepatic coma:* 4 gm/day PO in divided doses for 5-6 days.
streptomycin	Streptomycin	Give deep IM injection in large muscle mass. *Adults:* 1st wk: 1 gm parenterally twice daily; 2nd wk: 0.5 gm parenterally twice daily with penicillin. • *Enterococcal endocarditis* *Adults:* 0.5-1 gm parenterally twice daily with penicillin for 4 wk.
tobramycin	Nebcin	May be used in combination with penicillin or cephalosporin in the treatment of unidentified infections before results of sensitivity tests are known. Do not premix with other drugs. *Adults and children:* 3 mg/kg/day IM q8h.
CEPHALOSPORINS **First Generation**		
cefadroxil	Duricef	*Adults:* 1-2 gm/day in single or 2 divided doses. *Children:* 30 mg/kg/day in divided doses q12h.
cefazolin	Ancef Kefzol Zolicef	IM or IV use. *Adults:* 250 mg to 1 gm q8h.
cephalexin	Keflex	*Adults:* 1-4 gm/day in divided doses. *Children:* 25-50 mg/kg/day in divided doses.
	Keftab	*Adults:* 1-4 gm/day in divided doses. Do not use in children.
cephapirin	Cefadyl	IM or IV use. *Adults:* 500 mg to 1 gm q4-6h. *Children:* 40 mg/kg in 4 divided doses.
cephradine	Velosef	Give PO, IM, or IV. *Adults:* 250 mg q6h. *Children:* 25-50 mg/kg/day in divided doses.
Second Generation		
cefaclor	Ceclor	*Adults:* 250-500 mg PO q8h. *Children:* 20 mg/kg/day in divided doses.
cefmetazole	Zefazone	*Adults:* 2 gm IV q6-12h for 5-14 days.

Table **12-5**

Broad-Spectrum Antibiotics—cont'd

GENERIC NAME	TRADE NAME	COMMENTS AND DOSAGE
CEPHALOSPORINS—cont'd		
Second Generation—cont'd		
cefonicid	Monocid	*Adults:* 1 gm once daily IV or deep IM.
cefotetan	Cefotan	*Adults:* 1-2 gm IV or IM q12h for 5-10 days.
cefoxitin	Mefoxin	Recommended by CDC in treatment schedules for gonorrhea and acute pelvic inflammatory disease. *Adults:* 1-4 gm q6-8h.
cefprozil	Cefzil	*Adults:* 500 mg PO once daily for 10 days. *Children:* 15 mg/kg PO q12h for 10 days.
cefuroxime	Ceftin Kefurox Zinacef	*Adults:* 250-500 mg twice daily. See CDC treatment schedules for gonorrhea and acute pelvic inflammatory disease.
loracarbef	Lorabid	*Adults:* 200-400 mg PO q12h for 7 days. *Children:* 30 mg/kg/day in divided doses for 10 days.
Third Generation		
cefdinir	Omnicef	Used in community-acquired pneumonia, chronic bronchitis, acute bacterial otitis media, acute maxillary sinusitis, pharyngitis/tonsillitis, and uncomplicated skin infections. *Adults:* Give 300-600 mg q12h for 10 days. *Children:* See package insert.
cefepime	Maxipime	Used in urinary tract infection, pneumonia, skin infections. Give IV or IM according to dosing schedule in package insert.
cefixime	Suprax	*Adults:* 400 mg/day PO or 200 mg q12h. *Children:* 8 mg/kg/day PO or 4 mg/kg q12h.
cefoperazone	Cefobid	Give IM or IV. *Adults:* 2-4 gm/day in 2 divided doses.
cefotaxime	Claforan	Give IV or IM. Maximum daily dose is 12 gm. Dosage depends on severity.
cefpodoxime	Vantin	200 mg PO q12h for 14 days. Reduce dosage in renal impairment.
ceftazidime	Fortaz Tazidime Tazicef	*Adults:* 1 gm IV or IM q8-12h.
ceftibuten	Cedax	*Adults:* Give 400 mg once daily for 10 days. *Children:* See package insert.
ceftizoxime	Cefizox	*Adults:* 1 or 2 gm q8-12h.
ceftriaxone	Rocephin	*Adults:* 1-2 gm once daily IV or IM. *Children:* 50-75 mg/kg/day.
CHLORAMPHENICOL		
chloramphenicol	Chloramphenicol Chloromycetin	Give PO on empty stomach. Switch from IV to oral form as soon as possible. Chloramphenicol sodium succinate is effective only if administered IV and must not exceed 100 mg/mL. Administer over 1- to 2-min interval. Avoid repeated courses of therapy. *Adults:* 50-100 mg/kg/day in 4 divided doses. *Children:* 50 mg/kg/day in 4 divided doses.
LINCOSAMIDES		
clindamycin	Cleocin	Give deep IM injection. Single IM injections that total 600 mg or greater are not recommended. For IV therapy, do not administer as bolus. For oral administration, take on empty stomach with a full glass of water.

Continued

Table 12-5

Broad-Spectrum Antibiotics—cont'd

GENERIC NAME	TRADE NAME	COMMENTS AND DOSAGE
LINCOSAMIDES—cont'd		
clindamycin	Cleocin	• *Adults* PO: 150-300 mg q6h; more severe infections may require 300-450 mg q6h. *Parenterally:* 600-1200 mg/day in 2-4 divided doses; more severe infections may require 1200-2700 mg/day in 2-4 divided doses. • *Children* *PO:* 8-16 mg/kg/day in 3-4 divided doses; more severe infections may require 16-20 mg/kg/day in 3-4 divided doses. *Parenterally:* 15-25 mg/kg/day in 3-4 divided doses; more severe infections may require 25-40 mg/kg/day in 3-4 divided doses.
lincomycin	Lincocin Lincorex	*Adults:* 500 mg PO q8h, with more severe infections requiring 500 mg PO q6h; or 600 mg/day IM as a single dose; more severe infections may require 500 mg IM q12h; 600 mg to 1 gm IV q8-12h. Maximum dose is 8 gm/day.
MISCELLANEOUS		
bacitracin	Bacitin 🍁 Bacitracin	*Infants under 2.5 kg:* 900 units/kg/day IM in 2-3 divided doses. *Patients over 2.5 kg:* 1000 units/kg/day IM in 2-3 divided doses.
colistimethate	Coly-Mycin M	*Adults and children:* 2.5-5 mg/kg/day parenterally in 2-4 divided doses. Do not exceed 5 mg/kg/day in patients with normal renal function. Dosage must be altered in patients with impaired renal function.
colistin	Coly-Mycin S	*Adults and children:* 5-15 mg/kg/day PO in 3 divided doses.
novobiocin	Albamycin	*Adults:* 250 mg q6h or 500 mg q12h PO. *Children:* 15-30 mg/kg/day. Give for 48 hours after temperature returns to normal.
polymyxin B	—	Do not exceed 25,000 units/kg/day. IM administration not recommended because of severe pain at injection site. *Adults and children:* 15,000 units/kg/day IV in 2 divided doses.
spectinomycin	Trobicin	*Adults:* 2 gm IM as a single dose. *For antibiotic resistance:* 4 gm IM divided between 2 injection sites. *Disseminated gonococcal infections:* 2 gm IM twice daily for 3 days.
vancomycin	Vancocin Vancoled	Should be administered IV only for treating MRSA, not IM. Rapid IV administration may cause hypotension. Dilute solution in 200 mL of glucose or saline solution and infuse over a 30-min period. IV infusion may cause thrombophlebitis. Drug of choice in treating *Staphylococcus* bacteria. *Adults:* 500 mg Pulvules q6h or 1 gm PO or IV q12h, lower with renal impairment. *Children:* 20 mg/lb/day PO in divided doses; 44 mg/kg/day IV in divided doses.
FLUOROQUINOLONES		Medications are excreted primarily by renal mechanism. All dosages must be adjusted in patients with impaired renal function. Calculate serum creatinine levels to determine accurate dosage. Keep patients well hydrated.

ciprofloxacin	Cipro	Used in many infections. Also approved for treatment and prophylaxis of anthrax.
		Adults: Note: 200 mg IV = 250 mg PO
		Dosage and duration depends on severity of infection:
		   400 mg IV q12h = 500 mg PO q12h
		   400 mg IV q8h = 750 mg PO q12h

enoxacin	Penetrex	*Adults:* 200-500 mg q12h for 7-14 days. Take 1 hr before or 2 hr after a meal.

Table 12-5

Broad-Spectrum Antibiotics—cont'd

GENERIC NAME	TRADE NAME	COMMENTS AND DOSAGE
FLUOROQUINOLONES—cont'd		
grepafloxacin	Raxar	*Adults:* 400-600 mg once daily with or without food for 7-10 days.
levofloxacin	Levaquin	*Adults:* 500 mg once daily for 7 days IV or PO.
lomefloxacin	Maxaquin	*Adults:* 400 mg once daily for 10-14 days.
norfloxacin	Noroxin	*Adults:* 400 mg q12h for 3-10 days. Take 1 hr before or 2 hr after meals with glass of water.
ofloxacin	Floxin	*Adults:* 200-400 mg q12h for 7-10 days.
sparfloxacin	Zagam	*Adults:* Give two 200-mg tablets as a loading dose; then one 200-mg tablet daily for 10 more days with or without food.
trovafloxacin	Trovan	*Adults:* Give 100-200 mg IV or PO for 3-14 days depending on indication.
KETOLIDES		
telithromycin	Ketek	New product with low potential to produce macrolide-type resistance. Rapid bactericidal activity. *Adults:* 800 mg (tablets) once daily for 5 days. Community-acquired pneumonia may require 7- to 10-day treatment.
MACROLIDES		
azithromycin	Zithromax	500 mg as a single dose on the first day, followed by 250 mg once daily on days 2 through 5 for a total dose of 1.5 gm. Administer 1 hr before or 2 hr after a meal.
clarithromycin	Biaxin	*Adults only:* 250-500 mg q12h for 7-14 days.
dirithromycin	Dynabac	*Adults and children over 12 yr:* Give 500 mg PO daily for 5-14 days.
erythromycin	EES E-Mycin Ilosone	*Adults:* 250 mg (400 mg ethylsuccinate) PO q6h; 15-20 mg/kg/day parenterally. Dosage may be increased with the severity of the infection. Comes as base or as one of 5 other preparations. *Children:* 30-50 mg/kg/day PO in 3-4 divided doses; 15-20 mg/kg/day IM.
TETRACYCLINES		
demeclocycline	Declomycin	Frequently associated with photosensitivity and anaphylactoid reactions. *Adults:* 150 mg PO 4 times daily or 300 mg PO twice daily. *Children over 8 yr:* 3-6 mg/lb/day PO in 2 or 4 divided doses.
doxycycline	Vibramycin Periostat Doxychel	Used to prevent traveler's diarrhea. It may be taken with food. *Adults:* 200 mg PO in 2 divided doses for the first day; follow with 100 mg/day in 2 divided doses or as a single dose. *Children over 8 yr:* 2 mg/lb/day in 2 divided doses for the first day; follow with 1 mg/lb/day in 2 divided doses or as a single dose.
minocycline	Minocin Dynacin	Has delayed kidney excretion, as compared with other tetracyclines. Half-life is 11-20 hours. *Adults:* 200 mg PO initially, then 100 mg q12h. *Children over 8 yr:* 4 mg/kg initially, then 2 mg/kg q12h.
oxytetracycline	Terramycin Uri-Tet	Diarrhea common. Give deep IM injection in gluteal mass. If pain persists after injection, ice may be applied to the area. Avoid rapid IV administration. *Adults:* 1-2 gm/day PO; 100-250 mg IM q12h; 100-250 mg IV q12h. Do not exceed 500 mg q6h. *Children older than 8 yr:* 10-20 mg/lb/day PO in 4 divided doses; 15-25 mg/kg/day IM in 2 or 3 divided doses; 10-20 mg/kg/day IV in 2 doses.
tetracycline	Tetracap Panmycin Sumycin	*Adults:* 1-2 gm/day PO in 2 or 4 equal doses. *Children over 8 yr:* 10-20 mg/lb/day PO; or 12/mg/kg/day in 4 divided doses.

6. The patient should notify the nurse, physician, or other health care provider if diarrhea persists for more than 24 hours or if stools have blood or mucus.
7. The patient should not take tetracycline with any iron preparations, antacids, milk, or dairy products.
8. The patient should watch for dizziness; if it develops, it may be severe enough to limit driving or operating machinery.
9. Liquid medication should be kept in light-resistant containers.
10. The patient with diabetes should be made aware that many antibiotics change the results of a urine glucose test.
11. The patient should be alert to the possibility of bone marrow depression after therapy is completed and promptly report any bruising, petechiae, sore throat, or weakness.

SECTION TWO
Antitubercular Drugs

OVERVIEW

Tuberculosis is a disease still found among poor and undernourished people. It is most commonly seen in underdeveloped nations where living conditions are crowded and unsanitary. However, it is also increasingly found in the United States among drug users, alcoholics, and AIDS patients or others with lowered immunity. At present, most cases of infectious tuberculosis are found in people who have been previously incompletely treated with antitubercular medications and in people who, as a result of reduced immunity from human immunodeficiency virus (HIV) infection, have primary tuberculosis. In these cases, the organisms are often resistant to the antitubercular medications used in the normal treatment regimen.

Tuberculosis is caused by *Mycobacterium tuberculosis,* which infects animals as well as humans. Multiple-drug-resistant (MDR) organisms (strains that are resistant to current drugs) are now commonly found and require vigorous methods of treatment to control infection. New guidelines for treatment of tuberculosis are published by the Centers for Disease Control and Prevention (CDC) in Atlanta, Georgia, almost every year. Because there are many new cases of tuberculosis, as well as numerous untreated cases, many new state laws have been passed that take aggressive action against individuals who are infected with tuberculosis and who refuse to take or complete adequate drug therapy. In some states, patients may actually be sent to prison until they have completed the required drug therapy and have been rendered noninfectious.

ACTION

The main action of antitubercular drugs involves an intracellular or extracellular bacteriostatic effect against *M. tuberculosis.* Most drugs used to treat tuberculosis do not kill the bacterium, but they control the disease and prevent its spread through various organ systems in the infected patient or to other individuals. The drugs control the bacteria by preventing them from producing new cell walls, so new bacterial cell growth is limited. Some antitubercular drugs are bactericidal, killing the organism.

USES

Chemoprophylaxis, or taking a drug to prevent disease, is recommended when the patient is at high risk of developing active tuberculosis. The current duration of prophylactic treatment is 1 year. At present, isoniazid is the only drug recommended for prophylactic therapy. Isoniazid prophylaxis is not recommended for healthy individuals over the age of 35 because of their increased risk of developing hepatitis. Prophylaxis is recommended, however, if the patient is at special risk for developing tuberculosis, as indicated in Box 12-1. *Chemotherapy,* or taking a drug to treat disease, is recommended for patients with active tuberculosis.

Antitubercular drugs are classified as primary or secondary agents to describe the way they are used in treating tuberculosis. Most primary agents are bactericidal and are necessary to sterilize the tuberculosis lesions. Secondary agents are generally less effective and more toxic than the primary agents. They are used with primary agents for patients infected with partially or completely drug-resistant organisms or to treat lesions found outside the lungs.

ADVERSE REACTIONS

Mycobacterium tuberculosis is able to build up a resistance to antitubercular drugs. Use of a combination of drugs helps to slow the development of bacterial resistance. Most of the antitubercular medications cause only mild and infrequent symptoms such as nausea, vomiting, and diarrhea. Most of these symptoms stop when the dosage is reduced. Some of the drugs used to treat tuberculosis are toxic to various parts of the body (for example, the ears, kidneys, and liver). The patient must be watched closely to detect development of any of these more serious problems.

Box 12-1   High-Priority Candidates for Tuberculosis-Preventive Therapy

Patients of all ages with a positive tuberculin test, no previous therapy, and the following:
- Known or suspected HIV infection
- Close contact with individuals with infectious, clinically active tuberculosis (TB)
- Recent tuberculin skin test conversion
- Employment in a health care job with exposure to large numbers of individuals who may get TB
- Medical problems that increase the risk of TB (for example, diabetes, immunosuppressive therapy, IV drug use, end-stage renal disease, malignancies, hemodialysis)
- Abnormal chest x-ray studies that show old fibrotic lesions

Patients younger than 35 years old, with a positive tuberculin test and no additional risk factors, and the following:
- Being born in a high-prevalence country
- Residence in long-term care facilities (for example, nursing homes) or prisons
- Belonging to a medically underserved low-income population

Capreomycin may cause headache; ototoxicity (hearing loss, tinnitus, vertigo); nephrotoxicity (elevated BUN and nonprotein nitrogen, proteinuria, casts, hematuria, albuminuria, decreased creatinine clearance); changes in blood cells; abnormal liver function tests; maculopapular rash associated with febrile reaction; urticaria; muscle weakness; pain and swelling or excessive bleeding at the injection site; and sterile abscesses.

Ethambutol is associated with dizziness, headache, confusion, dermatitis, abdominal pain, anorexia, nausea, vomiting, joint pain and swelling, optic neuritis (loss of vision), and loss of visual acuity.

Ethionamide may produce severe postural hypotension (low blood pressure when a person suddenly stands up), mental depression, rash, anorexia, diarrhea, epigastric distress, jaundice, nausea, and vomiting.

Isoniazid may produce peripheral neuropathies, visual disturbances, optic neuritis, hyperglycemia (high blood sugar level), hyperkalemia (increased potassium in the blood), nausea, constipation, epigastric distress, vomiting, many changes in blood cells, arthritis symptoms, chills, fever, rash, dyspnea (uncomfortable breathing), headache, tachycardia (rapid heartbeat), and urinary retention in men. Severe and sometimes fatal hepatitis may develop even after many months of treatment. The drug also changes the results of a variety of laboratory tests. Symptoms of overdosage may occur anytime from 30 minutes to 3 hours after the isoniazid is administered. Nausea, vomiting, slurred speech, dizziness, impaired vision, and visual hallucinations may be among the early symptoms. Severe overdosage will result in central nervous system depression, respiratory distress, coma, and severe intractable seizures.

Pyrazinamide has been associated with photosensitivity, rashes, diarrhea, hepatocellular damage, nausea, vomiting, gout, decreased blood clotting time, and anemia.

Rifampin has produced drowsiness, headache, generalized numbness, transient low-frequency hearing loss, visual disturbances, abdominal pain or cramps, diarrhea, epigastric distress, hepatitis, nausea, sore mouth and tongue, vomiting, and many changes in blood cells. Symptoms of overdosage include nausea, vomiting, increasing lethargy, unconsciousness, liver enlargement and tenderness, and jaundice.

Streptomycin sulfate may produce dizziness, headache, paresthesia (numbness or tingling), vertigo, anorexia, nausea, stomatitis, vomiting, changes in blood cells, arthralgia (joint pain), hypertension (high blood pressure), hypotension (low blood pressure), myocarditis, hepatotoxicity, splenomegaly (enlarged spleen), ototoxicity, and nephrotoxicity.

DRUG INTERACTIONS

Many drugs should not be given at the same time as or right after antitubercular drugs, or put on the skin while the patient is on antituberculosis therapy, because of the significant risk for neurotoxicity and nephrotoxicity. All drugs taken by the patient should be checked closely for drug interactions, which are very common among the antitubercular drugs.

Nursing Implications and Patient Teaching

Assessment

A tuberculosis infection may develop in a patient's lungs, bones, bladder, or other organs. A patient with active tuberculosis may have symptoms such as productive cough, pain, fever, night sweats, and weight loss, or the patient may be without symptoms. The diagnosis of tuberculosis is made from the patient's history, physical examination, x-ray studies, and laboratory work. Once the diagnosis is made, the patient may be hospitalized while treatment is started. Long-term treatment is required, and much of the treatment will be carried out when the patient is at home.

Diagnosis

Patients with tuberculosis often have needs for financial, nutritional, and career counseling. These individuals may have other medical problems and may be taking multiple drugs, resulting in additional problems with side effects and scheduling of dosages. The nurse must be prepared to help analyze all the needs of the patient if effective treatment is to be offered. In particular, you should be involved in watching to see if the patient is compliant, because treatment programs in which you watch the patient taking the medication (directly observed therapy) may be required to protect the public from this disease.

Planning

Drug resistance is likely to develop if only one drug is given for active tuberculosis. Two or more drugs should always be given. Drugs that are highly ototoxic should not be given together. Two hepatotoxic drugs should not be given together when clinically active hepatitis is present.

To prevent the development of drug resistance, you should be aware of the following:
- Patient compliance
- Culture conversion (sputum cultures that gradually change from positive to negative)
- Selection of appropriate drugs

The CDC Advisory Council for the Elimination of Tuberculosis has issued its recommendations for initial therapy of tuberculosis. The regimen for children and adults who do not have HIV infection is as follows:
- Daily isoniazid (INH), rifampin (RIF), and pyrazinamide (PZA) and either ethambutol (EMB) or streptomycin (SM) sulfate for 8 weeks.
- EMB or SM can be added to the initial regimen if needed.
- INH and RIF daily or two to three times per week for 16 weeks or up to 6 months.
- Continue for 6 months beyond culture conversion.

You should directly observe the patient take the medication. The daily dose should be given in the morning before the patient eats or drinks anything else.

For tuberculosis patients with HIV infections, use the previous treatment schedule, but continue for 9 months beyond culture conversion.

Because of the long-term nature of the required treatment, drug toxicity is a special problem. Dosages for elderly patients, unusually small adults, and patients with renal impairment should be watched. All patients should be carefully asked about symptoms of adverse reactions. If toxic effects, adverse reactions, or allergic reactions occur, all drugs should be stopped and further evaluation should be done. Restarting drugs after toxic effects or adverse reactions have ceased should be done with caution.

In the event of an unsuccessful treatment regimen, you should evaluate for patient compliance and the presence of an MDR strain. If the problem is patient compliance, the same treatment regimen can be started again. With an MDR strain, two or more new drugs should be added to the regimen, never a single drug, because drug resistance may develop more easily with only one new drug. The drugs used for re-treatment for

an MDR strain include *para*-aminosalicylate, capreomycin, cycloserine, ethionamide, and kanamycin.

Guidelines for the treatment of tuberculosis are frequently updated by the CDC. The latest information should always be used in treating patients to avoid problems with drug resistance.

Implementation

Antitubercular drugs should be given in single daily doses unless contraindicated. All drugs, unless stated otherwise, should be taken at the same time each day, preferably in the morning. This is especially important with the combination of isoniazid and rifampin, to decrease the chance of drug resistance. When poor compliance is suspected, the care provider should directly observe the patient while he is taking the drugs.

If parenteral administration is required, the injection sites should be rotated and each site inspected for signs of tenderness, swelling, or redness. If a patient does not seem to be getting better, make sure she is taking the medicine.

Many of these drugs cause gastric irritation. This may be reduced by taking medication with food. Isoniazid is the only antitubercular medication that is best absorbed on an empty stomach. It should be taken either 1 hour before or 2 hours after a meal as a single daily dose. It should be taken with food only if it cannot be tolerated on an empty stomach.

The therapy of choice for uncomplicated pulmonary tuberculosis is the use of two drugs, isoniazid and rifampin, which are bactericidal both intracellularly and extracellularly. The duration of therapy is usually a minimum of 9 months. Sputum that is cultured 1 to 3 months after the initiation of isoniazid and rifampin therapy will usually be negative for the bacillus. The therapy usually continues for 6 months after sputum conversion takes place. When necessary, the combination of pyrazinamide and streptomycin sulfate may be used to substitute for either one of the bactericidal drugs above. However, there is some controversy over the effectiveness of this shorter, 9-month course of therapy when isoniazid is not used.

At present, intermittent therapy with isoniazid and rifampin is being investigated. The American Thoracic Society recommends that these two drugs be given daily for 2 to 8 weeks. Then the patient is switched to twice per week for a total of 39 weeks. The minimum duration of therapy is 9 months. The daily dosage recommendations for adults are isoniazid 300 mg and rifampin 600 mg. The twice-weekly dosage plan for adults is isoniazid 15 mg/kg of body weight and rifampin 600 mg. The American Thoracic Society recommends intermittent therapy only for uncomplicated pulmonary tuberculosis. See the new CDC guidelines for treatment of patients with MDR strains.

Whenever a combination of drugs does not have both an intracellular and an extracellular bactericidal effect, therapy must continue for the traditional 18 to 24 months. This usually occurs when bacteriostatic drugs are used.

See Table 12-6 for a summary of common antitubercular drugs.

Evaluation

Drug resistance should be suspected if the patient has been treated for tuberculosis in the past. Drugs used in the regimen for the earlier infection may be used again while waiting for the results of sensitivity studies, but at least two new drugs should also be added. Drug resistance is low in infections acquired in the United States, but high in tuberculosis infections acquired from Asian, South and Central American, and African sources. Drug resistance is less likely to occur when two bactericidal drugs are given together rather than when one bactericidal drug is given together with bacteriostatic drugs.

Vital signs should be monitored for recurrence of acute infection. Patients should be weighed at each visit to monitor their general health status. Weight loss

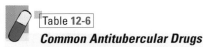

Table 12-6
Common Antitubercular Drugs

GENERIC NAME	TRADE NAME	COMMENTS AND DOSAGE
PRIMARY TREATMENT AGENTS		
ethambutol	Myambutol ♦	Give once every 24 hr. When one other bactericidal drug is used in combination with this medication, therapy generally lasts 18-24 months. It has been used in twice-weekly regimens. Ethambutol may be taken with food. Watch for optic neuritis, rash. • *Initial treatment:* 15 mg/kg PO in a single daily dose. • *Retreatment:* 25 mg/kg PO in a single daily dose for 60-90 days; dosage is then decreased to 15 mg/kg/day.
isoniazid	Isotamine ♦ Nydrazid PMS-Isoniazid ♦	Well absorbed after PO or IM administration. Dosage is determined by weight, with the usual adult dose being 5 mg/kg or 300 mg/day. Children require higher doses than adults. Give with pyridoxine to reduce incidence of peripheral neuropathies. Isoniazid is the drug of choice in the prophylactic treatment of tuberculosis infections. *Adults:* 300 mg/day for 1 yr. Watch for hepatic and neurologic toxicity.
pyrazinamide	Pyrazinamide ♦	Should be administered with at least one other antitubercular drug. *Adults:* 20-35 mg/kg/day in 3 or 4 divided doses. Maximum daily dose is 3 gm. Watch for hepatic toxicity and hyperuricemia, arthralgia, and arthritis.
rifampin	PMS Pyrazinamide ♦ Rifadin Rimactane	Used in combination with other antitubercular drugs. Usually given PO, in a single dose, 1 hr before or 2 hr after eating. Peak plasma concentrations occur 2-4 hr after ingestion. *Adults:* 600 mg/day PO in a single dose. Dosage range is 450-600 mg/day. This is the same whether the therapy is intermittent or daily. *Elderly and debilitated:* 10 mg/kg/day; not to exceed 600 mg/day. *Children 5 yr and older:* 10-20 mg/kg/day; not to exceed 600 mg/day. Watch for hepatic and hematologic toxicity.
rifapentine	Priftin	*Induction phase:* Give four 150-mg tablets twice weekly (every 3 days) for 2 mo with food as part of drug combination therapy. *Continuation phase:* Give 1 tablet each wk for 4 mo with other drugs.
streptomycin sulfate	—	Give in combination with other antitubercular agents, except capreomycin. Streptomycin should be given only IM. Limit quantity in one dose because injections are painful, and sterile inflammatory reactions may occur. Watch for renal and eighth cranial nerve toxicity. *Adults with normal renal function:* 1 gm/day IM (may be given 5 days/wk) for 2-3 mo; then 2-3 times/wk for 4-6 wk. *Elderly patients, unusually small adults, and individuals with renal impairment:* Give reduced dosages, usually 0.5 gm/day IM according to previous schedule.

Continued

Table 12-6

Common Antitubercular Drugs—cont'd

GENERIC NAME	TRADE NAME	COMMENTS AND DOSAGE
RETREATMENT AGENTS		
para-aminosalicylate (PAS)	Nemasol Paser	May produce nausea, vomiting, diarrhea, or abdominal pain. Dosage is usually 14-16 gm/day PO in 2-3 divided doses. Watch for GI distress, hepatitis.
capreomycin	Capastat Sulfate	Give deep IM. Watch for renal and eighth cranial nerve toxicity. *Adults:* 1 gm/day IM (not to exceed 20 mg/kg/day) for 60-120 days, then 1 gm IM 2-3 times/wk. The reduced dosage may continue for 18-24 mo.
cycloserine	Seromycin Pulvules	Usual dose is 500 mg to 1 gm/day PO in divided doses. Watch for psychoses, seizures, rash.
ethionamide	Trecator-SC	Take with meals or antacids to reduce GI distress. High percentage of patients cannot tolerate therapeutic dose. *Adults:* 250 mg PO twice daily. Every 5 days the dose may be increased by 125 mg/day, until 1 gm/day is given. Dosages should never exceed 1 gm/day. The usual dose is 0.5-1 gm/day PO. Watch for hepatitis, GI distress, hypersensitivity.
kanamycin	Kantrex	Give 15 mg/kg once daily IM for adults, 7.5-15 mg/kg once daily IM for children. Watch for renal and eighth cranial nerve toxicity.
PREVENTION IN HIV PATIENTS		
rifabutin	Mycobutin	Usual dose: 300 mg once daily. Divided dose, taken with food, may decrease GI distress.

should be reported to the physician or other health care provider. Diet changes and nutritional supplements may be indicated.

Some patients taking ethambutol develop psychologic changes. If the patient becomes depressed, anxious, or withdrawn or stops talking, or shows any changes in personality, these findings should be reported to the physician or other health care provider.

Because of marked toxicity of these drugs, it is essential to carefully and regularly monitor both the bacteriologic studies and the toxic side effects of the drugs. Baseline sputum smears, culture and sensitivity studies, chest x-ray studies, weight, and renal, hepatic, and hematopoietic studies should be obtained.

Patient and Family Teaching

Because patients must take their drugs for a long time, it is important to establish a good relationship with the patient. Clear instructions should be given about the importance of continuing to take the drugs as ordered and what problems to report to the nurse, physician, or other health care provider at the scheduled visits. It is important to stress the following instructions:

1. Laboratory and diagnostic tests and frequent office visits are necessary throughout the treatment of tuberculosis. The patient must continue to meet with the nurse, physician, or other health care provider so progress can be measured.

2. The drug must be taken exactly as directed. The dosage must not be altered without specific instructions from the nurse, physician, or other health care provider. It is very important to take these drugs as ordered. If a dose is missed, it should be taken as soon as it is remembered, unless it is almost time for the next dose. In that case, the missed dose should not be taken and the regular dosing schedule should be followed. Forgetting to take a dose or failing to continue with one of the drugs may cause the organisms to develop a resistance to the medication. This allows the disease process to continue, with continued risk for the patient, close family members, and contacts.

3. Tuberculosis is a disease that must be reported to the local health department. Family members and close contacts also need to be screened for tuberculosis.

4. During the initial period of illness, patients must remember that they are contagious. Every effort must be made to cover the mouth when coughing, to dispose of sputum and soiled tissues carefully, and to act to protect those nearby.

5. The patient should remember that the whole body is involved in fighting this disease. The body requires adequate rest, nourishing food, and as restful and quiet a recovery environment as possible.
6. Any adverse reactions should be reported promptly. Particular symptoms to report include any episodes of easy bruising; fever; sore throat; unusual bleeding; skin rashes; mental confusion; headache; tremors; severe nausea; vomiting; diarrhea; malaise; yellowish discoloration of the skin; visual changes; severe pain in knees, feet, or wrists; excessive drowsiness; or changes in personality or affect.
7. The patient should not take other drugs without the knowledge and permission of the nurse, physician, or other health care provider.
8. With the exception of isoniazid (which should be taken on an empty stomach), medication should be taken with food or milk. If an aftertaste occurs, a mouthwash, juice, or sugarless gum may be used after taking the medication.
9. The patient should establish a regular time each day to take medication.
10. The medication should be kept in a safe place, away from animals or children.
11. The patient should wear a Medic Alert bracelet or necklace or carry some other form of emergency identification indicating the medications being taken.

SECTION THREE
Antiparasitic Drugs

OVERVIEW

Parasites affecting humans are a world wide problem. Three major categories of drugs used to treat parasites are discussed in this section: amebicides, anthelmintics, and antimalarial products. Each major category is discussed in detail.

AMEBICIDES

ACTION

Amebiasis is caused by the parasite *Entamoeba histolytica*. In the United States or Canada, this infection is seen primarily in people who have traveled abroad. It is also found in those who have eaten unwashed fruits or vegetables imported from other countries, so this infection could be common. The main action of an amebicide is to destroy the invading ameba, which may be located within the GI tract or some other place in that body to which it has traveled (extraintestinal). Infections outside the intestinal tract are much more difficult to treat. The most common extraintestinal infection is a hepatic abscess.

USES

Amebicides are the primary therapy for both intestinal and extraintestinal amebiasis. The choice of drug depends on the location of the infection.

Diiodohydroxyquin and metronidazole are also used to treat *Trichomonas vaginalis*. Chloroquine is primarily an antimalarial agent and is also used for rheumatoid arthritis.

ADVERSE REACTIONS

All drugs used to treat amebiasis may cause nausea, vomiting, headache, anorexia, diarrhea, or GI distress.

Chloroquine may produce dizziness, irritability, pruritus, ototoxicity, tinnitus, vertigo, visual disturbances, or abdominal cramps.

Diiodohydroxyquin has been known to cause ataxia (poor coordination), neurotoxicity, peripheral neuropathy, optic neuritis, abdominal cramps, rectal and skin itching, constipation, and hair loss.

Metronidazole may cause changes in the electrocardiogram (ECG), ataxia, confusion, depression, insomnia, irritability, vertigo, flushing, pruritus, blurred vision, nasal congestion, abdominal cramps, constipation, dysuria (painful urination), polyuria (excretion of a large amount of urine), pyuria (increased white blood cells in the urine), fever, and metallic taste.

Paromomycin may produce vertigo, rash, ototoxicity, abdominal cramps, constipation, hematuria, and nephrotoxicity.

Symptoms of overdosage are also seen with all of these drugs.

DRUG INTERACTIONS

With the exception of metronidazole, there are no significant drug interactions. Combining metronidazole with alcohol can produce severe headache, flushing, cramps, nausea, and vomiting. If metronidazole is combined with disulfiram, acute psychosis may result.

Nursing Implications and Patient Teaching

Assessment

You should learn as much as possible about the health history of the patient, including any allergy to drugs; current use of alcohol or disulfiram; chronic renal, cardiac, thyroid, or liver disease; and the possibility of pregnancy. These conditions are contraindications or precautions to the use of amebicides.

Diagnosis

Does this patient have problems with severe diarrhea that may produce dehydration? Are there knowledge deficits about handling, washing, and storage of fruits and vegetables? Are there other problems that would limit the medication therapy for this patient?

Planning

Four major drugs are used as amebicides. The contraindications for drug use are somewhat different depending on the drug chosen. The specific product information should be consulted.

Implementation

The drug to be ordered depends on the location of the infection. Some of these drugs are specific for extraintestinal infections. Because these drugs are very toxic, the decision to treat the patient should be carefully made, and only the smallest therapeutic dosage possible should be given for the shortest period of time. If the initial drug is ineffective and another drug is more hazardous, retreatment with the initial drug may be advised.

You should teach the patient about the method of infection and review specific methods of personal hygiene to prevent reinfection and reduce the risk of spreading infection to others.

Table 12-7 provides a summary of amebicides.

Evaluation

After drug therapy, periodic stool tests will be required to make certain that the disease has been eliminated. These tests may be needed monthly for up to 1 year after therapy.

You should be alert to signs of toxicity. If severe symptoms appear, the drug may have to be stopped.

Patient and Family Teaching

You should tell the patient and family the following:
1. The patient should take all drugs as prescribed and not skip any doses or double the medication doses. The patient should not stop taking the medication without being advised to do so by a nurse, physician, or other health care provider.
2. The patient should take this drug with or after meals to decrease the chances of stomach upset.
3. Some patients experience side effects from this medication. The patient should report any new or troublesome symptoms to the nurse, physician, or other health care provider.
4. The GI system (mouth) is the point of entry for these parasites. Usually, infection comes from parasite feces getting into the food or by hand-to-mouth contamination. Food should be washed carefully before eating, and hands should be washed after going to the bathroom and before preparing foods. This is important to avoid spreading infection.
5. After drug therapy has been completed, it is essential that a stool examination be performed periodically to look for reinfection or for continuing infection in people who still have amebiasis but are not symptomatic.

ANTHELMINTICS

ACTION

Infestation by worms is called **helminthiasis.** It is most commonly caused by pinworms, roundworms, hookworms, tapeworms, or whipworms. The worm gains entrance to the body through unclean food, unwashed hands, or the skin. The diagnosis is made by finding the eggs or the parasite in the stool of the infected individual. Once the type of parasite has been identified, the health care provider may order the best medication for its destruction. The way the drug works depends on the product used.

The exact action of diethylcarbamazine citrate as an anthelmintic is not known. It is thought that it sensitizes the parasite's cuticle to allow phagocytosis by the macrophages of the host. Mebendazole blocks the glucose uptake of helminths. Piperazine paralyzes the muscles of parasites by blocking the effects of acetylcholine at the neuromuscular junction, and the parasite is removed by normal peristalsis during the bowel movement. The exact action of thiabendazole is not known, but it is thought to interfere with metabolic pathways essential for a variety of helminths.

USES

Thiabendazole is the drug of choice for cutaneous larva migrans (creeping eruption), pinworms, roundworms, *Strongyloides,* and mild cases of hookworm.

Niclosamide and paromomycin are used to treat cestodiasis (tapeworm infestation).

Piperazine and pyrantel pamoate are used to treat roundworms and pinworms. Pyrantel is also effective against hookworms.

Diethylcarbamazine citrate is used mostly in tropical areas, or in patients who have been in areas where filariae are endemic. It is used to treat Bancroft's filariasis, Malayan filariasis, dipetalonemiasis, or

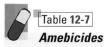

Table 12-7
Amebicides

GENERIC NAME	TRADE NAME	COMMENTS AND DOSAGE
chloroquine	Aralen	Watch for ototoxicity; obtain baseline audiometry tests. This drug is used primarily in combination with other amebicides to treat hepatic abscess. • *Hepatic abscess* *Adults:* Give 600 mg base (1 gm) daily for 2 days, then 300 mg base (500 mg) daily for 2-3 wk. At the same time, give diiodohydroxyquin 650 mg 3 times daily for 20 days. Reduce dosage for children.

diiodohydroxyquin or iodoquinol	Yodoxin	Drug of choice in asymptomatic intestinal amebiasis.
		Adults: 630-650 mg PO 3 times daily for 20 days.
		Children: 30-40 mg/kg/day PO in 3 doses for 20 days.
		• *Mild, moderate, or severe intestinal amebiasis*
		  Adults: In addition to metronidazole (750 mg 3 times daily for 5-10 days) give 630-650 mg PO 3 times daily for 20 days.
		  Children: In addition to metronidazole (35-50 mg/kg/day in 3 doses for 10 days) give 30-40 mg/kg PO in 3 doses for 20 days.

metronidazole	Flagyl
	Protostat
		Drug of choice in mild to severe intestinal amebiasis and in treatment of hepatic abscess. Patient should not take alcohol while on this medication and should not use with disulfiram.
		•*Mild, moderate, and severe intestinal amebiasis*
		  Adults: Give 750 mg 3 times daily for 5-10 days, plus diiodohydroxyquin 630-650 mg 3 times daily for 20 days.
		  Children: Give 35-50 mg/kg/day in 3 doses for 10 days, plus diiodohydroxyquin 30-40 mg/kg/day in 3 doses for 20 days.

paromomycin	Humatin	Used as alternative drug therapy for asymptomatic intestinal amebiasis and mild to moderate infections; may cause ototoxicity, so audiometry tests should be obtained; give medication with meals.
		• *Asymptomatic intestinal amebiasis*
		  Adults and *children:* As alternative to diiodohydroxyquin, give 25-30 mg/kg/day in 3 doses for 7 days.
		• *Mild-to-moderate intestinal amebiasis*
		  Adults and children: Give 25-30 mg/kg/day in 3 doses for 7-10 days.

infestation with loiasis (a filarial worm dwelling in tumors in subcutaneous connective tissue and often affecting the eyes).

Mebendazole is used in single or mixed infections to treat pinworm, roundworm, hookworm, and whipworm infestations.

ADVERSE REACTIONS

Each drug has different side effects. Headache, weakness, anorexia, nausea, vomiting, abdominal pain, arthralgia, lassitude (weariness), malaise, myalgia (widespread muscle pain), and skin rash are all common reactions. Allergic reactions may occur as a result of the dead microfilaria, and may be seen with fever, lymphadenitis (inflammation of the lymph nodes), pruritus, and pedal edema (foot swelling). The number of side effects increases with higher dosages and longer length of treatment.

DRUG INTERACTIONS

These anthelmintic drug work against each other (antagonistic) if they are given together. The drugs also may interfere with a number of specific drugs, such as heparin, and a variety of laboratory tests. Specific product information should be consulted for each drug.

Nursing Implications and Patient Teaching

Assessment

You should learn as much as you can about the health history of the patient, including the presence of hypertension; allergy; eye disease; intestinal obstruction; inflammatory bowel disease; severe hepatic, renal, or cardiac disease; malaria; and the possibility of pregnancy. These conditions are contraindications or precautions to treatment with anthelmintics.

The patient may have no symptoms or may be listless, fatigued, and irritable or have abdominal pain, diarrhea, and weight loss. The patient may also have edema (collection of large amounts of fluid in tissues), especially of the lower extremities, and a discharge from the eyes. If helminthiasis is seen commonly in your practice, you should learn the signs and symptoms of infestation by the various helminths.

Diagnosis

Has the patient developed skin lesions, dehydration, or other problems that require or would affect treatment? Is there lack of information that caused this problem? Are there teaching needs to prevent reinfection? Does the patient have other problems that would interfere with or limit therapy for this problem?

Planning

Severe pruritus may occur in the treatment of cutaneous larva migrans, and an antiinflammatory agent may be necessary.

Patients with a recent history of malaria should be treated with an antimalarial agent before giving them anthelmintics to prevent a relapse.

Because pinworm infections are easily transferred from person to person, all family members may have to be treated.

Piperazine can be used in the last trimester of pregnancy. However, this drug has potential neurotoxicity, so long or repeated treatment in excess of the recommended dosage should be avoided, especially in children.

Implementation

Thiabendazole therapy may cause an asparagus-like odor of the urine. The patient's skin may also have an unusual odor. This medication may cause drowsiness or dizziness; therefore, the patient should use caution in driving or doing tasks that require alertness.

Severe hookworm infestations may produce anemia, so iron supplementation and a diet rich in iron may be required.

The patient should store piperazine syrup and tablets in tightly closed containers to avoid evaporation or decomposition. Liquids are easier for children to take. Medication is usually given in the morning before breakfast.

Patients may develop allergic reactions to the dead microfilaria and may need treatment for symptoms. Antihistamines or corticosteroids may be necessary to reduce allergic effects, particularly in the treatment of ocular onchocerciasis.

Table 12-8 provides a summary of anthelmintics.

Evaluation

You should help determine if the patient is taking his medication as ordered and is doing other things that

might be ordered. Help collect stool specimens after every treatment to make sure the worms are gone. The patient should have an ophthalmologic (eye) examination if he is currently undergoing treatment for ocular onchocerciasis.

Teach the patient the hygienic measures that are necessary to prevent reinfestation.

If the patient develops neurologic complications with piperazine therapy, this medication should be stopped and another drug should be used.

Patient and Family Teaching

You should tell the patient and family the following:
1. The patient must take this medication as ordered. Therapy usually involves an initial treatment that should kill all worms, but in some cases, a second course must be taken. It is important to report any symptoms that do not disappear after treatment.
2. Worms passed in bowel movements are still alive and capable of infecting others. Care must be used to avoid transmission. For the week after treatment begins, the patient should do the following:
   • Wash the toilet seat daily with soap and water.
   • Once a week for 2 weeks, boil the sheets and underwear twice in water and disinfectant.
   • Use special precautions in handling food or drink around others.
3. Worm infestations are easily transmitted, and all family members may need to be tested to see if they have worms also.
4. Some people have diarrhea and abdominal discomfort while taking the medication.
5. If the patient develops any signs of headache, tremors, muscle weakness, or blurred vision, or if one eye does not align properly with the other eye, the nurse, physician, or other health care provider should be alerted.
6. The patient may require iron supplements and an iron-rich diet during hookworm treatment.

ANTIMALARIALS

ACTION

Malaria is a big problem in many countries where wetlands provide a good breeding ground for mosquitoes. Patients with malaria have periods of acute sickness followed by periods where they are symptom free. The antimalarial drugs suppress the infection but often do not cure it. Although malaria is not commonly seen in the United States or Canada, it is becoming more frequent in Florida, other areas of the South, and areas adjoining Mexico. You may also see cases among immigrants, migrant farmers, and travelers returning from areas where malaria is endemic (occurs in a regular pattern). People

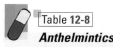

Table 12-8
Anthelmintics

GENERIC NAME	TRADE NAME	COMMENTS AND DOSAGE
albendazole	Albenza	For treatment of lesions from pork or dog tapeworm. Give 400 mg twice daily with meals for 28 days, followed by a 14-day cycle with no medications; repeat for 2 more cycles.
diethylcarbamazine citrate	Hetrazan	Start this oral medication at lowest recommended doses and then gradually increase dosage as needed. • *Wuchereriasis:* 2 mg/kg 3 times daily after meals for 7-14 days. • *Loiasis:* 2 mg/kg 3 times daily after meals for 10 days. • *Onchocerciasis:* 2 mg/kg 3 times daily after meals for 14-21 days.
ivermectin	Stromectol	For treatment of intestinal parasites and onchocerciasis. Give 200 mcg/kg as single dose with water. Usually no repeat dose needed.
mebendazole	Vermox ♦	No special diets, fasting, or purgation before administration is necessary. Medication is taken orally by chewing, crushing, and/or mixing with food. • *Pinworms:* 100 mg PO as a single dose. • *Roundworms, hookworms, and whipworms:* 100 mg PO in the morning and evening for 3 days; repeat treatment in 3-4 wk if infestation is still present.
piperazine	Entacyl ♦ Piperazine	• *Roundworm (ascariasis) infections* *Adults:* 3.5 gm PO as a single daily dose. *Children:* 75 mg/kg PO as a single dose; maximum daily dose 3.5 gm; give for 2 consecutive days. • *Pinworm (enterobiasis) infections* *Adults and children:* 65 mg/kg PO as a single daily dose.
praziquantel	Biltricide	Give 3 doses of 20 mg/kg as a 1-day treatment. Tablet very bitter if not swallowed promptly.
pyrantel	Antiminth Reese's pinworm Pin-Rid	Medication can be administered as a single dose for treating roundworms and pinworms; hookworms require longer therapy. No special fasting or diet is necessary before taking medication. Purging is not necessary. Taking drug with fruit juice or milk may make it more palatable. • *Roundworm and pinworm therapy* *Adults and children:* 11 mg/kg as a single dose; maximum dose 1 gm; this dose should be repeated after 2 wk for pinworms. • *Hookworms* *Adults and children:* 11 mg/kg for 3 consecutive days; treatment should be repeated after 1 mo if necessary.
thiabendazole	Mintezol	Chew tablets well before swallowing. Take drug after meals. *Adults and children over 150 lb:* 1.5 gm PO. *Adults and children under 150 lb:* 10 mg/lb PO. • *Pinworms (enterobiasis):* Give 2 doses in 1 day; repeat regimen in 7 days. • *Cutaneous larva migrans:* Give 2 doses/day for 2 days. If active lesions are still present after completion of therapy, a second course should be administered. • *Roundworms (ascariasis), Strongyloides, and hookworms:* Give 2 doses/day for 2 days.

in the military or those traveling to or living in areas where malaria is endemic can use antimalarials to prevent malaria and to treat the symptoms.

Malaria is caused by four species of the protozoan *Plasmodium*. These species are *P. falciparum*, *P. malariae*, *P. vivax*, and *P. ovale*. The protozoan parasites are transmitted to humans by the *Anopheles* mosquito.

When a mosquito bites a person infected with malaria, the protozoans enter the mosquito's stomach, where they reproduce. The resulting sporozoites make their way to the salivary glands of the mosquito. They are then transmitted to other individuals whenever the mosquito bites. The sporozoites grow and divide in the human host, entering the red blood cells of the person and maturing into the adult form of the protozoan, which then produces infection and the symptoms of malaria.

Antimalarial drugs interfere with the life cycle of *Plasmodium*, usually while it is in the red blood cells. These drugs reduce the ability of the deoxyribonucleic acid (DNA) to reproduce or serve as a template, thereby decreasing protein synthesis in susceptible organisms. Not all drugs are effective against all four species of *Plasmodium*. In addition, many strains of *Plasmodium* have developed resistance to commonly used drugs. The drugs used in treating malaria are not without risk, and you should study these drugs carefully.

Primaquine interferes with the metabolism of parasites. Folic acid antagonists affect the differential growth requirements and the demand for nucleic acid precursors between the host and the parasite. In sulfonamide products, there is a competitive antagonism of *para-aminobenzoic acid*, which is a component in folic acid synthesis. Quinine, the earliest known medication for malaria, reduces the effectiveness of *Plasmodium*'s DNA to act as a template in chloroquine-resistant strains of *P. falciparum*. It also decreases the parasite's oxygen use and carbohydrate metabolism, and is a skeletal muscle relaxant, antipyretic, and analgesic.

USES

Antimalarials are used to suppress and treat acute malaria attacks caused by erythrocytic forms of *P. ovale, P. malariae, P. vivax,* and most strains of *P. falciparum*. The 4-aminoquinoline drugs are ineffective against the gametocytes of *P. falciparum* but are used with primaquine to cure malaria caused by *P. malariae* and *P. vivax*.

ADVERSE REACTIONS

Synthetic 4- and 8-aminoquinolines may produce hypotension, ECG changes, mild and transient headaches, pruritus, abdominal cramps, anorexia, diarrhea, nausea, vomiting, blood dyscrasias, visual blurring, reduced hearing, and tinnitus.

Folic acid antagonists may produce anorexia, atrophic glossitis (loss of papillae of the tongue), vomiting, and anemias.

Quinine poisoning is called *cinchonism* and causes diarrhea, dizziness, headache, nausea, tinnitus, visual blurring, fearfulness, confusion, excitement, hypothermia (abnormally low body temperature), syncope (light-headedness and fainting), abdominal cramps, vomiting, anemias, pruritus, rash, urticaria, and night blindness.

All of these drugs may sometimes produce blood dyscrasias, as well as visual and neurologic changes. Overdosage may produce convulsions and cardiac collapse.

DRUG INTERACTIONS

Use of any antimalarials with other drugs that cause dermatologic, ototoxic, or neurologic symptoms may produce toxicity. There are isolated drugs that interact with these preparations, so read the manufacturers' information carefully.

Nursing Implications and Patient Teaching

Assessment

You should learn as much as possible about the patient's health history, including if the patient is pregnant or has a history of allergy, psoriasis, porphyria, or glucose-6-phosphate dehydrogenase deficiency. These conditions are contraindications or precautions to the use of antimalarials.

The symptoms of malaria include periodic fever and chills, profound sweating, headache, nausea, body pains, and exhaustion. The patient may report having been in an area where malaria is endemic. Objective signs of malaria include periodic diaphoresis (sweating) and periodic cycles of fever as high as 104° to 105° F.

Diagnosis

Is the patient dehydrated? What is the patient's state of nutrition? Are there other chronic diseases or problems that may interfere with this therapy? Is the patient taking other medications?

Planning

Because certain strains of *P. falciparum* are resistant to 4-aminoquinoline compounds, individuals infected with these strains should be treated with other antimalarial drugs such as quinine.

Individuals taking high dosages or going through prolonged antimalarial therapy may develop irreversible retinal damage of their eyes. Children are highly sensitive to 4-aminoquinoline compounds, primarily chloroquine.

Quinine should be used with care in patients with cardiac dysrhythmias. Cardiotoxicity may result with quinine use. In very sensitive individuals, reversible thrombocytopenia may occur with quinine use.

Clinical Goldmine

Active Base of Medicine

The amount of active base of a medicine varies from product to product. The dosage should be decided on the basis of the amount of active base in the product. The product package information lists the tablet's equivalence to the base.

Laboratory work to measure the glucose-6-phosphate dehydrogenase level in black patients and in those of Mediterranean ancestry may be required because antimalarial drugs may precipitate hemolysis in some vulnerable patients. The drug should be stopped if the patient develops any blood dyscrasia that is not part of the disease.

dose is usually followed by one-half that dose on the next 2 days. To prevent malaria, these drugs are usually started 2 weeks before the individual enters an area where malaria is endemic. The medication is taken once weekly on the same day of the week and is continued for 8 weeks after the individual has left the area.

Table 12-9 provides a summary of antimalarials.

Implementation

Chloroquine phosphate and hydroxychloroquine are administered orally. To treat malaria, an initial loading

Evaluation

You should watch for the malaria symptoms to go away. If the patient requires long-term therapy, you should

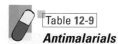

Table 12-9
Antimalarials

GENERIC NAME	TRADE NAME	COMMENTS AND DOSAGE
4-AMINOQUINOLINES		
chloroquine HCl	Aralen HCl	Parenteral drug of choice for treating acute malarial attacks when oral therapy is ineffective. *Adults:* 200-250 mg IM initially, and repeated q6h prn. *Children:* 5 mg/kg (base) initially, repeated in 6 hours prn.
chloroquine phosphate	Aralen Phosphate	• *Malaria suppression* *Adults:* 500 mg once weekly on same day of wk, beginning 2 wk before entering malaria-endemic area and continued for 8 wk after departure. *Children:* 5 mg/kg (base) once weekly on same day of wk, beginning 2 wk before entering malaria-endemic area and continuing for 8 wk after departure. • *Malaria treatment* *Adults:* 1 gm initially, then 500 mg in 6 hr and 500 mg daily for the next 2 days. *Children:* 10 mg/kg (base) initially, then 5 mg/kg (base) in 6 hr and 5 mg/kg (base) daily for the next 2 days.
hydroxychloroquine	Plaquenil	• *Malaria suppression* *Adults:* 400 mg once weekly on same day of wk, beginning 2 wk before entering malaria-endemic area and continued for 8 wk after departure. *Children:* 5 mg/kg (base) once weekly on same day of wk, not to exceed adult dosage, beginning 2 wk before entering malaria-endemic area and continued for 8 wk after departure. • *Malaria treatment* *Adults:* 800 mg initially, then 400 mg in 6 hr and 400 mg daily for the next 2 days. *Children:* 10 mg/kg (base) initially, then 5 mg/kg (base) in 6 hr and 5 mg/kg (base) daily for the next 2 days.
8-AMINOQUINOLONES		
primaquine phosphate	Primaquine Phosphate	Initiate primaquine therapy following a course of chloroquine phosphate suppressive treatment or during the last 2 wk of therapy with chloroquine phosphate. • *Malaria suppression* *Adults:* 26.3 mg once daily for 14 days, beginning immediately after leaving malaria-endemic area. *Children:* 0.3 mg/kg (base) once daily for 14 days, beginning immediately after leaving malaria-endemic area.

Continued

Table 12-9

Antimalarials—cont'd

GENERIC NAME	TRADE NAME	COMMENTS AND DOSAGE
FOLIC ACID AGONISTS		
pyrimethamine	Daraprim	• *Malaria suppression* Therapy should begin 2 wk before entering malaria-endemic area and be continued for 10 wk after departure. *Adults and children over 10 yr:* 25 mg once weekly. *Children 4-10 yr:* 12.5 mg once weekly. *Children younger than 4 yr:* 6.25 mg once weekly.
MISCELLANEOUS AGENTS		
doxycycline	Doxycycline	• *Malaria prophylaxis* *Adults:* 100 mg once daily for 1-2 days before travel to malaria-endemic area and daily during travel and for 4 wk after leaving the area. *Children:* 2 mg/kg/day up to adult dose of 100 mg/day.
halofantrine HCl	Halfan	*Adults:* Mild to moderate malaria. Give 500 mg every 6 hr for 3 doses; repeat this course 7 days later. Second course may be eliminated in patients with known previous infections or who have lived in malaria-endemic areas for their lifetime.
mefloquine	Lariam	• *Treatment* *Adults:* 5 tablets (1250 mg) as a single dose. • *Prophylaxis* *Adults:* 250 mg once weekly for 4 wk, then every other wk up to 4 wk after leaving travel area.
quinine sulfate	—	Concurrent use of pyrimethamine 50 mg daily for the first 3 days of quinine therapy plus sulfadiazine 2 gm daily for the first 6 days is recommended. • *Chloroquine-resistant malaria* *Adults:* 650 mg q8h for 10-14 days. *Children:* 25 mg/kg q8h for 10-14 days.

obtain a CBC and urinalysis every so often, and check for signs and symptoms of hemolysis. Also, you should occasionally check the knee and ankle reflexes to see if there is any weakness. An ECG may be obtained before starting quinine therapy and again during treatment if the patient develops any cardiac rhythm problems. Any report of visual problems makes a full eye examination necessary.

CASE STUDY

Bill Ethington, 64 years old, comes into the clinic with a temperature of 104° F. He is sweating profusely, feels nauseated, and says that he feels "horrible." He reports he has never felt this way before. He sits in the chair but twists and turns, rubbing his lower back as he talks. A urine specimen is positive for red blood cells and protein, and a microscopic specimen shows bacteria and urinary casts. The nurse practitioner confirms that he has a urinary tract infection.

1. What antibiotics are used primarily for urinary tract infections and why?

2. What special instructions would you give the patient if the nurse practitioner started the patient on Gantrisin?
3. What other problems does Mr. Ethington have that need nursing or medical care?
4. Would the medication ordered be any different if this patient was a pregnant woman?
5. What other types of drugs might Mr. Ethington need?

Patient and Family Teaching

You should tell the patient and family the following:

1. The patient should take all the medication as ordered and not stop when the symptoms disappear.
2. The nurse, physician, or other health care provider should be called as soon as possible if the patient has ringing in the ears, hearing difficulties, or any problems with vision.
3. Taking medication with meals can reduce GI upset. The nurse, physician, or other health care provider should be called if there is any severe nausea, vomiting, anorexia, abdominal cramps, or diarrhea.
4. This medication should be kept out of the reach of children.
5. Quinine products may cause the skin to appear somewhat yellow.
6. Quinine may cause dizziness and blurred vision. The patient should be very careful when driving.
7. Malaria may recur. The patient should watch for symptoms to develop again and call the nurse, physician, or other health care provider as soon as possible.

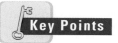

Key Points

- A wide range of drugs are available to treat infections.
- These drugs include broad-spectrum antibiotics, antitubercular drugs, antiparasitic medications, penicillins, sulfonamides, and antifungal drugs (discussed in Chapter 13).
- Because antiinfectives are so commonly used, you must be familiar with significant adverse reactions and drug interactions and should know what to teach the patient and family for each type of antibiotic.
- New antibiotics are continually being developed, partly because of research in this area and also because resistant strains of many organisms have developed (especially strains resistant to penicillin, which has been in wide use for many years).

Go to the free CD-ROM for an Audio Glossary, animations, video clips, and Review Questions for the NCLEX-PN® Examination.

evolve Be sure to visit the companion Evolve website at http://evolve.elsevier.com/Edmunds/LPN/ for WebLinks, a link to the top 200 drugs by prescription, and sign-up pages for newsletter drug updates.

DRUG CALCULATION REVIEW

1. A 10-year-old child has come to the family practice clinic with complaints of fever and right ear pain for 3 days. The physician diagnoses acute bacterial otitis media and orders an injection of ceftriaxone (Rocephin) 600 mg IM. The available vial of powder is marked ceftriaxone 1 gm, with the following instructions: "Reconstitute with 9.6 mL diluent to equal 100 mg/mL."

   A. How many milliliters will the nurse prepare?

   B. Where should this injection be given?

   C. Should the nurse divide the dose?

2. Order: Penicillin G 1,000,000 units intramuscular stat

   Available: Penicillin G 600,000 units/mL

   Question: How many milliliters of penicillin should be given?

3. Order: Infuse vancomycin 1.5 gm in 150 mL of D$_5$W IVPB (IV piggyback).

   Medication information: States that IV vancomycin should be infused using an IV infusion device at a rate of 1 gm/hr.

   Question: How many milliliters per hour should the nurse set the IV infusion device for?

4. Order: Kefzol 400 mg IM every 6 hours

   Reconstitution directions: Add 2 mL of 0.9% normal saline to a vial of Kefzol 500 mg to yield a total volume of 2.2 mL.

   Question: How many milliliters should be administered with each dose? (Round to the nearest tenth.)

CRITICAL THINKING ?

1. After a complete physical, Mrs. Johnson, age 87, has just been prescribed a broad-spectrum antibiotic, much to her surprise. Her physician has asked you to administer a first dose for her before she leaves your clinic to head for the pharmacist and then home. After the doctor leaves the room, Mrs. Johnson confides to you, "I'm worried, hon. He shouldn't have given me an antibiotic, should he? I don't have a sore throat. I have a virus." Explain to Mrs. Johnson the wide variety of indications for these drugs. Also explain why an antibiotic is sometimes ordered for a viral infection.

2. Mrs. Johnson asks you which antibiotic you will be giving to her and says, "That's not penicillin, is it? The last time I took penicillin, I got an awfully scratchy throat." Why is this significant?

3. What is the most important point to emphasize in a teaching plan for a patient newly diagnosed with tuberculosis?

4. While doing volunteer work overseas, Mr. Johannsen developed malaria and had to come home. His doctor has prescribed chloroquine phosphate. Write out a teaching plan to explain to Mr. Johannsen how to control infection and reinfection, the lifelong possibility of relapses, endemic reactions, how to take his medication, and the need for follow-up examinations.

5. Ms. Keaton thinks she is allergic to penicillin, although she says she has "never been tested." What are the signs and symptoms of hypersensitivity or allergy?

6. If Ms. Keaton tells you she thinks she is allergic to penicillin because it made her "stomach sick" when she was a child, what signs or symptoms is she describing?

7. Ms. Keaton comes back to the clinic, complaining that she still has the same bladder infection she came to you for the first time. Her doctor switches her to a sulfonamide. "What good will that do?" she asks you. Explain the actions and uses of sulfonamides. Draw up a teaching plan for this patient, stressing the importance of taking the medication properly, symptoms that should be reported immediately to the physician or other health care provider, and symptoms of hypersensitivity.

8. Ms. Keaton calls your clinic two weeks later, stating she has "another infection like the last time." "I guess those other pills didn't work, either," she says. After she makes another appointment with her doctor, Ms. Keaton asks you if she should "just start taking the pills that were left over" until she sees the doctor. What might you suspect has happened? What would be your most appropriate answer to her question?

13 Antivirals, Antiretrovirals, and Antifungal Medications

Objectives

After reading and studying this chapter, you should be able to do the following:

1. Describe how antiviral and antiretroviral medications work.
2. List common medications used in treating AIDS and AIDS-related fungal infections.
3. Outline Standard Precautions the nurse takes in limiting exposure to AIDS. (Review material in Chapter 10.)

Key Terms

Be sure to check out the bonus material on the free CD-ROM, including selected audio pronunciations.

acquired immunodeficiency syndrome (AIDS) (ă-KWĪ-ĕrd ĬM-ū-nō-dē-FĬSH-ĭn-sē, p. 197)
antifungal medications (ăn-tī-FŬN-găl, p. 205)
antiretrovirals (ăn-tī-RĔT-rō-vī-rălz, p. 197)
human immunodeficiency virus (HIV) (ĬM-ū-nō-dē-FĬSH-ĭn-sē, p. 197)
mycotic infections (mī-KŎT-ĭk, p. 205)
opportunistic infections (ŏp-ŏr-TŪN-ĭst-ĭk, p. 202)
retrovirus (RĔT-rō-vī-rŭs, p. 197)
virions (VĪ-rē-ŭnz, p. 197)

OVERVIEW

Acquired immunodeficiency syndrome (AIDS) is a disease that causes a breakdown in the immune system so that the patient is unable to fight infection. Because so many people who develop AIDS die, it is one of the most frightening diseases that we are now seeing. More than 98% of individuals who develop the most severe form of the disease die within 5 years of diagnosis. Advances in treatment have prolonged the life of patients who can get the needed medications.

AIDS is a viral disease that probably arose in central Africa in the 1950s but is now found throughout the world. In the United States, the groups at highest risk for developing AIDS include homosexual and bisexual men, although the fastest growing group to develop AIDS is heterosexual women. Intravenous (IV) drug abusers, people in prison, female sexual partners of people in AIDS risk groups, and children born to mothers at risk make up the other groups of people most likely to get AIDS. Minorities are overrepresented among the people who get AIDS. Recipients of blood products or of semen for artificial insemination also have developed AIDS. Because AIDS is an epidemic with a high mortality rate, it is important for you to understand what role medications play in slowing the advance of this disease and in treating the other diseases that may result from the patient's reduced immunity.

AIDS is caused by a **retrovirus** currently named **human immunodeficiency virus (HIV)**. Retroviruses are viruses that contain ribonucleic acid (RNA) rather than deoxyribonucleic acid (DNA) as their genetic material. The HIV attaches to the CD4 protein with the help of coreceptors (CXCR4 or CCR5) found on helper T lymphocytes and other cells such as macrophages and dendritic cells. The HIV then fuses its membrane with that of the host cell and inserts its genetic material into the cytoplasm. The viral genetic material is then transcribed into double-stranded DNA called proviral *DNA*. The HIV enzyme, reverse transcriptase, is responsible for creating the double-stranded DNA from the viral RNA. Once produced, this DNA often becomes integrated into the chromosomal DNA of the host cell. The HIV DNA is then able to use the host cell's genetic machinery to create new HIV RNA genetic material and messenger RNA. The messenger RNA codes for the development of HIV polyproteins, which must be cleaved, or separated, into individual proteins by the HIV enzyme protease in order for infectious **virions** (rudimentary virus particles) to be produced. Once this occurs, new virions are assembled and bud from the host cell's membrane and are able to infect new cells. This process is demonstrated in Figure 13-1. **Antiretrovirals** are an important group of drugs that slow the growth or prevent the duplication of retroviruses; they are used to limit the advance of HIV and AIDS.

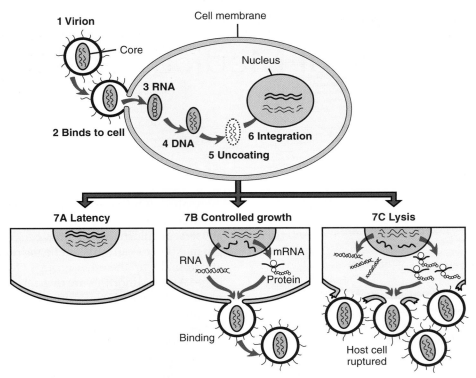

FIGURE **13-1** Infection and cellular outcomes of HIV. HIV infection begins when a virion *(1)*, or virus particle, binds to the outside of a susceptible cell and fuses with it *(2)*, injecting the core proteins and two strands of viral RNA *(3)*. Uncoating occurs, during which the core proteins are removed and the viral RNA is released into the infected cell's cytoplasm. The double-stranded DNA *(4)*, or provirus, migrates to the nucleus, uncoats itself *(5)*, and is integrated into the cell's own DNA *(6)*. The provirus then can do a couple of things: remain latent *(7A)* or activate cellular mechanisms to copy its genes into RNA *(7B)*, some of which is translated into virus proteins or ribosomes. The proteins and additional RNA then are assembled into new virions that bud from the cell. The process can take place slowly, sparing the host cell *(7B)*, or so rapidly that the cell is lysed or ruptured *(7C)*.

Antivirals

OVERVIEW

Viral infections are not suppressed by antibiotics. The advent of HIV infection, the greater incidence of herpes infections, and other common viral illnesses have led to the development of medications that are helpful in lessening the effects of these infections. Most of these drugs do not lead to cure, but only lessen the symptoms.

ACTION AND USES

These medications are used in the immunocompromised patient with HIV infection, or for adults and children at risk. Other uses are for patients with herpes zoster, herpes simplex, genital herpes, or varicella. Some antiviral medications are helpful in treating patients with cytomegalovirus (CMV) retinitis.

ADVERSE REACTIONS

These drugs are all associated with risk, and the risk-to-benefit ratio should be studied before they are given. Most of these products can cause damage to the liver or the kidney (hepatotoxic or nephrotoxic); many are associated with blood dyscrasias and peripheral neuropathies. Some of the drugs are quite new, and information about adverse effects is still being collected. All health care personnel involved with giving these drugs must read the latest product information before administering these products.

DRUG INTERACTIONS

These drugs also have many drug interactions, often with products not usually involved in drug reactions. If you are giving these drugs, you must read carefully about each of these products to determine if it can be given safely to your patient.

Nursing Implications and Patient Teaching

Assessment

You should understand clearly why the product is being ordered and what the physician or other health care provider hopes to accomplish with the drug plan. What do you know about the patient that you believe will help or hurt her ability to take the medicines?

Diagnosis

What other problems does this patient have that might limit the effectiveness of treatment? Because antivirals only lessen symptoms and cannot cure disease, the same viral infection often occurs many times, and pa-tients may need education, comfort, and basic teaching about how to reduce pain, itching, or discharge. These patients often experience weakness and muscle wast-ing. Do they have adequate nutrition? Can they afford the medicine? Will they be compliant?

Planning

The information about these products is growing every day. You should review the latest information from the package inserts before giving these products.

Implementation

Several of these products have special storage require-ments or instructions for mixing. You need to read the latest information to administer these products correctly.

Specific information about these products is given in Table 13-1.

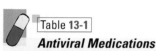

Table **13-1**

Antiviral Medications

GENERIC NAME	TRADE NAME	COMMENTS AND DOSAGE
acyclovir	Zovirax	For initial and recurrent mucosal and cutaneous HSV-1 and HSV-2 and varicella-zoster infections in immunocompromised individuals, and in severe acute and recurrent genital herpes in patients who are not immunocompromised. May also be used for acute treatment of herpes zoster and chickenpox lesions. Begin with parenteral infusion and follow with oral therapy. Dosage depends on condition, acuity, and severity.
amantadine HCl	Symmetrel	For prophylaxis of influenza A virus respiratory tract illnesses in patients at high risk because of underlying disease. *Adults:* 200 mg daily as a single dose or 100 mg twice daily. *Children 9-12 yr:* 100 mg twice daily. *Children 1-9 yr:* 2-4 mg/day. May need to treat for 30-90 days.
cidofovir	Vistide	Used in CMV retinitis in patients with AIDS. Give as an IV infusion over 1 hr. Give 2 gm probenecid PO 3 hr before each dose and 1 gm at 2 hr and again at 8 hr after infusion.
famciclovir	Famvir	For acute herpes zoster and recurrent genital herpes. • *Acute herpes zoster:* 500 mg q8h for 7 days • *Recurrent genital herpes:* 125 mg twice daily for 5 days.
foscarnet Na	Foscavir	For CMV retinitis and HSV infections. Give 90 mg/kg q12h or 60 mg/kg over a minimum of 1 hr q8h for 2-3 wk depending on response.
ganciclovir	Cytovene	For CMV retinitis and infection in AIDS patients. Begin parenteral therapy and follow with oral tablets. Watch for granulocytopenia and thrombocytopenia.
oseltamivir phosphate	Tamiflu	For treatment of uncomplicated acute illness from influenza in patients older than 1 yr who have been symptomatic for more than 2 days or for prophylaxis for people older than 13 yr.
ribavirin	Virazole	For severe lower respiratory tract infections in hospitalized infants and young children with severe infections from RSV. Powder for aerosol administration only.
rimantadine	Flumadine	For prophylaxis and treatment of illnesses caused by various strains of influenza virus. In children, used as prophylaxis against influenza A virus. *Adults:* 100 mg twice daily. *Children:* 5 mg/kg once daily.

Continued

Table 13-1

Antiviral Medications—cont'd

GENERIC NAME	TRADE NAME	COMMENTS AND DOSAGE
valacyclovir HCl	Valtrex	Used for herpes zoster and recurrent genital herpes. • *Herpes zoster:* 1 gm 3 times daily for 7 days • *Recurrent genital herpes:* 500 mg twice daily for 5 days
valganciclovir HCl	Valcyte	Used to treat CMV retinitis, particularly in patients with AIDS. May produce granulocytopenia, anemia, and thrombocytopenia. Give 900 mg twice daily with food for 21 days.
zanamivir	Relenza	Treatment of uncomplicated acute illness from influenza A and B in adults and children older than 7 years of age who have been symptomatic for more than 2 days.

HSV, Herpes simplex virus; *RSV,* respiratory syncytial virus.

Evaluation

Watch the patient for signs of improvement in symptoms. Watch particularly for signs of toxicity or adverse effects.

Patient and Family Teaching

You should tell the patient and the family the following:
1. Some of these products are quite new and are used in the treatment of problems for which there has been little treatment until recently.
2. This medication is usually able to reduce symptoms or suppress symptoms, but it does not cure disease.
3. The patient should be careful to follow any specific storage instructions for the medication.
4. The patient should learn the specific symptoms that would indicate the development of adverse effects. If these develop, the patient should telephone the nurse, physician, or other health care provider or return immediately to the clinic, depending on the symptoms.
5. Many medications should be taken with bottled water in order to protect the patient from pathogens in impure water.

SECTION TWO

Antiretroviral Agents

OVERVIEW

Research and clinical drug trials continue to make changes in what we know about AIDS. This will affect what drugs we use to treat AIDS patients and how we use them. You should rely on only the most current information.

ACTION

Antiretroviral agents act to stop more retroviruses from being made by interfering with the ability of a retrovirus to reproduce, or replicate. At present, there are two basic types of antiretrovirals in clinical use: reverse transcriptase inhibitors and protease inhibitors. Reverse transcriptase inhibitors act early in the life cycle of the virus, and protease inhibitors act later in the life cycle of the virus.

USES

These drugs are used to slow the advance of AIDS infection and keep whatever immunity the patient still has. They may also be used to prevent HIV in infants born to HIV-infected mothers or in health care workers who have been exposed to HIV. (The effectiveness of such treatment is shown when there is not a change in antibody test results from HIV-negative to HIV-positive, or seroconversion.) All of these medications are relatively new and fairly toxic, with many adverse effects and drug interactions.

Reverse transcriptase inhibitors prevent the HIV enzyme reverse transcriptase from creating HIV proviral DNA from the viral RNA. This in turn prevents more viruses from being produced. There are two categories of reverse transcriptase inhibitors: nucleoside analogue reverse transcriptase inhibitors and nonnucleoside analogue reverse transcriptase inhibitors.

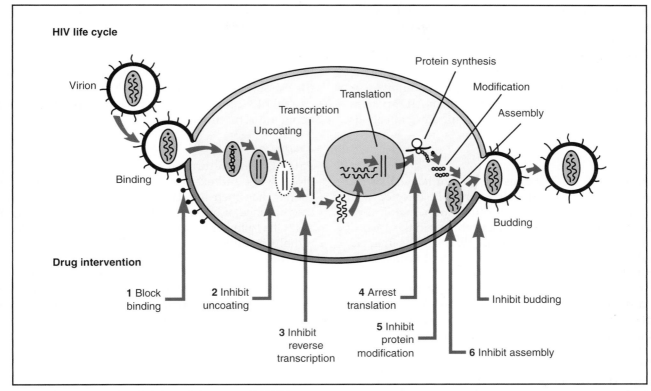

FIGURE 13-2 HIV is subject to attack by drugs at several stages during its life cycle. Certain agents could block the binding of HIV to the CD4 receptors on the surface of helper T cells *(1)*. Other agents might keep viral RNA and reverse transcriptase from leaving their protein coat *(2)*. Drugs such as AZT and other dideoxynucleosides prevent the reverse transcription of viral RNA into viral DNA *(3)*. Later, antisense oligonucleotides could block the translation of messenger RNA (mRNA) into viral proteins *(4)*. Certain compounds could interfere with viral assembly by modifying such processes *(5)*, and finally, antiviral agents such as interferon could keep the virus from assembling itself and budding out of the cell *(6)*.

The other type of medication used in AIDS patients is the protease inhibitors. One of the final stages of the HIV life cycle is the production of HIV polyproteins, which are coded for by the viral messenger RNA. These polyproteins must be cleaved, or separated into the individual proteins necessary for the production of more infectious virions, by the HIV enzyme called protease. Protease inhibitors block the HIV enzyme protease and therefore prevent these polyproteins from being cleaved. This causes noninfectious HIV virions to be produced.

Figure 13-2 illustrates different stages in which drugs attack HIV. These medications are given only under the direction of a specialist, but you may see patients getting these drugs who have other health problems.

ADVERSE REACTIONS

These medications often cause severe toxic reactions. You must constantly watch for symptoms of pancreatitis, peripheral neuropathy, and myopathies, as well as less serious conditions such as mouth ulcers, rash, headaches, diarrhea, and nausea.

DRUG INTERACTIONS

Most of these drugs inhibit the cytochrome P-450 enzyme system in the liver that is involved in the metabolism of medications. For this reason, they should not be taken at the same time as other drugs. It is important to check with the physician or other health care provider before any medications are given to patients taking antiretroviral medications.

Nursing Implications and Patient Teaching

Assessment

You should learn all you can about the history and course of the disease, the medications the patient has used, and his response to the medications. Most of the drugs used in the treatment of AIDS are toxic to the liver. Assess for past or present history of hepatitis or hepatomegaly (enlarged liver) plus current, as well as past, alcohol use or abuse. Assess for a history of pancreatitis and symptoms of peripheral neuropathy because these are frequently caused by medications.

You should also ask about AIDS-related **opportunistic infections**—infections that develop because the damage to the body's immune system leaves it unable to protect the patient against these organisms. Opportunistic infections would not ordinarily be a problem to an individual but, because of reduced immunity, they may cause great pain and suffering in an AIDS patient. Ask the patient specifically about respiratory infections, skin lesions, and *Candida* infections.

Diagnosis

What stage of disease does the patient have? Has she only been exposed to the virus, or is she infected with HIV and symptomatic? In addition to the medical diagnoses, does the patient have problems in the areas of hydration, nutrition, or hygiene? What are the financial needs, emotional concerns, and spiritual needs? Does the patient have a support system, or is she going through this illness alone? Does the patient engage in unsafe sexual or drug practices that present risk to other individuals? What deficits in knowledge does she have about HIV infection, prognosis, and treatment?

Planning

Compliance is required in helping patients with HIV infection. They must return frequently to their health care providers for tests and examinations. Because they are at risk for developing opportunistic infections as a result of their damaged immune system, patients must be taught the signs of such infections. They must be willing to take all the medicines that are prescribed. These drugs are often expensive and may have complicated directions for when they need to be taken. For patients who are trying to slow or halt their HIV infection, it is important to provide individual teaching and to help these patients with their specific problems if you want to succeed with the treatment goals.

Before beginning drug therapy with antiretrovirals, the helper T lymphocyte (CD4) count must be measured and plasma HIV RNA laboratory studies must be done. These results help assess a patient's immunologic status and severity of infection. They also provide a means of measuring how well the treatment is working. A complete blood cell count (CBC), including a white blood cell count (WBC) with differential, folate, vitamin B_{12}, ferritin, iron, and percentage of iron saturation, should also be obtained. Liver function tests and hepatitis B, C, and A serologies, as well as amylase, triglyceride, and lipase levels, will also be ordered. All of these laboratory studies are repeated during the treatment and help show treatment success or onset of adverse effects.

All of the protease inhibitors are potent inhibitors of the cytochrome P-450 enzyme system and have many contraindications to use of other drugs at the same time.

Implementation

In working with these patients, be certain to follow Standard Precautions. Wear gloves when necessary to avoid exposure to lesions or bodily fluids. Patients should be taught how to take care of minor problems and when they should return for care.

Table 13-2 provides a list of important information about antiretrovirals.

Evaluation

Patients must return on a frequent basis for further blood work and examinations. They must also return sooner than their regular schedule when they suspect the presence of opportunistic infections. Patients generally have fewer severe side effects with the protease inhibitors, although patients taking indinavir sulfate may develop "Crix belly." This is a syndrome characterized by elevated levels of triglycerides, cholesterol, and plasma glucose, with a weight gain of 40 lbs or greater. Fat accumulates in the lower abdomen and flanks and tissue is often lost in the arms and legs.

Clinical Landmine

Signs or Symptoms of Pancreatitis

Patients who develop any signs or symptoms of pancreatitis should have their medication stopped immediately until it is ruled out.

Patient and Family Teaching

You should tell the patient and family the following:
1. Compliance is essential. Patients must take their medications as ordered. With many of these drugs, taking too little medication, following the drug schedule only part of the time, or not taking the medication may result in a resistant strain of HIV that cannot be treated.
2. Antiretrovirals do not cure HIV infection. Also, the use of these medications does not stop the need to prevent transmission through safe sex practices and Standard Precautions.

Clinical Landmine

Prescribed Doses

Taking less than the prescribed dose can be more harmful than not taking the drug at all.

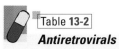

Table 13-2

Antiretrovirals

DRUG	CLINICAL TOXICITIES	DOSAGE	NURSING IMPLICATIONS
REVERSE TRANSCRIPTASE INHIBITORS			
Nucleoside Analogues			
didanosine (ddl) (Videx)	Pancreatitis, peripheral neuropathy, retinal depigmentation, diarrhea, headache, dry mouth, insomnia, nervousness	≤60 kg: 125 mg twice daily or 167 mg twice daily sachet; >60 kg: 200 mg twice daily or 250 mg twice daily sachet	Do not take medication with food; do not mix with acidic beverages; separate other drugs from ddl by 2 hr.
lamivudine (3TC) (Epivir HBV)	Peripheral neuropathy, headache, pancreatitis (in children)	150 mg twice daily; reduce dosage with renal impairment	Use in combination with zidovudine.
stavudine (d4T) (Zerit)	Peripheral neuropathy, diarrhea, nausea, vomiting	≤60 kg: 30 mg twice daily; >60 kg: 40 mg twice daily	Do not use with zidovudine.
zalcitabine (ddC) (Hivid)	Peripheral neuropathy, oral ulcers, rash, esophageal ulceration, pancreatitis (rare)	0.75 mg 3 times daily; reduce dose in renal impairment	Concomitant use with ddl is not recommended.
zidovudine (ZDV, AZT) (Retrovir)	Headache, nausea, myopathy, myositis, malaise, hepatic stenosis	200 mg 3 times daily or 300 mg twice daily; reduce dose in renal impairment	Nausea and headaches often resolve after 4-6 weeks of therapy; 60% CNS penetration; drug of choice for HIV CNS disease.
REVERSE TRANSCRIPTASE INHIBITORS			
Nonnucleoside Analogues			
abacavir sulfate (Ziagen)	Fatal hypersensitivity reactions have been associated with this drug. Discontinue immediately if any signs of hypersensitivity.	Give 300 mg twice daily in combination with other antiretroviral drugs.	Question patient about any new symptoms that may suggest hypersensitivity.
delavirdine (DLV) (Rescriptor)	Rash (pruritus), headaches	400 mg 3 times daily	When used as monotherapy, resistance can rapidly develop; antacids decrease absorption. If used with ddl, separate by 1 hr.
efavirenz (Sustiva)	Used in treating HIV along with other antiretroviral agents	600 mg daily in addition to other protease inhibitors or nucleoside analogue reverse transcriptase inhibitors	May be taken with food. Avoid high-fat meals.
nevirapine (NVP) (Viramune)	Rash (Stevens-Johnson syndrome)	200 mg daily × 2 wk, then increase to 200 mg twice daily	When used as monotherapy, resistance can rapidly develop; once-daily dosing during first 2 wk may lessen incidence of rash.

Continued

Table 13-2

Antiretrovirals—cont'd

DRUG	CLINICAL TOXICITIES	DOSAGE	NURSING IMPLICATIONS
PROTEASE INHIBITORS			
amprenavir (Agenerase)	There are no long-term studies evaluating long-term suppression.	*Adults:* 1200 mg bid in combination with other antiretroviral agents.	May be taken with or without food; however, high-fat meals reduce absorption of drug. Do not take supplemental vitamins that contain vitamin E because RDA would be exceeded.
indinavir (Crixivan)	Nephrolithiasis, nausea, abdominal pain, "Crix belly," hematuria	800 mg 3 times daily	Should be taken 1 hr before or 2 hr after meals; drink >1.5 L/day to avoid renal stones; decrease rifabutin dose by 1/2. Concurrent use with St. John's wort and other CYP3A substrates contraindicated.
nelfinavir mesylate (Viracept)	Diarrhea, nausea	750 mg 3 times daily	Should be taken with food.
ritonavir (Norvir)	Nausea, diarrhea, taste changes, circumoral paresthesias, thrombocytopenia	600 mg twice daily	Should be taken with food; has numerous drug interactions.
saquinavir mesylate (Invirase, Fortovase)	Diarrhea, nausea, abdominal pain, ataxia, neutropenia, hemolytic anemias	600 mg 3 times daily	Should be taken with high-fat meals.
PROTEASE INHIBITOR COMBINATION			
lopinavir/ritonavir (Kaletra)	Used in treating HIV infection. No results from controlled trials evaluating the effect on clinical progression of HIV.	Give a capsule = 400/100 mg twice daily with food.	

CNS, Central nervous system.

3. All HIV-positive women should be warned of the high risk of HIV transmission in breast milk. The Centers for Disease Control and Prevention advises all HIV-infected women not to breastfeed.

4. The patient should report all other medications he is taking, including over-the-counter (OTC) medications and those medications that were obtained outside of the traditional medical settings, or illegal drugs.

5. The patient should learn the signs and symptoms of pancreatitis.

6. The patient should report signs and symptoms of peripheral neuropathy. The peripheral neuropathy caused by several of the reverse transcriptase inhibitors is sensorimotor in character. Initially the patient feels numbness and burning, usually involving the toes. Patients may have decreased light touch, pinprick, temperature, and vibration sensation in the feet and up to the midcalf. These symptoms may be followed by sharp, shooting pains, which progress to severe, continuous burning pain that is often worse at night and requires narcotic analgesics.

Clinical Landmine

Peripheral Neuropathy

This neuropathy is usually reversible if the medication is promptly discontinued.

SECTION THREE
Antifungals

ACTION AND USES

A fungus is a plant that produces yeastlike or moldlike diseases called **mycotic infections** in humans. These can be either superficial infections, such as in the skin or nail, or systemic infections, such as in the lung or liver. Because fungi are found almost everywhere—in most water supplies, in the air, and in the soil—they pose a real risk for immunocompromised patients.

Antifungal medications are medications used orally, intravenously, topically, and vaginally to treat mycotic infections. There are a variety of antifungals; some are used primarily for vaginal yeast or fungal infections and others are used to treat superficial or systemic infections. The actions and uses of the most common medications used in treating general fungal infections are described in Table 13-3.

Because AIDS destroys the body's immune system, patients with AIDS are prey to many opportunistic infections. Fungi that the body would usually keep under control now cause some of the most problematic infections. You should understand how antifungal medications may be helpful in improving the general well-being of AIDS patients.

Clinical Landmine

Adverse Reactions

Many of the adverse reactions to antifungals are similar to the symptoms of the disease they are intended to cure. It is sometimes difficult to determine if the patient needs more or less medication.

ADVERSE REACTIONS

See Table 13-3 for adverse reactions to common antifungal medications.

Symptoms of overdosage include severe nausea, vomiting, and diarrhea.

Clinical Landmine

Antifungal Drug Interactions with Alcohol

Because of severe drug interactions with alcohol products, you should assess the patient's alcohol intake patterns.

DRUG INTERACTIONS

Severe superinfection may result when antifungals are given along with prolonged corticosteroid therapy. Activity of oral anticoagulants is decreased when they are used at the same time as griseofulvin; it may be necessary to adjust the anticoagulant dosage. Griseofulvin activity is decreased when used at the same time as barbiturates, requiring dosage adjustments of griseofulvin. Use of alcohol while taking antifungals potentiates, or increases, the effect of the alcohol. Because antacids, anticholinergics, and H_2 blockers change gastrointestinal (GI) pH, the patient should not take ketoconazole for at least 2 hours after taking any H_2 blockers.

Toxicity can result when flucytosine is used along with other drugs that depress bone marrow or when used during radiation therapy. Use of flucytosine with hepatotoxic or nephrotoxic drugs should be avoided. The use of flucytosine also decreases leukocyte and platelet counts and hemoglobin levels.

Metronidazole and alcohol cause severe disulfiram-like reactions with severe nausea, vomiting, tachycardia (rapid heartbeat), flushing, and confusion. It is very important to warn patients not to take anything containing alcohol if they are taking metronidazole.

Nursing Implications and Patient Teaching

Assessment

You should learn as much as you can about the patient's health history, including any allergy, bone marrow depression, use of alcohol or other drugs that may produce drug interactions (particularly corticosteroids),

Table **13-3**

Actions, Uses, and Adverse Effects of Common Antifungal Medications

DRUG	ACTION	USES	ADVERSE EFFECTS
flucytosine	Synthetic, fluorinated antifungal agent with fungistatic activity. The antifungal activity is evident when drug is converted to 5-fluorouracil in the fungus cell, thereby inhibiting nucleic acid synthesis. It acts as a fungicidal agent when used in high doses.	Used to treat serious systemic fungal infections caused by susceptible strains of *Candida* and *Cryptococcus*.	Headache, drowsiness, confusion, vertigo (feeling of dizziness or spinning), macular rash, urticaria (hives), nausea, vomiting, diarrhea, blood cell changes, and abnormal liver function tests.
griseofulvin	Fungistatic or fungicidal antibiotic derived from *Penicillium griseofulvin*. It deposits in keratin precursor cells, where it becomes tightly bound, leaving new keratin cells that are highly resistant to fungal infection as exfoliation occurs.	Used to treat fungal infections involving the hair, skin, and nails caused by susceptible species of *Epidermophyton, Microsporum,* and *Trichophyton.*	Headache, vertigo, dizziness, irritability, sore throat, nausea, vomiting, epigastric distress, dryness of mouth, oral thrush, black furry tongue, anorexia, diarrhea, photosensitivity, rash, urticaria, changes in blood cells, angioedema (swelling of the skin and mucous membranes), arthralgia (joint pain), blurred vision, proteinuria (large amounts of protein in the urine), fever, malaise (weakness), and vaginal discharge.
ketoconazole	Broad-spectrum antibiotic with fungistatic or fungicidal activity. It impairs the synthesis of the fungus cell membrane, producing increased membrane permeability, which causes the cellular components to leak out.	Used to treat systemic fungal infections caused by candidiasis, chronic mucocutaneous candidiasis, oral thrush, candiduria, blastomycosis, paracoccidioidomycosis, coccidioidomycosis, histoplasmosis, and chromomycosis. It has also been used to treat pityriasis versicolor and vaginal candidiasis.	May produce abdominal pain, diarrhea, dizziness, fever, headache, gynecomastia (enlargement of the breasts in men), impotence, nausea, photophobia (sensitivity to light), pruritus (itching), and vomiting. Oligospermia (low sperm count) has been reported in patients taking excessively high doses.
nystatin	Polyene antibiotic with fungistatic or fungicidal activity. The drug may allow intracellular components to leak through the fungal cell membrane by binding to sterols in the cell membrane.	Used to treat intestinal, vaginal, and oral fungal infections caused by susceptible strains of *Candida albicans* and other *Candida* species.	Nausea, vomiting, diarrhea.

and the possibility of pregnancy. Some of the drugs may be teratogenic (causing deformities in the fetus).

The patient may have a history of fever and chills at the onset of infection. Itching is a common finding. A history of recent antibiotic therapy is common. The nurse may observe the classic signs of white discharge and erythema (redness or irritation) associated with thrush (*Candida* infection). The patient may also have a history of multiple scaly or blistered red patches on the skin, itching and soreness of infected areas, and brittle nails with yellow discoloration and separation from the nail bed.

Memory Jogger

Antifungals

ketoconazole: This medication has been associated with hepatic toxicity, so the patient must be monitored closely.

flucytosine: Close monitoring of hematologic, renal, and hepatic status is essential.

metronidazole (Flagyl) and alcohol: Counsel patients not to drink alcohol or eat alcohol-containing products while taking this medication because a severe GI and cardiovascular response may develop.

Diagnosis

In addition to the medical diagnoses, what additional problems does the patient have? Are there difficulties in maintaining adequate nutrition or cleanliness or in paying for medications? Consider the need for education of the patient or family.

Planning

Individuals allergic to penicillin may exhibit cross-sensitivity to antifungal agents, although this is rare. The patient may experience photosensitivity (abnormal response to exposure to sunlight) when taking these drugs.

Hepatotoxicity (usually reversible) and a few cases of hepatitis in children have been reported with ketoconazole. Liver function studies must be monitored so that any liver damage may be noted. The product should be discontinued if even a minor elevation in the liver function studies develops.

Implementation

The absorption rate of griseofulvin is increased after the patient eats a fatty meal. Ketoconazole requires stomach acidity for dissolution and absorption. In patients with achlorhydria (lack of hydrochloric acid), tablets should be dissolved in a small amount of aqueous 0.2 N HCl solution. The patient should drink the solution with a straw to avoid staining the teeth and should follow the medication with a full glass of water. You should explain to the patient how and why this is done.

Because griseofulvin is absorbed over a long period, single daily doses are often adequate. The patient must keep using the medication until the fungal infection is gone, as shown by both clinical and laboratory tests. This process may require several weeks or many months of therapy, depending on the organism that is causing the infection and the site of the infection. Use of both oral and topical antifungal agents may be required to treat some fungal infections, primarily tinea pedis.

Clinical Goldmine

Exposure to HIV

Patients who have recurrent vaginal infections that do not easily clear up and who have been exposed to HIV should be evaluated further.

Table 13-4 presents a summary of antifungal medications.

Evaluation

You should observe the patient for therapeutic effects, such as the disappearance of shaking chills and fever, and watch for signs of GI distress. The patient should continue to take the medication until the laboratory tests show that normal function has returned.

Nausea, vomiting, and diarrhea are symptoms of overdosage of most of the antifungal medications.

Clinical Landmine

Liver or Renal Changes

Watch carefully for signs of liver or renal changes. These drugs are very toxic. Report all patient complaints promptly.

Patient and Family Teaching

You should tell the patient and family the following:

1. The patient should take all medication as ordered and not stop treatment when the symptoms disappear. The therapy may have to continue for many weeks before lab tests show that the infection is gone.
2. The nurse, physician, or other health care provider should be called if the patient has any nausea, vomiting, or diarrhea, or any bruising, sore throat, or fever. These drugs are very toxic, and no adverse effects should go unreported.

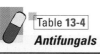

Table 13-4

Antifungals

GENERIC NAME	TRADE NAME	COMMENTS AND DOSAGE
amphotericin B	Amphotec Fungizone IV	Give 0.25 mg/kg slow IV. Gradually increase if patient tolerates medication. For use only in patients with progressive and potentially fatal fungal infections.
fluconazole	Diflucan	Give 200 mg PO or IV on first day, then 100 mg daily for 2-3 weeks.
flucytosine	Ancobon Ancotil	*Adults and children:* 50-150 mg/kg daily in divided doses q6h.
griseofulvin microsize	Grifulvin V Grisactin	Divided doses are recommended for those patients unable to tolerate single doses. • *Fungal infection* *Adults:* 500 mg PO daily in single or divided doses after meals. *Children:* 10 mg/kg PO daily in single or divided doses after meals.
griseofulvin ultramicrosize	Fulvicin P/G Grisactin-Ultra Gris-PEG	Griseofulvin ultramicrosize has approximately 1.5 times the biologic activity of griseofulvin microsize, with no advantage in effectiveness or safety. • *Fungal infection* *Adults:* 250 mg daily in single or divided doses after meals. *Children:* 5 mg/kg daily in single or divided doses after meals.
ketoconazole	Nizoral	*Adults:* Initially, give 200 mg daily. May increase up to 400 mg daily, depending on seriousness of the disease and clinical response. *Children over 2 yr:* Give 3.3-6.6 mg/kg PO daily. Duration of treatment is not specific and should be based on clinical response. Minimum treatment for candidiasis is 10 days to 2 weeks. May require therapy for up to 6 months.
miconazole	Monistat-Derm	Give 200-3600 mg IV or as bladder instillation, depending on organism.
nystatin	Mycostatin	Shake oral suspension well before use. Available for many routes. • *Oral thrush* *Adults and children:* 400,000-600,000 units (4-6 mL) 4 times daily; one half of dose is held in each side of mouth a short time before swallowing. *Older infants:* 200,000 units (2 mL) 4 times daily; one half of dose is held in each side of the mouth a short time before swallowing. *Neonates:* 100,000 units (1 mL) 4 times daily; one half of dose is held in each side of mouth a short time before swallowing. • *Intestinal candidiasis* *Adults:* 500,000-1,000,000 units 3 times daily, continued for at least 2 days after absence of symptoms. • *Vaginitis:* 1-2 tablets intravaginally for 2 wk. Can also be treated with oral doses as in intestinal candidiasis.
Terbinafine HCl	Lamisil	• *Onychomycosis:* For fingers, give 250 mg/day PO for 6 wk. For toenails, give 250 mg/day PO for 12 wk. Optimal clinical effect is seen several months after fungus is cured and healthy nail has grown. Keep tablets cool and protect from light.
RELATED DRUG		
Metronidazole	Flagyl	Give IV or PO. Dosage varies, depending on site of infection. See package insert. Not an antifungal agent but used for patients with mixed fungal and bacteria or protozoa infections.

3. The oral suspension of nystatin should be shaken thoroughly before use.
4. Griseofulvin should be taken with meals that are high in fat; this causes more of the medication to be absorbed. Sometimes people taking this drug develop photosensitivity, or an intolerance to the sun. Alcoholic beverages should be avoided while taking griseofulvin or metronidazole.
5. Cleanliness of hair, skin, and nails will help control or limit the spread of infection.
6. If skin rash occurs or if nausea, vomiting, or diarrhea becomes severe in patients taking flucytosine,

they should tell the nurse, physician, or other health care provider. When several capsules must be taken, they should be taken over a period of 15 minutes to avoid or reduce nausea and vomiting. If symptoms do not resolve within 2 to 3 days, the nurse, physician, or other health care provider should be called.
7. Patients may be asked to use only bottled water to decrease exposure to community water supplies that may have a level of organisms that may be dangerous to immunocompromised patients.

CASE STUDY

Ms. Lucille Betts, a patient who has AIDS, comes into the clinic complaining of numbness and a burning sensation in her feet and lower legs. A physical examination shows her reflexes to be intact, but she has decreased sensation of light touch, pinprick, temperature, and vibration in the feet and midcalf. She has been under treatment with a reverse transcriptase inhibitor.
1. What do you believe is going on?
2. If the symptoms are ignored, what is the usual course?
3. What is the treatment?
4. Lucille discovers she is pregnant. What special requirements for treatment are there for pregnant women?
5. Lucille reports a thick white vaginal discharge and severe perineal itching. What is the probable diagnosis?

6. Why are infections of this type common in immunocompromised individuals?
7. What type of precautions should health care providers use in performing the vaginal examination on Lucille?
8. Lucille has an allergy to penicillin. Why might this be a problem for her?
9. Lucille is started on a vaginal antifungal medication. The nurse warns her that _____ is a common skin reaction associated with many antifungal medications.
10. Most vaginal infections are cured within 3 to 4 days. Is there any reason to suspect that this will not be the case with Lucille?
11. Lucille is at risk for fungal infections at what other sites?

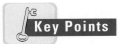

Key Points

- This category of drugs is undergoing constant change as new products are added to the market. It is an area of intense research interest, and new information is being discovered every day that will help patients with immune deficiency problems.
- These are important but powerful and dangerous drugs.
- Although they are drugs ordered by specialists, these products are being used by more and more patients being seen in clinics and primary care practices. Thus you will need to know specifics about these drugs and what you need to tell your patients about them.

Go to the free CD-ROM for an Audio Glossary, animations, video clips, and Review Questions for the NCLEX-PN® Examination.

evolve Be sure to visit the companion Evolve website at http://evolve.elsevier.com/Edmunds/LPN/ for WebLinks, a link to the top 200 drugs by prescription, and sign-up pages for newsletter drug updates.

DRUG CALCULATION REVIEW

1. Order: Acyclovir 10 mg/kg IV over 1 hour every 8 hours

   Question: How many milligrams of acyclovir will be given for a 110-lb person?

2. Order: Amphotericin B 30 mg IV daily over 30 minutes

   Supply: Amphotericin B 30 mg in 100 mL 0.9% normal saline

   Question: How many milliliters per hour should the IV pump be set for?

CRITICAL THINKING ?

1. Mr. Delavan, a patient in the hospital where you work, has been given metronidazole for a systemic mycotic infection; he also has AIDS and is taking several other medications as well. Why is it so important to check the ingredients of all other medications Mr. Delavan is taking? What unpleasant interaction can result otherwise?

2. Mr. Delavan had had a number of adverse reactions to a series of treatment trials. He confides in you that he has become wary of ever taking a drug again, saying, "All they do is make me sicker, I think. If I take this drug, how do I know it isn't just hurting me in some way?" What adverse reactions should you observe for in Mr. Delavan because he is taking a fungicide? Write up a treatment and evaluation plan for this patient.

3. A few months later, Mr. Delavan is back. His AIDS has progressed slightly, but a more immediate problem is the discovery that he now has tuberculosis. Mr. Delavan is having trouble believing his diagnosis, and is even a little panicky. He tells you that he is anxious to "get rid of it quick before it makes me sicker! How did this happen? I thought this disease was eradicated a long time ago!" Explain to Mr. Delavan why and how tuberculosis is easy to contract now. Also explain that tuberculosis requires a long-term treatment plan and why compliance is so important. Revise your treatment and teaching plan for this patient.

4. Mr. Harris has HIV and comes to the clinic because of a severe *Candida* infection of his mouth (thrush). He is started on an antifungal medication. He returns several days later with nausea, vomiting, and severe diarrhea. What do you believe is the source of the symptoms? What other interventions might be indicated?

5. Mr. Harris has a large, open, weeping lesion on his leg. The doctor says that this lesion is common in HIV-infected patients and is known as Kaposi's sarcoma. What precautions would you take in cleaning and dressing this lesion?

6. Mrs. Blake has had HIV for some time. She is 8 months pregnant. What are some of the special things you would want to discuss with this prospective mother?

7. Ms. Lizz has had a bad fungal infection of her toenails. She has been taking the medication terbinafine for a couple of months. She is upset that she sees no improvement. What can you tell her?

8. Ms. Sorenson comes in for her doctor's appointment complaining of a "white itchy" vaginal discharge. While you are taking her history, you check her medical records and note that this is a follow-up appointment for her. She was seen by her doctor 10 days ago for strep throat, for which her physician prescribed penicillin. Ms. Sorenson tells you that she finished the antibiotics, and was "fine until yesterday, when it began to get itchy. Can penicillin cause this? Or do I need more?" What would you tell her?

9. Mr. Lopez arrives for his physician's appointment quite upset. He tells you he is "really embarrassed by the pimple on his lip," which appears inflamed. He states it "tingles a lot and is getting bigger every day...it feels like it's going to pop." While you are asking him how long this has been going on, he mentions he "just got over a bad cold." What might be Mr. Lopez's problem?

14 Antineoplastic Medications

Objectives

After reading and studying this chapter, you should be able to do the following:

1. List the types of drugs used to treat neoplastic disease or cancer.
2. Identify the major adverse reactions associated with antineoplastic agents.
3. Develop a teaching plan for a patient taking an antineoplastic drug.

Key Terms

Be sure to check out the bonus material on the free CD-ROM, including selected audio pronunciations.

alkylating agents (ĂL-kă-lā-tĭng, p. 211)
antibiotic preparations (ăn-tĭ-bī-ŎT-ĭk, p. 211)
antimetabolites (ăn-tĭ-mĕ-TĂB-ō-līts, p. 212)
chemotherapeutic agents (kē-mō-thĕr-ă-PŪ-tĭk, p. 211)
male or female hormones (HŎR-mōnz, p. 212)
malignancy (mă-LĬG-năn-sē, p. 211)
metastasis (mă-TĂS-tă-sĭs, p. 211)
mitotic inhibitors (mī-TŎT-ĭk ĭn-HĬB-ĭ-tŏrs, p. 212)
neoplasms (NĒ-ō-plăzmz, p. 211)

medications are used to treat neoplastic diseases: alkylating agents, antibiotic preparations, antimetabolites, hormones, and mitotic inhibitors.

The types and sites of malignancies vary, and some agents are more effective in treating certain types of malignancies than are other products. The ideal antineoplastic agent damages the malignant cells of the patient while keeping the normal cells as healthy as possible.

Normal cells in the body do not all grow at the same rate. The cells in the gastrointestinal (GI) tract, bone marrow, hair follicles, lymph tissue, mouth, and testes or ovaries are rapidly dividing and growing. Antineoplastic drugs affect rapidly growing tumor cells, but also affect all these other rapidly growing normal cells, thus producing many of the adverse reactions caused by these drugs (diarrhea, alopecia [hair loss], infertility, and the like).

There are many new, highly toxic products on the market in cancer treatment, including interferon, mitotane, and asparaginase. Antineoplastic drugs are strong and may be toxic, and should be ordered by a cancer or oncology specialist. Adverse reactions are common with this group of medications, so you will need to carefully watch the patient.

OVERVIEW

Most cells in the body grow slowly at a rate that can be predicted. When cell growth becomes rapid and uncontrolled, **neoplasms** (abnormal growths or tumors that may be benign or malignant) may be found. These cells often have the ability to travel throughout the body, spreading this unusually rapid cell growth into other areas (**metastasis**) and robbing other tissues of the nutrients (substances that support life and growth) required for normal health. We call this out-of-control cell growth **malignancy**.

Antineoplastic agents, also called **chemotherapeutic agents**, are used to treat malignant diseases. They slow cell growth or delay the spread of the malignant cells into other parts of the body. Antineoplastic agents are most often used with other forms of treatment such as surgery and radiation. The following five types of

ACTION AND USES

The five major types of antineoplastic agents may be used in combination or alone. There are often specific research protocols or rules that govern the use of these medications. It is important for you to accurately report all reactions and adverse effects that the patient might have so that the action of these products can be understood.

Alkylating agents are used to interfere with the normal process of cell division. This effect occurs in both malignant and normal cells, although malignant cells seem to be affected much more by the medications.

Specific **antibiotic preparations** are used, not for their antiinfective properties, but to delay or prevent cell division of the malignant cells. This action is caused by interference with deoxyribonucleic acid (DNA) and ribonucleic acid (RNA) synthesis.

Antimetabolites disrupt normal cell functions by interfering with various metabolic functions of the cells. This action is most effective in cells that are the most rapidly dividing.

Some tumors may depend on **male or female hormones**, the chemicals produced by the sex glands. In patients who have these types of tumors, various hormones that counteract the effects of the hormones used by the tumors may be effective in treatment. The mechanism of action is unclear.

Mitotic inhibitors are a special group of medications that directly interfere with or stop cell division.

A mix of other drugs, most of which have been developed in the last few years, now make up the largest category of antineoplastic drugs, the miscellaneous agents. These products are used for treatment of a wide variety of conditions. Many of them have unlabeled uses, whereas, for others, clinical trials are being done to determine if they are effective and safe.

ADVERSE REACTIONS

The action of the antineoplastic agents on normal cells causes many of the adverse reactions. Some of these reactions depend upon the dose given. Nausea, vomiting, anorexia, and diarrhea are seen with almost all products. Other common reactions include alopecia and bone marrow depression. (Patients with bone marrow depression are more likely to get infections and may show bruising or bleeding.) Renal toxicity, hepatic toxicity, ototoxicity, ocular effects, peripheral neurotoxicity, and hypersensitivity are common among these drugs, and patients must be monitored carefully.

 Clinical Landmine

Antineoplastic Agents

These are some of the most dangerous drugs given to patients. However, they may save the patient's life, so the benefit outweighs the risk. You must always watch the patient and look for changes that might be the onset of serious adverse reactions.

Some reactions are so severe that the patient feels worse with therapy than with the malignancy. There may be no cure for the adverse effects except to stop therapy and not treat the malignancy. Knowledge about the most common adverse effects will help you develop a care plan to prevent or reduce as many symptoms as possible.

DRUG INTERACTIONS

Most antineoplastic drugs interact with other medications the patient may be taking. It is very important to consult the manufacturer's guidelines before starting treatment.

Nursing Implications and Patient Teaching

Assessment

You should learn all you can about the patient's history, the type of malignancy and current status, medications taken, surgeries, allergies, and response. Many patients have numerous hospital admissions for treatment of a malignancy. Old hospital records should be read whenever possible to find accurate information and avoid the need for the patient to repeat information. The patient who comes into the hospital several times should be asked to review her progress since the last time she was hospitalized. It is important to find out about the patient's emotional and physical responses to the illness, her cultural beliefs, spiritual and family support, and acceptance of the problem.

Diagnosis

What other problems does this patient have that may interfere with treatment? Are there adverse effects or disease progression that must be treated? Is the patient fearful or worried? Is money an issue?

Planning

You should read the latest product information about the preparation, storage, and administration of antineoplastic medications. You should understand and follow all warnings, precautions, and contraindications. Some preparations should be given only by a physician or other health care provider or a specially trained chemotherapy nurse. New information is common.

The initial dosage of antineoplastic medication is often calculated in milligrams per kilogram (mg/kg) or milligrams per square meter of body surface area (mg/m^2 BSA). These calculations are based on surface nomograms, which are provided in the drug maker's product insert. The starting dosage will be calculated by the specialist, with future adjustments based on the patient's response as measured by laboratory tests and x-ray studies.

Implementation

You should carefully follow the dosage, frequency, and administration procedures as outlined for any drugs you are authorized to give. Administration of these toxic products may pose a safety hazard to the nurse, as well as the patient, if the products are not administered properly. The syringes, bottles, and needles must be handled and disposed of carefully. There should be a special area designated for mixing these preparations.

Table 14-1 presents the product information for the major antineoplastic agents. Additional detailed information on hormones may be found in Chapter 20.

Evaluation

You should check the patient closely for adverse effects, regularly noting subjective complaints or objective findings on the chart so that the physician or other health care provider may follow the patient's progress. Teach the patient which symptoms to report to the nurse, physician, or other health care provider when the patient goes home and medications are given on an outpatient basis. Table 14-1 includes a listing of common adverse effects for many of these drugs.

Nursing or pharmacologic interventions are often needed to reduce adverse effects. Antiemetics may be given for nausea; special skin care may be needed; and analgesics or narcotics may be required. Patients

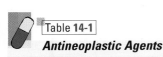

Table 14-1
Antineoplastic Agents

GENERIC NAME	TRADE NAME	COMMENTS AND DOSAGE
ALKYLATING AGENTS		
altretamine	Hexalen	Used for palliative treatment of patients with persistent or recurrent ovarian cancer.
busulfan	Busulfex Myleran	Used in chronic myelogenous leukemia; may produce leukopenia, anemia, thrombocytopenia, hyperpigmentation of skin, and cataracts. Give 1-8 mg/day PO.
carboplatin	Paraplatin	Used in ovarian carcinoma. Give 360 mg/m^2 IV on day 1 every 4 wk.
carmustine	BiCNU	Used in patients with brain tumors, Hodgkin's disease, and multiple myeloma; may produce leukopenia, thrombocytopenia, azotemia, nausea, and vomiting; causes burning at injection site. Give 100-200 mg/m^2 IV.
	GLIADEL Wafer	This is a wafer that is inserted into the cavity after surgery. Use up to 8 wafers at a time.
chlorambucil	Leukeran 🍁	Used in Hodgkin's disease, chronic lymphocytic leukemia, and malignant lymphomas; may produce hyperuricemia and bone marrow depression. Give 0.03-0.2 mg/kg/day PO.
cisplatin	Platinol-AQ 🍁	Used in advanced bladder cancer and some metastatic testicular and ovarian tumors; may produce nausea, vomiting, leukopenia, thrombocytopenia, ototoxicity, and nephrotoxicity. Give 50-70 mg/m^2 IV for bladder cancers and ovarian tumors; 20 mg/m^2 for testicular tumors.
cyclophosphamide	Cytoxan Neosar	Used in Hodgkin's disease, leukemia, carcinoma of ovary and breast, malignant lymphomas, multiple melanoma, and neuroblastoma; may produce anorexia, nausea, vomiting, diarrhea, cystitis, alopecia, leukopenia, thrombocytopenia, or anemia.
dacarbazine	DTIC-Dome	Used in metastatic malignant melanoma, Hodgkin's disease.
ifosfamide	Ifex 🍁	Used in multiple myeloma. Give 6 mg/day IV in one dose.
lomustine	CeeNu	Used in Hodgkin's disease, some brain tumors; may produce nausea, vomiting, alopecia, anemia, leukopenia, thrombocytopenia. Give 100-130 mg/m^2 PO.
mechlorethamine	Mustargen 🍁	Used in Hodgkin's disease, bronchogenic carcinoma, and lymphosarcoma; may produce nausea, vomiting, jaundice, alopecia, skin rash, diarrhea, lymphocytopenia, granulocytopenia, and thrombocytopenia. Give 0.4 mg/kg IV as a total dose for a course of therapy. Give as a single dose, or divide.
melphalan	Alkeran 🍁	Used in carcinoma of ovary and for multiple myeloma; may produce nausea, vomiting, skin rash, and bone marrow depression. Give 6-10 mg/day PO.
streptozocin	Zanosar	Used in carcinoma of the pancreas; may produce severe nausea, vomiting, and renal toxicity. Give 500-1000 mg/m^2 IV.

Continued

Table **14-1**

Antineoplastic Agents—cont'd

GENERIC NAME	TRADE NAME	COMMENTS AND DOSAGE
ALKYLATING AGENTS—cont'd		
thiotepa	Thioplex	Used in lymphosarcomas or carcinoma of breast, ovary, or urinary bladder; may produce nausea, vomiting, and bone marrow depression; causes pain at injection site. Give 0.3-0.4 mg/kg IV. May infiltrate the tumor directly.
ANTIBIOTICS		
bleomycin	Blenoxane	Used in testicular carcinoma, lymphomas, and squamous cell carcinomas of head and neck; may cause vomiting, rash, erythema, fever, chills, pulmonary fibrosis, and pneumonitis. Give 0.25-0.5 units/kg IV, IM, or subcutaneously.
dactinomycin	Cosmegen	Used in testicular or uterine carcinoma, Wilms' tumor, and Ewing's sarcoma; may produce anorexia, nausea, vomiting, alopecia, and bone marrow depression. Give 0.5 mg/day IV. Very corrosive to soft tissue.
daunorubicin	—	Used in adult leukemias; may produce nausea, vomiting, fever, chills, alopecia, and bone marrow depression. Give 45 mg/m^2/day IV. Use under strict protocols.
doxorubicin	Adriamycin Rubex	Used in acute leukemias, Wilms' tumor, carcinomas of breast, ovary, and bladder, lymphomas, neuroblastomas, and soft tissue and bone sarcomas; may cause anorexia, nausea, vomiting, alopecia, fever, and bone marrow depression. Give 30-75 mg/m^2 IV.
epirubicin	Ellence	Used as a component of adjuvant therapy in patients with evidence of axillary node tumor involvement after resection of primary breast cancer. Severe local tissue necrosis develops with extravasation during administration. Watch for myocardial toxicity.
idarubicin	Idamycin	Used in adult acute monocytic lymphoma. Give 12 mg/m^2 daily for 3 days slow IV.
mitomycin	Mutamycin	Used in adenocarcinoma of the stomach and pancreas; may cause anorexia, nausea, vomiting, headache, blurred vision, fever, and bone marrow depression. Give 20 mg/m^2 IV as a single dose, or 2 mg/m^2/day IV for 5 days.
mitoxantrone	Novantrone	Used in combination with other drugs in initial therapy for acute nonlymphatic leukemia; may cause petechiae, nausea, vomiting, diarrhea, stomatitis, sepsis, fungal infections, dyspnea, fever, and alopecia. Give 12 mg/m^2 day on day 1 and day 3; follow with a course of cytosine.
plicamycin	Mithracin	Used to treat hypercalcemia and hypercalciuria associated with neoplasms and malignant testicular tumors; may produce anorexia, nausea, vomiting, diarrhea, stomatitis, hematemesis, and hemorrhaging of GI tract. Give 25-30 mcg/kg/day IV for 3-4 days.
teniposide	Vumon	Used in acute lymphoblastic leukemia. Watch to avoid extravasation during IV therapy because severe tissue necrosis may occur.
valrubicin	Valstar	Used in treating intravesical therapy of BCG-refractory carcinoma in situ of the urinary bladder in patients for whom immediate cystectomy would be associated with morbidity or mortality.
ANTIMETABOLITES		
allopurinol	Zyloprim	Used in the management of patients with leukemia, lymphoma, and solid tumor malignancies who are receiving cancer therapy that causes elevation of serum uric acid levels. May be given orally or by injection.
capecitabine	Xeloda	Prodrug of 5-fluorouracil with complex dosing schedule used in metastatic breast cancer.

Table 14-1

Antineoplastic Agents—cont'd

GENERIC NAME	TRADE NAME	COMMENTS AND DOSAGE
ANTIMETABOLITES—cont'd		
cladribine	Leustatin	Used in treating hairy cell leukemia and unlabeled uses in a wide variety of other conditions.
cytarabine	Cytosar-U	Used in acute myelocytic or lymphocytic leukemia; may cause nausea, vomiting, anorexia, diarrhea, and bone marrow depression. Give 200 mg/m^2/day IV or subcutaneously. Duration of treatment varies with patient response.
floxuridine	FUDR	Used in GI adenocarcinoma metastatic to liver; may produce anorexia, nausea, vomiting, diarrhea, alopecia, and bone marrow depression. Give 0.1-0.6 mg/kg/day IV.
fludarabine	Fludara	Used in chronic lymphocytic leukemia. Give 25 mg/m^2 IV over 30 min for 5 consecutive days every 28 days.
fluorouracil	Adrucil	Used in carcinoma of breast, stomach, colon, and pancreas; may cause anorexia, nausea, vomiting, diarrhea, alopecia, and bone marrow depression. Give 3-12 mg/kg/day IV.
gemcitabine	Gemzar	Used in adenocarcinoma of the pancreas.
mercaptopurine	Purinethol	Used in acute lymphatic leukemia and acute or chronic myelogenous leukemia; may produce hyperuricemia, hepatotoxicity, and bone marrow depression. Give 1.5-2.5 mg/kg/day PO maintenance.
methotrexate	Folex PFS	Used in breast cancer, lymphosarcoma, and severe psoriasis; may cause nausea, vomiting, headache, rash, pruritus, stomatitis, bone marrow depression, leukopenia, and renal failure. Give 10-50 mg/wk IV, IM, or PO or up to 6.5 mg/day PO standard. Dosage varies depending on specific treatment requirements.
pentostatin	Nipent	Used in hairy cell leukemia. Give 4 mg/m^2 IV every other week in well-hydrated patient.
thioguanine	Thioguanine	Used in acute nonlymphocytic leukemias and chronic myelogenous leukemia; may produce nausea, vomiting, stomatitis, hyperuricemia, hepatotoxicity, and bone marrow depression. Give 2-3 mg/kg/day PO.
HORMONES		
anastrozole	Arimidex	First-line treatment of postmenopausal women when they have either hormone receptor–positive or hormone receptor–unknown classification of locally advanced or metastatic breast cancer.
bicalutamide	Casodex	A nonsteroidal antiandrogen used in advanced prostate cancer along with LHRH. Take 50 mg PO at same time once a day.
diethylstilbestrol diphosphate	Honvol Stilphostrol	Used in inoperable prostatic carcinoma; may produce pruritus, rash, gynecomastia, thrombophlebitis, and cerebral or pulmonary emboli. Give 50-200 mg PO 3 times daily; may give IV.
estramustine	Emcyt	Used in metastatic prostatic carcinoma; may cause nausea, vomiting, diarrhea, anorexia, fluid retention, edema, leukopenia, rash, and thrombocytopenia. Give 15 mg/kg/day PO in 3 or 4 divided doses.
exemestane	Aromasin	For the treatment of advanced breast cancer in postmenopausal women whose disease has progressed after tamoxifen therapy. Also used in the prevention of prostate carcinogenesis.
flutamide	Eulexin	Used in metastatic prostatic carcinoma. Give 250 mg PO 3 times daily.
goserelin acetate	Zoladex	Used in palliative treatment of carcinoma of prostate. Give 3.6 mg subcutaneously every 28 days in upper abdominal wall.
letrozole	Femara	Used in treatment of advanced breast cancer in postmenopausal women with disease progression after antiestrogen therapy.
leuprolide	Lupron	Used in advanced prostatic carcinoma; may produce nausea, vomiting, anorexia, dizziness, headache, edema, and bone pain. Give 1 mg/day subcutaneously.

Continued

Table **14-1**

Antineoplastic Agents—cont'd

GENERIC NAME	TRADE NAME	COMMENTS AND DOSAGE
HORMONES—cont'd		
medroxyprogesterone	Depo-Provera	Used in renal or endometrial carcinoma; may cause pruritus, breast tenderness, and cerebral or pulmonary emboli. Give 400-1000 mg/wk IM.
megestrol acetate	Megace	Used in endometrial or breast carcinoma. Give 40 mg PO 4 times daily for breast carcinoma; 40-320 mg/day PO for endometrial cancer.
nilutamide	Nilandron	An antiandrogen used for metastatic prostate cancer along with surgical castration. Give 300 mg for 30 days and then 150 mg/day with or without food.
tamoxifen	Nolvadex	Used in breast cancer in postmenopausal women; may produce hypercalcemia and ophthalmic changes. Give 10-20 mg PO twice daily.
testolactone	Teslac	Used in breast cancer in postmenopausal women; may cause anorexia, nausea, vomiting, edema, paresthesia, and hypertension. Give 250 mg PO 4 times daily.
toremifene citrate	Fareston	Used in treatment of metastatic breast cancer in postmenopausal women with estrogen receptor-positive or estrogen receptor-unknown tumors.
triptorelin pamoate	Trelstar	Used in palliative treatment of advanced prostate cancer.
MITOTIC INHIBITORS		
docetaxel	Taxotere	Used in patients with advanced breast cancer.
etoposide	VePesid	Used in testicular tumors; may produce anorexia, nausea, vomiting, alopecia, and granulocytopenia. Give 50-100 mg/m^2/day IV. Duration of treatment varies with patient response.
paclitaxel	Taxol	Used in ovarian carcinoma, breast carcinoma, AIDS-related Kaposi's sarcoma.
teniposide	Vumon	Used in childhood acute lymphocytic lymphoma patients in combination with other products. Extremely corrosive to soft tissue. Give slow IV.

undergoing chemotherapy and/or radiation frequently explore herbal preparations to help control adverse effects. You should ask the patient about any of these products that he or she may be using, because many may be dangerous or toxic to an immunocompromised patient. Dehydration must be avoided, and bowel regularity must be maintained. You will need to be thorough in your evaluation of the patient's response.

You and the patient must cooperate in getting needed follow-up laboratory work and x-ray studies to determine the response to medication. Provide opportunities for patients to discuss with you their feelings and attitudes about the disease and their therapy.

Patient and Family Teaching

You should tell the patient and family the following:
1. Antineoplastic agents may be toxic and must be taken as ordered. The patient should learn the reason for their use, what they will do, and the possible adverse reactions. The patient may be required to sign a written consent form before many of these drugs can be administered.
2. The patient should learn in detail about the possible adverse effects of these drugs. Specific plans for preventing or reducing symptoms should be developed. The patient should know which symptoms to report to the nurse, physician, or other health care provider.
3. The patient's meals should be made as palatable and attractive as possible because most antineoplastic agents produce anorexia, nausea, and vomiting. The patient may be unable to eat anything at times but may find holding ice chips in the mouth to be helpful.
4. The patient should learn the signs of dehydration caused by diarrhea.

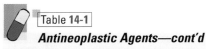

Table 14-1

Antineoplastic Agents—cont'd

GENERIC NAME	TRADE NAME	COMMENTS AND DOSAGE
MITOTIC INHIBITORS—cont'd		
vinblastine	Velban Velsar	Used in Hodgkin's disease, Kaposi's sarcoma, lymphoma, and testicular carcinoma; may cause nausea, vomiting, malaise, headache, numbness, paresthesias, weakness, depression, and leukopenia. Give 3.7 mg/m^2/wk IV as determined by WBC counts.
vincristine	Oncovin Vincasar PFS	Used in Hodgkin's disease, Wilms' tumor, acute leukemia, lymphosarcoma, neuroblastoma; may produce nausea, vomiting, diarrhea, fever, weight loss, ataxia, headache, and mouth ulcers. Give 1.4 mg/m^2/week IV.
vinorelbine tartrate	Navelbine	IV product used in non–small cell lung cancer. Unlabeled uses in breast cancer, ovarian carcinoma, and Hodgkin's disease.
MISCELLANEOUS AGENTS		
aldesleukin	Proleukin ◆	Used in metastatic renal cell carcinoma.
asparaginase	Elspar	Used with other drugs in acute lymphocytic leukemia.
hydroxyurea	Hydrea ◆	Used in melanoma and squamous cell carcinoma. Unlabeled use for sickle cell anemia, thrombocythemia, HIV, psoriasis. Dosage is calculated on actual weight.
interferon alfa-2a	Roferon-A	Used in hairy cell leukemia, AIDS-related Kaposi's sarcoma, chronic myelogenous leukemia.
interferon alfa-2b	Intron-A	Used in hairy cell leukemia, malignant melanoma, condyloma acuminatum, AIDS-related Kaposi's sarcoma, chronic hepatitis C and B.
levamisole	Ergamisol	Used as adjunct therapy in colon cancer.
mitotane	Lysodren	Used for inoperable adrenal cortical carcinoma.
pegaspargase	Oncaspar	Used in acute lymphoblastic leukemia.
porfimer	Photofrin	A photosensitizing agent used in the treatment of esophageal cancer.
procarbazine HCl	Matulane	Used with other drugs in combination to treat Hodgkin's disease. Dose is calculated on patient's actual weight.
rituximab	Rituxan	Used in treatment of Hodgkin's disease.

AIDS, Acquired immunodeficiency syndrome; *BCG,* B-cell growth; *HIV,* human immunodeficiency virus; *LHRH,* luteinizing hormone–releasing hormone; *WBC,* white blood cell.

5. Hair loss is usually of great concern to the patient. Patients should be given information on wigs and toupees that might be worn until their own hair grows back. Patients with long hair might want to save the hair and have a wig made from their own hair. There are shops that specialize in this service in many large cities.

6. Patients who have had surgery for cancer, such as mastectomy or amputation, should be provided with information about strengthening of muscles after surgery, postoperative recovery period, and prosthesis use.

7. There are many support groups available for specific types of cancer, and former patients may visit the hospital and talk to the patient about their colostomy or mastectomy. The patient can be referred to community resources for further information.

8. The patient should keep any medication that is taken home in a locked cabinet away from children or pets.

CASE STUDY

Bonnie Taylor, 48 years old, is admitted to the hospital with a diagnosis of acute lymphoblastic leukemia (ALL) and *Salmonella* sepsis. She has had four other admissions for chemotherapy and supportive care. She has lost weight and currently weighs 110 pounds. She is to receive platelets and a whole blood transfusion. The medications prescribed include:

- Acetaminophen (Tylenol) 650 mg PO q4h for fever.
- Gentamicin (Garamycin) 50 mg IV q8h.
- 6-Mercaptopurine (Purinethol) 200 mg PO daily.
- Trimethobenzamide HCl (Tigan) 200 mg suppository q6h prn.

1. The usual adult daily dose of 6-mercaptopurine is 2.5 mg/kg/day. How does this compare with what is ordered?

2. The usual adult daily dose of gentamicin is 3 mg/kg/day in three equal doses, given every 8 hours by IV. If the product comes in doses of 40 mg/mL, how much medication will be drawn up to be injected?
3. Why is gentamicin ordered?
4. Why is 6-mercaptopurine ordered?
5. Why is trimethobenzamide HCl ordered?
6. Why might this patient have an elevated temperature? What would you give her and when?
7. What other chemotherapeutic agents might be used for the treatment of leukemia?
8. Because of her condition and all of the medications she is taking, what are some of the things you would monitor?

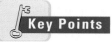

- The five types of agents commonly used to treat neoplastic disease are alkylating agents, antibiotic preparations, antimetabolites, hormones, and mitotic inhibitors.
- Because these drugs are highly toxic, it is especially important for you to monitor adverse reactions in the patient.
- Dosages must be precisely followed and care must be taken in the preparation and disposal of syringes, bottles, and needles.

Go to the free CD-ROM for an Audio Glossary, animations, video clips, and Review Questions for the NCLEX-PN® Examination.

evolve Be sure to visit the companion Evolve website at http://evolve.elsevier.com/Edmunds/LPN/ for WebLinks, a link to the top 200 drugs by prescription, and sign-up pages for newsletter drug updates.

DRUG CALCULATION REVIEW

1. The physician orders an IV solution of cisplatin (Platinol) 10 mg in 1000 mL of dextrose 5% in 0.9% saline solution (D_5NS). This solution is to infuse at a rate of 1.25 mg/hr. If the drop factor is 20 gtt = 1 mL, what is the flow rate in drops per minute?

2. Order: Bleomycin 45 units IV

   Supply: Bleomycin 15 units per vial

   Question: How many vials of bleomycin are needed for each dose?

3. Order: Cytoxan 10 mg/kg IV

   Question: How many mg of Cytoxan are needed for a person weighing 65 kg?

4. Order: Interferon alfa 3,000,000 international units (IU) subcutaneously 3 times per week

   Supply: Interferon alfa 6,000,000 IU/mL

   Question: How many milliliters of interferon alfa are needed with each dose?

CRITICAL THINKING ?

1. What common action do all antineoplastic agents share? Are they usually used alone? Why or why not? Describe how treatments (chemotherapy, radiation, or surgery) might be combined and in what order, depending on the circumstances.

2. What healthy, or normal, cells are also affected by antineoplastic agents? Describe the adverse reactions associated with these cells. Why does this occur?

3. What is the importance of baseline evaluation in determining therapeutic progress? What factors are taken into consideration? What types of evaluation might be done?

4. What exactly is the nurse's responsibility in each type of evaluation discussed in question 3?

5. Write out a teaching plan for explaining to a patient the correct administration of these powerful agents and what to reasonably expect for both therapeutic and adverse effects.

6. Ms. Reynolds is a 30-year-old postmastectomy patient who is currently undergoing chemotherapy. She tells you her 5-year-old daughter will be starting kindergarten in a few months and will need "all her shots for school soon." What points will you need to include in your patient education?

7. What would you explain to Mr. Sorrento, who asks you why, if he "has cancer, the doctor doesn't think he's ready for chemo"?

8. What laboratory results would be significant in evaluating patient response to chemotherapy? Why?

Objectives

After reading and studying this chapter, you should be able to do the following:

1. Identify the approved way to give different forms of antianginal therapy.
2. Discuss the uses and general actions of cardiac drugs used to treat dysrhythmias.
3. Describe the common treatment for various types of lipoprotein disorders.
4. Explain the actions of different categories of drugs used to treat hypertension.
5. List the general uses and actions of cardiotonic drugs.
6. Identify indications for electrolyte replacement.

Key Terms

action potential duration (p. 230)
chronic heart failure (CHF) (p. 241)
chronotropic (KRŌ-nō-TRŌP-ĭk, p. 241)
compelling indications (p. 250)
dehydration (dē-hī-DRĀ-shŭn, p. 260)
depolarization (dē-pō-lăr-ĭ-ZĀ-shŭn, p. 231)
digitalis toxicity (dĭj-ĭ-TĂL-ĭs, p. 241)
digitalizing dose (DĬJ-ĭ-tăl-īz-ĭng, p. 243)
dromotropic (DRŌM-ō-TRŌP-ĭk, p. 241)
dysrhythmia (dĭs-RĬTH-mē-ă, p. 228)
ectopic beats (ĕk-TŌP-ĭk, p. 230)
edema (ĕ-DĒ-mă, p. 241)
effective refractory period (rē-FRĂK-tŏr-ē, p. 230)
electrocardiogram (ECG) (ĕ-lĕk-trō-KĂR-dē-ō-gram, p. 229)
end-organ damage (p. 250)
fluid and electrolyte mixtures (ĕ-LĔK-trō-lĭt, p. 260)
hyperlipidemia (hī-pĕr-lĭp-ō-DĒ-mē-a, p. 236)
hyperlipoproteinemia (hī-pĕr-lĭp-ō-PRŌT-ĕ-NĒ-mē-ă, p. 235)
myocardial infarction (mī-ō-KĂR-dē-ăl ĭn-FĂRK-shŭn, p. 237)
myocardium (mī-ō-KĂR-dē-ŭm, p. 228)
normal sinus rhythm (SĪ-nŭs RĬTH-ĭm, p. 229)
pacemaker (p. 228)
positive inotropic action (ĭ-nă-TRŌP-ĭk, p. 241)
primary hypertension (hī-pĕr-TĔN-shŭn, p. 246)
secondary hypertension (p. 246)

OVERVIEW

This chapter is divided into six major sections, each with a focus on an important job of the cardiovascular or circulatory system. Some cardiovascular drugs have more than one action and are used for several reasons in the patient with cardiovascular problems. However, they are usually classed into one of the major drug categories.

Section One, Antianginals and Peripheral Vasodilators, focuses on the drugs used to treat chest pain from angina and problems with diseases causing blockage of the arteries, mostly in the legs. These drugs are widely prescribed, and you will have a major role in teaching the patient how to properly store and use them. Section Two discusses the four major classes of medications used for dysrhythmias (irregular heartbeats). The antidysrhythmics are powerful drugs, and there may be many adverse reactions from some of these medications. Section Three looks at lipids (fats) and the problem of lipoprotein abnormalities. Antihyperlipidemic agents are discussed as a part of the overall therapy for lipoprotein problems. Section Four focuses on the drugs that make the heartbeat stronger—the cardiotonics, such as digitalis and related products. These are some of the most common drugs for patients both in and out of the hospital, and you must clearly understand how the drugs work and be able to teach patients about them. Antihypertensives, diuretics, and urinary system drugs are explored in Section Five. Because hypertension (high blood pressure) is so common, you will want to understand everything about how these drugs reduce the blood pressure. The latest guidelines for antihypertensive therapy are listed, as well as common adverse reactions to these types of drugs. Although most of the drugs acting on the kidney are diuretics, other agents that affect the urinary tract are also presented here. Section Six covers fluid and electrolytes.

These sections give basic information about each drug category. If you review the anatomy and physiology of the cardiovascular and urinary systems at the same time, it will help you understand both the problems that occur in these systems and how the different drugs act to solve those problems.

CARDIOVASCULAR AND URINARY SYSTEMS

The cardiovascular system is made up of the heart, blood vessels (Figure 15-1), and blood. This system moves nutrients (substances that support life and growth), waste products, gases, and hormones through the body. It also plays a role in the immune response and changes in the body temperature.

Using special cardiac muscle and nerve systems, electrical impulses tell the heart muscle when to contract, forcing blood from the heart and through blood vessels and out through the body. Arteries move blood from

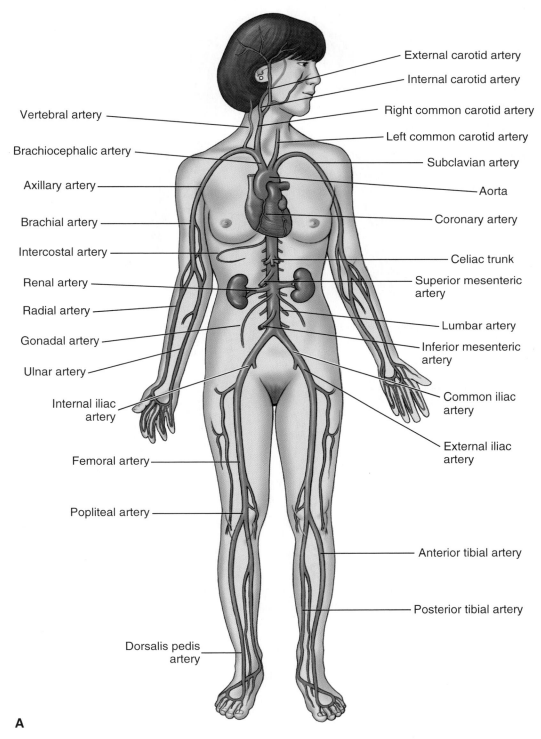

A

FIGURE **15-1** Cardiovascular system. **A,** Major arteries.   *Continued*

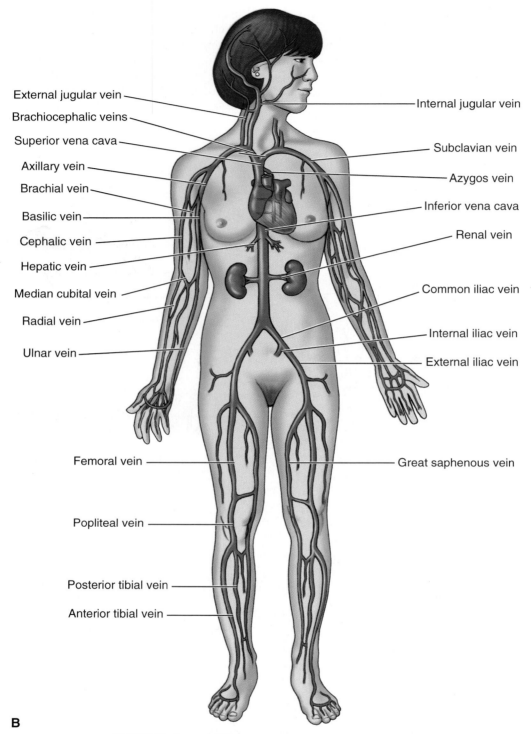

External jugular vein

Brachiocephalic veins

Superior vena cava

Axillary vein

Brachial vein

Basilic vein

Cephalic vein

Hepatic vein

Median cubital vein

Radial vein

Ulnar vein

Internal jugular vein

Subclavian vein

Azygos vein

Inferior vena cava

Renal vein

Common iliac vein

Internal iliac vein

External iliac vein

Femoral vein

Popliteal vein

Posterior tibial vein

Anterior tibial vein

Great saphenous vein

B

FIGURE 15-1—cont'd Cardiovascular system. **B,** Major veins.

the heart to tissues using smaller branches called *arterioles*. Veins move blood from tissues back toward the heart, beginning with their smaller branches called *venules*. Capillaries are very small vessels that link arterioles and venules.

The heart is the pump of the circulation. The heart itself is fed by small coronary arteries that send nutrients to it during the resting phase of the cardiac cycle. The heart may weaken with disease and age and become less efficient. In patients with hypertension, the blood vessels become less elastic and the increased pressure against which the heart has to pump causes the heart to work harder. Thus diseases or abnormal conditions of the heart, arteries, or veins produce more stress on the heart itself.

Many of the cardiovascular drugs also have either direct or indirect action on the urinary system (Figure 15-2). The kidneys, urinary bladder, and ducts that carry urine work together to remove waste products from the circulatory system, to regulate blood pH and ion levels, and to keep water balance. Strong pumping of the heart, good circulation through the vessels, and the full removal of waste products through the urinary system are all needed to keep the body's fluid and electrolyte balance.

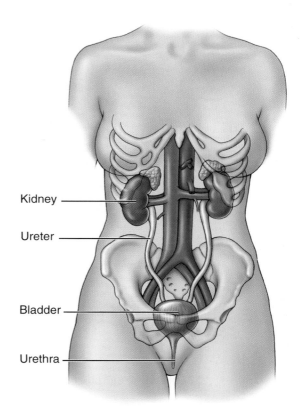

FIGURE **15-2** Urinary system.

Antianginals and Peripheral Vasodilators

ACTION

Narrowing or constriction of the smooth muscle in the coronary arteries and the peripheral vascular system (vessels in the arms and legs) reduces the amount of blood carried to the heart and the peripheral tissues (Figure 15-3). When there is a lack of blood supply to bring oxygen and nutrients to the heart or to peripheral tissues, the pain of angina or peripheral vascular disease is felt. Nitrates are the best drugs for treating coronary artery disease, whereas vasodilating agents (agents to open up the vessels) are used for peripheral vascular disease. The use of beta blockers in treating angina has also increased over the years even though there is not agreement about their effectiveness. Calcium channel blockers may also play a role in treating angina, although concern about their possible role in changes in the heart (which may lead to chronic heart failure) in patients who have had a myocardial infarction (heart attack) has limited their use. (Additional information on some of these drugs can be found in the discussion of antihypertensives and diuretics in Section Five.)

Microcirculation

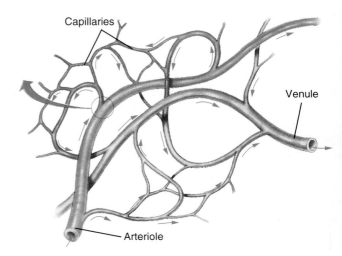

FIGURE **15-3** Main components of the microcirculation. An arteriole supplies a capillary bed, which drains into a venule.

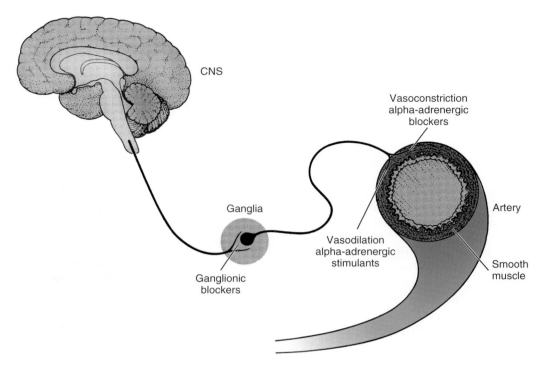

FIGURE **15-4** Site of action of peripheral vasodilators. *CNS,* central nervous system.

NITRATES

Nitrate products have a direct action on vascular smooth muscle and cause it to relax. This effect is felt in both the arterial and venous circulation. Arterial relaxation reduces the pressures the heart has to pump against, whereas venous relaxation helps in venous pooling of blood, thereby decreasing venous return to the heart. These effects work together to decrease myocardial oxygen use. In addition, nitrates increase the use of the other small blood vessels in the heart (collaterals) so that there is better oxygen supply to the inner layers of the heart muscle. Nitrates are readily absorbed under the tongue, through the skin, and orally, but products taken orally are rapidly changed in the liver to inactive products. The half-life for nitroglycerin given sublingually (under the tongue) is only 1 to 4 minutes. Newer forms of the medication can be applied directly to the skin or used as a patch and allow nitrates to pass directly into the bloodstream, thus reaching the heart before being destroyed by the liver.

CALCIUM CHANNEL BLOCKERS

Calcium is an electrolyte that helps move electrical impulses through cardiac tissue. Calcium channel blockers are drugs that help slow down the flow of calcium ions across the cell membrane, thus reducing the amount of calcium available to move electrical impulses. The drugs in this group are used for different actions. Some calcium channel blockers act directly on vascular smooth muscle to dilate (open up) coronary arteries and arterioles, which relieves anginal pain because more oxygen can go to the cardiac tissue. Other calcium channel blockers are used to reduce the response of the cardiac conduction system to electrical impulses and treat cardiac dysrhythmias. They are also used with other drugs to treat hypertension. (See the sections on antidysrhythmics and antihypertensives for additional information on calcium channel blockers.)

PERIPHERAL VASODILATORS

Patients with occlusive arterial disease (blockage of the arteries that makes them smaller) have been treated with vasodilating drugs (drugs that help expand or open up the arteries), but with only limited success. These patients often have swollen, painful feet with ulcers around the ankles. Vasodilator drugs relax the smooth muscles of peripheral arterial blood vessels, and help lead to better circulation to the arms and legs (Figure 15-4).

USES

Rapid-acting nitrates (such as amyl nitrite, sublingual nitroglycerin, and sublingual or chewable isosorbide dinitrate) are used mostly to relieve pain in acute angina. The long-acting nitrates and topical, transdermal, transmucosal, and oral sustained-release nitroglycerin products are used to prevent or treat anginal attacks when they are likely to occur (for example, with exercise) and to reduce the severity and frequency of anginal attacks. They are also used to reduce the work of the heart in cases of myocardial infarction (MI), in chronic heart failure, and for relief of gallbladder, gastrointestinal (GI), urethral, and bronchial smooth muscle pain.

It is not known if it is safe to use nitroglycerin in patients with acute MIs. When it is used in patients with recent MIs, the transdermal patch systems work the best, but patients must be closely evaluated. Intravenous (IV) nitroglycerin is used to control severe angina in an acute MI and also to control acute pain during procedures on the heart, such as cardiac catheterization. This IV nitroglycerin requires careful monitoring of the patient in a cardiac care or critical care unit.

Peripheral vasodilating agents are used to treat pain in the legs caused by problems such as intermittent claudication, arteriosclerosis obliterans, Raynaud's disease, nocturnal leg cramps, and vasospasm caused by blood clots.

ADVERSE REACTIONS

There are many common adverse reactions to nitrates, including flushing, postural hypotension (low blood pressure when a person suddenly stands up), tachycardia (rapid heartbeat), confusion, dizziness, fainting, headache, light-headedness, vertigo (feeling of dizziness or spinning), weakness, drug rash, localized pruritus (itching), skin lesions, eye and mouth edema, local burning in the mouth, nausea, and vomiting.

Some of these cardiac preparations contain tartrazine, a chemical that may cause an allergic type of reaction with symptoms similar to asthma. Patients who are allergic to aspirin have a greater chance of reacting to tartrazine.

When nitrate products are used for long periods, tolerance (increased resistance caused by repeated use) may develop and the drugs may become less helpful. High doses may cause violent headaches. All nitrates should be given with care to patients with a recent history of stroke or cerebrovascular accident (CVA), because these conditions cause widening of the cerebral arteries.

Peripheral vasodilating agents may cause dizziness, headache, weakness, tachycardia, flushing, postural hypotension, dysrhythmias, confusion, severe rash, nervousness, tingling, and sweating. Some side effects disappear within a few weeks if they are mild and if the patient can keep taking the medication.

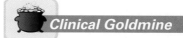

Clinical Goldmine

Tolerance to Nitrates

Tolerance to nitrates may develop over time with repeated use. If the patient develops tolerance to one nitrate, it is likely that he will develop tolerance to other nitrates (cross-tolerance). Other coronary vasodilators may have to be used.

DRUG INTERACTIONS

Nitrates increase the effects of atropine-like drugs and tricyclic antidepressants, and decrease the effects of all choline-like drugs. The action of anticholinergic drugs, especially antihistamines, may be made stronger. Nitrates should not be taken at the same time as prazosin because of the possibility of interaction. Taking alcohol, beta blockers, antihypertensives, narcotics, and vasodilators with nitrates and nitrites (especially amyl nitrite) may produce severe hypotension (low blood pressure) and cardiac collapse. Nitrates may antagonize (interfere with) the vasopressor actions of sympathomimetic drugs. A cold environment or the use of tobacco reduces the action of nitroglycerin. Nitroglycerin also increases urine vanillylmandelic acid (VMA) and catecholamine levels, and this may interfere with some laboratory tests.

The action of peripheral vasodilating agents is made stronger by antihypertensives and alcohol, leading to hypotension.

Nursing Implications and Patient Teaching

Assessment

You should learn as much as possible about the health history of the patient in order to find out if she has heart disease, other health problems, the possibility of pregnancy, or allergy, or is taking other drugs that may cause interactions. Get a full description of the angina pain so that the best drug can be prescribed.

Diagnosis

What other problems does this patient have that may interfere with treatment? Can he understand what has happened to him? Does he have any problems with his weight? What kind of diet does he eat? Is there any problem with his kidneys?

Planning

In reviewing the medicines that might be ordered, refer to the information in Table 15-1, which compares the action of various nitrate and nitrite products.

Table 15-1			
Comparison of Nitrate-Nitrite Products			
PRODUCT	**ONSET**	**DURATION**	**PREPARATION**
AGENTS FOR ACUTE ANGINA			
amyl nitrite	30 sec	3-5 min	Inhalant
isosorbide dinitrate	2-5 min	1-2 hr	Sublingual/chewable
nitroglycerin	1-3 min	3-5 min	Sublingual
	3 min	4-6 hr	Transmucosal
	Immediately	3-5 min	Intravenous
AGENTS FOR ANGINA PROPHYLAXIS			
isosorbide dinitrate	15-30 min	4-6 hr	Oral
	Slow	12 hr	Sustained release, PO
isosorbide mononitrate	30-60 min	Not determined	Oral, sustained release
nitroglycerin	Slow	8-12 hr	Sustained release, PO
	30-60 min	4-6 hr	Topical ointment
	30-60 min	24 hr	Transdermal

Implementation

Review the ways to administer different types of nitroglycerin products in Chapter 10. Overdosage may produce bad headaches; these often go away by lowering the dose and giving analgesics. As the patient continues to take the nitroglycerin product, these headaches will gradually go away.

Table 15-2 provides a list of antianginal and peripheral vasodilating medications.

Evaluation

The drug should be stopped if blurring of vision or dry mouth occurs. If the patient says that some of the sustained-release medication is being passed in the stool, it is likely that food moves through the patient's GI tract too fast to allow the drug to be absorbed. These patients should take oral or sublingual medication.

Elderly patients may have postural hypotension with these drugs and need to be watched very carefully. They may need to have someone with them when they take the medication.

The patient must learn the uses and limits of the nitrate being taken. The patient should understand the schedule of when to take the drug and be given information about when to call for help if she has chest pain that does not go away after taking the drug. There are many important things to learn about giving this medication by its various routes. Very high doses may produce severe headaches, so patients must be taught what to take and when to take it. A person who has been using a nitrate for a long time should gradually cut down the amount taken in order to avoid causing more anginal attacks, which may happen if the drug is stopped suddenly.

 Clinical Landmine

Anginal Attacks

For acute angina, the patient should put one tablet under the tongue as soon as the pain begins. The medication should not be chewed or swallowed; it should be left to dissolve under the tongue. The patient should lie down and rest. If the pain is not relieved within 3 to 5 minutes, a second pill may be taken. If the pain is not relieved within another 3 minutes, a third pill may be taken. If the pain is still not relieved, the patient must be taken to an emergency room immediately to be checked to see if he is having an acute myocardial infarction.

Patient and Family Teaching

You should tell the patient and family the following:
1. Nitroglycerin is very fragile and chemically breaks down rapidly; sunlight speeds up this process. Even under the best conditions, these drugs lose their strength 3 months after the bottle has been opened. The patient will need a new prescription every 3 months, and any old drugs should be thrown away. A burning feeling under the tongue, which is a normal finding, does not tell you if the medication is still good. However, medication that is still active will produce a throbbing headache. If the patient fails to feel the throbbing in the head, usually the medication has lost its potency (strength).
2. Common and expected side effects of nitroglycerin include flushing of the face, brief throbbing headache, increased heart rate, dizziness, and

Table 15-2
Antianginal and Peripheral Vasodilating Medications

GENERIC NAME	TRADE NAME	USES	ADVERSE REACTIONS	DOSE RANGES
ANTIANGINALS				
amyl nitrite	Amyl Nitrite	Angina pectoris	Flushing, headache, dizziness, tachycardia, weakness, vertigo	0.18-0.3 mL by inhalation
isosorbide dinitrate (PO, sublingual [SL], and chewable)	Coradur ✦ Isordil Sorbitrate	Prophylaxis of angina, acute angina	Same as above	5-30 mg PO 4 times daily; 2.5-30 mg SL; 5 mg chewable and increase as needed
isosorbide mononitrate	ISMO Imdur	Prophylaxis of angina	Same as above	20 mg PO twice daily
nitroglycerin (SL)	Nitrostat Nitro Quick	Prophylaxis, treatment, and management of angina	Same as above	1 tablet SL; repeat in 5 min 3 times, as needed
nitroglycerin (sustained release)	Nitro-Time Nitroglyn Nitrong	Prophylaxis or management of angina	Same as above	1 capsule or tablet q8-12h
nitroglycerin (topical)	Nitro-Bid Nitrol	Prevention and treatment of angina caused by CAD	Same as above	1-2 inches q4-8h (1 inch equals 15 mg nitroglycerin)
nitroglycerin (transdermal patch)	Nitrodisc Nitro-Dur Transderm-Nitro	Prevention and treatment of angina caused by CAD	Same as above	Apply pad daily; leave on for 12-14 hr; take off for 10-12 hr
nitroglycerin (translingual)	Nitrolingual	Prophylaxis and treatment of acute angina	Same as above	1 or 2 metered doses sprayed onto oral mucosa
nitroglycerin (transmucosal)	Nitrogard	Prophylaxis and treatment of angina	Same as above	Insert buccally 1 mg q3-5h during waking hours
PERIPHERAL VASODILATORS				
cyclandelate	Cyclospasmol ✦	Intermittent claudication, arteriosclerosis obliterans	Headache, flushing, GI distress, tachycardia, weakness	200-600 mg/day PO before meals and at bedtime
hydralazine	Apresoline	Essential hypertension, CHF from high afterload	Angina, tachycardia, peripheral neuritis, blood dyscrasias, constipation, paralytic ileus, nausea, vomiting, diarrhea	10 mg 4 times daily; increase to 25-50 mg 4 times daily; 300 mg/day maximum
isoxsuprine	Vasodilan Voxsuprine	Peripheral vascular disease, cerebral vascular insufficiency	Dizziness, hypotension, rash, tachycardia, nausea, vomiting, GI distress, nervousness, weakness, sweating	10-20 mg PO 3-4 times daily; 5-10 mg IM 2-3 times daily
papaverine	Papaverine Pavabid Pavagen	Peripheral vascular disease, cerebral ischemia	GI distress, nausea, flushing, vertigo, rash, drowsiness, headache, sedation, sweating	100-300 mg PO, IM, IV 1-5 times daily; 3-12 mg IM or IV slowly q3h prn

CAD, Coronary artery disease.

light-headedness when sitting up rapidly. The headache usually lasts no longer than 20 minutes and may be relieved with analgesics. The patient should rest for 10 to 15 minutes after the pain is relieved. The doctor should be notified if blurring of vision, persistent headache, or dry mouth occurs.

3. The medication should be taken on an empty stomach when possible.

4. The patient must not drink alcoholic beverages while taking nitrate products.

5. The active ingredient in nitroglycerin is very easily destroyed. Storage in plastic or in a cardboard box allows the nitrate to escape. Placing cotton in the top of the container or storing other drugs with nitroglycerin (such as in a pillbox) will absorb the nitrate. The medication should be stored in the original dark glass container. All cotton should be removed, and the container should be kept tightly capped and out of sunlight; for topical ointment, the tube should be kept tightly closed. Store nitroglycerin in the refrigerator.

6. Patients using inhalant medication should take it only when lying or sitting down. Because this is a product that will catch fire easily, the patient must not smoke and should avoid using the drug around fire or sparks.

7. Transmucosal nitroglycerin tablets should not be chewed or swallowed. The patient should put the tablet inside the cheek or under the lip and let it slowly dissolve.

8. The topical ointment should be spread in a thin layer on the skin, using an applicator and a ruler. The ointment should not be rubbed or massaged into the skin. The patient should wash off any medication that might have gotten on the hands.

9. For transdermal application, the patient should select a hairless spot (or clip hair) and apply the adhesive pad to the skin. Washing, bathing, or swimming does not affect this system. If the pad does come off, it should be discarded and a new one should be placed on a different site.

10. If the medication does not seem to be as effective after the patient has taken it for a while (requiring the patient to take several pills before getting relief), the patient may be developing a tolerance to the drug or the product may have lost its potency. Stopping the drug for several days may be long enough to make the body sensitive to it again. The smallest possible dose should be taken to reduce the risk of tolerance.

11. In the hospital, the patient's blood pressure should be taken before giving sublingual nitroglycerin and also between doses. Nitroglycerin may cause hypotension. Because the coronary arteries receive their blood supply during diastole, hypotension also decreases the blood flow to the coronary arteries, thus making the blood pressure even lower if the patient is having an MI.

12. The patient should keep a record of every anginal attack, the number of pills taken, and any side effects. The patient should bring this record each time he goes to see his health care provider.

13. The patient should use nitroglycerin when anginal attacks are likely; taking the medication before the activity may prevent or reduce the degree of pain.

14. This medication is only part of the therapy for angina. The patient should try to avoid things that cause pain (stress, heavy exercise, overeating, and smoking), reduce calorie intake if weight loss is desirable, and develop a program of regular and sensible exercise.

15. The patient should not eat large amounts of foods that stimulate the heart (coffee, tea, caffeinated soft drinks, and chocolate).

16. This medication must be kept out of the reach of children and others for whom it is not prescribed.

SECTION TWO

Antidysrhythmics

ACTION

A person with heart disease or another problem that has an affect on the heart muscle is at risk of developing irregular beating of the heart, or cardiac **dysrhythmia.** Because the term *dysrhythmia* (irregular rhythm) explains what happens to the patient better than the older term *arrhythmia* (without rhythm), it is now commonly used. Dysrhythmias may be fast or slow, with an irregular or regular pattern. The most common causes of dysrhythmias are irritation to the heart tissue after the patient has suffered an MI, fluid and electrolyte imbalances, diet, hypoxia (reduced blood oxygen), and reactions from drugs.

The middle layer of the heart wall, or **myocardium,** is made up of special muscle cells. These muscle cells work together under the direction of a special group of nerve fibers called the **pacemaker** that is located in the sinoatrial (SA) node. The pacemaker cells direct the rest of the cardiac cells by sending electrical impulses through a special nerve system known as the cardiac conduction system. These impulses cause atrial and ventricular contraction (pumping). A person's heart rate is based on how fast the pacemaker cells direct the heart to pump, and by how fast this information is spread through the heart. The usual path of this information flow begins in the SA node, passes through the atrium to the atrioventricular (AV) node, through the bundle of His, through the right and left bundle branches, and out through the Purkinje fibers of the myocardium. When the electrical impulse has spread along this pathway, the heart will contract, forcing blood out into the arteries. After a brief rest, the cycle will begin again. This is called **normal sinus rhythm.**

The electrical message directing the heart to contract depends on a special balance of electrolytes (such as calcium and sodium) in the cardiac tissues and on good function of the cardiac conduction system. This electrical message is what is recorded on the **electrocardiogram (ECG).** Figure 15-5 illustrates the conduction system of the heart and the ECG pattern that it makes.

When the cells in the conduction system do not have enough oxygen or are destroyed or damaged through disease, or when the electrolytes are not present in the right balance, irregular heart action is found. Some patients may describe very slow, regular or irregular heartbeats; some patients may have fast, irregular heartbeats. Some individuals may only feel a little dizzy or report that their heart has "skipped a beat." You may feel an irregular pulse or hear the irregularity with the stethoscope. The exact type of irregular rhythm can only be determined by taking an ECG. Some patients may wear a heart monitor strapped to their chest, or they may be placed in a coronary care unit so they may be closely watched. The goal of any treatment plan or therapeutic regimen is for the patient's heart to regain a normal rate and rhythm.

Medications that act to make the heart rhythm normal are called antidysrhythmic medications. They act on the individual cells of the heart. Each individual heart cell might be thought of as a gun. With each heartbeat, the cell (gun) has to get ready to shoot (fire), fire,

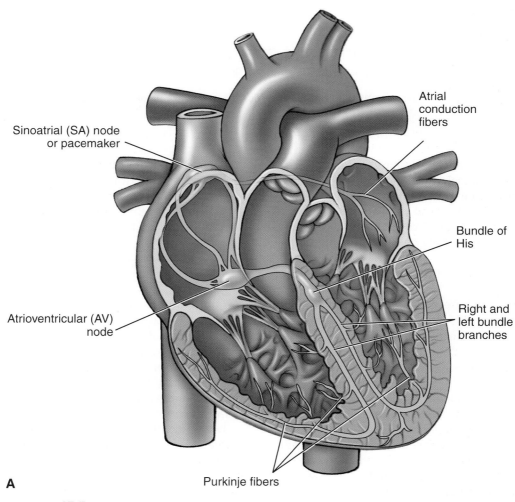

A

FIGURE **15-5 A,** Conduction system of the heart.

Continued

Labels on figure: Sinoatrial (SA) node or pacemaker; Atrial conduction fibers; Bundle of His; Right and left bundle branches; Atrioventricular (AV) node; Purkinje fibers

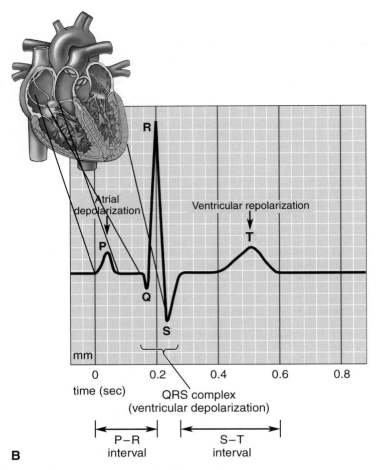

B

FIGURE **15-5—cont'd B,** Normal electrocardiogram showing one cardiac cycle.

and then reload. As one cell discharges (fires), it triggers the next cell to discharge. After passing the electrical message to the next cell, and each conduction cell must rest (reload) before it can pass another electrical signal. The antidysrhythmic drugs affect the cells that are beating (firing) irregularly by action during each of those phases of cell activity.

1. Class I drugs (quinidine, procainamide, disopyramide):
   a. Lengthen the **effective refractory period** (the time period during which the cells cannot discharge their electrical activity [slow the reloading of the cell]) of atrial and ventricular myocardium by slowing the fast inward current caused by the sodium electrolyte.
   b. Make the heart less excitable.
2. Class II drugs (beta blockers such as propranolol, esmolol, and acebutolol) reduce sympathetic excitation to the heart (affect the loading of the cell).
3. Class III drugs (amiodarone) lengthen the **action potential duration,** or the length of time it takes for one cell to fire and recover (slow the firing); class III drugs are currently investigational.

4. Class IV drugs (including calcium channel blockers such as verapamil) selectively block the ability of calcium to enter the myocardium and prolong the effective refractory period (or resting period) in the AV node (affect the reloading of the cell).

USES

It is important to find the cause of the dysrhythmia in order to decide which drug will be most helpful. The two basic actions within the heart that cause dysrhythmias are (1) increased sensitivity of electrical cells in the heart, resulting in irregular or early **ectopic beats** (the cell fires before it should); and (2) electrical activity moving through abnormal conduction pathways (the trigger that causes the cell to fire does not always work properly).

Two drugs that are often used to treat rapid and irregular dysrhythmias are quinidine and procainamide. These drugs are chemically different, but both act to quiet the myocardial cells and make them less excitable and less likely to fire. This not only decreases the heart rate, but also stops some of the extra or irregular beats.

Table 15-3

Acute Treatment and Chronic Prophylaxis of Dysrhythmias

| | TYPE OF TREATMENT INDICATED* | |
DYSRHYTHMIA	ACUTE	CHRONIC PROPHYLAXIS
Sinus tachycardia (rarely treated)	Propranolol	Propranolol
Premature atrial contractions (usually in patients with history of atrial fibrillation)	Digoxin	Digoxin, quinidine, disopyramide, procainamide, propranolol
Premature ventricular contractions (multifocal, on vulnerable part of T wave, or in symptomatic patient)	Lidocaine Procainamide	Quinidine, disopyramide, procainamide, digoxin, propranolol
Atrial flutter/atrial fibrillation	Cardioversion Digoxin	Digoxin, propranolol quinidine, disopyramide, procainamide, verapamil
Paroxysmal supraventricular tachycardia	Carotid massage Cardioversion Propranolol Digoxin Verapamil Adenosine	Propranolol, digoxin, quinidine, disopyramide, procainamide, verapamil

*Listed in order of suggested use.

Bretylium is a drug used to slow the conduction rate of the electrical impulse in the ventricular muscle. This drug also acts to slow the release of norepinephrine, a powerful chemical in the cardiac cells, so the heart muscle beats more slowly.

Disopyramide slows the depolarization of the cardiac cells. **Depolarization** is the movement of electrolytes into and out of the cell as it gets ready to send another electrical message. The heart rate is slowed because each cell is slower in recovering from sending the message to the next cell (the reloading time takes longer).

A widely used IV medication is lidocaine. The electrical impulse sent to the cardiac muscles must be of certain strength or it cannot pass along the conducting nerve fibers. Lidocaine increases the strength of the impulse. A diseased heart may have many electrical impulses trying to move at the same time, but some impulses are very weak. By increasing the strength that the impulse must reach before it may be conducted, many weak impulses will be screened out, and the overall heart rate will be slower.

Adenosine is a powerful drug that may cause the heart to stop beating for several seconds when a very rapid heartbeat is changed to normal (normal sinus rhythm). This is very upsetting for patients, who often refuse to take it more than once.

Other drugs that affect heart activity are the beta-adrenergic blockers, of which propranolol is the most well known. Drugs in this category act very much like quinidine, but they also decrease the response of the heart muscle to epinephrine and norepinephrine (other chemical neurotransmitters) by blocking the stimulation

of the heart's beta receptors. (Again, the reloading of the cell is affected).

You can see that many of the antidysrhythmic drugs are so powerful that they should only be used in critical care units where the patient may be closely monitored. Some of these drugs are often given as an IV injection followed by an IV solution filled with the medication. As the patient's condition becomes more stable, she may be changed to other antidysrhythmic drugs that are better for long-term therapy.

There are many different antidysrhythmic medications. Table 15-3 lists drugs that may commonly be used in the treatment of acute and chronic dysrhythmias.

ADVERSE REACTIONS

Most drugs given to control dysrhythmias may also cause other dysrhythmias. All patients receiving these drugs should have their heart carefully monitored by ECG for any change.

Specific symptoms to watch for with each medication include the following:

- Bretylium may cause hypotension (especially postural hypotension), vertigo, light-headedness, nausea, and vomiting.
- Disopyramide may cause dry mouth, constipation, urinary hesitancy, urinary retention, urinary frequency, blurred vision, dryness of mucous membranes, dizziness, headache, hypokalemia (decreased potassium in the blood), and fatigue.
- Lidocaine may cause drowsiness, dizziness, fear, euphoria (excessive happiness), tinnitus (ringing

in the ears), blurred or double vision, hypotension, cardiac collapse, respiratory depression or arrest (slow or stopped breathing), bradycardia (slow heartbeat), convulsions, and hallucinations.

- Procainamide may cause anorexia (lack of appetite), rash, pruritus, nausea, severe hypotension, and ventricular dysrhythmias.
- Propranolol may produce bradycardia, dizziness, vertigo, rash, bronchospasm, hyperglycemia or hypoglycemia (high or low blood sugar level), hypotension, agranulocytosis (very low number of white blood cells), visual disturbances, fatigue, chest pain, arthralgia (joint pain), and pruritus.
- Quinidine may cause cardiac dysrhythmias, hypotension, diarrhea, tinnitus, headache, vertigo, confusion, delirium, disturbances in vision, and abdominal pain. Toxic effects are called *cinchonism,* and the patient will complain of tinnitus, light-headedness, headache, fever, vertigo, nausea, vomiting, and dizziness. The first time the patient takes the medicine, a test dose should be given to check for quinidine syncope—a condition in which the body reacts to quinidine by reducing blood flow to the brain, producing syncope (light-headedness and fainting), loss of consciousness, and sometimes death.
- Verapamil forms a cloudy mixture that cannot be injected if it is mixed in the same syringe or bottle with sodium bicarbonate or nafcillin.

Clinical Landmine

Patient History of Chronic Heart Failure

The antidysrhythmic drugs often cause or worsen chronic heart failure or urinary retention. Patients with a past history of heart failure should be watched carefully.

DRUG INTERACTIONS

Quinidine's effect is increased by potassium and is reduced by hypokalemia. Verapamil actions are stronger when used at the same time as digitalis and beta blockers. Beta blockers have many interactions with other drugs, and you must read about every drug the patient is taking when he is to receive a beta blocker.

Nursing Implications and Patient Teaching

Assessment

You should learn everything you can about the patient's health history, including any drug allergies, other drugs being taken that may cause drug interactions, and other medical problems, including factors such as hypoxia (reduced blood oxygen), acid-base imbalance, increased or decreased potassium, or drug toxicity.

Diagnosis

Does the patient have other health problems that will affect therapy? Does the patient drink lots of caffeine? Smoke? Exercise? Is the patient overweight?

Planning

An ECG should be obtained before medications are started. This will determine the status of the heart before treatment so that changes can be seen.

Implementation

Vital signs must be taken before giving any antidysrhythmic medication. Hospitalized patients often continue their antidysrhythmia medications when they go home. You should take every chance you have to teach the patient about the medications she is taking.

Table 15-4 presents information about the antidysrhythmics.

Evaluation

If the patient's heart is not being watched with a cardiac monitor, the results from ECGs must be closely watched for changes. Electrolyte levels and other laboratory data should also be obtained.

Patient and Family Teaching

You should tell the patient and family the following:
1. The patient must take this medication exactly as ordered and not skip doses or double the doses.
2. Some people have side effects from these drugs. The patient should report any new or distressing symptoms to the nurse, physician, or other health care provider, especially any sudden weight gain, trouble breathing, or increased coughing.
3. The patient must return regularly for visits to the nurse, physician, or other health care provider for checkups to see how the medicine is affecting his heart.
4. The drug may cause dizziness or blurred vision, so the patient should be careful if driving or doing tasks for which she needs to be alert. The patient should avoid drinking alcohol because this makes her even less alert and increases adverse symptoms.
5. The patient must not take any other drugs without telling the nurse, physician, or other health care provider to make sure that the combination is safe. This would include aspirin, laxatives, cold and sinus products, or other over-the-counter (OTC) drugs.

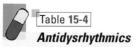

Table 15-4

Antidysrhythmics

GENERIC NAME	TRADE NAME	USES	ADVERSE REACTIONS	DOSE RANGES
CLASS I DRUGS				
A				
disopyramide	Norpace	Treat ectopic ventricular dysrhythmias	Constipation, urinary hesitancy, headache, dry mouth, blurred vision, nausea	100-200 mg 4 times daily
procainamide	Procan SR Pronestyl	PVCs, ventricular tachycardias, atrial fibrillation, PAT	Ventricular dysrhythmias, anorexia, urticaria (hives), chills, hypotension	Give IV bolus and then 1-4 mg/min IV drip or 500-1000 mg q4-6h; or 50 mg/kg/day PO
quinidine (gluconate, sulfate, or poly-galacturonate)	Cardioquin Quinalan Quinate 🍁 Quinora	PACs, PVCs, PAT, atrial flutter, atrial fibrillation	Tinnitus, disturbed vision, headache, nausea, dizziness	0.2-0.6 mg PO or 330 or 600 mg IM, depending on product; reserve for hospitalized patient
B				
lidocaine (without preservatives)	Xylocaine	Life-threatening ventricular dysrhythmias	Bradycardia, drowsiness, hypotension, light-headedness, convulsions	50-100 mg IV push, 1-4 mg/min IV drip
mexiletine	Mexitil	Symptomatic ventricular dysrhythmias	GI distress, tremor, light-headedness, incoordination, hepatic and hematologic effects	600-1200 mg/day
tocainide	Tonocard	Symptomatic ventricular dysrhythmias	Light-headedness, dizziness, nausea, vomiting, paresthesia (numbness and tingling), tremor, blood dyscrasias	200-400 mg q8h
C				
encainide	Enkaid	Life-threatening ventricular dysrhythmias	Anorexia (lack of appetite), dizziness, nervousness	75-200 mg PO daily
flecainide acetate	Tambocor	Life-threatening ventricular dysrhythmias	Anorexia, dizziness, nervousness, blurred vision, chest pain	100 mg PO q12h
ibutilide fumarate	Corvert	For rapid conversion of atrial fibrillation of recent onset.	May provoke other life-threatening arrhythmias and so requires patient to be hospitalized and carefully monitored.	Give 1 vial (1 mg) infusion over 10 min. If arrhythmia does not terminate within 10 min, a second 1-min infusion of equal strength may be administered 10 minutes after completion of the first infusion.

Continued

Table 15-4

Antidysrhythmics—cont'd

GENERIC NAME	TRADE NAME	USES	ADVERSE REACTIONS	DOSE RANGES
CLASS I DRUGS—cont'd				
C—cont'd				
propafenone	Rythmol	Life-threatening ventricular dysrhythmias	Dizziness, unusual taste, AV block, nausea, vomiting	150 mg q8h
D				
moricizine (does not belong to A, B, or C category but shares some characteristics of each)	Ethmozine	Severe ventricular dysrhythmias	May provoke other dysrhythmias	600-900 mg/day in 3 divided doses
CLASS II DRUGS: BETA BLOCKERS (See section on antihypertensives)				
acebutolol	Sectral	Ventricular tachycardia	Bradycardia, dizziness	200 mg twice daily
esmolol	Brevibloc	Supraventricular tachycardia	Bradycardia, dizziness	50-200 mcg/kg/min
propranolol	Inderal	Cardiac dysrhythmias, migraine, angina, MI, pheochromocytoma	Bradycardia, dizziness, vertigo, rash, bronchospasm, hyperglycemia, hypertension, agranulocytosis	10-30 mg PO 3 times daily
CLASS III DRUGS				
amiodarone	Cordarone Pacerone	Life-threatening ventricular dysrhythmias	GI distress, CNS symptoms, photosensitivity (abnormal response to exposure to sunlight)	800-1000 mg/day PO
bretylium	Bretylate	Prophylaxis and treatment of ventricular fibrillation	Hypotension, postural hypotension, nausea, vomiting, lightheadedness, vertigo	5-10 mg/kg IV over 10-30 min as bolus and then 1-4 mg/min IV drip
dofetilide	Tikosyn	Used to convert atrial fibrillation/atrial flutter and maintain normal sinus rhythm	May precipitate other fatal dysrhythmias	Give 500 mcg twice daily. Monitor carefully and have resuscitation equipment available for 3 days after starting medication.
sotalol	Betapace	Life-threatening ventricular tachycardia	Life-threatening ventricular tachycardia	80 mg twice daily, up to 240 mg/day
CLASS IV DRUGS				
adenosine	Adenocard	Supraventricular tachycardia	Facial flushing, shortness of breath	6 mg rapid IV bolus
Calcium Channel Blockers				
verapamil	Calan Isoptin	Supraventricular tachydysrhythmias	Cardiac dysrhythmias, CHF, hypotension	80-120 mg PO q6-8h; may be given IV push for acute SVT

PAC, Premature atrial contraction; *PAT,* paroxysmal atrial tachycardia; *PVC,* premature ventricular contraction; *SVT,* supraventricular tachycardia.

SECTION THREE

Antihyperlipidemics

OVERVIEW

Cholesterol and other fatty acids are called *lipids*. The body needs a certain amount of cholesterol and triglycerides, which are both normal and vital parts of blood plasma. Like other lipids, they are not soluble in liquid and so they are carried in the plasma by linking to lipoproteins (albumin and globulins). Lipoproteins are described by how thick or dense they are (high-density lipids and low-density lipids). The four major types of lipoproteins are as follows:

1. *Chylomicrons.* These are the largest and lightest of the lipoproteins. They are formed from the absorption of dietary fat in the intestine and are mostly triglycerides. Chylomicrons are normally present in plasma for only 1 to 8 hours after the last meal, and they make the plasma look cloudy. If a tube of blood from a fasting patient shows a thick layer of fat or cloudy plasma after several hours, the patient may have an inability to handle dietary fat.

2. *Very low-density lipoproteins (VLDLs).* These are made up of large amounts of triglycerides that were made in the liver and are called pre-beta lipoproteins. The pre-beta form is a carrier state for moving triglycerides that have been produced in the liver into the plasma. Nearly all the triglycerides in plasma that are not in chylomicrons are considered to be VLDLs.

3. *Low-density lipoproteins (LDLs).* When VLDLs break down and link with cholesterol and protein, very little triglyceride is left. What remains is then called beta lipoprotein. About 75% of the cholesterol in plasma is moved in this form. High serum levels of LDLs indicate cholesterol levels that are higher than the body needs. Patients with high LDL levels are at high risk for developing atherosclerosis.

4. *High-density lipoproteins (HDLs).* These small, dense lipoproteins are called alpha lipoproteins and contain very small parts of triglycerides. They are mostly made up of protein and cholesterol. They serve as the vacuum cleaners of the tissues, clearing out excess cholesterol. They may prevent atherosclerotic activity by blocking uptake of LDL cholesterol by vascular smooth muscle cells.

Chylomicrons and VLDLs are seen as triglyceride-rich lipoproteins, whereas LDLs and HDLs are viewed as cholesterol-rich lipoproteins. These two lipoproteins differ in several respects, including their cholesterol transporting activities. Simply stated, LDLs move cholesterol from the liver to peripheral tissues and HDLs remove cholesterol from the periphery and transport it to the liver. Figure 15-6 shows the normal physiology of lipoprotein transport. Chylomicrons are the largest and least dense of the lipoproteins; as size decreases and density increases, the next type is the VLDLs (pre-beta lipoproteins), then the intermediate-density lipoproteins (IDLs, or broad beta lipoproteins), then the LDLs (beta lipoproteins), and finally the HDLs (alpha lipoproteins, the smallest and most dense).

Patients with defects in lipid transport or metabolism have one of several types of **hyperlipoproteinemia.** These patients can be classed on the basis of the types of lipoproteins that are elevated in the plasma. The type of hyperlipoproteinemia refers to the abnormal

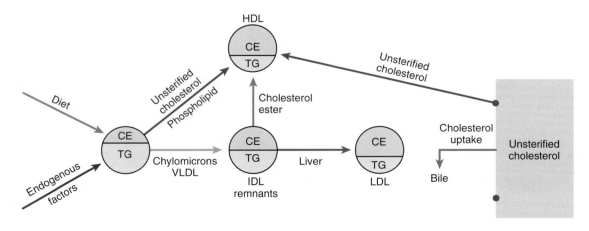

FIGURE **15-6** Normal pathway of lipid metabolism. *CE,* Cholesterol esters; *HDL,* high-density lipoproteins; *IDL,* intermediate-density lipoproteins or remnants; *LDL,* low-density lipoproteins; *TG,* triglycerides; *VLDL,* very-low-density lipoproteins.

lipoprotein pattern but does not indicate the specific disease. Accurate diagnosis and treatment plans may be made if these classes are used. Types of hyperlipoproteinemia are as follows:

Type I: Loss of an enzyme in one step of the removal of chylomicrons. This relatively rare disorder is seen in infancy and is marked by abdominal pain. It results in high levels of both cholesterol and triglycerides but does not lead to atherosclerosis. It has also been called fat-induced or exogenous (produced by outside causes) hyperlipoproteinemia.

Type II: Increased production or inadequate clearance of LDLs. In this inherited disorder, yellowish lipid deposits called xanthomas may be found on knees, feet, elbows, and ears. Patients in subgroup A have high levels of LDLs, with normal VLDL levels and a slight increase in triglycerides. Type IIA is fairly common and carries with it an increased risk for having atherosclerosis. It is also known as familial hypercholesterolemia. Patients in subgroup B have high levels of LDLs and VLDLs, hypercholesterolemia, and hypertriglyceridemia.

Type III: Block in metabolism of VLDL to LDL, causing an abnormal "intermediate" form of lipoprotein to circulate in the plasma. Elevated LDL, VLDL, cholesterol, and triglyceride levels are found. This is a recessively inherited disorder and is not as common as some other types. It is also marked by xanthomas and does carry a risk of producing atherosclerosis. It is also known as broad beta disease.

Type IV: Increased production or inadequate clearance of VLDLs. Triglycerides are increased, but LDLs and cholesterol are normal or slightly increased. This is also called carbohydrate-induced or endogenous (produced by inside causes) hyperlipoproteinemia, and it is the most common form. A definite risk for atherosclerosis exists with this type.

Type V: VLDL excess combined with poor chylomicron removal. High levels of VLDLs, triglycerides, and chylomicrons are found. It is not linked with a risk of atherosclerosis, and it is a relatively uncommon type. It has also been called mixed hyperlipoproteinemia.

Hyperlipidemia is the term used to describe an increase in levels of lipoproteins in the blood. This may mean high amounts of triglycerides, high amounts of cholesterol, or both. Hyperlipidemia leads to atherosclerosis, a process that begins slowly and without symptoms. Patients with damage to the lining of their vascular walls (which occurs in most people in the process of aging and may be made more rapid by other factors) have a gradual buildup of fatty deposits within the lining of the vessel walls of the arterial system. This process leads to narrowing of the blood vessel lumen so that blood flow is slowed (Figure 15-7). The clinical results of these lipid deposits include the onset of angina that results from ischemic heart disease (lack of oxygen in the cells of the myocardium), cerebrovascular disease (including stroke), peripheral ischemia (lack of oxygenated blood in the legs caused by problems in the circulation of the legs), and renovascular hypertension.

Atherosclerosis in the coronary arteries causes coronary heart disease (CHD). The coronary arteries that feed and nourish the heart become smaller because the inner wall of the arteries are narrowed as they fill with plaques, or patches of atherosclerotic tissue. Although the narrowing of the coronary artery may decrease the blood supply to the heart, it is only when a plaque is broken or torn and platelets cling to the torn area and produce a blockage that the blood supply is decreased

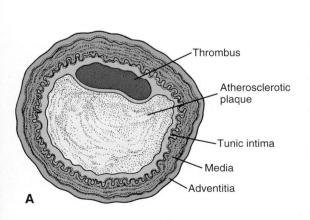

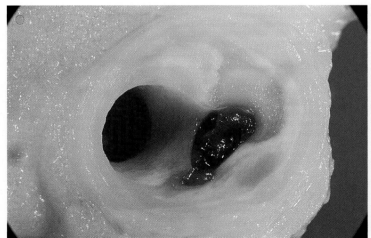

FIGURE **15-7** **A,** Occlusion of an atherosclerotic coronary artery by a thrombus. **B,** Plaque disruption. The cap of the lipid-rich plaque has become torn and a thrombus has formed, mostly inside the plaque.

Table 15-5
Diet and Drug Therapy for the Hyperlipidemias

TYPE	DIET	DRUGS
I	Low fat; no other restrictions	None is effective
IIa	Low cholesterol, low in saturated fats; increased intake of polyunsaturated fats	HMG-CoA reductase inhibitors, bile acid sequestrants, nicotinic acid
IIb	Same as above	HMG-CoA reductase inhibitors, bile acid sequestrants, gemfibrozil, nicotinic acid, clofibrate, fenofibrate
III	Low cholesterol, low calorie, low in saturated fats; high protein	Nicotinic acid, gemfibrozil, clofibrate, fenofibrate
IV	Low carbohydrate, low alcohol, low cholesterol, low calorie; maintain protein intake	Gemfibrozil, nicotinic acid, clofibrate, fenofibrate
V	Low fat, low carbohydrate, low alcohol; high protein	Gemfibrozil, nicotinic acid, clofibrate, fenofibrate

enough to cause a heart attack. When the heart does not get enough blood to its muscle cells, those cells die. This is called **myocardial infarction.**

Research suggests that high blood LDL cholesterol levels lead to CHD. There is an opposite link between HDLs and CHD risk—that is, high levels of HDL cholesterol are viewed as protecting the patient against CHD. This is why LDLs are sometimes called "bad cholesterol" and HDLs are called "good cholesterol." Evaluation of LDL and HDL levels is of primary importance because research has now shown that lowering serum lipids or cholesterol can help reduce the risk of atherosclerotic disease. Although the average cholesterol level for people in the United States has dropped, there are still many people with levels that place them at risk for CHD.

Guidelines for the diagnosis and treatment of hyperlipidemia have been issued by the National Cholesterol Education Program. These guidelines emphasize the following:

1. *Establish therapy based on risk of CHD.* Those who have CHD, men over 45 years old, and women over 55 years old are now considered high-risk patients who would benefit from cholesterol-lowering drug therapy. Young adult men (under 35 years old) and premenopausal women with elevated total and LDL cholesterol levels are at risk, regardless of their overall health, but should try diet and exercise before resorting to drug therapy.
2. *Take a closer look at HDL levels.* HDL levels should be recorded at the first cholesterol test and should be noted when choosing a cholesterol-lowering therapy. Higher HDL levels (>60 mg/dL) may in fact be a negative CHD risk factor; that is, patients with higher HDL levels are at lower risk for CHD.
3. *View physical activity and diet (reducing intake of saturated fat) as important parts of any cholesterol-lowering therapy.* In young patients this may be the only therapy necessary.

As you can see, both diet therapy and drug therapy are important. In patients anxious to reduce elevated levels of lipids, behavior changes to reduce other risk factors and diet should always be a part of the treatment plan. Four classes of drugs are used to treat hyperlipidemia: hydroxymethylglutaryl coenzyme A (HMG-CoA) reductase inhibitors, the fibric acid derivatives, bile acid sequestrants, and niacin. A list of the usual diet and drug therapy regimens in the various types of hyperlipidemias is provided in Table 15-5.

ACTION

HMG-COA REDUCTASE INHIBITORS

Several HMG-CoA reductase inhibitors are used to treat hyperlipidemia. They are the most costly drugs for treating hyperlipidemia, but patients also tolerate them best and they are highly effective at lowering LDL levels. The ability of the six drugs in this class to lower LDL levels can be roughly ranked in the following order, with the most powerful drug first: atorvastatin > simvastatin > pravastatin = lovastatin > cerivastatin = fluvastatin. Adverse effects are similar for all six of these agents. A switch from one drug to another may be needed if adverse reactions occur. Liver function tests (LFTs) should be monitored in patients taking these products.

FIBRIC ACID DERIVATIVES

Gemfibrozil and fenofibrate are the preferred drugs of this class because they are more effective and have fewer adverse effects compared with clofibrate. Both are highly effective at lowering triglycerides and increasing HDL levels, but are less effective than the HMG-CoA reductase inhibitors at lowering LDL levels. Gemfibrozil and fenofibrate are well tolerated but can cause liver toxicity and cholelithiasis (gallstones).

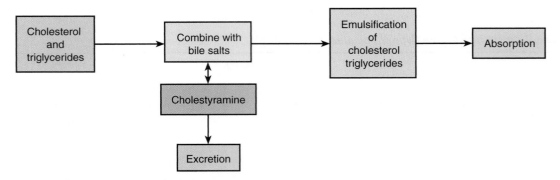

FIGURE **15-8** Mechanism of action of bile acid sequestrants.

BILE ACID SEQUESTRANTS

Cholestyramine and colestipol work to reduce serum cholesterol levels by forming an insoluble compound with bile salts and thus increasing bile loss through the feces (stool). This loss of bile, which would normally be recycled through the liver and bowel, causes increased oxidation of cholesterol to form bile. This results in a decrease in LDL plasma levels and a decrease in serum cholesterol levels (Figure 15-8). These drugs are usually used to treat type II hyperlipoproteinemia and are mostly used for lowering LDL levels. They are the only antihyperlipidemics that increase triglyceride levels. Patients may not be willing to use these drugs because of adverse GI effects such as constipation, bloating, and nausea. Both of these resin agent drugs are equally effective. Because they remain in the bowel and are not absorbed, there is no need to do tests to watch for adverse effects.

NIACIN

Niacin is one of the most effective antihyperlipidemics at lowering triglyceride levels and increasing HDL levels, and is similar to the bile acid sequestrants in its ability to lower LDL levels. The main limit to the use of niacin is its adverse effect of flushing (red color in the face and neck), although patients generally develop an ability to tolerate this problem with continued use. Flushing occurs shortly after the drug is taken and can be reduced by taking aspirin (30 minutes before) and increasing the niacin dosage very slowly over 3 to 4 weeks from 500 to 1000 mg three times daily. Niacin reduces glucose tolerance and may cause hyperuricemia (high uric acid levels), so it should be used with caution in patients with diabetes or gout. It remains the cheapest antihyperlipidemic and is probably underused in practice.

ADVERSE REACTIONS

All these medications may affect liver function, and LFTs should be ordered regularly. You should also be aware of the following:

- Cholestyramine and colestipol hydrochloride may cause constipation.
- Clofibrate may cause GI upset.
- Lovastatin (Mevacor) should not be given to pregnant women.

DRUG INTERACTIONS

Because these drugs act by binding, giving the drug with other medications may cause those drugs to be bound to the product. Cholestyramine, colestipol, and gemfibrozil may make warfarin anticoagulants more effective. Clofibrate interacts with probenecid, warfarin, and sulfonylureas.

Normal absorption of fat-soluble vitamins may be reduced with bile acid sequestrants, and the patient may show symptoms of vitamin deficiency if the dosage is at a high level or the drugs are taken for a long time. You should watch for bleeding problems that may result from hypoprothrombinemia caused by vitamin K deficiency. Normal fat digestion may be disturbed. Some patients, especially very young or small patients, are more likely to develop hyperchloremic acidosis because of the chloride anion exchange.

These drugs will delay the absorption of cephalexin, clindamycin, chlorothiazide, digitalis preparations, folic acid, iron, penicillin G, phenylbutazone, phenobarbital, thyroid and thyroxine preparations, and trimethoprim. If the patient has been placed on a regular dose of any of these drugs and then bile acid sequestrant therapy is discontinued, toxic levels of the other drugs may develop once the bile acid resin no longer binds the drug. This would be especially important to consider in digitalis therapy. Mild increases of alkaline phosphatase and serum glutamic-oxaloacetic transaminase, serum phosphorus, and chloride have been seen, with a decrease in serum sodium and potassium levels.

Nursing Implications and Patient Teaching

Assessment

You should learn as much as possible about the health history of the patient, including any allergies, other medications that are being taken that may lead to drug interactions, diet, other things the patient has done to try to reduce cholesterol levels, and the possibility of pregnancy.

Diagnosis

Does this patient have other problems that will interfere with this therapy? Does the patient have a family history that causes him to feel anxious about early death? Does the patient have problems with exercise, diet, or stress that make it more difficult for him to follow the treatment plan?

Planning

You should encourage weight reduction when necessary, because the patient should be as healthy as possible. The patient must be taught about the long-term nature of this disease and the need for lifelong diet changes. Your ability to work with the patient, win her confidence, be aware of her reactions, and encourage her will be important in getting her to try to comply with diet, medication, and life style changes that may save her life. She will need to return to see her health care provider frequently, so you may have many chances to encourage and support her.

Implementation

If antihyperlipidemic drugs are taken for a long period of time, extra or supplemental doses of vitamins A, D, and K should be given. These should be given orally or through intramuscular (IM) injection.

Bile acid sequestrant preparations should be taken three times a day before meals. (Although there is no evidence that taking these drugs more than twice daily is helpful or therapeutic, the patient should get in the habit of taking the medication with each meal as a part of the total dietary change.) These drugs come as a powder that will need to be added to a liquid. They may be taken with milk, water, juice, or carbonated beverages; made into gelatin; or put into soups, cereals, or fruits with high moisture content, such as applesauce, nectars, fruit cocktail, or pineapple. The packet or a level scoopful of the powder should be added into the full glass or bowl. Allow the powder to dissolve slowly, without stirring, for at least 1 minute (stirring makes lumps). When dissolved, the patient should stir it and make sure it is all mixed and then drink it all. He should rinse the empty glass or bowl with water to make sure he is taking the full amount of medicine.

Table 15-6 provides a summary of antihyperlipidemics.

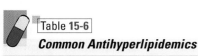

Table 15-6
Common Antihyperlipidemics

GENERIC NAME	TRADE NAME	DOSAGE
BILE ACID SEQUESTRANTS		
cholestyramine resin	Questran Prevalite	1 tsp PO 3-4 times daily with meals; mix with 8 oz water or juice.
colestipol	Colestid	5-30 gm PO daily in 2-4 doses with meals; mix with 8 oz water or juice.
colesevelam	Welchol	3 tablets twice daily with food or 6-7 tablets daily with a meal; may be used alone or with other antihyperlipidemics; mix with 8 oz water or juice.
HMG-COA REDUCTASE INHIBITORS		
atorvastatin Ca	Lipitor	Take 10 mg initially; increase up to 80 mg/day as needed; may take any time
fluvastatin	Lescol	Take 10-20 mg once daily at bedtime initially; may increase to 20-80 mg/day
lovastatin	Mevacor	20 mg PO once daily at PM meal; increase as needed at 4-wk intervals; do not exceed 80 mg/day
pravastatin	Pravachol	Give 10-20 mg once daily at bedtime; may increase to 40 mg daily
simvastatin	Zocor	Start with 5-10 mg once daily in the evening; may go up to 40 mg/day; adjust dose at intervals of at least 4 wk
OTHER PRODUCTS		
clofibrate	Atromid-S	2 gm PO once daily in 2-4 doses with meals
fenofibrate	Tricor	67 mg/day given with meals; maximum dose 201 mg/day
gemfibrozil	Lopid	600 mg PO 30 min before AM and PM meals; do not exceed 1500 mg daily
nicotinic acid or niacin	Niaspan Niacor	1-2 gm PO 3 times daily; maximum 6 gm/day

Evaluation

The patient may have constipation or hemorrhoids. Use of a high-bulk diet and a laxative may allow the patient to stay on the drug plan. The patient should be watched carefully to prevent bad constipation and impaction.

 Geriatric Considerations

Antihyperlipidemic Drugs

- Geriatric patients may be taking other medications in addition to the antihyperlipidemia medications. You should be aware that diuretics such as hydrochlorothiazide and chlorthalidone can increase cholesterol levels by 10% and that beta blockers such as propranolol and estrogen may increase triglyceride serum levels by 25% to 50%.
- Dietary modifications and/or recommendations are vital to a successful lipid reduction program. When goals cannot be met by diet alone, drug therapy may be prescribed.
- Constipation, a common (sometimes severe) side effect, has been reported in geriatric patients taking cholestyramine and colestipol. Encourage the patient to increase daily fluid intake to help reduce the constipating effects of this drug.
- The antihyperlipidemic drugs should be administered before or with meals (follow the manufacturer's instructions) because these drugs are generally not effective if they are not administered with food. Lovastatin is often given with supper to obtain its maximum beneficial effects, because the highest rate of cholesterol production occurs from midnight to 5 AM.

Modified from McKenry LM, Salerno E: Mosby's pharmacology in nursing, ed 21, St Louis, 2003, Mosby.

Patient and Family Teaching

You should tell the patient and family the following:
1. The patient should take the medication as ordered and not change the dose or stop taking it without telling the nurse, physician, or other health care provider.
2. The most important thing that can be done in learning to live with this problem is to follow the special diet. Lowering dietary intake of cholesterol and saturated fats, reducing calories, and increasing fluids and fiber content are very helpful. The patient should follow the diet that lists the foods that should and should not be eaten.
3. Some of the antihyperlipidemics come as a powder that must be mixed with liquid before being taken. It may be mixed with beverages, soups, fruits, cereals, or gelatin. The powder should be added to the liquid and not stirred until it is completely dissolved. The container should be rinsed with water so that the patient gets all of the medication in each dose.
4. The patient should take any other medicine 1 hour before or 4 to 6 hours after taking antihyperlipidemics. That is because these medicines are like glue and will delay the absorption of other drugs if taken at the same time.
5. Some patients experience side effects from these drugs. The patient must tell the nurse, physician, or other health care provider if any new or troublesome symptoms occur, especially frequent stomach upset, constipation, gas, bloating, heartburn, nausea, vomiting, or bleeding of any type.
6. The patient should keep this medication out of the reach of children and all others for whom it is not prescribed.
7. To decrease constipation, the patient should eat a high-bulk diet (fruit, raw vegetables, bran) and drink at least 2 quarts of fluid per day.

SECTION FOUR

Cardiotonics

OVERVIEW

Cardiotonics make the heart beat stronger and slower. These drugs are also called cardiac glycosides (glycosides are sugar-containing substances made from plants). The major cardiac glycoside is the digitalis preparation digoxin. It has been used for many years.

ACTION

All cardiotonics have the following two actions:
1. They increase the strength or force of the contraction (or pumping) of the heart muscle (myocardium).
2. They slow the heart rate.

These actions are especially important in hearts that may be weakened by age or disease.

Table 15-7	*Symptoms of Weakened Heart or Chronic Heart Failure*
ORGAN AFFECTED	**SYMPTOMS**
Brain	Dizzy, less alert
Heart	Enlarged heart, murmurs or abnormal heart sounds, dysrhythmias
Lungs	Productive cough, shortness of breath
Kidneys	Edema of tissues of hands and feet
General	Rapid weight gain, weakness, lethargy (sleepiness)

The normal heart pumps oxygenated blood from the left ventricle out through the body. If the heart is weak, less oxygenated blood can be pumped out with each contraction or beat of the heart.

When cardiac output (the amount of blood pumped out with each heartbeat × the heart beat) decreases, other organs are affected. For example, the brain reacts to receiving less blood by becoming dizzy, drowsy, or less alert. The kidneys become less effective at removing waste products, electrolytes, and extra water from the bloodstream. This extra fluid may then pool in the spaces between cells or organs or in other dependent tissues **(edema).** Sometimes the heartbeat itself becomes irregular or too fast. As the body attempts to deal with these changes, the blood pressure may increase or a more rapid heart rate may develop. These actions may place further strain on the heart. We call these symptoms of weak or inadequate heart action **chronic heart failure (CHF)** (Table 15-7).

All cardiotonics have the same basic drug action. They differ only in the speed and length or duration of their action. A drug that affects the rate of rhythmic movements, such as the heartbeat, is called a **chronotropic** drug. A **dromotropic** drug influences the velocity (speed) of the passage of an electrical impulse in nerve or cardiac muscle fibers.

INCREASING STRENGTH OF MYOCARDIAL CONTRACTION

The first action of the cardiotonic drugs is to increase the strength of each heartbeat or the force of the contraction. The stronger heartbeat pumps more blood, and increases the cardiac output. This effect of the drug is called a **positive inotropic action.** As more blood reaches the brain, lungs, kidneys, and other tissues, the signs of inadequate heart action decrease or go away (Figures 15-9 and 15-10).

SLOWING HEART RATE

The second action of the cardiotonic drugs is to slow the heartbeat. They do this by slowing down the rate at which the pacemaker in the SA node begins the electrical cycle, and also by slowing the rate at which that information is passed through the rest of the heart. (See the discussion of cardiac conduction in Section Two of this chapter.)

USES

Cardiotonics are used to treat CHF and rapid or irregular heartbeats, such as atrial fibrillation, atrial flutter, and (sometimes outside the hospital) frequent premature ventricular contractions or paroxysmal atrial tachycardia.

ADVERSE REACTIONS

Cardiotonics are very powerful and can act as poisons on the heart.

Many things may happen that make even a safe dose of digitalis harmful to a patient. When a patient begins to show toxic or harmful reactions from too much medication, **digitalis toxicity** has developed. The symptoms of digitalis toxicity may begin slowly and are often easy to overlook. Some symptoms are included in Table 15-8.

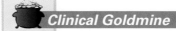 **Clinical Goldmine**

Medication Amounts

The amount of medicine that is helpful (therapeutic) and the amount that is harmful (toxic) are not very different.

Treatment of digitalis toxicity begins by stopping the drug and beginning treatment of symptoms as needed. The physician or other health care provider may order blood tests to measure the serum blood digitalis level. The serum level of digoxin that is needed to help the patient (be therapeutic) is 0.5 to 2 ng/mL (nanograms per milliliter), and the toxic serum level is 2.5 ng/mL. Digoxin has a rapid onset and a short length of action. Antidotes for digitalis toxicity (drugs that work opposite digitalis) include phenytoin, potassium chloride, activated charcoal, lidocaine, atropine, colestipol, and cholestyramine. Medication such as atropine may be ordered to speed up the pulse if the rate is very slow. Potassium may also be given to help the heart's ability to beat regularly.

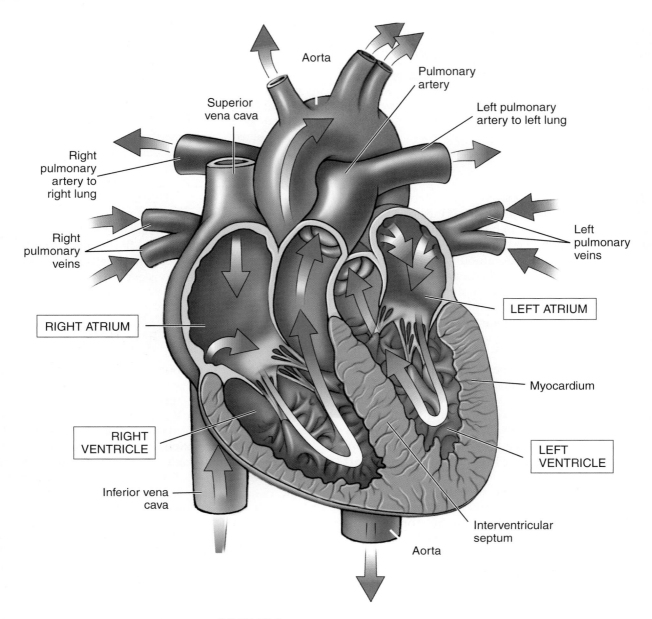

FIGURE **15-9** Internal anatomy of the heart.

Table 15-8   *Common Signs and Symptoms of Digitalis Toxicity*

SYSTEM	SYMPTOMS
Cardiac	Bradycardia, dysrhythmia, tachycardia
Central nervous system	Apathy, confusion, delirium, disorientation, drowsiness, headache, mental depression, visual changes (blurred vision, yellow/green vision, halos around dark objects)
Gastrointestinal	Anorexia, diarrhea, nausea, vomiting
Musculoskeletal	Severe weakness

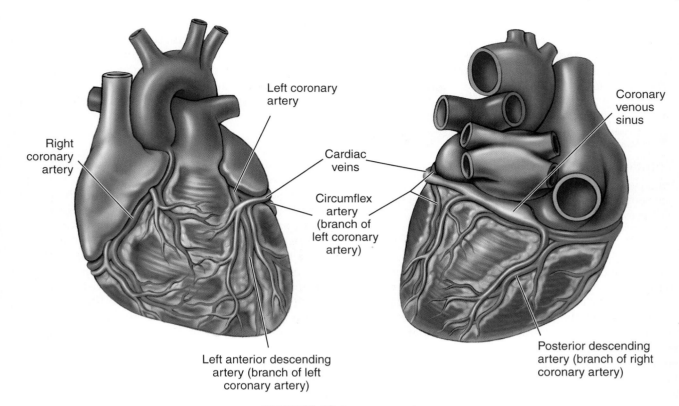

FIGURE **15-10** Coronary arteries.

DRUG INTERACTIONS

Beta-adrenergic blocking agents, calcium gluconate, calcium chloride, succinylcholine, and verapamil increase both the therapeutic and the toxic effects of cardiotonics.

Cholestyramine reduces the therapeutic effects.

Any medication that changes the electrolyte balance may also lead to digitalis toxicity.

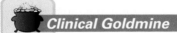

Clinical Goldmine

Cardiotonics

Cardiotonics are some of the most common medicines. Because these drugs may reach toxic levels very quickly, it is important for you to closely watch the patient receiving these drugs.

Nursing Implications and Patient Teaching

Assessment

Before beginning the medication, you should check the patient for the following:
1. History of nausea, vomiting, diarrhea, weakness, shortness of breath, confusion, or depression.

2. Presence on physical examination of muscle weakness, confusion, hypertension, bradycardia, tachycardia, dysrhythmias, abnormal heart sounds or murmurs, unusual lung sounds produced during inspiration or expiration, cyanosis (blue color to the skin), peripheral edema, or distended jugular veins; the patient should also be weighed.
3. Abnormal laboratory results may be found with ECGs, chest x-ray studies, complete blood counts, serum enzymes, serum electrolytes, and renal and hepatic studies.

Diagnosis

What other problems does this patient have that interfere with therapy? Is the patient overweight? Anxious? Unwilling to accept that she has cardiac problems?

Planning

You should know about two different types of dosages for patients taking digoxin: the initial **digitalizing dose** (or loading dose) and maintenance (regular daily) doses. More frequent and higher digitalizing doses are given when a patient begins taking digoxin so that a specific level of medication can be reached in the blood. When the amount of drug in the patient's blood reaches the desired level, smaller maintenance doses are given once a day to maintain the blood level. How fast the desired drug level is reached is based on the dosage, the diagnosis of the patient, and many other factors.

Because of the risk for overdosage, great care must be taken not to confuse two common cardiotonic medications: digitoxin and digoxin. Confusing these medications may hurt the patient. Extra care must also be taken in checking the correct dosage.

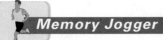

Memory Jogger

Withholding Medication

When you withhold (do not give) a patient's medication, you should always contact the physician or other health care provider immediately.

Implementation

Before giving each dose of a cardiotonic drug, the apical pulse rate (using a stethoscope and listening to the chest) should be taken for 60 seconds. If the apical pulse rate is below 60, the medication should not be given and the physician or other health care provider should be notified unless there is a written order giving different directions. The drug should also be withheld if there are any symptoms of digitalis toxicity or if the patient's condition has worsened since the last time the medication was given. Do not withhold the medicine without notifying someone in authority.

IM injection of cardiotonic drugs is painful. If these injections are necessary, you should take special care to change or rotate the site where you give the injection. Warm packs applied to the area may be necessary to reduce painful swelling.

Table 15-9 gives a summary of cardiotonic medications.

Evaluation

Patients must be watched very closely for symptoms of digitalis toxicity. Changes from the first time the patient is seen should be written down in the patient record. Vital signs, including daily weights, are very important to record. Patients with other lung, GI, kidney, or central nervous system (CNS) problems, patients taking many other medications (especially diuretics and electrolytes), and confused patients who are not eating or drinking well are all at risk for digitalis toxicity. Digitalis toxicity may cause life-threatening dysrhythmias. These may be treated with digoxin immune Fab (Digibind), which has antigen-binding fragments that come from specific antidigoxin antibodies. This product may save lives, but it requires careful monitoring of the patient's vital signs and potassium levels and special plans for slowly reducing the amount of drug that is given to avoid causing other life-threatening events.

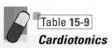

Table 15-9

Cardiotonics

GENERIC NAME	TRADE NAME	USES	ADVERSE REACTIONS	DOSE RANGES
digoxin	Lanoxicaps Lanoxin	Atrial flutter, atrial fibrillation, PAT, CHF	Digitalis toxicity	*Digitalizing:* 0.4-0.6 mg IV or 500-750 mcg PO; individualize according to age, weight, renal status *Maintenance:* based on serum digoxin level; usually 0.125-0.5 mg PO daily
dobutamine	Dobutrex	Short-term treatment of cardiac decompensation	Ectopic activity, hypotension, tachycardia, and hypertension	Give 2.5-15 mcg/kg/min by IV drip
inamrinone	—	For the short-term management of CHF patients who can be closely monitored and have not responded to digitalis	Ectopic activity, GI distress, hypersensitivity (allergy) reactions, and hepatotoxicity (damage to the liver)	Give 0.75 mg/kg slowly by IV bolus over 2-3 min initially; then 5-10 mcg/kg/min as maintenance infusion
milrinone	Primacor	CHF—short term	Ventricular dysrhythmias	Loading dose followed by continuous IV infusion for severe CHF

PAT, Paroxysmal atrial tachycardia.

Pediatric Considerations

Digitalis

- Digitalis is reported to be a leading cause of accidental toxicity in children.
- Individualized dosing with very close monitoring is necessary, especially in premature and immature infants.
- Early signs of toxicity in infants and children may include a slow heart rate (less than 60 beats/minute) and irregular heart rhythms.

Modified from McKenry LM, Salerno E: Mosby's pharmacology in nursing, ed 21, St Louis, 2003, Mosby.

Geriatric Considerations

Digitalis

- The elderly often have a reduced tolerance for this drug; lower doses of digitalis may be necessary to reduce the potential for drug toxicity.
- Decreased libido and impotence have been reported in approximately 35% of male users because of digoxin's estrogen-type effects. Also, gynecomastia (enlargement of the breasts in men) and breast tenderness have been reported. The earliest symptom of digitalis toxicity is extreme fatigue. Almost 100% of patients also experience anorexia. Weakness, irregular pulse, and visual disturbances are also common signs of digitalis toxicity.

Modified from McKenry LM, Salerno E: Mosby's pharmacology in nursing, ed 21, St Louis, 2003, Mosby.

Patient and Family Teaching

The patient usually continues to take this medication once she leaves the hospital. You should tell the family and patient the following:

1. The patient or a dependable family member must be taught to look for the same things that you have been watching. This may require teaching the patient or family member how to take the pulse. Before the patient goes home, the nurse, physician, or other health care provider should tell the patient what to do when the pulse is below 60 beats/minute.
2. The patient should tell the nurse, physician, or other health care provider if lack of appetite, nausea, vomiting, diarrhea, unusual weakness, fatigue, vision changes, depression, confusion, or dizziness occurs.
3. The medication must be kept in a safe place, away from animals or small children.
4. The medication must not be stopped unless the patient is told to stop by the nurse, physician, or other health care provider. It is very important that the patient does not run out of medicine. The nurse, physician, or other health care provider should be called if the patient has no medication.
5. It is important to keep office visits with the nurse, physician, or other health care provider so that changes in the patient's health can be determined. The patient should have lab tests done as soon as possible when they are ordered.
6. The patient should not take other prescription drugs or OTC drugs without the approval of the nurse, physician, or other health care provider. Some drugs interfere with the action of cardiotonic drugs and may cause very serious problems.
7. The patient should take the medication at the same time every day, as directed by the nurse, physician, or other health care provider; digitalis products are usually taken after meals.
8. The patient should wear a Medic Alert bracelet or necklace or have other emergency identification indicating the medication being taken.
9. The patient taking cardiotonic drugs may be advised to eat foods rich in potassium. Good sources of potassium include bananas and citrus fruits, dried fruits, dried beans and lentils, all-bran cereal, and decaffeinated coffee (if the patient is not permitted to take caffeine products).

SECTION FIVE

Antihypertensives, Diuretics, and Other Drugs Affecting the Urinary Tract

OVERVIEW

Hypertension is a disorder in which the patient's blood pressure is elevated above normal values for his age. Research has shown that blood pressures above 150/90 mm Hg are associated with accelerated vascular damage of the heart, the brain, and the kidneys, leading to an increased risk of early death. Lowering the blood pressure below 150/90 mm Hg has been demonstrated to dramatically reduce the chance of myocardial infarction, stroke, and other target organ damage.

Primary hypertension (or essential hypertension) accounts for 80% to 90% of all cases of high blood pressure, but in most cases the cause is unknown. In some cases, high blood pressure results from another disease or other problem and is then called **secondary hypertension.**

Approximately 40 million people in the United States have hypertension, a disorder that cannot be cured but can be controlled. Risk factors for hypertension include increasing age, black race, male sex, family history of hypertension, obesity, diabetes mellitus, hypercholesterolemia, smoking, and previous history of vascular disease.

ACTION

Many types of drugs are available to treat hypertension. They act at many sites in the body and through several different ways. These drugs fall roughly into the following five main categories:
1. *Diuretics* indirectly reduce blood pressure by producing sodium and water loss and lowering the tone or rigidity of the arteries.
2. *Adrenergic antagonists* are nervous system stimulants and inhibitors that assist in lowering cardiac output and/or peripheral resistance.
3. *Angiotensin-related drugs* affect the renin-angiotensin system of the kidney. Angiotensin-converting enzyme (ACE) inhibitors act on the renin-angiotensin system to promote a decrease in the work of the heart (vascular afterload and preload) through vasodilation (vascular opening) when angiotensin II is inhibited. Angiotensin II receptor antagonists block the vasoconstrictive (narrowing) and aldosterone-secreting effects of angiotensin II by selectively blocking the binding of angiotensin II to angiotensin receptors in many tissues.
4. *Vasodilators* lower the pressure out in the tissues of the arms and legs or the peripheral resistance.
5. *Channel calcium blocking agents* reduce peripheral resistance (in the arms and legs) through smooth muscle relaxation and vasodilation.

Because each of these five drug categories works in a different manner and is also useful in treating problems other than hypertension, the action of each drug category is discussed separately. Figure 15-11 shows the different places where these antihypertensive medications may act.

Many of these drugs can be mixed together to produce a new combination drug with many actions. Some of these products combine potassium-sparing and potassium-losing drugs. These drugs may be good for some patients, so that they do not need to take so many

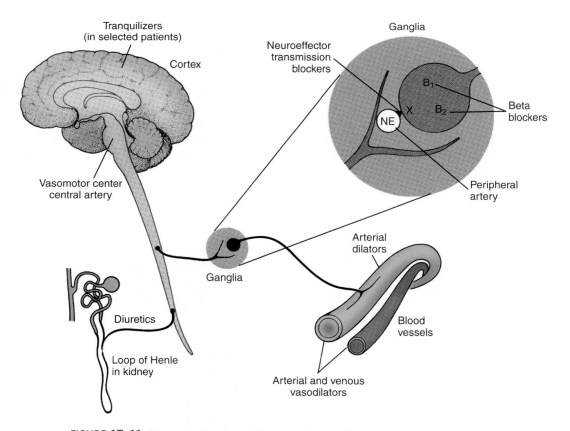

FIGURE **15-11** Sites of action for antihypertensive medications. *NE,* Norepinephrine.

pills, but the ability to increase or decrease one of the drugs in the combination product to meet the specific needs of a patient is lost.

DIURETICS

The action of all diuretics is to increase fluid loss from the body. Diuretics have been the main drugs used in antihypertensive therapy for the past 40 years. They are popular because they work quite well, are quite safe, are well tolerated, and are not very expensive. Diuretics may be classed into four related groups: thiazides (for example, chlorothiazide, hydrochlorothiazide, and polythiazide), the thiazide-like sulfonamides (for example, chlorthalidone, metolazone, quinethazone, and indapamide), loop diuretics (for example, furosemide, ethacrynic acid, and bumetanide), and the potassium-sparing diuretics (for example, amiloride, triamterene, and spironolactone).

Thiazides and Sulfonamide Diuretics

Thiazides and sulfonamide diuretics have similar actions. They work to prevent the reabsorption of sodium and chloride through direct action on the end of the ascending loop and the beginning of the distal tubule of the loop of Henle in the distal kidney tubule. They act to block sodium and chloride reabsorption and slightly limit carbonic anhydrase. Their long half-life may lead to the loss of large amounts of potassium.

The thiazides also act directly to dilate the smooth muscles in the arterioles, the smallest vessels in the arterial system. Because the arterioles are made larger, the heart does not have to pump so hard to get blood into them. This helps keep blood pressure lower. Thiazides also work to promote reabsorption of calcium, which may make them good for use in older adults with osteoporosis.

Geriatric Considerations

Diuretics

- Elderly patients are more susceptible to the development of the adverse reactions of postural hypotension, impaired mentation, hypokalemia (except with potassium-sparing diuretics), and increased serum glucose levels.
- Lower doses are advised in the elderly population, with dosage increases based on the patient's individual therapeutic response and/or the development of adverse reactions.
- When a diuretic is to be discontinued, it is recommended that the drug be reduced gradually to avoid the development of serious edema.

From McKenry LM, Salerno E: Mosby's pharmacology in nursing, ed 21, St Louis, 2003, Mosby.

Loop Diuretics

Loop diuretics act by blocking active transport of chloride, sodium, and potassium in the thick ascending loop of Henle. These drugs often work well in patients with very low glomerular filtration rates, because they are so efficient in limiting the reabsorption of sodium. The peak diuretic effect is much greater for loop diuretics than that seen with any other type of diuretic. They are often used in patients with kidney disease and to treat CHF, cirrhosis of the liver, and kidney diseases in which a powerful diuretic is required.

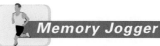

Memory Jogger

Fluid Balance

In understanding fluid and electrolyte balance, a good rule to remember is that water tends to follow sodium; thus with sodium loss, water also is pulled out and lost through the urine.

Potassium-Sparing Diuretics

Potassium-sparing diuretics increase the excretion of water and sodium but save potassium. These drugs act by binding at receptor sites in the distal renal tubular cell nucleus, resulting in changes in the creation of proteins that affect the exchange of sodium and potassium. These drugs are used in patients with kidney disease, in elderly patients with poor kidney function who have hypokalemia, or in those patients with the risk for having hypokalemia, often because of treatment with other medications such as digitalis. (Refer to Figure 15-12 for a review of the different parts of the kidney nephron.)

ADRENERGIC INHIBITORS

Adrenergic inhibitors are also divided into five different categories of drugs:

1. Beta-adrenergic blockers
2. Central adrenergic inhibitors
3. Peripheral adrenergic antagonists
4. Alpha$_1$-adrenergic inhibitors
5. Combined alpha- and beta-adrenergic blockers

The sympathetic nervous system relies on two adrenergic neurohormones or neurotransmitters, epinephrine and norepinephrine, to send its messages. These adrenergic inhibitors occupy the adrenergic receptors so that the neurohormones cannot make contact with the receptors, thus preventing stimulation. Adrenergic nerve fibers have either alpha or beta receptors. Thus the blocking can be of alpha, beta, or both alpha and beta receptor sites. If the medication blocks all adrenergic receptor sites, we say it is nonselective in its blocking. Alpha receptor blockers are an important drug group.

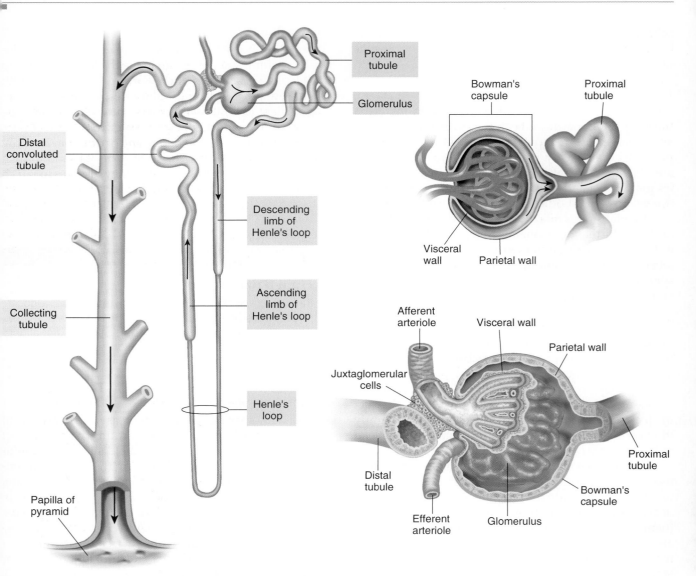

FIGURE **15-12** Components of a nephron and direction of flow of fluid.

Beta Blockers

Beta blockers are classed into two groups: nonselective and selective beta antagonists. The nonselective agents block both beta$_1$ and beta$_2$ sites. The selective beta$_1$ blocking agents stop the action of the beta$_1$ receptors of the heart, but have less influence on the beta$_2$ receptors of the bronchi in the lung. There are no selective beta$_2$ inhibitors.

Nonselective beta blockers reduce the heart rate and the force of the contraction, prevent renin release, and slow the outflow of sympathetic nervous system messages from the brainstem to the vasomotor center telling the body to narrow the blood vessels and increase the heart rate. Because these drugs block both beta$_1$ and beta$_2$ impulses, they have a wide range of side effects.

Central Adrenergic Inhibitors

Central adrenergic inhibitors stimulate peripheral alpha-adrenergic receptors, and thus cause brief vasoconstriction, and then stimulate the presynaptic alpha$_2$-adrenergic receptors in the centers in the brainstem that coordinate cardiovascular function. As a result of this, the total number of sympathetic nervous system messages from the brain are decreased, leading to vascular relaxation and lower blood pressure.

Peripheral Adrenergic Antagonists

Peripheral adrenergic antagonists work as adrenergic neuron blocking agents that prevent sympathetic nervous system vasoconstriction by limiting norepinephrine release from storage sites in the neurons and by using up all the norepinephrine at nerve endings. Total peripheral resistance to blood flow is thus decreased because the vascular smooth muscle is relaxed.

Alpha₁-Adrenergic Inhibitors

Alpha₁-adrenergic inhibitors work through selective blocking of postsynaptic alpha-adrenergic receptor sites, leading to a lowering of peripheral vascular resistance and blood pressure. Both arterioles and venules are dilated by this relaxation of the arteriolar and venous smooth muscles.

Labetalol hydrochloride has a combination of alpha- and beta-adrenergic blocker action. It works as selective alpha₁-adrenergic blocker but is also a nonselective beta-adrenergic blocker.

ANGIOTENSIN-RELATED AGENTS

Angiotensin-Converting Enzyme Inhibitors and Angiotensin II Receptor Antagonists

When the juxtaglomerular apparatus of the kidneys is stimulated, renin is released into the bloodstream to produce angiotensin I. Angiotensin I is then changed to angiotensin II in the liver and the lungs by ACE. Angiotensin II is a powerful vasoconstrictor that acts on the adrenal cortex to increase aldosterone secretion. This renin-angiotensin reaction is important in saving sodium and water when needed in an emergency to keep the blood pressure up when the patient is in shock, but at other times, it may help lead to the high blood pressure found in hypertension. Figure 15-13 shows a review of the renin-angiotensin system.

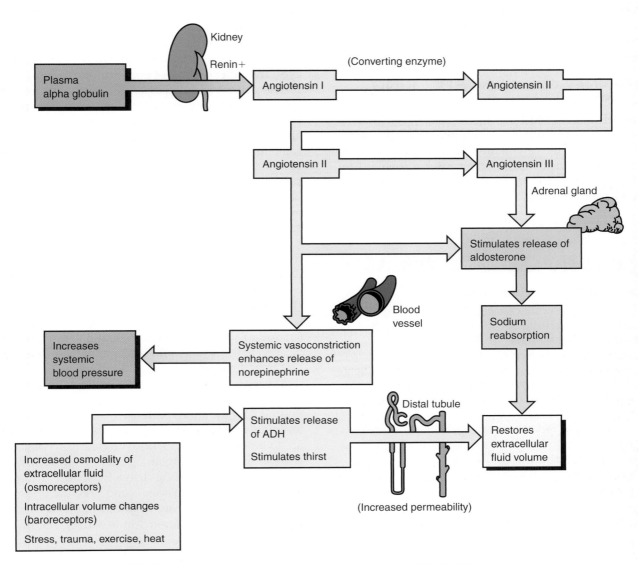

FIGURE **15-13** Physiologic effects of renin-angiotensin system. *ADH,* Antidiuretic hormone.

Although we do not know everything about the action of ACE inhibitors, they are thought to stop the change of angiotensin I to angiotensin II by preventing the action of ACE in the plasma and vascular endothelium. There may be other complex actions of these drugs that also help reduce blood pressure. ACE inhibitors are not to be given to pregnant women in the second and third trimesters.

Angiotensin II receptor antagonists block the vasoconstrictor and aldosterone-secreting effects of angiotensin II by selectively blocking the binding of angiotensin II to the angiotensin receptor found in many tissues. ACE inhibitors often produce a cough in patients. Angiotensin II antagonists do not produce cough.

VASODILATORS

Vasodilators reduce systolic and diastolic blood pressure by direct relaxation of vascular smooth muscle, thus lowering peripheral vascular resistance. The exact way these drugs work is not known, but they appear to block calcium from moving through the cell membrane.

CHANNEL CALCIUM BLOCKING AGENTS

Channel calcium blocking agents selectively limit the passage of extracellular calcium ions through specific ion channels of the cell membrane in cardiac, vascular, and smooth muscle cells. This causes a lowered peripheral vascular resistance and a fall in systolic and diastolic blood pressure.

Geriatric Considerations

Calcium Channel Blockers

- The elderly are more susceptible to these agents and the side effects of increased weakness, dizziness, fainting episodes, and falls.
- Although nitroglycerin (or other nitrates) may be taken at the same time as these agents, the patient should be advised to report any increase in frequency or intensity of angina attacks to her health care provider.
- Nicotine may reduce the effectiveness of these agents; thus reduction or avoidance of tobacco smoking is advisable.
- Alcohol consumption may result in hypotensive episodes in some patients. Whenever possible, the use of alcohol should be avoided.
- These agents should not be suddenly stopped because severe rebound angina attacks may result; gradual drug withdrawal is required.

From McKenry LM, Salerno E: Mosby's pharmacology in nursing, ed 21, St Louis, 2003, Mosby.

USES

Antihypertensives and diuretics (Table 15-10) are used alone or in combination to decrease elevated systolic and/or diastolic blood pressure. *Blood pressure* may be defined as pressure of the blood against the walls of the various vessels. The blood pressure is highest at the moment the ventricles contract (systole) because the heart has to push very hard to get the blood out into the circulation. This is called *systolic pressure.* Pressure during ventricular relaxation is known as *diastolic pressure* and is the pressure at the lowest part of the cardiac cycle. These pressures are written as a fraction, with the systolic as the numerator (the number on top of the fraction) and the diastolic as the denominator (the number on the bottom of the fraction). Respected clinical studies suggest that it is beneficial to use a combination of diet, drug therapy, and reduction of risk factors to treat hypertension. The therapeutic goal in the hypertensive patient is to reduce the blood pressure to normal or near normal with few adverse effects. Reduction of both systolic and diastolic pressure has been associated with decreased risk of damage to the vascular tissues of the heart, kidneys, brain, eyes, and other organs, or **end-organ damage.**

The patient with hypertension may have no symptoms or may complain of not feeling well in general. Headaches, frequently associated with hypertension, are often produced by stress, tension, or other reasons, rather than being related to high blood pressure, unless very severe blood pressure elevations are present. In cases of secondary hypertension, there may be reports of getting up at night to go to the bathroom (nocturia), history of renal trauma (producing renal artery stenosis), or a family history of hypertension.

Hypertension is classified according to the stages listed in Table 15-11. The choice of antihypertensive drug to use depends on many factors: how severe the hypertension is, the presence of **compelling indications** (other diseases for which a specific class of antihypertensives has been shown to improve the patient's condition), the use of other drugs, and the patient's willingness to accept the mild but unavoidable side effects that may develop.

The Joint National Committee on the Detection, Evaluation, and Treatment of High Blood Pressure has indicated how the antihypertensive drugs should be used for initial therapy and when and what additional drugs are to be used (Table 15-12). The treatment plan starts with a single mild agent, gradually increasing the dosage, and then adding drugs from other drug categories to bring the diastolic blood pressure under control. The drug effects are balanced in this approach to take advantage of different kinds of drug action.

STAGE I: LIFESTYLE CHANGES

Before starting drug therapy for patients with hypertension, a lot of effort should be made to help patients

Table 15-10

Antihypertensive Agents and Their Dosage Ranges

MEDICATION CATEGORY AND DRUGS	DOSAGE RANGE (mg/day)	
	INITIAL	MAXIMUM
DIURETICS		
Thiazide and Related Sulfonamide Diuretics		
bendroflumethiazide (Naturetin)	2.5	5
benzthiazide (Exna)	25	200
chlorothiazide (Diuril)	250	500
chlorthalidone (Hygroton)	25	50
hydrochlorothiazide (HydroDiuril, Esidrix)	25	50
hydroflumethiazide (Saluron)	25	50
indapamide (Lozol)	2.5	5
methyclothiazide (Enduron)	2.5	5
metolazone (Zaroxolyn, Mykrox)	2.5	5
polythiazide (Renese)	2	4
quinethazone (Hydromox)	50	100
trichlormethiazide (Naqua)	2	4
Loop Diuretics		
bumetanide (Bumex)	0.5	10
ethacrynic acid (Edecrin)	50	200
furosemide (Lasix)	80	480
torsemide (Demadex)	10	200
Potassium-Sparing Agents		
amiloride (Midamor)	5	10
spironolactone (Aldactone)	50	100
triamterene (Dyrenium)	50	100
ADRENERGIC INHIBITORS		
Peripheral Adrenergic Antagonists		
guanadrel (Hylorel)	10	150
guanethidine (Ismelin)	10	300
Rauwolfia Alkaloids		
reserpine	0.05	0.25
Central Adrenergic Inhibitors		
clonidine (Catapres)	0.2	1.2
guanabenz (Wytensin)	8	32
methyldopa (Aldomet)	500	2000
Alpha$_1$-Adrenergic Blockers		
doxazosin (Cardura)	1	16
prazosin (Minipress)	2	15
terazosin (Hytrin)	1	5
Beta-Adrenergic Blockers		
acebutolol (Sectral)	400	1200
atenolol (Tenormin)	25	100
betaxolol (Kerlone)	10	40
bisoprolol (Zebeta)	5	20
carteolol (Cartrol)	2.5	5
metoprolol (Lopressor)	50	300
nadolol (Corgard)	20	120
pindolol (Visken)	20	60
propranolol (Inderal)	40	480
sotalol (Betapace)	160	320
timolol (Blocadren)	20	60

Continued

Table 15-10

Antihypertensive Agents and Their Dosage Ranges—cont'd

| MEDICATION CATEGORY AND DRUGS | DOSAGE RANGe (mg/day) | |
	INITIAL	MAXIMUM
Combined Alpha- and Beta-Adrenergic Blocker		
labetalol (Normodyne)	200	1200
VASODILATORS		
hydralazine (Apresoline)	30	150
minoxidil (Loniten)	5	40
ACE INHIBITORS		
benazepril (Lotensin)	10	40
captopril (Capoten)	37.5	150
enalapril (Vasotec)	10	40
fosinopril (Monopril)	10	80
lisinopril (Zestril)	10	40
moexipril (Univasc)	3.75	15
quinapril (Accupril)	10	80
ramipril (Altace)	2.5	20
trandolapril (Mavik)	1 (2 in African Americans)	8
ANGIOTENSIN II RECEPTOR ANTAGONISTS		
candesartan (Atacand)	2	8
irbesartan (Avapro)	150	300
losartan (Cozaar)	50	100
valsartan (Diovan)	80	320
CHANNEL CALCIUM BLOCKING AGENTS		
amlodipine (Norvasc)	5	10
bepridil (Vascor)	200	400
diltiazem (Cardizem)	120	360
felodipine (Plendil)	5	20
isradipine (DynaCirc)	5	20
nifedipine (Procardia)	30	60
verapamil (Calan)	240	480

Table 15-11 ## Classification and Management of Blood Pressure (BP) for Adults

| BP CLASS | SYSTOLIC BP (mm Hg) | DIASTOLIC BP (mm Hg) | INITIAL DRUG THERAPY | |
			WITHOUT COMPELLING INDICATION	WITH COMPELLING INDICATION
Normal	<120	and <80	None indicated	Drugs for compelling indications
Prehypertension	120-139	or 80-89		
Stage 1 HTN	150-159	or 90-99	Thiazide-type diuretics for most. May consider ACEI, ARB, BB, CCB or combination	Drug(s) for compelling indications. Other antihypertensive drugs (diuretics, ACEI, ARB, BB, CCB) as needed
Stage 2 HTN	≥160	or ≥100	Two-drug combination for most (usually thiazide-type diuretic and ACEI or ARB or BB or CCB)	

Modified from National Heart, Lung, and Blood Institutes, National High Blood Pressure Education Program: *The Seventh Report of the Joint National Committee on the Prevention, Detection, Evaluation, and Treatment of High Blood Pressure.* Bethesda, MD, 2003, National Institutes of Health.
CEI, Angiotensin-converting enzyme inhibitors; *ARB,* angiotensin II receptor blockers; *BB,* beta blockers; *CCB,* calcium channel blockers; *HTN,* hypertension.

Table 15-12 *Management of Hypertension Based on Risk Stratification*

BLOOD PRESSURE STAGES (mm Hg)	RISK GROUP A (NO RISK FACTORS AND NO TOD/CCD)	RISK GROUP B (AT LEAST ONE RISK FACTOR, NOT INCLUDING DM; NO TOD/CCD)	RISK GROUP C (TOD/CCD AND/OR DM, WITH OR WITHOUT OTHER RISK FACTORS)
High-normal (130-139/85-89)	Lifestyle modification*	Lifestyle modification	Drug therapy†
Stage 1 (140-159/90-99)	Lifestyle modification (up to 12 mo)	Lifestyle modification (up to 6 mo)	Drug therapy
Stages 2 and 3 (>160/>100)	Drug therapy	Drug therapy	Drug therapy

*Should be adjunctive therapy for all patients recommended for pharmacologic therapy.
†For those patients with heart failure, renal insufficiency, or diabetes.
DM, Diabetes mellitus; *TOD/CCD,* target organ damage/clinical cardiovascular disease.

reduce their risk factors. Life style changes to help patients lose weight, increase physical activity, and reduce fat, salt, and calories in the diet are helpful in lowering blood pressure. Behavior change to assist them to stop smoking and reduce alcohol intake is also important.

STAGE II: DRUG THERAPY

The drug of choice in starting antihypertensive therapy is an oral thiazide—or thiazide-like sulfonamide drug—or an adrenergic beta blocker. Other drugs are added if needed based on how the patient responds to the first drug (Figure 15-14). Most thiazides or beta blockers are effective when given once a day. The drug is started in a low dosage and increased as needed until the maximum dose is reached. In many cases, one of the drugs by itself will reduce the diastolic blood pressure to the desired level. Because these drugs commonly produce hypokalemia, a potassium supplement may also be required. Loop diuretics are used when hypertension is severe and the blood pressure must come down quickly. An anti-adrenergic agent may be added to the treatment plan if the maximum doses of diuretics or beta blockers fail to lower the blood pressure to the desired level. These two categories of drugs work well together to bring down blood pressure and lower the chance of side effects, and they are better than using an antiadrenergic agent alone. There are a variety of antiadrenergic drugs, so the patient can try different combinations to find the ones that work best. The patient should move on to the next level of drug treatment only if the drugs he has tried fail to control the blood pressure. It should be noted that beta blockers seem to be less effective in blacks and very elderly patients. Captopril is another drug that seems to be less effective in black patients.

Other drugs that might be added to the therapeutic plan are the vasodilators. Vasodilators are most effective when used with a beta-adrenergic blocking agent to control the rapid heartbeat that often results from lowering peripheral resistance.

Guanethidine, another adrenergic-inhibiting agent, can also be used in refractory (resistant to treatment) hypertension. This drug almost always has dramatic side effects, so it is used in only severe cases of hypertension. The initial dose should be small, with doses carefully increased as the patient is watched.

There has been a lot of research on antihypertensive drugs in therapy in recent years; new drugs have entered the market and more research findings have been published. Some drugs are particularly helpful in certain conditions. See Table 15-13 for drugs used in other diseases.

ADVERSE REACTIONS

Each category and each drug have many important adverse reactions. Hypokalemia and drowsiness are commonly seen, and many drugs produce impotence in men. Table 15-14 provides a list of the most common adverse reactions to the antihypertensive and diuretic drugs. For example, prazosin may cause severe syncope after the first dose, so the patient should take the first dose when someone can be with her.

DRUG INTERACTIONS

Frequently a patient with high blood pressure has to take many different medicines because he may have other medical problems. All of the antihypertensive drugs may have drug interactions. You must check each drug that the patient is taking in order to prevent effects that would lower the blood pressure too much or that might make the blood pressure go even higher.

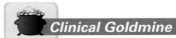 *Clinical Goldmine*

Collecting Data

It is important to collect and record a good initial database (history, physical, and laboratory findings) to evaluate the progression of end-organ damage over the years.

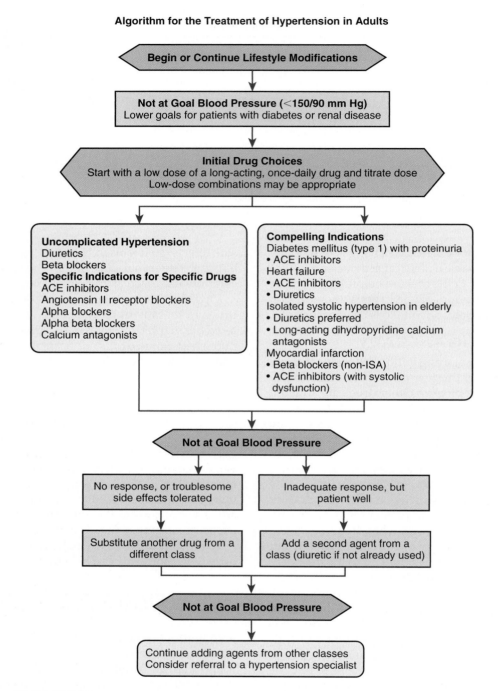

Algorithm for the Treatment of Hypertension in Adults

Begin or Continue Lifestyle Modifications

Not at Goal Blood Pressure (<150/90 mm Hg)
Lower goals for patients with diabetes or renal disease

Initial Drug Choices
Start with a low dose of a long-acting, once-daily drug and titrate dose
Low-dose combinations may be appropriate

Uncomplicated Hypertension
Diuretics
Beta blockers
Specific Indications for Specific Drugs
ACE inhibitors
Angiotensin II receptor blockers
Alpha blockers
Alpha beta blockers
Calcium antagonists

Compelling Indications
Diabetes mellitus (type 1) with proteinuria
• ACE inhibitors
Heart failure
• ACE inhibitors
• Diuretics
Isolated systolic hypertension in elderly
• Diuretics preferred
• Long-acting dihydropyridine calcium
  antagonists
Myocardial infarction
• Beta blockers (non-ISA)
• ACE inhibitors (with systolic
  dysfunction)

Not at Goal Blood Pressure

No response, or troublesome
side effects tolerated

Inadequate response, but
patient well

Substitute another drug from a
different class

Add a second agent from a
class (diuretic if not already used)

Not at Goal Blood Pressure

Continue adding agents from other classes
Consider referral to a hypertension specialist

FIGURE **15-14** Treatment regimen for hypertension. *ACE,* Angiotensin-converting enzyme; *ISA,* intrinsic sympathomimetic activity.

Table **15-13**

Antihypertensive Drug Classes Used in Other Diseases

COMPELLING INDICATION	DIURETIC	BETA BLOCKER	ANGIOTENSIN-CONVERTING ENZYME INHIBITOR	ALPHA RECEPTOR BLOCKER	CALCIUM CHANNEL BLOCKER	ALDOSTERONE ANTAGONIST
Heart failure	X	X	X	X		X
Post MI		X	X			X
High risk for CAD	X	X	X		X	
Diabetes	X	X	X	X	X	
Chronic kidney disease			X	X		
Recurrent stroke prevention	X		X			

Modified from National Heart, Lung, and Blood Institutes, National High Blood Pressure Education Program. *The Seventh Report of the Joint National Committee on the Prevention, Detection, Evaluation, and Treatment of High Blood Pressure.* Bethesda, MD, 2003, National Institutes of Health.
CAD, Coronary artery disease.

Table **15-14**

Adverse Drug Effects of Antihypertensive and Diuretic Drugs

MEDICATION	SIDE EFFECTS	PRECAUTIONS
DIURETICS		
Alpha-adrenergic blockers	"First-dose" syncope with prazosin; postural hypotension, weakness, palpitations, dizziness	Use cautiously in elderly patients because of hypotension.
Beta-adrenergic blockers	Bradycardia, insomnia, fatigue, sexual dysfunction, bizarre dreams, decreased HDL cholesterol	Do not use in patients with asthma, COPD, CHF, heart block, and sick sinus syndrome. Use with caution in patients with diabetes and peripheral vascular disease.
Central-acting adrenergic blockers	Drowsiness, fatigue, sexual dysfunction, dry mouth	Clonidine and guanabenz may produce rebound hypertension if abruptly stopped. Methyldopa may cause liver damage and a positive direct Coombs' test.
Combined alpha- and beta-adrenergic blockers	Nausea, fatigue, dizziness, asthma, headache	Do not give with sick sinus syndrome or heart block; use with caution in CHF, bronchial asthma, COPD, diabetes mellitus.
Loop diuretics	Same as for thiazides	Effective in chronic renal failure; use caution regarding hypokalemia and hyperuricemia; may cause hyponatremia, especially in the elderly.
Peripheral-acting adrenergic inhibitors	Sexual dysfunction, nasal congestion, postural hypotension, diarrhea, lethargy	Use very cautiously in elderly patients because of the hypotension. Rauwolfia and reserpine are not to be given to patients with a history of mental depression.
Potassium-sparing agents	Hyperkalemia, sexual dysfunction, gynecomastia, mastodynia	Monitor fluid and electrolytes
Thiazides and thiazide-related sulfonamides	Hypokalemia, hyperuricemia, glucose intolerance, hypercholesterolemia, sexual dysfunction	May be ineffective in renal failure; hypokalemia increases digitalis toxicity; hyperuricemia may precipitate acute gout.

Continued

Table 15-14		
Adverse Drug Effects of Antihypertensive and Diuretic Drugs—cont'd		
MEDICATION	**SIDE EFFECTS**	**PRECAUTIONS**
VASODILATORS		
Vasodilators	Headache, tachycardia, and fluid retention Hydralazine may produce positive ANA Minoxidil may produce abnormal growth of hair, ascites (intraperitoneal pooling of large amount of fluid)	May produce angina in patients with coronary artery disease. Lupus-like syndrome may occur with higher doses of hydralazine. May cause or aggravate pleural and pericardial effusions.
ANGIOTENSIN-CONVERTING ENZYME INHIBITORS		
ACE inhibitors	Hyperkalemia, nonproductive cough (frequent)	Can cause neutropenia with autoimmune-collagen disorders. May cause proteinuria or reversible acute renal failure in patients with bilateral renal artery stenosis.
CALCIUM CHANNEL BLOCKING AGENTS		
Calcium channel blockers	Headache, hypotension, nausea, dizziness, flushing, edema, constipation	Use with caution in patients with CHF or heart block; do not administer immediately after MI.

ANA, Antinuclear antibody; *COPD,* chronic obstructive pulmonary disease.

Nursing Implications and Patient Teaching

Assessment

You should learn as much as possible about the health history of the patient. Although the cause for most high blood pressure is unknown, the health care provider will look for any disease that might also cause hypertension, such as Cushing's disease, Addison's disease, renal artery stenosis, coarctation of the aorta, or pheochromocytoma. You will want to ask about whether the patient has other diseases, allergies, or medications that may affect antihypertensives and diuretics.

The number of drug side effects and problems that occur when hypertension is not treated well enough is high, and good record keeping is important in learning if the patient is getting well.

Diagnosis

Does the patient understand that she may need to take high blood pressure drugs for the rest of her life? Does the patient understand that she will need to change her life style in order to reduce high blood pressure? What factors does the patient have that will make therapy difficult?

Planning

Because there is no cure for high blood pressure, a lot of patient teaching and education is needed to help the patient understand what is happening to him and to gain his help in successful treatment. Although taking the medication is important, it is also important to work on other things in the patient's life, such as removing risk factors and changing the diet.

Implementation

Many patients with hypertension do not feel sick, so they have a hard time being compliant with the treatment regimen. High blood pressure is a "silent disease" because it has no symptoms. Because patients may only have symptoms as a result of side effects from their medication, they may not want to take drugs. It is important to teach patients about what is really happening to them to help them understand their disease.

Because of the high costs for antihypertensive drugs and the desire of patients to have control over their therapy, many patients explore the use of herbal medications to lower blood pressure. The Complementary and Alternative Therapies box describes some of the more common herbal products that patients may use. Little research has been done to show if herbal products are safe or helpful.

You should help encourage patients to lose weight, lower sodium intake, avoid stress and emotional pressures, develop regular and reasonable exercise routines, and have hobbies or activities that make them feel good about themselves (improve self-esteem). Remind them that taking their medications is only a small part of the total treatment plan.

Evaluation

In addition to taking the patient's blood pressure, a good eye examination can tell if the patient is keeping her

Complementary and Alternative Therapies

Hypertension

HERBAL PREPARATION	COMMENTS
Coleus	Potential interactions with anticoagulants, aspirin, NSAIDs, antiplatelet agents
Garlic	Potential interaction with anticoagulants, aspirin, NSAIDs, antiplatelet agents; may potentiate antihypertensives, antihyperlipidemics
Hawthorn	May interact with antidysrhythmics, antihypertensives, cardiac glycosides, ACE inhibitors, angiotensin II receptor blockers

Modified from Krinsky DL, Lavella JB, Hawkins EB, et al: *Natural therapeutics pocket guide*, ed 2, Hudson, Ohio, 2003, Lexi-Comp, Inc.
NSAIDs, Nonsteroidal antiinflammatory drugs.

blood pressure down. The blood vessels of the eye can be seen by looking through the pupil into the eye with an ophthalmoscope. By examining the fundus of the eye, it is possible to tell whether the blood pressure has been high even if it is low when the patient is seen. Many parts of the body are damaged by high blood pressure: the heart, the lungs, the eyes, and the kidneys. You will want to ask if the patient has any complaints that might suggest that she has problems in any of these areas (end-organ damage). Find out what side effects she might be experiencing as she takes the medications. Men should always be asked about their sexual functioning because impotence is often caused by these medications. They usually will not tell anyone this information unless asked, and they may not even realize that sexual problems may be caused by their medication.

Patient and Family Teaching

You should tell the patient and family the following:
1. The patient should take this medication just as ordered by the nurse, physician, or other health care provider. If a dose is missed, it should be taken as soon as it is remembered, if it is within an hour or two of the scheduled time. If it is close to the next scheduled dose, the next dose should be taken at the regular time; the doses should not be doubled.
2. The patient should take medication with a full glass of orange juice (unless not permitted by diet). Other potassium-rich foods should be eaten daily, including citrus foods (especially oranges and tomatoes), bananas, dried fruits, apricots, cantaloupe, watermelon, nuts, dried beans, beef, and fowl.
3. The patient should know that taking the medication is only one part of the treatment plan. Getting rid of other risk factors is also important, such as losing weight (if overweight), lowering sodium intake, stopping smoking, increasing exercise, and avoiding extra stress and emotional pressures. The patient should avoid foods high in sodium, such as lunch meats, smoked meats, Chinese food, processed cheese, and snack foods. The patient should not salt food when cooking or add salt to food after it is cooked.

4. Numerous side effects could occur from use of these drugs. The patient must notify the nurse, physician, or other health care provider of any new or uncomfortable symptoms that develop. Changing drugs may be necessary to find the best drugs. The patient and all the people working to help him get better should have a good relationship. It is very important for the patient to keep appointments and to want to come back for care.
5. This medication must be kept out of the reach of children and others for whom it is not prescribed because it is very dangerous for them. The patient should not leave it lying on night tables or low dressers where young children might take it accidentally.
6. The goal of therapy is to help the patient feel as healthy as possible and to avoid any long-term problems. There is no cure for most high blood pressure, and therapy lasts a lifetime. Taking medication and getting rid of other risk factors will help lower the chance of serious problems in the future. It is important to keep taking the medicine, even when the patient feels well, and to keep seeing the health care provider regularly.
7. Patients should wear a Medic Alert bracelet or necklace and carry a medical identification card saying that they have high blood pressure and listing the drugs that they are taking.

OTHER NONDIURETIC DRUGS USEFUL IN TREATING URINARY PROBLEMS

OVERVIEW

There are many problems that might produce urinary tract symptoms. Drugs used for these problems usually involve giving relief for symptoms. These include drugs that are used to treat urinary incontinence (wetting) and benign prostatic hyperplasia (BPH) and drugs for urinary tract analgesia (pain relief) that are used for urinary tract infections.

ACTION AND USES

Drugs for Urinary Incontinence

Urinary incontinence is when patients wet themselves or leak urine, and this problem may have many causes. Medications used in treating this problem include some anticholinergics/antispasmodics, alpha-adrenergic agonists, estrogens, cholinergic agonists, and alpha-adrenergic antagonists. The anticholinergic agents stop contraction of the bladder and decrease the response of some of the bladder muscles. Antispasmodic drugs have a direct action on smooth muscle relaxation. Estrogen used either orally or vaginally may help restore urethral mucosa and increase vascularity, tone, and the ability of the urethral muscle to respond.

Benign Prostatic Hyperplasia

This is a noncancerous growth of the prostate gland; if this gland becomes large enough, it can cause voiding problems. Drugs used in the management of BPH are the alpha$_1$-adrenergic receptor blockers (these have already been discussed for the treatment of hypertension). Tamsulosin (Flomax) is an alpha-adrenergic receptor blocker used only for the treatment of symptoms of BPH. Finasteride is also used for treatment of BPH.

Short-Term Analgesia

Phenazopyridine is a drug used to control pain in the urinary tract, usually from acute urinary tract infection.

Nursing Implications and Patient Teaching

Assessment

Talk with the patient to make certain you understand the patient's symptoms. The patient may be nervous about talking about these problems.

Diagnosis

Find out the reason why the medication is being given. Are the symptoms because of another problem, or do they represent the major problem? (Is there other gynecologic or genitourinary disease present?) Read any medical records kept by the patient about her urinary incontinence or voiding problems. This may be helpful in learning the cause of the symptoms.

Planning

Teach the patient about why he has the problem and how the medication will help.

Implementation

Sometimes the patient is asked to keep a bladder diary. If so, explain clearly how to keep the records about her accidents and why. Give the patient a lot of support so they will be compliant.

Drug action and uses, adverse effects, drug interactions, and important patient teaching points are given in Table 15-15.

Table 15-15

Miscellaneous Nondiuretic Drugs Used to Treat Urinary Problems

ACTION AND USES MEDICATION	ACTION AND USES	ADVERSE EFFECTS	DRUG INTERACTIONS	NURSING IMPLICATIONS AND PATIENT TEACHING
DRUGS FOR URINARY INCONTINENCE				
Anticholinergics/Antispasmodics				
flavoxate (Urispas)	Antispasmodic action for dysuria, nocturia, urgency, suprapubic pain, frequency, incontinence caused by detrusor instability, and hyperreflexia	Headache, confusion, nervousness, nausea, vomiting	Enhances anticholinergic effects of other anticholinergic drugs	
oxybutynin chloride (Ditropan)	Used to relieve symptoms associated with detrusor instability, hyperreflexia, or involuntary bladder contractions	Drowsiness, dry mouth, blurred vision, constipation; may aggravate symptoms of heart disease, hyperthyroidism, GI problems	May increase digoxin serum concentrations; may decrease action of haloperidol and enhance development of tardive dyskinesia (repeated involuntary muscle movements); avoid alcohol	Requires careful patient teaching concerning response and side effects; monitor clinical effectiveness through use of a bladder diary documenting voiding activity

Table 15-15

Miscellaneous Nondiuretic Drugs Used to Treat Urinary Problems—cont'd

ACTION AND USES MEDICATION	ACTION AND USES	ADVERSE EFFECTS	DRUG INTERACTIONS	NURSING IMPLICATIONS AND PATIENT TEACHING
DRUGS FOR URINARY INCONTINENCE—cont'd				
Anticholinergics/Antispasmodics—cont'd				
propantheline (Pro-Banthine)	Treats involuntary ureteral and bladder contractions by competitively blocking action of acetylcholine at postganglionic parasympathetic receptor sites	Dry mouth, constipation, urinary retention	Increases effect of narcotic analgesics, class I antidysrhythmics, antihistamines, phenothiazines, TCAs, corticosteroids, CNS depressants, beta blockers, and amoxapine	
tolterodine (Detrol)	For urinary frequency, urgency, and urge incontinence caused by bladder overactivity	Less dry mouth than with oxybutynin; dyspepsia, headache, constipation, dry eyes	None noted	Avoid tolterodine in patients with glaucoma, ulcerative colitis, megacolon, GI or urinary obstruction; use with care in individuals with BPH
Cholinergic Agonist				
bethanechol chloride	Used in nonobstructive urinary retention	Hypotension, dizziness, flushing, sweating	With other cholinergics, additive cholinergic effects and toxicity may occur	Dosage highly individualized
DRUGS FOR BENIGN PROSTATIC HYPERPLASIA				
Alpha-Adrenergic Antagonists				
finasteride (Proscar)	Symptoms of BPH	Impotence, decreased libido, decreased volume of ejaculate, breast tenderness and enlargement, hypersensitivity reactions including lip swelling and skin rash	None noted	May be taken with or without food; 6-12 mo of therapy may be required to assess response
tamsulosin (Flomax)	Treats symptoms of BPH by selective inhibition of alpha$_{1A}$ receptors	Postural hypotension, dizziness, somnolence, rhinitis, diarrhea, abnormal ejaculation	Potentiates other alpha-adrenergic blocking agents	Take at the same time every day, approximately ½ hr after eating; may take 2-4 wk before response is seen
DRUG FOR URINARY TRACT ANALGESIA				
phenazopyridine (Pyridium) ✦	Symptomatic relief of pain, burning, urgency, frequency associated with UTI	Headaches, rash, vertigo, GI disturbance, anaphylactic (shock)-like reactions	None noted	Stains the urine orange or red and may stain fabrics; notify doctor if patient develops jaundice (yellow color of skin or eyes); available OTC

TCA, Tricyclic antidepressant; *UTI,* urinary tract infection.

Evaluation

All of these medications should reduce symptoms. Explain to patients how they will know when the medication is working. For medications related to BPH, explain that treatment may be required for weeks or months before their symptoms go away.

Patient and Family Teaching

You should tell the patient and family the following:
1. The patient and family should learn the causes of urinary incontinence or BPH.
2. The embarrassment some patients feel can be eased by talking about how common these problems are for patients.
3. The patient should be taught any special things he needs to know about taking the medication with food or after meals.
4. Patients may be asked to keep records to help show the results of treatment; these should be reviewed at each patient visit.
5. The patient who is taking medication for urinary pain should know that the drug will change the color of the urine. Patients should return for further treatment if symptoms return after they have taken all the medication.

SECTION SIX

Fluid and Electrolytes

OVERVIEW

Strong pumping of the heart, good circulation through the vessels, and the full removal of by-products through the urinary system are all needed to keep the body's fluid and electrolyte balance. Lack of body fluid may be due to inadequate intake, excess loss, or both. This imbalance may be treated by administration of fluids and electrolyte mixtures.

ACTION AND USES

Fluid and electrolyte mixtures are solutions of water and calories in the form of carbohydrates, with minerals and electrolytes such as sodium, potassium, chloride, calcium, and phosphorus. These are given when oral food intake has been stopped or to prevent **dehydration** (loss of a large amount of water from the body tissues, along with loss of electrolytes), especially in patients with diarrhea.

Causes of dehydration include vomiting, bowel obstruction (which causes a pooling of fluid and electrolytes), diarrhea, and fever (which increases the use of fluid and electrolytes). The body attempts to adjust to the reduced circulating volume by pulling in first extracellular fluid and then intracellular fluid. This causes an imbalance of both fluid and electrolytes that must be corrected.

Fluid and electrolytes may be given either orally or parenterally to prevent dehydration when oral intake is briefly halted and to replace moderate losses of fluids and electrolytes (Table 15-16 and Box 15-1).

Electrolyte solutions are especially useful in managing dehydration in infants caused by diarrhea.

Nursing Implications and Patient Teaching

Signs of dehydration include weight loss, dry skin, lack of sweat, dry mucous membranes, decreased urinary output, hypotension, tachycardia, and increased respirations. In infants, dehydration may also include sunken fontanelles and loss of skin turgor (strength and mass). Fluid and electrolytes are also required in the comatose or acutely ill patient who is unable to take oral substances for a long time.

These solutions are contraindicated when the patient has severe or continuing diarrhea or other major fluid loss that requires IV replacement or has vomiting that cannot be stopped. They should not be used in patients with intestinal obstruction or bowel perforation (opening), or decreased renal function, or when the homeostatic mechanism of the body is damaged.

The prescribed amount should not be exceeded. If the patient is still thirsty after taking the recommended dose, extra fluids in the form of water or other fluids that do not contain electrolytes should be given.

 Clinical Landmine

Electrolyte Deficiency

Electrolyte deficiency may also result if the patient increases intake of liquids with a low mineral content (such as drinking distilled water after vigorous exercise and sweating).

Table 15-16

Fluid and Electrolytes for Oral Administration

PRODUCT	COMMENTS AND DOSAGE
ORAL ELECTROLYTE SOLUTIONS	
Pedialyte	Dosage should be based on water requirements calculated on the basis of total body surface area for infants and young children. A general guide uses 1500 mL/m^2 for maintenance during illness and 2400 mL/m^2 for maintenance and replacement of mild to moderate fluid losses (as in diarrhea or vomiting). *Replacement in mild to moderate fluid losses:* *Children 5-10 years of age:* 1-2 quarts/day *Older children and adults:* 2-3 quarts/day
SALT SUBSTITUTES	
Adolph's salt substitute Morton salt substitute Neocurtasal NoSalt Nu-Salt	OTC preparations that can be used in both cooked and uncooked foods to make food more palatable for patients with sodium restrictions. These potassium chloride preparations come in a salt shaker dispenser and are used in amounts slightly less than normal amounts of NaCl. Contraindicated in patients with severe kidney disease or oliguria. Long-term use may require iodine supplements in some patients.
SALT SUBSTITUTES	
sodium bicarbonate	Used as gastric, systemic, and urinary alkalinizer. May relieve symptoms of occasional overeating and indigestion. Give 325 mg to 2 gm 2-4 times daily. Daily maximum intake should not exceed 16 gm.

Box 15-1 | **Fluid and Electrolytes for Parenteral Administration**

- Products are available in a variety of concentrations, volumes, and combinations
- See the physician or other health care provider's order and the package insert

AMINO ACIDS
- Amino acid substrates with electrolytes in a variety of combinations

CARBOHYDRATES
- Dextrose in water with 2.5% to 70% concentrations
- 5% or 10% alcohol in 5% dextrose infusions
- 10% fructose in water
- 10% invert sugar in water

ELECTROLYTES
- 0.2% to 5% sodium chloride solutions
- Potassium chloride or potassium acetate for injection

ELECTROLYTES—cont'd
- Calcium chloride for injection
- Calcium gluconate for injection
- Calcium gluceptate for injection
- Calcium products—combined
- Magnesium sulfate or magnesium chloride for injection
- Sodium bicarbonate for injection
- Sodium lactate for injection
- Sodium acetate for injection
- Tromethamine for slow infusion
- Sodium phosphate for injection
- Potassium phosphate for injection
- Ammonium chloride for injection

TRACE METALS (FOR SLOW INFUSION)
- Zinc, copper, manganese, molybdenum, chromium, selenium, and iodine

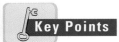

Key Points

- The major classes of cardiovascular medications are antianginals, peripheral vasodilators, antidysrhythmics, antihyperlipidemics, antihypertensives, cardiotonics, and diuretics. (Other miscellaneous drugs affecting the urinary tract are also included in the last section.)
- Each major class deals with an important part of the circulatory and renal systems.
- Cardiovascular medications are commonly used by patients, and you have an important teaching job in helping the patient understand the proper storage and use of medications.
- In addition, a thorough understanding of the anatomy and physiology of the heart is important, because this will help you understand both the cardiovascular problem and the action of the various medications.
- Electrolytes are given in the event that oral food intake has been suspended or are given to prevent dehydration and electrolyte loss.

Go to the free CD-ROM for an Audio Glossary, animations, video clips, and Review Questions for the NCLEX-PN® Examination.

evolve Be sure to visit the companion Evolve website at http://evolve.elsevier.com/Edmunds/LPN/ for WebLinks, a link to the top 200 drugs by prescription, and sign-up pages for newsletter drug updates.

CASE STUDY

A 50-year-old African American man comes to the clinic with a 1-week history of occipital headache that he describes as "a constant ache in the back of my head." The 650-mg Tylenol that he has taken regularly four to five times daily over the past week often has not cured his headache. Approximately 7 months ago, the patient was told that his blood pressure was "up" during a yearly employment physical. He has a history of asthma, gout, and angina. His father and sister have high blood pressure. His diet is high in fat and salt.

    Physical examination: Blood pressure: right arm sitting, 160/105 mm Hg; left arm sitting, 162/104 mm Hg. The heart is not enlarged; there are no murmurs or abnormal rhythms. Apical pulse, 84 beats/minute.

1. Assuming the patient's blood pressure remained at the same level after two subsequent blood pressure checks, what factors, specific to this patient, should be considered before placing the patient on antihypertensive medications?

2. What class of medication would most likely be of greatest help in controlling this patient's blood pressure with the fewest adverse reactions?
  a. Thiazide or loop diuretic.
  b. Beta blocker.
  c. Alpha blocker.
  d. Centrally acting agent.
  e. Adrenergic neuron blocking agent.
  f. Direct-acting vasodilating agent.
  g. Angiotensin-converting enzyme inhibitor.
  h. Calcium channel blocker.
3. Which of the drugs listed in question 2 would not be indicated?
4. The doctor orders hydrochlorothiazide 12.5 mg daily. What would you tell the patient about this drug?
5. Assuming the drug was ineffective in reducing the patient's blood pressure after 4 weeks, what could be done to achieve adequate control of the blood pressure?

DRUG CALCULATION REVIEW

1. Procainamide (Pronestyl) IV bolus of 0.1 gm has been ordered by the physician for a patient with frequent premature ventricular contractions. The vial is labeled 200 mg/mL. How many milliliters should the nurse prepare for this bolus?
2. Order: Inderal 30 mg by mouth 4 times per day
   Supply: Inderal 20 mg per tablet

Question: How many tablets of Inderal should be given with each dose?
3. Order: Lasix 60 mg by gastrostomy tube daily
   Supply: Lasix 20 mg/5 mL

Question: How many milliliters of Lasix should be given with each dose?

CRITICAL THINKING ?

1. Ms. Henson, age 70, was admitted to the hospital yesterday with acute angina pectoris. She is a heavy smoker and says that most evenings she drinks either wine or beer with her dinner and coffee with dessert every night. Her physician prescribes sublingual nitroglycerin for anginal pain. Describe major points to teach this patient, especially regarding medication storage and administration and the results she may expect. Draw up a plan of action for teaching and reviewing with Ms. Henson what she needs to know about contacting her physician if she has taken three nitroglycerin tablets and continues to have pain.

2. Point out some key distinctions between class I, class II, class III, and class IV antidysrhythmics. Consult Table 15-4 if you require additional information.

3. Explain the need for careful ECG monitoring of patients taking antidysrhythmic medications. Include what you should be sure to teach about each drug.

4. Identify nursing strategies and patient teaching points associated with bile acid sequestrants and antihyperlipidemic agents. Describe how to make these medications more palatable, methods for reducing unpleasant side effects, and the need for long-term medication and diet therapy and for regular medical follow-up.

5. Develop a generalized, introductory patient teaching plan for the patient with recently diagnosed hypertension. As a first step, be sure to break essential information down into several short lessons to avoid overwhelming the patient with information. Stress what the patient can do, rather than focusing only on what the patient should not do.

6. Describe the signs and symptoms of CHF and of the various dysrhythmias. Why might a dysrhythmia cause CHF?

7. Create a teaching plan for the patient taking a digitalis product. Be sure to include the following elements: (1) why the drug is needed, (2) why it is important to take the drug regularly, (3) what adverse effects to watch out for, (4) how to take a radial pulse, and (5) what to do if the radial pulse falls below 60 beats/minute.

8. Using the information from Question 7, explain the reasons for the nursing interventions that should be used when a patient exhibits signs and symptoms of digitalis toxicity.

9. Miss Green comes in for treatment of a urinary tract infection. She is in great pain, and the doctor tells her to buy Pyridium, an OTC product. What information does Miss Green need to know in taking this product?

10. When obtaining a nursing history from a patient taking a newly prescribed diuretic, what information would be a priority? What questions would you ask the patient to obtain this information?

11. Referring to your data obtained in Question 10, what information would you want to emphasize in a teaching plan for this patient?

12. You are asked to monitor a new patient, Ms. Falk, for dehydration. Review the signs and symptoms of dehydration. When is dehydration most likely to occur?

13. Ms. Falk has been told she needs fluid and electrolyte supplementation. Explain to her the reasons for such therapy and how it will help her.

16 Central and Peripheral Nervous System Medications

Objectives

After reading and studying this chapter, you should be able to do the following:

1. Identify the major classes of drugs that affect the central nervous system.
2. Explain the major actions of drugs used to treat disorders of the central nervous system.
3. List different actions of antimigraine products.
4. Identify the role of psychotropic drugs in psychotherapeutic intervention.
5. Compare and contrast different categories of medications used to treat depression.

Key Terms

Be sure to check out the bonus material on the free CD-ROM, including selected audio pronunciations.

acetylcholine (ăs-ē-tĭl-KŌ-lēn, p. 265)
adrenergic blocking agents (ăd-rĕn-ĔRJ-ĭk, p. 265)
adrenergic drugs (p. 265)
adrenergic fibers (p. 265)
anticholinergics (ăn-tĭ-kō-lĭn-ĔRJ-ĭk, p. 265)
barbiturates (băr-BĬ-chŭr-āts, p. 269)
catecholamines (kăt-ē-KŌ-lă-mēnz, p. 265)
central nervous system (p. 264)
cholinergic drugs (ko-lĭn-ĔRJ-ĭk, p. 265)
cholinergic fibers (p. 265)
hypnotic agent (hĭp-NŎT-ĭk, p. 306)
idiopathic (ĭd-ē-ō-PĂTH-ĭk, p. 269)
initial insomnia (ĭn-ĬSH-ăl ĭn-SŎM-nē-ă, p. 306)
intermittent insomnia (ĭn-tĕr-MĬT-ĕnt ĭn-SŎM-nē-ă, p. 306)
neurotransmitters (nŭr-ō-TRĂNS-mĭt-ĕrz, p. 265)
norepinephrine (NŌR-ĕp-ĭn-ĔF-rĕn, p. 265)
Parkinson's disease (p. 282)
peripheral nervous system (pĕ-RĬF-ĕr-ăl, p. 264)
receptor (rē-SĔP-tŏr, p. 265)
sedative agent (SĔD-ă-tĭv, p. 306)
seizures (SĒ-zhŭrz, p. 269)
status epilepticus (STĂT-ŭs ĕp-ĭ-LĔP-tĭ-kŭs, p. 271)
terminal insomnia (TŬR-mĭn-ăl ĭn-SŎM-nē-ă, p. 306)

OVERVIEW

This chapter has six sections discussing drugs that act on various parts of the central nervous system (CNS). Although many drugs are used in treating CNS diseases, the principles of drug usage, actions of the medications, and adverse reactions are very similar. You will benefit from learning how these drugs are the same and how they are different for the various categories of drugs. Although narcotic and nonnarcotic analgesics are also CNS drugs, they will be discussed in Chapter 17.

Section One of this chapter explores antimigraine agents. Section Two covers the medications used to treat various types of seizures. Section Three discusses drugs for vertigo (feeling of dizziness or spinning), and Section Four presents drugs used to treat Parkinson's disease. Section Five introduces all the psychotropic drugs and includes subsections dealing specifically with medications used to treat anxiety, depression, and psychosis, and with lithium, a unique medication. Section Six discusses sedative-hypnotics and their use in anxiety and sleep disorders.

NERVOUS SYSTEM

The major structures of the nervous system include the brain, spinal cord, nerves, and sensory receptors (Figure 16-1). The nervous system regulates and coordinates the body's activities, including the senses, controls movement, and coordinates physiologic and intellectual functions.

The nervous system has two divisions, the central and the peripheral. The **central nervous system,** made up of the brain and the spinal cord, is located within the cranial cavity of the skull and the vertebral canal of the spinal column. The **peripheral nervous system** includes all nervous structures (ganglia and nerves) that lie outside the cranial cavity and the vertebral canal. These include the cranial and spinal nerves and the sympathetic division of the autonomic nervous system.

Pathology located in the brain may produce either local or general symptoms; abnormalities in the

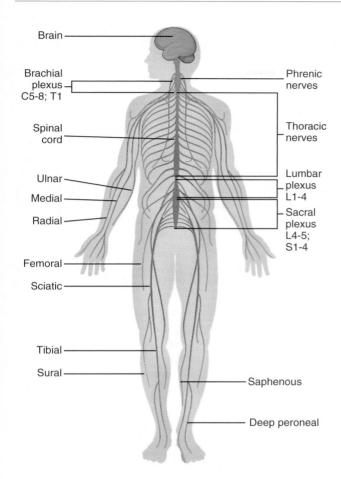

FIGURE **16-1** Central nervous system. *C*, Cervical; *L*, lumbar; *S*, spinal; *T*, thoracic.

peripheral system usually cause only local symptoms. Because the nerve and muscle systems are mixed together so closely, it is often difficult to tell if disease lies within the nerves or the structures activated by the nerves.

Although the drugs covered in this chapter focus on the actions of the CNS, or those actions controlled by the brain and spinal cord, many of these agents act through the peripheral nervous system (PNS). The PNS produces changes or activity in the body through the nerves and chemicals of the motor nervous system and the autonomic nervous system as they carry out directions from the CNS.

To learn how drugs act on the CNS, you should understand how nerves send or transmit information from the brain through chemical messengers or **neurotransmitters.** The neurotransmitter chemical is released at the end of one neuron and passes across a small gap to activate the next neuron in the chain. At the end of the nerve chain, it stimulates an organ, smooth muscle, or gland to produce a physiologic response.

The two major neurotransmitters in the body are **norepinephrine,** which acts on the sympathetic nerves, and **acetylcholine,** which acts on the parasympathetic nerves. There are several other important neurotransmitters, especially in the brain. Nerve fibers that release norepinephrine are called **adrenergic fibers.** Nerve fibers that release acetylcholine are called **cholinergic fibers.** Most organs in the body are influenced by both types of fibers, which have opposite effects. For example, adrenergic activity speeds up the heart rate, and cholinergic activity slows it down. It is possible to compare this system to a car that is influenced by an accelerator and a brake.

There are several names for the types of drugs that act on the CNS. Drugs that produce effects in the body similar to those produced by norepinephrine are called **adrenergic drugs,** or sympathomimetic drugs. These drugs are also referred to as **catecholamines.** There are three naturally occurring catecholamines in the body: norepinephrine, which is secreted from nerve terminals; epinephrine, which is secreted from the adrenal medulla; and dopamine, which is found at selected sites within the brain, kidneys, and gastrointestinal (GI) tract.

Those drugs whose action is similar to acetylcholine are called **cholinergic drugs,** or parasympathomimetic drugs. Agents that block the release of acetylcholine and inhibit cholinergic activity are called **anticholinergics.** Agents that block the release of epinephrine and norepinephrine and inhibit the adrenergic system are called **adrenergic blocking agents.** An overdose of cholinergic drugs can cause a "cholinergic crisis." These basic terms are used throughout this chapter. Remembering these terms and definitions will help you understand drug actions.

When neurotransmitters release their chemicals, the chemicals are targeted to act at certain parts of the body. Each neurotransmitter has a certain chemical shape (like a key), which produces an action only when it "fits into" a specific **receptor** (lock) for that chemical. These receptors are classified as alpha, beta, or dopaminergic. The alpha and beta receptors are further divided into types 1 and 2. When stimulated, alpha and beta receptors often have opposite effects on the heart, blood vessels, GI tract, or eye muscles. The text will often refer to a medication as having alpha or beta properties. For example, some medications are called *beta blockers* because of their selective action in blocking only the beta-adrenergic effects in the body.

Many of the drugs discussed in the following sections act on more than one type of receptor. Each agent acts differently, making it possible for certain drugs to be given for specific actions without many adverse reactions. It should be clear that, if dosages are exceeded, many receptors may be overly stimulated, causing widespread and serious effects. Thus, accuracy is very important in giving these drugs.

Antimigraine Agents

ACTION

Antimigraine agents block nerve impulses in the receptors of the sympathetic nervous system. The ergot alkaloids used in the prophylaxis and treatment of vascular headaches are adrenergic-blocking agents. Adrenergic-blocking agents dilate the veins in smooth muscle tissue in the peripheral vascular system and the uterus. This reduces cerebral blood flow and arterial pulsing, which reduces the headache pain. Other actions include an increase in contractions of the uterus (oxytocic effect) and a decrease in blood pressure.

The process that produces migraine headaches is thought to be local dilation of the blood vessels in the cranium or the release of sensory neuropeptides through nerve endings in the trigeminal system. The vascular 5-hydroxytryptamine (5-HT) receptor is present on the human basilar artery and in the vessels of human dura mater. Use of the 5-HT, or serotonin, receptor antagonists results in cranial vessel constriction (narrowing) and blocking of neuropeptides that cause inflammation, which happens at the same time the patient feels the relief from migraine headache. Some of these products also cross the blood-brain barrier, produce central activity on the trigeminovascular system, and stop nerve depolarization at peripheral sites in the cranium.

USES

Antimigraine agents are used in both the prevention and the treatment of vascular headaches. They relieve the pain of vascular headaches by narrowing dilated cerebral arteries. They are also used, although less commonly, in pregnant women for oxytocic and other smooth muscle spasmogenic effects. The action of 5-HT agonists is not affected by whether or not the migraine has an aura, length of attack, sex or age of the patient, relationship to menstrual period, or use of other common migraine prevention drugs.

ADVERSE REACTIONS

Adverse reactions to antimigraine agents include heart murmurs, brief tachycardia (rapid heartbeat), confusion, depression, dizziness, drowsiness, fixed miosis (constriction) of the pupil of the eye, paresthesias (numbness and tingling) in the toes, weakness (especially in legs), nausea and vomiting, leg cramps, localized pruritus (itching) and edema (fluid buildup in the body tissues),

and neutropenia of the blood. Symptoms of overdosage include numb, cold, pale extremities; constant muscle pain even at rest; decreased or absent arterial pulses; drowsiness; confusion; depression; convulsions; hemiplegia; and fixed miosis. Because of the potential for 5-HT agonists to cause coronary vasospasm, patients with ischemic heart disease or other major cardiovascular disease, or uncontrolled hypertension (high blood pressure) should not use these products.

DRUG INTERACTIONS

When antimigraine agents are used with other vasoconstrictors, vasoconstriction may be increased. The 5-HT agonists may not be used within 24 hours of taking an ergotamine-containing preparation and may not be used at the same time with monoamine oxidase (MAO) inhibitor therapy (given for depression).

Nursing Implications and Patient Teaching

Assessment

You should learn as much as possible about the health history of the patient in order to identify the type of headache (whether tension, migraine, or cluster) and to rule out things that might prevent the use of these drugs, such as coronary artery disease or conditions in which a sudden change in blood pressure may be dangerous.

The patient may have a history of migraine headaches, vascular headaches, or headache pain of a periodic, throbbing, severe nature. The pain may be one-sided (unilateral) and is commonly felt over one eye. Photophobia (sensitivity to light) and sensitivity to sound may be present, as well as nausea and vomiting. A family history of vascular headaches or history of motion sickness as a child, series of headaches in clusters, history of hypertension, a food allergy, or use of birth control pills may be present. The headache may be relieved or eased by sleeping or vomiting or drinking a caffeinated drink.

You should ask about whether the patient uses any herbal products or vitamins to control headache or migraines, because some of these products may interact adversely with other drugs, including nonsteroidal antiinflammatory drugs (NSAIDs). The Complementary and Alternative Therapies box summarizes herbal preparations the patient may be using and their drug interactions. You may observe signs of sweaty hands and feet, scalp tenderness, autonomic dysfunction (such as miotic pupil), red eye, and unilateral nasal congestion.

Complementary and Alternative Therapies

Headache

PRODUCT	COMMENTS
Feverfew	Potential interaction with anticoagulants, aspirin, NSAIDs, antiplatelet agents
Gingko	Potential interaction with anticoagulants, aspirin, NSAIDs, antiplatelet agents; may interact with MAO inhibitors, acetylcholinesterase inhibitors
White willow	Potential interaction with aspirin, anticoagulants, methotrexate, metoclopramide, phenytoin, probenecid, spironolactone, valproic acid, NSAIDs, antiplatelet agents

Modified from Krinsky DL, Lavella JB, Hawkins EB, et al: *Natural therapeutics pocket guide,* ed 2, Hudson, Ohio, 2003, Lexi-Comp, Inc.

Diagnosis

In addition to the medical diagnosis, what other symptoms does this patient have that require nursing action? Are there needs for patient education, nutrition information, and quiet time away from people? Sometimes identifying the migraine triggers leads to the diagnosis of other emotional or physical problems.

Planning

The diagnosis of vascular headaches can be made if the patient's pain is relieved after an intramuscular (IM) injection of 1 mL (0.5 mg) of ergotamine.

Ergot alkaloids increase uterine contraction and may be harmful to the pregnant patient. These migraine medications are slowly and incompletely absorbed from the GI tract. Traces of ergotamine remain in various tissues; this accounts for its long-lasting and toxic actions.

Implementation

If migraine agents are used at the onset of an attack, the ability of the drugs to relieve migraine pain and symptoms is increased.

These products are available in oral, sublingual, parenteral, and rectal forms, and as a solution for inhalation. Deciding which form to use requires you to think about many factors, including whether the purpose of the agent is to prevent or to treat migraine.

Oral and rectal preparations are absorbed slowly and incompletely from the GI tract. To speed up this absorption, caffeine is included with oral and rectal preparations of ergot alkaloids. Persons who are vomiting and cannot tolerate oral preparations are given rectal forms of the agent. Inhalant methods are preferred by some patients. Sublingual tablets are more quickly absorbed than either rectal or oral preparations. IM and subcutaneous preparations are commonly used, but absorption is often incomplete and slow.

A list of important dosage information about antimigraine products is presented in Table 16-1.

Evaluation

You should monitor the patient to see if the drug is helping: there should be a decrease in number and severity of migraine headaches. To determine if overdosage, toxicity, or adverse reactions are developing, you should monitor the patient's blood pressure in standing, sitting, and lying positions and check for peripheral pulses.

Long-term use of migraine agents can lead to acute overdosage or chronic toxicity because of the wide variability in their absorption, metabolism, and excretion. Because patients often treat themselves, they may not realize that they are overdosing themselves.

Abruptly stopping migraine agents after long-term use can result in rebound (or new-onset) migraine headaches; therefore, they should be stopped very slowly.

Patient and Family Teaching

You should tell the patient and family the following:

1. The patient should take the medication as ordered and not increase the dosage without talking to the nurse, physician, or other health care provider because acute poisoning or overdosage may result.
2. The patient should not allow his arms and legs to get cold after taking this medication.
3. The nurse, physician, or other health care provider should be contacted immediately if numbness, coldness of extremities, or pain in the legs during walking occurs.
4. Oral antimigraine agents may produce stomach upset. The medicine should be taken with milk or meals if possible to decrease this effect.
5. Common side effects of antimigraine agents include headache, nausea, vomiting, diarrhea, dizziness, and light-headedness when rapidly changing positions.
6. After taking this drug, the patient should lie down immediately in a quiet, dark room to help obtain relief of symptoms. Soft music or relaxation techniques may also benefit the patient.
7. The nurse, physician, or other health care provider should be contacted immediately if more than 8 mg of oral ergotamine is needed to relieve migraine pain.
8. This drug should not be used by a female patient who suspects she is pregnant.

Table **16-1**

Antimigraine Preparations

GENERIC NAME	TRADE NAME	COMMENTS AND DOSAGE
ERGOTAMINE DERIVATIVES		
dihydroergotamine	DHE 45 Migranal	An alpha-adrenergic blocking agent with pharmacologic and toxic properties similar to ergotamine used to treat migraine headaches. The drug causes cerebral vasculature to constrict, but it does not have an oxytocic effect and can be used during pregnancy. • *Migraine treatment:* 1 mg IM to be repeated at hourly intervals, not to exceed a total of 3 mg; or 1 mg IV to be repeated once. The total weekly dose should not exceed 6 mg or 1 spray in each nostril; repeat in 15 min as needed.
ergotamine tartrate	Ergomar	An alpha-adrenergic blocking agent that exerts direct vasoconstriction on cranial blood vessels, relieving pulsations thought to be responsible for vasoconstriction. Dependence on ergotamine may develop, necessitating gradual withdrawal from this product. • *Migraine treatment:* 2 mg PO or sublingually at the start of an attack, followed by 1 mg every 30 min as needed for full relief, up to 6 mg per migraine attack or 10 mg/wk; the total amount is then used for subsequent attacks.
Combination products	Cafergot Cafetrate supps Ercaf Midrin Wigraine	Cafergot is a combination of ergotamine, caffeine, and other products used to treat migraine and vascular headaches. Caffeine is included in these products to increase absorption of ergot alkaloids. Small amounts of belladonna alkaloids and barbiturates may also be included to control nausea and produce sedation. • *Migraine treatment:* 2 tablets PO at the start of an attack, followed by 1 tablet every 30 min to a maximum of 6 tablets per attack or 10 per week; or 1 suppository at the start of an attack. This dosage may be repeated 1 hr later if needed. Do not exceed 2 suppositories per attack, or 5 per week.
methysergide maleate	Sansert	Used as a migraine prophylactic for patients suffering from one or more severe vascular headaches per week. Thought to block serotonin activity in the CNS, which may be related to vascular headaches. This drug can produce highly toxic effects. Therefore, continuous administration should not exceed 6 mo. After each 6-mo course of therapy, 3-4 wk should be drug-free, followed by another 6-mo course of medicine. Monitor weight and watch for signs of edema, toxicity, and fibrosis at regular 3-mo intervals. Because of significant adverse effects in some individuals, reserve this drug for patients with severe, frequent, uncontrollable headaches. • *Migraine prophylaxis:* 4-8 mg daily in divided doses with meals or milk.
SEROTONIN (5-HT) RECEPTOR AGONISTS		
almotriptan	Axert	Give 6.25 or 12.5 mg for acute treatment of migraine in adults; may repeat after 2 hr.
naratriptan	Amerge	Single doses of 1 or 2.5 mg taken with fluid are effective in relieving acute pain; if headache returns or patient has only partial response, repeat dose in 4 hr. Higher doses do not produce better results.
rizatriptan benzoate	Maxalt	Take 5 or 10 mg; may be repeated after at least 2 hr. Do not exceed more than 30 mg in any 24-hr period. Comes as a tablet or an orally disintegrating tablet that does not require liquid but must not be opened until just before dosing.

Table 16-1

Antimigraine Preparations—cont'd

GENERIC NAME	TRADE NAME	COMMENTS AND DOSAGE
sumatriptan succinate	Imitrex	*Oral:* 25 mg taken with fluids as early as possible. Maximum single dose is 100 mg. Additional doses may be taken every 2 hr up to total of 200 mg/day. *Injection:* Maximum single dose 6 mg subcutaneously; may repeat once in 1 hr. *Intranasal:* Single dose of 5, 10, or 20 mg administered in one nostril. Dose may be repeated once after 2 hr, not to exceed total daily dose of 40 mg.
zolmitriptan	Zomig	Break a 2.5-mg tablet in half for initial dose. Repeat in 2 hr if headache returns. Do not exceed 10 mg within 24 hr. Use care in patients with liver dysfunction.

SECTION TWO

Anticonvulsants or Antiepileptic Drugs

ACTION

Seizures are sudden muscle contractions that happen without conscious control. They are a symptom of abnormal and excessive electrical discharge in the brain. A variety of diseases and disorders can produce seizures. One of the most common causes of chronic and recurring seizures is epilepsy, which is frequently of an unknown cause (**idiopathic**). Head injury, brain tumor, stroke, meningitis, temperature elevation, and poisoning, especially from excessive alcohol intake or drugs, are also common causes of seizure activity. The most frequent cause of a seizure is the failure to take medication to control previously diagnosed seizure activity. It is estimated that as many as 10% of all people will have a seizure during their lifetime, although this percentage may rise as more people abuse drugs. The diagnosis of epilepsy often has legal consequences, which vary among states, including restriction of driver's licenses and restriction from operation of heavy machinery or doing other activities that require alertness. You can see how it might be a problem if someone were driving a bulldozer and suddenly had a seizure.

The terms *epilepsy, convulsions,* and *seizures* are commonly used for the same thing, although they each have a slightly different medical meaning. A variety of terms have been used over the years to describe types of seizures, including *grand mal (tonic-clonic), petit mal (absence), psychomotor, myoclonic, atonic,* and *jacksonian*. More recently, there has been agreement to group seizures into two broad categories (generalized or focal), based on their clinical presentation and electroencephalographic (EEG) patterns. This chapter will continue to use both terms.

Sometimes surgery or dietary treatment may be used to control symptoms in a patient with a seizure disorder. More commonly, epileptic seizures are treated with medication. The goal of this type of therapy is to suppress or reduce the number of patient seizures.

A number of drugs control seizures through depression or slowing of abnormal electrical discharges in the CNS. These products work in a variety of ways. There is usually one drug that is more effective than another for a patient, depending on the type of seizure activity. Patients with newly diagnosed seizure disorders are usually started on parenteral injection therapy; when seizure activity has come under control, oral therapy is started.

There are four major anticonvulsant or antiepileptic drug groups: barbiturates, benzodiazepines, hydantoins, and succinimides. A list of anticonvulsants and their uses is presented in Table 16-2. In addition, a variety of miscellaneous drugs and herbal products used to treat seizure disorders. The Complementary and Alternative Therapies box provides a list of common herbal products that patients may use in the treatment of seizures and their drug interactions.

USES

Barbiturates, which have a long duration of action, are the primary category of prescription anticonvulsants and are used for their sedative effect on the brain. They may be used in combination with medications from the other three groups. Benzodiazepines are useful with some problems but also have a lot of serious

Table 16-2

Anticonvulsants and Their Primary Uses

GENERIC NAME	TRADE NAME	COMMENTS AND DOSAGE
BARBITURATES		
amobarbital sodium	Amytal Sodium	All forms of epilepsy, status epilepticus, eclampsia, tetanus, drug reactions
mephobarbital	Mebaral	Grand mal and petit mal seizures
phenobarbital	Phenobarbital	All forms of epilepsy, status epilepticus, severe recurrent seizures, eclampsia
secobarbital	Seconal	Status epilepticus, drug reactions, tetanus
BENZODIAZEPINES		
clonazepam	Klonopin	Petit mal, myoclonic seizures
clorazepate	Tranxene	Focal seizures
diazepam	Valium	All forms of epilepsy, status epilepticus, severe recurrent seizures, tetanus
HYDANTOINS		
ethotoin	Peganone	Tonic-clonic and psychomotor seizures
fosphenytoin	Cerebyx	Status epilepticus
mephenytoin	Mesantoin	Grand mal, psychomotor, focal, jacksonian seizures
phenytoin	Dilantin Diphenylan	Grand mal and psychomotor seizures, status epilepticus
OXAZOLIDINEDIONES		
trimethadione	Tridione	Petit mal seizures
SUCCINIMIDES		
ethosuximide	Zarontin	Petit mal seizures
methsuximide	Celontin Kapseals	Petit mal seizures
phensuximide	Milontin Kapseals	Petit mal seizures
OTHER DRUGS		
acetazolamide	Diamox	Grand mal, petit mal, myoclonic, mixed seizures
carbamazepine	Tegretol	Grand mal, mixed, psychomotor seizures
felbamate	Felbatol	Partial seizures, Lennox-Gastaut syndrome (associated with aplastic anemia and hepatic failure)
gabapentin	Neurontin	Partial seizures in adults
lamotrigine	Lamictal	Partial seizures in adults
levetiracetam	Keppra	Partial seizures in adults
oxcarbazepine	Trileptal	Partial seizures in adults and children
primidone	Mysoline	Grand mal, psychomotor, focal seizures
tiagabine	Gabitril	Adjunctive therapy for partial-onset seizures in adults
topiramate	Topamax	Adjunctive therapy for partial-onset seizures in adults
valproic acid	Depakene Depakote	Petit mal seizures

Complementary and Alternative Therapies

Epilepsy

PRODUCT	COMMENTS
Bitter melon	Potential interactions with insulin, oral hypoglycemics
Ginkgo	Potential interaction with anticoagulants, aspirin, NSAIDs, antiplatelet drugs; may interact with MAO inhibitors, acetylcholinesterase inhibitors
Gymnema	Potential interactions with insulin, oral hypoglycemics

Modified from Krinsky DL, Lavella JB, Hawkins EB, et al: *Natural therapeutics pocket guide,* ed 2, Hudson, Ohio, 2003, Lexi-Comp, Inc.

adverse effects. Hydantoins have a wide range of uses, and phenytoin (Dilantin) is by far the most commonly used anticonvulsant. Succinimides are used to control petit mal seizures. Each of these four groups, along with a variety of other miscellaneous anticonvulsants, will be discussed in this section.

Because of the variety of drugs and the many possible side effects, the choice of an anticonvulsant tends to be a trial or experiment for each patient. When seizures are not stopped with one drug, another may be added, or the first drug may be stopped and another product used instead.

Pediatric Considerations

Anticonvulsants

* The young patient (under age 23) is more susceptible to gingival hyperplasia, especially with phenytoin or mephenytoin therapy. Gingivitis, or gum inflammation, usually starts during the first 6 months of drug therapy, although severe hyperplasia is unlikely with dosages under 500 mg/day. A dental program of teeth cleaning and plaque control started within 7 to 10 days of initiating drug therapy helps to reduce the rate and severity of this condition.
* Coarse facial features and excessive body hair growth are more frequently reported in young patients.
* Chronic use of clonazepam may result in impaired physical or mental functions in the developing child. This may not become apparent until years later.
* Impaired school performance is reported with long-term, high-dose hydantoin therapy (especially at high or toxic serum levels).
* Children receiving valproic acid, especially those under 2 years old or those receiving multiple anticonvulsant drugs, are at a greater risk for serious hepatotoxicity. This risk decreases with advancing age.

Modified from McKenry LM, Salerno E: *Mosby's pharmacology in nursing,* ed 21, St Louis, 2003, Mosby.

Geriatric Considerations

Anticonvulsants

* The elderly population tends to metabolize anticonvulsants more slowly; thus drug accumulation and toxicity may occur. Monitor closely because dosage adjustments (lower doses) may be necessary.
* Serum albumin levels may be lower in geriatric patients, resulting in decreased protein binding of drugs such as phenytoin and valproic acid. Monitor closely because lower drug doses may be necessary.
* Administer intravenous doses at a rate slower than the recommended rate for an adult. The rate of administration of phenytoin to elderly patients should be 5 to 10 mg/min, up to a maximum of 25 mg/min.

Modified from McKenry LM, Salerno E: *Mosby's pharmacology in nursing,* ed 21, St Louis, 2003, Mosby.

BARBITURATES

ACTION

Barbiturates are CNS depressants. They act primarily on the brainstem reticular formation, reducing nerve impulses that go to the cerebral cortex. Barbiturates depress the respiratory system and slow the activity of nerves and muscles (smooth, skeletal, and cardiac). Barbiturates also raise the seizure threshold, or the level of electrical activity that must be produced before a seizure will occur. Barbiturates may be short-acting, intermediate-acting, or long-acting.

USES

Long-acting barbiturates are used as anticonvulsants to control and prevent grand mal seizures. They are sometimes used to treat **status epilepticus,** a condition in which a series of severe grand mal seizures occur one after another without stopping. They may also be used to treat seizures caused by tetanus, fever, or drugs.

ADVERSE REACTIONS

Adverse reactions to barbiturates include worsening of symptoms of certain organic brain disorders in elderly patients, dizziness, drowsiness, hangover, headache, lethargy (sleepiness), paradoxic restlessness or excitement, unsteadiness, photosensitivity (abnormal response to exposure to sunlight), rash, diarrhea, nausea, hepatitis with jaundice, vomiting, anemia, decreased platelet counts, unusual bleeding or bruising, urticaria (hives), joint and muscle pains, tolerance (increased resistance to the drug caused by repeated use), and withdrawal symptoms when discontinued.

In cases of acute overdose, the patient may show exaggerated CNS depression, slow shallow respirations, miosis, tachycardia, areflexia (absence of reflexes), shock, or coma. Death may occur as a result of cardiorespiratory failure.

DRUG INTERACTIONS

Because barbiturates increase metabolism, they reduce the activity of anticoagulants, corticosteroids, and digitalis preparations. MAO inhibitors may increase the depressant effects of the barbiturates. There may be significant additive effects if barbiturates are used along with alcohol, antihistamines, benzodiazepines, methotrimeprazine, narcotics, and tranquilizers.

BENZODIAZEPINES

ACTION

Benzodiazepines are CNS depressants. Their exact mechanism of action is not known, but they are thought to act on the hypothalamus and limbic system of the brain, decreasing the vasopressor response and increasing the arousal threshold. Benzodiazepines suppress the electrical spike-and-wave brain discharge in seizures and decrease the frequency, amplitude, duration, and spread of the discharge in minor motor seizures.

USES

Benzodiazepines are used to treat minor motor seizures and also to treat Lennox-Gastaut syndrome (petit mal variance) and patients who have failed to respond to succinimide. Three benzodiazepines are approved for use as anticonvulsants. Diazepam is used intravenously to control seizures and is the drug of choice for treatment of status epilepticus. Clonazepam is used for oral treatment of petit mal seizures in children, and clorazepate is used with other antiepileptic agents to control partial seizures.

ADVERSE REACTIONS

Adverse reactions to benzodiazepines include hypotension (low blood pressure), shortness of breath, difficulty focusing or blurred vision, confusion, drowsiness, flushing (red color in the face and neck), headaches, lightheadedness, paradoxic reactions (excitement, stimulation, hyperactivity), slurred speech, sweating, anorexia (lack of appetite), bitter taste, dry mouth, diarrhea, heartburn, nausea, vomiting, pruritus, rash, joint pains, and burning eyes.

Overdosage may produce marked drowsiness, weakness, impairment of stance and gait, confusion, and coma.

DRUG INTERACTIONS

Alcohol, other sedatives and hypnotics, antidepressants, anticonvulsants, and narcotics may produce additive sedative effects if used with benzodiazepines. Some combinations of anticonvulsants may result in an antidepressant effect or provoke additional seizures.

HYDANTOINS

ACTION

Hydantoins act primarily on the motor cortex, where they stop the spread of seizure activity by either increasing or decreasing the sodium ion movement across the motor cortex during the generation of nerve impulses.

USES

Hydantoins are used to treat grand mal and psychomotor seizures. Sometimes they are used to treat status epilepticus, migraine, and trigeminal neuralgia. They are also used in some nonepileptic psychotic patients.

ADVERSE REACTIONS

Adverse reactions to hydantoins include ataxia (poor coordination), dizziness, drowsiness, hallucinations, inattentiveness, nystagmus (rhythmic movement of the eyes), ocular disturbances, poor memory, slurred speech, constipation, nausea, vomiting, blood cell disturbances, purpura (bruising), acne-like eruptions, gingival hyperplasia, lupus erythematosus, hepatitis with jaundice, and lymph node hyperplasia. Hydantoins are also teratogenic.

Overdosage may produce ataxia, coma, dysarthria, hypotension, nystagmus, and unresponsive pupils.

DRUG INTERACTIONS

Hydantoin drug interactions are frequent and often substantial. You should carefully monitor the administration of this drug when it is used with any other medication or vitamins. It may also alter the results of various laboratory tests.

SUCCINIMIDES

ACTION

Succinimide-type anticonvulsants elevate the seizure threshold in the cortex and basal ganglia and reduce synaptic response to low-frequency repetitive stimulation.

USES

Succinimides are used to control petit mal seizures. Methsuximide is used for refractory petit mal cases.

ADVERSE REACTIONS

Adverse reactions to succinimides include dizziness, headaches, hiccups, hyperactivity, lethargy, mood or mental changes, rashes, blurred vision, photophobia, anorexia, abdominal pain, diarrhea, nausea, vomiting, urinary frequency, vaginal bleeding, blood cell changes, alopecia (hair loss), muscular weakness, systemic lupus erythematosus, disturbances of sleep, inability to concentrate, mental slowness, and night terrors.

DRUG INTERACTIONS

If succinimides are used with other anticonvulsants, they can result in increased sex drive (libido) or increased frequency of grand mal seizures. Bone marrow–depressing drugs used with succinimides can result in significant and fatal blood dyscrasias.

OTHER DRUGS

A variety of other products that are chemically unrelated have been in use for years in the treatment of seizures. New products continue to be developed in efforts to obtain better seizure control with reduced side effects. These products and their uses are listed in Table 16-2.

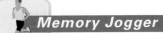

Memory Jogger

Drug Dependence
Dependence can develop with indiscriminate use, and abrupt withdrawal is dangerous.

Nursing Implications and Patient Teaching

Assessment

You should learn as much as possible about the health history of the patient, including drugs she is currently taking that may produce drug interactions, other anti-convulsants, response to anticonvulsants taken in the past, hypersensitivity (allergy), and the possibility of pregnancy. Cardiac, respiratory, hepatic, or renal diseases are contraindications or precautions to the use of anticonvulsants.

Diagnosis

For patients who are just starting on an antiseizure medication, you should find out what particular fears or concerns they have, as well as specific learning deficits. The diagnosis of these problems will help you develop an appropriate nursing care plan to meet those needs. If the patient has alcohol and drug abuse problems, there may be problems with drug withdrawal, legal problems, or difficulties with compliance that will need to be part of the care plan.

Planning

Elderly or weakened patients may be more sensitive to barbiturates and should be started on lower dosages. These patients are more likely to have hangover, confusion, and delirium.

Several of the anticonvulsant medications may produce blood dyscrasias or systemic lupus erythematosus. Benzodiazepines are changed by the liver into long-acting forms that may remain in the body for 24 hours or more and produce increased sedation; liver function may be damaged with long-term use. In addition, there is a risk of congenital malformations and neonatal depression with most anticonvulsants if used during pregnancy.

Implementation

Barbiturates are legally controlled substances. They should not be given to patients with a history of abuse or addiction. Barbiturates should not be given to patients in pain because these drugs may worsen the pain. When barbiturates are given parenterally, you should use great caution to avoid accidentally injecting into an artery or tissues because serious ischemia or gangrene could result.

When benzodiazepines are used in patients who have a mixed type of seizure activity, the drugs may increase or cause the onset of generalized tonic-clonic seizures. These drugs should also be used with caution in patients with poor or reduced renal function. Stopping the drugs quickly can produce status epilepticus. These drugs may cause drooling or increased secretions in patients with some types of respiratory problems.

The dosage of benzodiazepines must be decided for each patient, depending on the patient's response. The onset of action is about 30 to 60 minutes and the effects last 7 to 8 hours. The drug should be given 15 to 30 minutes before bedtime. Elderly or weakened patients should receive reduced dosages of all anticonvulsants. It is important to very slowly increase or decrease dosages.

Oral hydantoin suspension is often difficult to give accurately. The oral suspension should be shaken well before being given, and the liquid should not be frozen. Chewable tablets should not be used for once-a-day treatment.

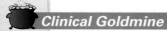

Clinical Goldmine

Oral Hydantoin Therapy

There are two types of oral hydantoin therapy: "prompt" and "extended" capsules. Capsules labeled "extended" are given only once a day. Capsules labeled "prompt" are given two or three times a day.

Subcutaneous or perivascular injection of hydantoins should be avoided because of the highly alkaline nature of the solution. Hydantoins should be administered very slowly when given intravenously (IV).

You should talk to the patient and family about the chance of brief but short-term personality changes with succinimide therapy. These should be reported to the nurse, physician, or other health care provider if they occur.

Once the patient is seizure-free with a particular drug, changing to hydantoin products should be avoided. All dosages must be determined for the individual. The dosage for children is usually larger by weight than for adults. The patient is usually given a single dose within the therapeutic range, and then the amount is gradually increased until the seizures are controlled, or until symptoms of overdosage or toxicity indicate that no further increases can be made.

Table 16-3 provides a list of important information about anticonvulsants, including dosages. A variety of miscellaneous anticonvulsants are also available. See Tables 16-2 and 16-3 for brief information about those products. Felbamate (Felbatol) has been used for partial seizures and Lennox-Gastaut syndrome. Enough cases

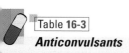

Table 16-3
Anticonvulsants

GENERIC NAME	TRADE NAME	COMMENTS AND DOSAGE
BARBITURATES		
Long Acting		
mephobarbital	Mebaral	Converts to phenobarbital in body. Onset in 1 hr; effective 10-16 hr; give 100-200 mg PO daily.
phenobarbital	Luminal	Give IM in large muscle mass because injection is very painful. Give slowly IV. Give 100-300 mg IM.
	Phenobarbital	Some forms come in sustained-release capsules. Onset in 1 hr, effective for 16 hr; give 50-100 mg 2 or 3 times daily.
Intermediate Acting		
amobarbital sodium	Amytal Sodium	For IV or IM injection; do not exceed 1 mg/min. Onset in 30-60 min; effective 8-10 hr. Give 65-200 mg in divided doses daily.
secobarbital	Seconal	Short-acting (3-6 hr), so not often used orally. Give 100 mg PO daily.
secobarbital sodium	Seconal Sodium	Give slowly, 50 mg/15 sec IV; give 100 mg PO; 120-200 mg per rectum; 50-250 mg parenterally.
BENZODIAZEPINES		
clonazepam	Klonopin	*Adults:* Initial dose is 1.5 mg PO divided into 3 doses/day. After 4-9 days, dosage may be increased by 0.5-1.5 mg/day every 3 days until the seizures stop or until the side effects prevent any further increase. Maximum recommended daily dose is 20 mg. *Infants and children up to 10 yr or 30 kg:* Initial dosage between 0.01 and 0.03 mg/kg/day PO; however, not to exceed 0.05 mg/kg/day, given in 2 or 3 divided doses. Dosage should be increased by not more than 0.25-0.5 mg every third day until a daily maintenance rate of 0.1-0.2 mg/kg is reached. Whenever possible, give in 3 equally divided doses; if this is not possible, give the largest dose before bedtime.
clorazepate	Tranxene	*Adults and children over 12 yr:* Initial dose is 7.5 mg tid. Increase by no more than 7.5 mg every week. Maximum dose not to exceed 90 mg/day. *Children 9-12 yr:* Initial dose is 7.5 mg bid. Increase by no more than 7.5 mg every week. Maximum dose not to exceed 60 mg/day.

Table 16-3

Anticonvulsants —cont'd

GENERIC NAME	TRADE NAME	COMMENTS AND DOSAGE
BENZODIAZEPINES—cont'd		
diazepam	Valium	• *Oral therapy:* *Adults:* 2-10 mg PO 2 to 4 times daily. Give 15-30 mg sustained-release capsules daily. *Geriatric or debilitated patients:* 2-2.5 mg PO daily or twice daily; gradually increase dose as needed. *Children over 6 months:* 1-2.5 mg PO 3 to 4 times daily initially; gradually increase dose as needed. • *Parenteral therapy:* Inject IV medication slowly only into large veins, 1 min for each 5 mg. *Adults:* Give 5-10 mg IV initially, repeated as necessary at 10- to 15-min intervals; maximum IV dose is 30 mg; therapy may be repeated in 2-4 hr as needed. *Children 5 yr and older:* Give 1 mg q2-5min; maximum IV dose is 10 mg; repeat in 2-4 hr as needed. *Children 30 days to 5 yr:* Give 0.2-0.5 mg slowly q2-5min; maximum IV dose is 5 mg.
HYDANTOINS		
ethotoin	Peganone	Give <1 gm daily in 4-6 evenly spaced and divided doses. Take after food. Usual adult dose is 2-3 gm/day. Calculate pediatric dose based on age and weight.
fosphenytoin	Cerebyx	Give loading dose of 15-20 mg phenytoin sodium equivalents (PE)/kg administered at 100-150 mg PE/min. Continuously monitor ECG and vital signs.
mephenytoin	Mesantoin	*Adults and children:* 50-100 mg PO daily; can be increased by an additional 50-100 mg in 3 or 4 divided doses at 1-wk intervals. Maximum dosage is 800 mg, 400 mg for children.
phenytoin	Dilantin	*Children:* 5 mg/kg/day PO in 2 or 3 equally divided doses initially; gradually increase to achieve level desired, up to 300 mg; maintenance dosage is 4-8 mg/kg/day. *Adults:* 100 mg PO 3 times daily initially; gradually increase to achieve level desired; maintenance dosage is 300-400 mg.
SUCCINIMIDES		
ethosuximide	Zarontin	*Adults and children 6 yr and older:* 250 mg twice daily initially, increase by 250 mg every 4-7 days until seizures are controlled or total daily dosage reaches 1.5 gm. The optimal dosage for most children is 20 mg/kg daily. *Children 3-6 yr:* 250 mg PO daily initially, increase by 250 mg every 4-7 days until seizures are controlled or total daily dosage reaches 1 gm.
methsuximide	Celontin Kapseals	*Adults:* 300 mg daily initially; increase by 300 mg at weekly intervals until seizures are controlled or total daily dosage reaches 1.2 gm. *Children:* Usual adult dosage. Small children may require adjustment using 150-mg capsule.
phensuximide	—	*Adults and children:* 500 mg twice daily initially, increased by 500 mg at weekly intervals until seizures are controlled or total daily dosage reaches 3 gm. Shake suspension well before pouring. Take drug with meals to decrease gastric discomfort. Efficacy of the drug decreases with long-term use.

Continued

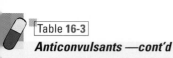

Table 16-3

Anticonvulsants —cont'd

GENERIC NAME	TRADE NAME	COMMENTS AND DOSAGE
MISCELLANEOUS ANTICONVULSANTS		
acetazolamide	Diamox	8-30 mg/kg/day in divided doses.
carbamazepine	Tegretol	200 mg twice daily initially, increasing gradually by 200 mg/day in divided doses at 6- to 8-hr intervals; do not exceed 1200 mg daily.
gabapentin	Neurontin	Add-on therapy for patients older than 12 years. Effective dose is 900-1800 mg/day in divided doses. Titrate to effective dose over a few days.
lamotrigine	Lamictal	Consult package insert for complex dosing instructions.
primidone	Mysoline	250 mg daily, with weekly increases of 250 mg until therapeutic response or tolerance develops. Usual dosage is 750-1500 mg daily; do not exceed 2000 mg daily.
topiramate	Topamax	Total daily dose as adjunctive therapy is 400 mg/day in 2 divided doses.
valproic acid	Depakene	15 mg/kg/day PO. Increase by 5-10 mg/kg/day at weekly intervals; do not exceed 30 mg/kg/day.

of aplastic anemia and hepatic failure have developed from use of this drug that it carries a warning regarding ts use.

Evaluation

t takes several weeks before the success of an anticonvulsant dosage plan can be seen. The therapeutic effects should be monitored, and you should note whether the degree of sedation is fitting into the patient's lifestyle. Blood levels may be needed to see if the drug is in the therapeutic range.

The patient's compliance should be followed in regard to the amount and times the drug is taken, any pattern of abuse, and drinking of alcohol. In addition, the patient should be asked about any paradoxic reactions, and evaluated for tolerance, dependence, withdrawal, and toxicity. Toxicity is indicated by jaundice (yellow color of skin, eyes, and mucous membranes), rash, and sore throat.

The patient should keep a record of uncontrolled seizures: the time, length, characteristics, and reaction.

Complete blood cell counts (CBCs) and liver function tests should be followed as a baseline and repeated on a set schedule for patients on long-term barbiturate therapy.

Tolerance is usually related to the total amount of drug received. Dependence and withdrawal symptoms may occur if these drugs are used for very long periods. Do not stop the drug quickly if the patient has been taking the drug for a long time.

Hydantoins are metabolized at various rates by patients; therefore, you should be alert to symptoms of toxicity. The patient should avoid alcohol while taking most anticonvulsants.

Adverse effects are common in long-term therapy. Gum overgrowth around the teeth (hyperplasia) is a typical finding with hydantoins and may cause distress to the patient and family. The patient and family must be educated about how to prevent and treat this problem.

Prescriptions should be written for a particular brand of medication. Once a patient's seizures are controlled with a certain brand, the patient should continue to receive that brand. Not all brands are the same and so the products cannot be substituted for each other (they are not interchangeable).

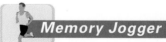

Memory Jogger

Oral Hygiene

The importance of good oral hygiene, especially of gums, should be emphasized when teaching patients taking hydantoins.

Patient and Family Teaching

You should tell the patient and family the following:

1. The patient should be aware that problems with tolerance, dependence, and addiction may occur with anticonvulsant medications.
2. The patient should take the medication exactly as prescribed and not discontinue taking it even if he has no seizures and may be feeling well. If a dose is forgotten, it should be taken as soon as it

is remembered, if it is within 1 to 2 hours of the regular dosage time. If it is later than 2 hours, the patient should skip the dose and take the next dose at the regular time. Double doses should not be taken. The regular medication schedule should be continued.

3. This medication should be kept in a locked cabinet or out of the reach of children and all others for whom the drug is not prescribed. The medication should not be shared with anyone.

4. Barbiturates may cause drowsiness, and the patient must be cautious when driving, using hazardous machinery, or performing tasks that require alertness.

5. Some medications produce daytime sedation that may interfere with the patient's job or home and child care responsibilities.

6. The nurse, physician, or other health care provider should be notified immediately if the patient experiences any rash, fever, unusual bleeding, bruising, sore throat, jaundice, or abdominal pain. Some people experience side effects while taking these drugs, so the health care provider should be notified of any new or uncomfortable symptoms.

7. The patient may have excessive dreaming when barbiturates are discontinued; this should lessen each night.

8. Tablets and capsules should be kept in a dry, tightly closed container.

9. Elixirs should be kept in a tightly closed, brown glass bottle.

10. A hangover feeling may sometimes be experienced the day after taking a benzodiazepine. It is dangerous to drink alcohol within 24 hours after taking this drug. The patient who takes this medication must not drink any alcohol.

11. Smoking may decrease the length of time benzodiazepines are effective.

12. Succinimides may be taken with food or milk to decrease stomach upset.

13. The liquid form of succinimides should be shaken well before the dose is measured.

14. The patient should maintain good oral hygiene: brushing teeth and gums with a soft toothbrush twice daily and rinsing the mouth well is important. The patient should see a dentist every 6 months; this is especially true if the patient is taking a hydantoin.

15. The patient should wear a Medic Alert bracelet or necklace or other identification that states the medical problem and the medication being taken.

16. Succinimides may make the urine appear pink, red, or red-brown.

17. Chewable tablets must be chewed or crushed before they are swallowed.

18. The patient must not change the brands or dosage forms unless ordered to do so by the nurse, physician, or other health care provider. Not all brands of these medications are interchangeable.

19. When undergoing any kind of surgery, including dental work, the patient should alert the nurse, physician, or other health care provider or dentist that she is taking an anticonvulsant medication.

20. The use of anticonvulsants is not advised in pregnancy. The patient and the nurse, physician, or other health care provider should discuss questions about becoming pregnant.

21. The patient should keep regular follow-up appointments with the nurse, physician, or other health care provider; this is essential to evaluate reactions to anticonvulsants.

SECTION THREE

Antiemetic-Antivertigo Agents

ACTION

Some drugs, metabolic disorders, radiation, motion, gastric irritation, vestibular neuritis, or increases in central trigger zone dopamine levels or vomiting center acetylcholine levels may provoke nausea and vomiting. Antiemetics and antivertigo agents act by one or more mechanisms to stop or limit this response. These drugs reduce indirect stimulation of the vomiting center and reduce the levels of dopamine and acetylcholine, which cause vomiting.

USES

Vomiting may be produced by direct action on the vomiting center of the brain, by indirect action through stimulation of the chemoreceptor trigger zone, and through increased activity of chemical neurotransmitters. Nausea and vomiting resulting from motion are probably caused by impulses to the vestibular network of the labyrinth system of the ear, which is located near the vomiting center. The impulses are conducted to the vomiting center by cholinergic nerves. Thus drugs that inhibit cholinergic nerve impulses should be effective in treating motion sickness.

Antiemetic or antivertigo agents usually are used to prevent and treat motion sickness or the nausea and vomiting that occur with anesthesia and surgery or with cancer treatment. They are also used to treat severe vomiting and hiccups that are intractable (cannot be stopped by the usual treatment methods).

Antidopaminergic agents are used almost exclusively to control nausea and vomiting. Anticholinergic medications are used to control motion sickness. Meclizine, dimenhydrinate, and diphenidol are the only products used to control vertigo. 5-HT agonists are routinely used prophylactically in patients expected to have nausea (e.g., patients undergoing chemotherapy).

ADVERSE REACTIONS

Drowsiness is the most common side effect of the anticholinergics, but tolerance to this reaction usually develops with long-term therapy. Patients may also feel dry mouth, stuffy nose, blurred vision, constipation, urinary retention, and other anticholinergic reactions.

DRUG INTERACTIONS

The sedative effect of some antiemetic medications is increased or potentiated by other CNS depressants. Anticholinergic antiemetics can increase the anticholinergic side effects of many other drugs. The drug interactions may vary, depending on the type of antiemetic-antivertigo drug, but would be similar to other anticholinergic or antidopaminergic products.

Nursing Implications and Patient Teaching

Assessment

You should learn as much as possible about the health history of the patient, including motion sickness, extrapyramidal reactions caused by antipsychotic therapy, labyrinthitis, vertigo, Ménière's disease, radiation therapy, or diabetes. Nausea and vomiting are common adverse reactions to drug therapy, and may occur after taking almost any medication.

You should also find out whether the patient has a history of allergy, is currently using drugs that would cause drug interactions (especially MAO inhibitors), or is pregnant. In all cases the underlying cause of vomiting, nausea, or vertigo should be found. In women of childbearing years, the possibility of pregnancy should always be considered by the nurse. These drugs should not be used for treating morning sickness because many drugs are not safe for the fetus.

Peppermint and ginger have been used in the treatment of motion sickness. Ask patients about the use of these herbs, because ginger has the potential to interact with anticoagulants, aspirin, NSAIDs, antiplatelet agents, and cardiac glycosides (digoxin).

Diagnosis

For patients who have been vomiting for a long time or who have vertigo, other problems may develop. Is the patient dehydrated? Is he getting enough good food? Are there problems related to work or family because of the patient's vomiting? You should explore these areas to determine if there are problems that require action.

Planning

Antiemetic and antivertigo agents should be used with extreme caution in patients doing tasks that require them to be mentally alert, because some of these products produce drowsiness. These agents are not recommended for use in children because they may contribute to the development, the misdiagnosis, or the severity of symptoms in Reye's syndrome, a brain encephalopathy that is often fatal in children.

Vomiting is often an important diagnostic clue and may point to a serious underlying problem. The cause of the vomiting or nausea should be found so that the best treatment can be given to get rid of the problem. Antiemetic drugs should not be the only form of therapy in cases of nausea or vomiting. Attempts to maintain hydration, restore electrolyte balance, and reduce other symptoms should be made.

 Pediatric Considerations

Antiemetic Agents

Pediatric patients with chickenpox, CNS infections, measles, dehydration, gastroenteritis, or other acute illnesses will be at special risk for adverse reactions and possibly Reye's syndrome. Avoid use of phenothiazine antiemetic therapy in such patients.

From McKenry LM, Salerno E: *Mosby's pharmacology in nursing*, ed 21, St Louis, 2003, Mosby.

Implementation

Phenothiazine derivatives all turn the urine pink or reddish-brown. They also may produce photosensitivity, so the patient should avoid exposure to sunlight. Antiemetic and antivertigo agents generally come in tablets, sustained-release capsules, and concentrates for oral use. For patients who are vomiting or so nauseated that they are unable to take oral medications, injection or suppository forms are usually given.

The dose should be as low as possible, and therapy should be stopped as quickly as possible. IV prepara-tions should be reserved for severe cases in patients in the hospital. Medications given IM should be switched when the patient can tolerate oral agents.

Table 16-4 summarizes important information about antiemetic-antivertigo agents.

Table 16-4

Antiemetic and Antivertigo Agents

GENERIC NAME	TRADE NAME	COMMENTS AND DOSAGE
ANTIDOPAMINERGICS		
Phenothiazines		
chlorpromazine	Ormazine Thorazine	A phenothiazine derivative used to control nausea and vomiting and to treat intractable hiccups. *Adults:* 10-25 mg PO q4-6h prn; 50-100 mg per rectum (PR) q6-8h prn; or 25 mg IM. If no hypotension develops, IM dose may be increased to 50 mg q3-4h. *Children over 6 months:* 0.5 mg/kg (0.25 mg/lb) orally 2-3 hr before operation or 0.5 mg/kg (0.25 mg/lb) IM 1-2 hr before operation. Children up to 5 years should not receive more than 40 mg/day. Children 5-12 years should not receive more than 75 mg/day unless vomiting is severe.
perphenazine	Trilafon	A phenothiazine derivative used to control severe nausea and vomiting, and for therapy of intractable hiccups in adults. IV use should be reserved for hospitalized patients and given in a slow drip. • *Nausea, vomiting, or hiccups:* 8-16 mg PO daily in divided doses. Occasionally, as much as 24 mg may be needed. For rapid control of vomiting, 5 mg IM may be given. Higher dosages and IV therapy should be reserved for hospitalized patients.
prochlorperazine	Compazine	A phenothiazine derivative used to treat vomiting. *Adults:* 5-10 mg PO 3 to 4 times daily; or 15 mg sustained-release tablet may be ordered every AM; or a 10 mg sustained-release tablet may be given q12h. Medication may be given PR, 25 mg twice daily; or 5-10 mg IM, repeated in 3-4 hours prn. Do not exceed 40 mg/day IM. *Children 40-85 lbs:* 2.5 mg 3 times daily or 5 mg twice daily; do not exceed 15 mg/day. *Children 30-39 lbs:* 2.5 mg PO or PR 2 or 3 times daily; do not exceed 10 mg/day. *Children 20-29 lbs:* 2.5 mg PO or PR daily or twice daily; do not exceed 7.5 mg/day. If IM medication is indicated, give 0.06 mg/lb.
promethazine	Phenergan	A phenothiazine derivative used to treat motion sickness and to prevent and control nausea and vomiting associated with surgery and anesthesia. Subcutaneous injection may cause tissue necrosis; intraarterial injection may produce gangrene of the extremity. • *Motion sickness* *Adults:* 25 mg 30-60 min before travel, repeat 8-12 hr later prn. On succeeding days, take 25 mg on arising and again before the evening meal. *Children:* 12.5-25 mg twice daily. • *Nausea and vomiting* *Adults:* 12.5-25 mg PO, IM, or PR q4-6h prn. If parenteral medication is indicated, give 25 mg deep IM. IV medication should be given to hospitalized patients only. *Children:* 0.25-0.5 mg/kg IM or PR q4-6h prn. For parenteral medication, do not give more than one half the adult dose. Preoperatively, may give equal doses of promethazine and a barbiturate or narcotic, and an atropine-like drug.

Continued

Table 16-4

Antiemetic and Antivertigo Agents—cont'd

GENERIC NAME	TRADE NAME	COMMENTS AND DOSAGE
ANTIDOPAMINERGICS—cont'd		
Other		
metoclopramide	Clopra Octamide Reglan	10 mg IV or PO before meals and at bedtime.
thiethylperazine	Torecan	A phenothiazine derivative that probably acts directly on the trigger zone and the vomiting center to reduce nausea and vomiting. IV use of drug is to be avoided because it will produce severe hypotension. IM use should be limited to deep IM injection, at or shortly before the termination of anesthesia. • *Nausea and vomiting:* 10-30 mg daily in divided doses.
triflupromazine	Vesprin	Phenothiazine derivative used to control severe nausea and vomiting. Medication may also change urine color to pink or reddish brown. Activity of drug may last for up to 12 hours after IM administration in children. *Adults:* 20-30 mg PO total daily dose for prophylaxis; for vomiting, 5-15 mg IM, repeated q4h prn up to 60 mg; or 1 mg IV, up to 3 mg total daily dose. *Children over 2½ yr:* 0.2 mg/kg PO, not to exceed 10 mg/day in 3 divided doses; may give 0.2-0.25 mg/kg IM, not to exceed 10 mg/day.
ANTICHOLINERGICS		
Antihistamines		
buclizine	Bucladin-S	Antiemetic with central anticholinergic activity; used for nausea and vomiting associated with motion sickness. *Adults:* 50 mg 3 times daily with a maintenance dose of 50 mg twice daily.
cyclizine	Marezine	Antiemetic, anticholinergic, and antihistaminic agent that also reduces the sensitivity of the labyrinthine apparatus; used primarily for motion sickness. *Adults:* 50-mg tablets PO 30 min before travel; repeat q4-6h; maximum 200 mg/day. Administer 50 mg IM q4-6h.
dimenhydrinate	Dimetabs Dramamine	Antiemetic and antivertigo agent used in motion sickness, in radiation sickness, or following anesthesia. It appears to depress motion-induced stimulation of the labyrinthine structures; may alter blood counts. *Adults:* 50-400 mg/day PO in divided doses; or 50 mg IM or IV prn. *Children over 3 yr:* 1.25 mg/kg 3 to 4 times daily with a maximum dosage of 300 mg/day PO or IM.
diphenhydramine	Benadryl Genahist	Antihistamine that blocks histamine receptors on peripheral effector cells. It has anticholinergic, antitussive, antiemetic, and sedative properties. With IV use, blood pressure should be carefully monitored. *Adults:* 50 mg PO 3 to 4 times daily or 10-50 mg IM or IV; maximum daily dose 400 mg. *Children over 20 lbs:* 12.5-25 mg PO 3 to 4 times daily; or 5 mg/kg PO or IM daily.
meclizine	Antivert Bonine	Antiemetic, anti–motion sickness, and antivertigo agent with anticholinergic properties. • *Motion sickness:* 50 mg 1 hr before departure; repeat q24h prn. • *Vertigo:* 25-100 mg/day in divided doses prn.

Table 16-4

Antiemetic and Antivertigo Agents—cont'd

GENERIC NAME	TRADE NAME	COMMENTS AND DOSAGE
ANTICHOLINERGICS—cont'd		
Other		
dronabinol	Marinol	Antiemetic primarily used for nausea and vomiting from chemotherapy. Give 5 mg/m^2 1-3 hr before the administration of chemotherapy, then every 2-4 hr after chemotherapy is given, for a total of 4-6 doses/day. May be increased by 2.5 mg/m^2 if dose is ineffective and no side effects have occurred. Use cautiously because disturbing psychiatric symptoms develop with higher dosages. May also be used as an appetite stimulant: give 2.5 mg before lunch and supper.
phosphorated carbohydrate sol	Emetrol (OTC)	Hyperosmolar carbohydrate solutions that relieve nausea and vomiting by a direct local action of the wall of the GI tract that reduces small muscle contraction. • *Antiemetic:* *Adults:* 15-30 mL every 15 minutes until distress subsides for 1 hr or 5 doses. *Children 2-12 yr:* 5 or 10 mL in same pattern. • *Morning sickness:* 15-30 mL on arising, and repeat every 3 hr or when nausea threatens. • *Motion sickness:* 15 mL in adults; 5 mL in children.
scopolamine	Transderm-Scop	Comes as a transdermal patch, which is placed behind the ear and releases medication at a constant rate over a 3-day interval. The transdermal mechanism allows for lower dosage and produces fewer adverse anticholinergic effects than the oral forms. Scopolamine is used to control motion sickness in adults. Many contraindications. • *Motion sickness:* 0.25-0.8 mg PO 1 hr before anticipated travel. • *Long-term therapy:* Apply 1 patch behind ear at least 4 hours before the antiemetic effect is desired; replace every 3 days for continued therapy.
trimethobenzamide	Tigan	Antiemetic that inhibits the chemoreceptor trigger zone in the medulla; used to control nausea and vomiting. Drug has been linked to the development of Reye's syndrome in children. Give deep IM only because solution is highly irritating to the tissues. *Adults:* 250 mg PO 3 to 4 times daily; or 200 mg IM 3 to 4 times daily; or 200 mg PR 3 to 4 times daily. *Children between 30 and 90 lbs:* 100 mg PO 3 to 4 times daily; or 100-200 mg PR 3 to 4 times daily. *Children under 30 lbs:* 100 mg PR 3 to 4 times daily.
5-HT RECEPTOR ANTAGONISTS		
dolasetron	Anzemet	Used in controlling nausea and vomiting associated with chemotherapy. Give 100 mg within 1 hr before chemotherapy. Lower dosages may be given to control postoperative vomiting.
granisetron	Kytril	Used for prevention of nausea and vomiting associated with initial and repeat courses of chemotherapy.
ondansetron	Zofran	Used in controlling nausea and vomiting associated with chemotherapy. See package insert for complex dosing instructions. May be given IV, suppository, solution, or tablet.

Evaluation

The nurse should monitor for therapeutic effectiveness and side effects.

Patient and Family Teaching

You should tell the patient and family the following:

1. The patient should take this medication as instructed by the health care provider and not double the dosage or alter the medication schedule.
2. If the drug is taken for motion sickness, the patient should take it 30 to 60 minutes before departure and 30 minutes before meals thereafter.
3. The patient should not drive, operate dangerous machines, or do anything that requires alertness while taking these drugs.
4. The patient should not take any other medications without the knowledge of the nurse, physician, or other health care provider. It is especially important for the patient to avoid other CNS depressants, including alcohol, because of the sedative effect.
5. Although some patients get very sleepy while taking these medications, this is usually a brief problem and will disappear if they keep taking the drug.
6. This medication should be kept out of the reach of children and others for whom it is not prescribed. Overdosage of this medication may be toxic.

SECTION FOUR

Antiparkinsonian Agents

ACTION

Antiparkinsonian agents are anticholinergic and dopaminergic drugs used to control the symptoms of Parkinson's disease by changing the neurotransmitters produced in the brain. The two main actions of the antiparkinsonian agents are (1) to block the uptake of acetylcholine at postsynaptic muscarinic cholinergic receptor sites and (2) to elevate the functional levels of dopamine in motor regulatory centers. These drugs exert a wide range of effects on all the tissue affected by the autonomic nervous system, including the eyes, respiratory tract, heart, GI tract, urinary bladder, nonvascular smooth muscle, exocrine glands, and CNS. Antiparkinsonian agents reduce muscle tremors and rigidity and improve mobility, muscular coordination, and performance.

USES

Paralysis agitans, or **Parkinson's disease,** is a chronic disorder of the CNS. The cause is unknown, but it is thought to involve an imbalance in chemical neurotransmitters within the brain in which too much acetylcholine and not enough dopamine is present in the basal ganglia. Common symptoms are fine muscle tremors, slowness of movement, rigidity, muscle weakness, a characteristic shuffling, forward-pitched gait, and resulting changes in posture and balance. There is no known cure for Parkinson's disease. Treatment goals are designed to relieve symptoms and to maintain movement and activity of the patient.

ADVERSE REACTIONS

Dopaminergic agents may produce dysrhythmias (irregular heartbeats), muscle twitching, psychotic reactions, rigidity, diarrhea, epigastric distress, GI bleeding, nausea, vomiting, blurred vision, alopecia, bitter taste, hot flashes, rash, and urinary retention.

Anticholinergic agents may cause postural hypotension (low blood pressure when a person suddenly stands up), tachycardia, agitation, confusion, depression, headache, memory loss, muscle cramping, constipation, vomiting, diplopia (double vision), increased intraocular pressure, decreased sweating, flushing, and skin rash.

Early signs of toxicity in the patient taking dopaminergic agents include muscle twitching and blepharospasm. Overdosage is a common phenomenon, particularly with long-term drug therapy. It is recognizable because the patient experiences a sudden onset of progressively worsening parkinsonian symptoms. These drugs should be tapered gradually.

DRUG INTERACTIONS

Common drug interactions differ according to whether the preparation is an anticholinergic or a dopaminergic agent. These drugs commonly interact with many types of medications; product information must be closely studied. Two herbal products, gingko and grape seed, are commonly used to treat symptoms of Parkinson's disease. The Complementary and Alternative Therapies box summarizes these products and their drug interactions.

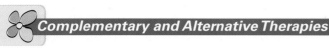

Complementary and Alternative Therapies

Parkinson's Disease

PRODUCT	COMMENTS
Ginkgo	Potential interaction with anticoagulants, aspirin, NSAIDs, antiplatelet agents; may interact with MAO inhibitors, acetylcholinesterase inhibitors
Grape seed	Potential interaction with anticoagulants, aspirin, NSAIDs, antiplatelet agents, methotrexate

Modified from Krinsky DL, Lavella JB, Hawkins EB, et al: *Natural therapeutics pocket guide,* ed 2, Hudson, Ohio, 2003, Lexi-Comp, Inc.

Nursing Implications and Patient Teaching

Assessment

You should learn as much as possible about the health history of the patient, including hypersensitivity; drugs currently being taken that may produce drug interactions; asthma, renal, liver, and cardiovascular disease, and epilepsy; other contraindications for the drug; and the possibility of pregnancy.

The patient may have a history of Parkinson's disease, drooling, or difficulty with coordination and walking. The patient may be taking an antipsychotic drug; with long-term use, these drugs can cause tardive dyskinesia, with symptoms similar to those of Parkinson's disease. The patient may be middle-aged or elderly and may have tremors at rest that are made worse by emotional stress. The arms may fail to move when walking, with rigidity first occurring in the proximal musculature, and the patient may be unable to perform activities of daily living.

Diagnosis

These patients frequently have other problems as a result of their medical diagnosis. Ataxia frequently leads to falls and soft-tissue and bone injuries. They may have deterioration of the skin, poor hygiene, deficits in nutrition, or other problems related to immobility. Their intelligence and ability to understand may be underestimated when they are unable to communicate well. They are frequently angry, depressed, and lonely. If you are willing to spend the time learning to communicate with the patient, you will gain a clear picture of the multitude of problems relevant to the patient.

Planning

Antiparkinsonian agents are contraindicated for persons with known hypersensitivity, acute narrow-angle glaucoma, asthma, history of epilepsy, peptic ulcer disease, and skin lesions. Persons on CNS stimulants, those exposed to rubella, those with acute psychoses, those with a history of melanoma, or patients receiving MAO inhibitor therapy should not take these medications. These drugs are known to aggravate many other diseases and must be used with caution.

The anticholinergics and some dopaminergics must be withdrawn slowly because many of these drugs have a long half-life. When withdrawing one preparation and beginning a new preparation, the new drug should be started in small doses and the old drug should be withdrawn gradually. These agents are usually initiated at the lowest dosage possible and the dosage is increased gradually until the maximum therapeutic effect has been obtained.

Implementation

These drugs are available in tablets, sustained-release capsules, syrup, elixir, and IV and IM injections. They are generally well absorbed from the GI tract. Peak blood levels are achieved in 1 to 6 hours, depending on the route of administration and the type of drug administered, except for the sustained-release capsules, which reach peak plasma blood levels in 8 to 12 hours. Sustained-release capsules are not recommended for initial therapy because they do not allow enough flexibility in dosage regulation. IV injection of anticholinergics can cause hypotension and incoordination.

Although dopamine cannot cross the blood-brain barrier, levodopa can move into the brain, where it is converted into dopamine. However, levodopa alone becomes less effective over time, and side effects are related to the dose. Therefore, carbidopa and levodopa are often administered together, usually as a fixed-combination product. Carbidopa is added to prevent peripheral breakdown of levodopa and reduce the overall dose of levodopa required.

If this combination drug is administered after levodopa therapy, the levodopa should be discontinued at least 8 hours before initiating therapy with carbidopa-levodopa. The carbidopa-levodopa combination should be substituted at a dosage level that provides 25% of the previous levodopa dose. When the fixed-combination dose is excessive, carbidopa can be given separately with levodopa so that each drug can be titrated individually.

Table 16-5 summarizes the important medications used to treat Parkinson's disease.

Evaluation

Long-term use of dopaminergic and anticholinergic agents often leads to akinesia (loss of movement), tardive dyskinesia (difficulty in performing voluntary movements), and dystonia (impairment of muscle tone)

Table 16-5

Antiparkinsonian Drugs

GENERIC NAME	TRADE NAME	COMMENTS AND DOSAGE
ANTICHOLINERGIC DRUGS		
belladonna alkaloids	Bellafoline	Competes with acetylcholine for muscarinic receptors at the postganglionic fibers of the parasympathetic nervous system; also used to control GI disturbances. Give 0.25-0.5 mg PO 3 times daily; 0.5-1 mL daily to twice daily parenterally.
benztropine	Cogentin	Contains anticholinergic and antihistamine properties. Pharmacologically, the drug inhibits excessive cholinergic activity in the striatal fibers. Used to treat extrapyramidal symptoms (except tardive dyskinesia) induced by antipsychotic agents. IM injection provides rapid (15 min) relief from acute dystonic reactions. Oral doses of the drug are cumulative; therefore, therapy should begin with a low dose and increase gradually at 5- to 6-day intervals as necessary. • *Parkinsonian symptoms:* 1-2 mg/day PO with meals or parenterally; range is 0.5-6 mg. • *Drug-induced extrapyramidal side effects:* 1-4 mg twice daily with meals.
biperiden	Akineton	Blocks central cholinergic receptors, restoring the balance between cholinergic and dopaminergic activity in the basal ganglia. IV or IM administration may produce incoordination. • *Parkinsonism symptoms:* 1-2 mg PO 3 to 4 times daily; give with meals. • *Drug-induced extrapyramidal symptoms:* 2 mg PO daily to 3 times daily. Administer 2 mg IM or IV for acute symptoms; repeat q30min to a maximum of 4 doses a day.
diphenhydramine	Benadryl	Blocks receptors on peripheral effector cells. *Adults:* 50 mg PO 3 to 4 times daily or 10-15 mg IM or IV as needed daily *Children over 20 lbs:* 12.5-25 mg PO 3 to 4 times daily; or 5 mg/kg PO or IM daily.
procyclidine	Kemadrin	A synthetic antiparkinsonian agent that inhibits hyperactive cholinergic activity in the striatal fibers. It is more effective in the relief of rigidity than tremor, and relieves excessive salivation. • *Parkinsonism:* 8-10 mg PO in 3-4 divided doses daily. Dosage may range from 6 to 15 mg daily. • *Extrapyramidal symptoms:* 10-20 mg in 3 divided doses daily.
trihexyphenidyl	Artane Trihexy-2	Exerts a direct inhibitory effect on the parasympathetic nervous system. Decreases rigidity, but most other symptoms improve to some degree. • *Idiopathic parkinsonism:* 6-10 mg PO in 3-4 divided doses; 1 mg initially and increased in 2-mg increments at intervals of 3-5 days until a total dosage of 6-10 mg is reached. Once maintenance dose is reached, sustained-release capsule may be used; 5 mg daily to twice daily.
DOPAMINERGIC DRUGS		
amantadine	Symmetrel	This drug enhances the release of dopamine from presynaptic nerve endings. The drug has no anticholinergic activity. • *Parkinsonism:* 100 mg daily to twice daily up to a maximum of 400 mg daily. • *Drug-induced extrapyramidal reactions:* 100 mg twice daily up to a maximum of 300 mg daily.

Table 16-5

Antiparkinsonian Drugs—cont'd

GENERIC NAME	TRADE NAME	COMMENTS AND DOSAGE
DOPAMINERGIC DRUGS—cont'd		
bromocriptine	Parlodel	Directly stimulates the dopamine receptors in the corpus striatum; this medication is especially helpful in patients who are beginning to deteriorate or develop tolerance to levodopa. Initiate therapy with 1.25-mg tablet, twice daily with meals. Increase after 2-4 wk prn by 2.5 mg/day; do not exceed 100 mg/day.
carbidopa	Lodosyn	Used with levodopa to slow the breakdown of levodopa; has no therapeutic action itself. Used when treatment requires separate titration of each drug.
carbidopa-levodopa	Sinemet-10/100 Sinemet-25/100 Sinemet-25/250 Sinemet-50/200	This is a fixed-combination antiparkinsonian agent used in all types of treatment of Parkinson's disease, and is composed of both carbidopa and levodopa. Tablet strength is indicated by numbering (mg carbidopa/mg levodopa). *For patients not receiving levodopa:* 1 tablet (10/100 or 25/100) 3 times daily initially; increase by 1 tablet daily until a maximum of 8 tablets is given. *For patients receiving levodopa:* Discontinue levodopa at least 8 hr before initiating therapy with this product. Administer 1 tablet (25/250) 3 to 4 times daily to patients previously requiring 1500 mg or more of levodopa each day.
entacapone	Comtan	Used as adjunct to carbidopa-levodopa to treat patients with idiopathic Parkinson's disease who experience the signs and symptoms of end-of-dose "wearing-off." Give 200-mg tablet with each carbidopa-levodopa dosage.
levodopa	Dopar Larodopa	A metabolic precursor of dopamine. It enters the CNS by crossing the blood-brain barrier and is converted to dopamine. Give 0.5-1 gm PO daily in 2 or more doses. Dosage may be increased gradually in increments of 0.75 gm every 3-7 days as tolerated. The usual optimum dose should not exceed 8 gm.
pergolide	Permax ♦	Adjunctive to carbidopa-levodopa therapy. Many adverse effects. Give 0.05 mg for 2 days, then gradually increase over 12 days.
selegiline	Eldepryl Carbex	Irreversible MAO inhibitor. Give 5 mg at breakfast and lunch; allows carbidopa-levodopa dosages to be reduced.
tolcapone	Tasmar	May cause hallucinations and tardive dyskinesia. Give 100 or 200 mg 3 times daily without food and always as adjunctive therapy to carbidopa-levodopa therapy.
DOPAMINE RECEPTOR AGONISTS, NONERGOT		
pramipexole	Mirapex	Binds with high affinity to dopamine D_3 receptors. May stimulate dopamine receptors in the striatum. Follow precise dosing schedule in package insert.
ropinirole	Requip	Give 0.25 mg 3 times daily as initial dose. Titrate weekly according to precise dosing schedule listed in package insert.

The dosage should be reduced to the minimum effective level to counteract these effects, and dosages should be tapered as necessary to avoid excessive medication.

Numerous laboratory tests may be altered by these medications; this should be taken into account when monitoring patient status.

Patient and Family Teaching

You should tell the patient and family the following:

1. The patient should take the medication exactly as ordered by the nurse, physician, or other health care provider. Clinical improvement may take 2 to 3 weeks, so the patient should not stop taking the medication unless advised to do so by the health care provider.
2. Antiparkinsonian agents should be taken after meals to avoid stomach upset.
3. The patient should avoid taking vitamin preparations with vitamin B_6 (pyridoxine).
4. The nurse, physician, or other health care provider should be contacted immediately if parkinsonian symptoms become suddenly worse, if intermittent winking or muscle twitching occurs, or if abdominal pain, constipation, distention, or urinary problems occur.
5. Common side effects include dry mouth, dizziness, drowsiness, and GI symptoms. Some patients experience dizziness or light-headedness, especially as they move from lying to standing positions. The patient should avoid driving or tasks requiring alertness or rapid changes of movement.
6. The patient's urine, sweat, and saliva may darken after exposure to air.
7. The patient should avoid overexertion during hot weather.
8. Periodic ophthalmologic examinations are necessary when taking anticholinergic drugs.

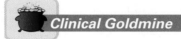 **Clinical Goldmine**

Controlling Adverse Effects

Decreasing the dosage can control the numerous adverse effects of these drugs.

SECTION FIVE

Psychotherapeutic Agents

OVERVIEW

Many of the drugs introduced in the following subsections act on more than one type of receptor. Each agent acts differently, making it possible for certain drugs to be given for specific actions without many adverse reactions. It should be clear that, if dosages are exceeded, many receptors may be excessively stimulated, causing widespread and serious effects.

ANTIANXIETY AGENTS

OVERVIEW

Anxiety is a common problem associated with many medical and surgical conditions, as well as a primary symptom in many psychiatric disorders. Anxiety is a normal human emotion, but when it is felt too frequently or interferes with a person's ability to perform activities of daily living, it is considered abnormal. Anxiety creates subjective feelings of helplessness, indecision, worry, apprehension, and irritability. Patients may complain of headache, gastric distress, insomnia, and inability to concentrate. It may also produce objective symptoms of restlessness, tremor, constipation, diarrhea, nausea, and muscle tension.

When anxiety is so severe that it must be treated with medication, antianxiety medications or tranquilizers are used to reduce some of the symptoms. They do not prevent the anxiety because the feelings or problems that produce the anxiety are still there. Therefore, antianxiety medication should be used for only a short time until other remedies can be found. It is especially important to view the use of these medications as a short-term solution because of the potential for addiction caused by them.

The major products used today for anxiety are the benzodiazepines, accounting for about 75% of the antianxiety prescriptions written today. Although benzodiazepines have a variety of uses, there are particular drugs in this category that are used primarily for treating anxiety. Other antianxiety agents are briefly included in this discussion.

ACTION

Benzodiazepines apparently act at the limbic, thalamic, and hypothalamic levels of the CNS, producing a calming effect. Benzodiazepines are used to relieve anxiety, tension, and fears that occur by themselves or as the

Pediatric Considerations

Psychotherapeutic Agents

- Buspirone has not been studied in persons under 18 years; therefore it is not recommended for use in that age group.
- Although diazepam (Valium) may be used in infants 6 months and over, this drug and other benzodiazepines should not be used to treat a hyperactive or psychotic child.
- The tricyclic antidepressants are usually not recommended for the treatment of depression in children under 12 years old. However, some agents, such as amitriptyline, desipramine, and imipramine, have been used in children over the age of 6 for major depression. Several of these agents are also used in the treatment of enuresis and attention deficit disorder. Be aware that children are very sensitive to an acute overdose, which should always be considered very serious and potentially fatal. Adolescents often require a decreased dose because of their sensitivity to this drug category.
- All adolescents taking antidepressants must be closely monitored for suicidal ideation because research suggests they are at higher risk for suicide than some other groups.
- Adverse effects reported in children receiving the tricyclic antidepressants include changes in electrocardiogram patterns, increased nervousness, sleep disorders, complaints of tiredness, hypertension, and mild stomach distress.
- Children are at a greater risk for neuromuscular or extrapyramidal side effects, especially dystonias. Monitor closely if antipsychotic agents are administered.
- Lithium may decrease the bone density or bone formation in children. If it is necessary to use this drug, monitor closely serum levels and for signs of toxicity.

Modified from McKenry LM, Salerno E: *Mosby's pharmacology in nursing*, ed 21, St Louis, 2003, Mosby.

Geriatric Considerations

Psychotherapeutic Agents

- The elderly population tends to have higher serum levels of the antipsychotic and antidepressant drugs because of changes in drug distribution resulting from a decrease in lean body mass, less total body water, less serum albumin, and usually an increase in body fat. Therefore, these patients require a lower drug dose and a more gradual drug dose titration than those of the adult patient.
- Geriatric patients are more prone to have orthostatic hypotension, anticholinergic side effects, extrapyramidal side effects, and sedation. They should be carefully evaluated before starting antipsychotic agents. If such potent medications are necessary, close supervision and the prescribing of the lowest dose possible are recommended.
- The elderly patient generally should receive half the recommended adult dose of the benzodiazepines. The patient with organic brain syndrome should receive only 33% to 50% of the usual adult dose with increases in dosage at 7- to 10-day periods. When clinical improvement is noted, attempts at tapering and discontinuing the drug should be instituted.
- The tricyclic antidepressants may cause increased anxiety in the geriatric patient. If the patient has cardiovascular disease, the use of the tricyclic antidepressants increases the risk of inducing dysrhythmias, tachycardia, stroke, congestive heart failure, or myocardial infarction.

Modified from McKenry LM, Salerno E: *Mosby's pharmacology in nursing*, ed 21, St Louis, 2003, Mosby.

result of illness. Other indications include management of delirium tremens after alcohol withdrawal; premedication for surgical and endoscopic procedures or electric cardioversion; treatment of convulsive disorders (diazepam only); and relief of muscle spasm.

ADVERSE REACTIONS

Adverse reactions to antianxiety agents include hypotension, tachycardia, clumsiness, confusion, depression, drowsiness, fatigue, headache, insomnia, paradoxic reactions (excitement, hallucinations, agitation, hostility, or rage), syncope (light-headedness and fainting), unsteadiness, visual disturbances, weakness, anorexia, constipation, difficulty swallowing, dry mouth, hiccups, jaundice, nausea, vomiting, urinary retention, blood cell changes, pruritus, skin rash, joint pain, and unexplained sore throat and fever.

Overdosage may produce sleepiness, confusion, coma, diminished reflexes, and hypotension. Tolerance is easily developed.

DRUG INTERACTIONS

Simultaneous administration of benzodiazepines with any of the following substances may increase either agent's effect: alcohol, anesthetics, MAO inhibitors, or CNS depressants such as antihistamines, barbiturates, phenothiazines, narcotics, sedatives, tranquilizers, hypnotics, anticonvulsants, or tricyclic antidepressants. Caffeinated products and excessive cigarette smoking can antagonize the anxiolytic effect of these drugs. Herbal products are also often used by patients to treat stress and anxiety. The Complementary and Alternative Therapies box summarizes herbal preparations the patient may be using and their drug interactions.

Complementary and Alternative Therapies

Stress/Anxiety

PRODUCT	COMMENTS
Chamomile	No reported toxicities
Kava kava	Potential interactions with ethanol, CNS depressants
St. John's wort	Potential interactions with antidepressants (including selective serotonin reuptake inhibitors, tricyclics, MAO inhibitors), narcotics, other CNS depressants, reserpine, digoxin
Valerian	Increased effect/toxicity with CNS depressants, sedative-hypnotics (barbiturates), antidepressants, anxiolytics, antihistamines

Modified from Krinsky DL, Lavella JB, Hawkins EB, et al: *Natural therapeutics pocket guide*, ed 2, Hudson, Ohio, 2003, Lexi-Comp, Inc.

Nursing Implications and Patient Teaching

Assessment

You should learn as much as possible about the health history of the patient, including hypersensitivities, underlying systemic disease (especially pulmonary, cardiac, liver, or renal disease, epilepsy or seizures, myasthenia gravis, mental illness, and drug abuse or dependence), possibility of pregnancy, breastfeeding, or whether the patient is currently taking any medications (both prescribed and over-the-counter [OTC]) that may produce drug interactions. These conditions are contraindications or precautions to the use of antianxiety agents.

Memory Jogger

Benzodiazepines

The patient should be given the smallest dosage possible to reduce the opportunity for overdose, particularly in those patients with a history of drug addiction or dependence.

The patient may have a history of feelings of apprehension, uncertainty, fear, an unpleasant state of tension, a sense of impending doom, insomnia (inability to sleep), irritability, hypersensitivity to stress, difficulty in concentrating, or nightmares.

Diagnosis

In addition to the medical diagnosis, what other problems does the patient experience? Does he have family support, or is he isolated and lonely? Is the patient able to work and take care of his daily needs, or is he incapacitated with anxiety?

Planning

Elderly patients (over age 60) and those with chronic illnesses may require a decreased initial dosage and may need careful monitoring of individual response before alterations in dosage are made. Benzodiazepines generally have a long half-life and can have cumulative effects. Patients with a history of seizures or epilepsy should have their dosages of benzodiazepines tapered slowly.

Implementation

Administering the benzodiazepines during or immediately after meals decreases the incidence of GI side effects. The manufacturers' instructions for diluting and slowly injecting parenteral medications should be followed to prevent the possibility of respiratory failure.

Depression commonly accompanies anxiety, so patients must be questioned and observed for suicidal tendencies.

Treatment with antianxiety agents should proceed slowly in the elderly, the debilitated, those with limited pulmonary reserve, and those in whom a hypotensive episode might precipitate heart problems.

Table 16-6 summarizes important dosage information about antianxiety medications.

Clinical Landmine

Benzodiazepines

Benzodiazepines accumulate in adipose tissue, which substantially increases their half-life, making them dangerous particularly for older patients.

Evaluation

Mental alertness, cognitive functions, and physical abilities may be impaired with the use of antianxiety agents. These drugs should be given in conjunction with counseling or psychotherapy for maximum benefit.

Abrupt termination of these agents may cause delayed withdrawal symptoms (up to 1 week later) of

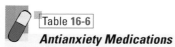

Table 16-6
Antianxiety Medications

GENERIC NAME	TRADE NAME	COMMENTS AND DOSAGE
BENZODIAZEPINES		
alprazolam	Xanax	Action peaks in 1-2 hr; half-life is 12-15 hr. Effectiveness and safety in children under the age of 18 have not been determined. *Adults:* 0.25-0.5 mg PO 3 times daily initially; titrate to maximum dose of 4 mg PO daily in divided doses. *Elderly, debilitated patients:* 0.25 mg PO 2 to 3 times daily initially.
chlordiazepoxide	Libritabs Librium Mitran	Peak levels in 1-4 hr; half-life is 5-30 hr. Food or antacids slow absorption. Injection IV must be very slow to avoid producing respiratory arrest. *Adults:* 5-25 mg 3 to 4 times daily; 5-10 mg 3 to 4 times daily may be given several days preoperatively to allay anxiety. *Elderly, debilitated patients:* 5 mg 2 to 4 times daily
clorazepate	Tranxene	Peak effect is in 60 min; half-life is 2 days. Some reports indicate a fall in hematocrit with long-term use. Can be given once each day. *Adults:* 30 mg daily; adjust gradually with a range of 15-60 mg daily. *Elderly, debilitated patients:* 7.5-15 mg daily initially.
diazepam	Valium	Peak blood levels are reached within 1-2 hr; half-life is 20-50 hr. • *Anxiety and management of convulsive disorders:* 2-10 mg 2 to 4 times daily. Sustained- release capsules, 15-30 mg daily. • *Skeletal muscle spasm:* 2-10 mg 3 to 4 times daily. Sustained-release capsules, 15-30 mg daily. *Elderly, debilitated patients:* 2-2.5 mg daily or twice daily, then gradually increase as tolerated. *Children:* 1-2.5 mg 3 to 4 times daily initially, then gradually increase.
halazepam	Paxipam	Action peaks in 1-3 hr; half-life is 14 hr. Individualize dosages as needed and tolerated. *Adults:* 20-40 mg PO 3 to 4 times daily. Optimal range is 80-160 mg PO daily. *Elderly, debilitated patients:* 20 mg PO 2 to 4 times daily.
lorazepam	Ativan	Action peaks in 2½ hr; half-life is 10-15 hr. Patients may experience withdrawal manifested as insomnia 2 or 3 nights after cessation of therapy. IM injection is used as a preanesthetic agent for adults only. It is also given IV for sedation and relief of anxiety. • *Anxiety:* 2-3 mg PO 2 to 3 times daily initially; usual range is 2-6 mg daily in divided doses, with the largest dose before sleep. • *Insomnia:* Single bedtime dose of 2-4 mg PO. *Elderly, debilitated patients:* 1-2 mg PO daily in divided doses.
oxazepam	Serax	Peak blood levels at 2-4 hr; half-life is 5-20 hr. The incidence of toxicity is low. • *Anxiety:* 10-30 mg PO 3 to 4 times daily. *Elderly, debilitated patients:* 10 mg PO 3 times daily initially, then increase gradually to 15 mg 3 to 4 times daily.
NONBENZODIAZEPINE ANTIANXIETY AGENTS		
buspirone	BuSpar	Approved for short-term use in anxiety disorders. Mechanism of action unknown; chemically unrelated to other antianxiety medications. *Adults:* 5 mg 3 times daily, increased by 5 mg every 2-3 days prn; maintenance, 20-30 mg daily in divided doses.
doxepin	Sinequan	*Adults:* 75-150 mg/day. For oral concentrate, do not mix with grape juice.

Continued

Table 16-6

Antianxiety Medications—cont'd

GENERIC NAME	TRADE NAME	COMMENTS AND DOSAGE
NONBENZODIAZEPINE ANTIANXIETY AGENTS—cont'd		
hydroxyzine	Atarax Vistaril	Antihistamine for the symptomatic relief of anxiety, especially in psychoneurosis. Also has analgesic activity that may be helpful in relieving pruritus caused by allergies. Medication may be used preoperatively for surgery or obstetric patients to permit decrease in narcotic dosages, reduce anxiety, and control emesis. Product also helps control acutely disturbed or hysterical patients. This product is for IM use only. Subcutaneous, intraarterial, or IV use may produce tissue necrosis and hemolysis. • *Anxiety* *Adults:* 50-100 mg PO 4 times daily. *Children over 6 years of age:* 50-100 mg/day PO in divided doses. *Children under 6 years of age:* 50 mg/day PO in divided doses. • *Sedative* *Adults:* 50-100 mg PO, or 25-100 mg IM. *Children:* 0.6 mg/kg PO, or 1.1 mg/kg IM.
meprobamate	Equanil Miltown	Antianxiety and mild skeletal muscle relaxant, acts on numerous sites in CNS to produce mild sedation; used for short-term relief of anxiety. *Adults:* 400 mg 3 to 4 times daily; smaller doses in elderly or debilitated patients; do not exceed 2400 mg daily.

abdominal or muscle cramps, vomiting, diaphoresis (sweating), tremor, or convulsions. Tapering the dosage for patients on long-term therapy helps prevent this problem.

You should take lying, sitting, and standing blood pressures when monitoring hypotensive changes.

Alternatives for coping with stress and change should be discussed with the patient. For example, increased regular physical activity, muscle relaxation exercises, and participation in hobbies may be helpful.

Patient and Family Teaching

You should tell the patient and family the following:

1. The patient should take this medication exactly as ordered and not stop taking the medication unless advised to do so by the nurse, physician, or other health care provider. If a dose is forgotten, it should be taken as soon as it is remembered, if it is within 1 to 2 hours of the regular dosage time. If it is later than 2 hours, the patient should skip the dose and take the next dose at the regular time. The patient should not double the dosage.

2. The patient must keep regular appointments with the nurse, physician, or other health care provider so that progress can be checked and side effects of the drug can be monitored.

3. Antianxiety agents can cause dizziness, lightheadedness, drowsiness, and unsteadiness. They may decrease the patient's ability to think or react clearly and quickly. The patient should not drive, operate hazardous machinery, or perform activities requiring alertness until response to the drug has been determined. These symptoms will often disappear after the patient has taken the medication for several weeks. Additionally, the patient should change to sitting or standing positions slowly to minimize these symptoms and prevent falls.

4. The patient should notify the nurse, physician, or other health care provider if any new or troublesome symptoms occur while she is taking this medication, such as ulcers or sores in the mouth, hallucinations, feelings of confusion, difficulty sleeping, skin rash, jaundice, bradycardia (slow heartbeat), difficulty with breathing, sore throat and fever, unusual nervousness, excitement, irritability, depression, or eye pain.

5. This medication must be kept out of the reach of children and all others for whom it is not prescribed.

6. The nurse, physician, or other health care provider should be informed if the patient begins taking any new prescription or nonprescription drugs. Many different medications have interactions with antianxiety agents; therefore, the health care provider may want to increase or decrease the dosage.

7. The patient should not drink any alcohol while taking this medicine.

8. The patient should be aware that cigarette smoking and the use of caffeinated beverages (coffee, tea, cola) can decrease the effect of antianxiety agents.

9. Benzodiazepines are not intended for use by pregnant women. If the patient is pregnant or breastfeeding, or if the patient should become pregnant while taking this medicine, the nurse, physician, or other health care provider should be informed immediately.

10. This drug may be habit forming; the patient should use it for the least time possible.

ANTIDEPRESSANTS

OVERVIEW

Depression, whether mild or so severe that it interferes with activities of daily living, has been recognized for centuries. Many types of therapy have been explored, but only in the last 30 years have medications been discovered that significantly help to improve a patient's mood without extensive side effects. Although all medications are equally effective in treating depression if they work, not all patients respond to all medications, and patients may experience different side effects with each drug.

MAO inhibitors were initially used to treat other diseases. The antidepressant effect was discovered as an unexpected side effect of that therapy. They were then used to treat depressed patients until tricyclic antidepressant therapy became available in the 1960s. MAO inhibitors are now used primarily when tricyclic therapy is unsatisfactory or when other therapy is inappropriate or refused. In the last few years, a number of chemically related selective serotonin reuptake inhibitors (SSRIs) have entered the field for treatment of depressed patients. Each of these groups will be discussed separately.

TRICYCLIC ANTIDEPRESSANTS

Action

The antidepressant effect of tricyclics is not completely understood. It is thought that tricyclic antidepressants inhibit the uptake of norepinephrine and/or serotonin (biogenic amines) by the presynaptic neuronal membrane in the CNS, thereby increasing the concentration of these biogenic amines at the synapse.

Uses

Tricyclic antidepressants are used primarily to relieve the symptoms of severe depression that has internal biological causes (endogenous depression). They may also be used to treat mild depression caused by factors in the patient's life (exogenous or reactive depression),

which is not self-limiting and does not interfere with usual activities of daily living. They are less commonly used for manic-depressive disorders as adjunctive or additional therapy.

Adverse Reactions

Adverse reactions to tricyclic antidepressants include dysrhythmias, postural hypotension, confusion, headache, drowsiness that lasts a long time, constipation, nausea, vomiting, blood dyscrasias, fever, photosensitivity, pruritus, skin rash, muscle twitching, tremors, urinary hesitancy or retention, altered liver function tests, blurred vision, and nervousness.

Overdosage may initially produce stimulation of the CNS, resulting in irritability, agitation, hallucinations, delirium, twitching, hypertonia, hyperreflexia, nystagmus, hyperpyrexia (very high body temperature), hypertension, and seizures (more commonly seen in children). This initial CNS stimulation is followed by CNS depression, causing drowsiness, areflexia, hypothermia (abnormally low body temperature), hypotension, dysrhythmias, respiratory depression, coma, or cardiorespiratory arrest.

Drug Interactions

Tricyclic antidepressants increase the CNS depressant effect of alcohol and other CNS depressants, particularly ethchlorvynol. The effects of anticonvulsants may be decreased when used with tricyclic antidepressants. The antihypertensive effects of guanethidine and clonidine may be blocked when used with most tricyclic antidepressants, with the exception of doxepin. There may be a reduction in the antidepressant effect of tricyclics and an increase in their side effects when used concurrently with estrogen, including oral contraceptives containing estrogen. An increased incidence of cardiac dysrhythmias has been found with concurrent use of thyroid medication and tricyclic antidepressants. Severe hypertension or hyperpyrexia may result when tricyclic antidepressants are used with MAO inhibitors or sympathomimetics.

Nursing Implications and Patient Teaching

Assessment

You should learn as much as possible about the health history of the patient; allergy, disease, and other medications the patient may currently be taking, including OTC preparations, must be considered. Many diseases present contraindications or precautions for the use of tricyclic drugs. The Complementary and Alternative Therapies box provides a summary of herbal products that patients may be taking to help with symptoms of depression and their drug interactions.

The patient may have a history of insomnia, early morning awakening, anorexia, constipation, loss of motivation, and fatigue. He may talk about feelings of

Complementary and Alternative Therapies

Depression

PRODUCT	COMMENTS
St. John's wort	Potential interaction with antidepressants (including SSRIs, tricyclics, MAO inhibitors), narcotics, other CNS depressants, reserpine, digoxin
Ginkgo	Potential interaction with anticoagulants, aspirin, NSAIDs, antiplatelet agents, MAO inhibitors, acetylcholinesterase inhibitors

Modified from Krinsky DL, Lavella JB, Hawkins EB, et al: *Natural therapeutics pocket guide,* ed 2, Hudson, Ohio, 2003, Lexi-Comp, Inc.

hopelessness and pessimism, say negative things about himself, respond slowly to questions, and have slowed motor movements, decreased facial expression, and stooped posture. You should assess the patient thoroughly for any suicidal feelings.

Diagnosis

What other problems does the patient have? Often a depressed patient does not eat, bathe, or dress appropriately. She may cut off contact with other people, and may be unable to work. Any of these problems may be addressed with the patient when she is starting to feel better.

Planning

Tricyclic antidepressants should not be given if the patient has a history of hypersensitivity to a tricyclic antidepressant. A patient who is hypersensitive to one type of tricyclic will likely be sensitive to all tricyclics (cross-sensitivity). Patients with a history of recent myocardial infarction, narrow-angle glaucoma, or severe hepatic or renal failure also should not take these drugs. Tricyclic antidepressants should be used very carefully with MAO inhibitors. You should discuss importance of contraception with women of childbearing age who are taking tricyclics.

Antidepressants may cause manic-depressive patients to go into the manic phase of their illness; exaggerated symptoms of paranoid ideation and schizophrenia may develop in patients who have these disorders. This may be avoided or treated by reducing the dosage of the tricyclic antidepressant or by using a tranquilizer.

Only the smallest reasonable amount of antidepressants should be given to patients who are possibly suicidal.

Implementation

Because the plasma concentrations of tricyclic antidepressants vary widely and may not correspond well with the dosage or therapeutic effects, the initial and maintenance dosages of these drugs must be carefully determined, based on the patient's age, physical health status, and response to the drug.

The initial dose may cause sedation, especially when the patient is taking a tricyclic known to have moderate to strong sedative effects. Therefore, tricyclic antidepressant therapy may be started with a single bedtime dose, especially for depressed patients with a sleep disturbance. The drug dosage can then be varied or titrated to achieve the best response with the lowest dosage and minimal side effects. A maintenance dosage, administered in divided doses or as a single bedtime dose, may be continued for 6 months to 1 year.

Table 16-7 summarizes the important information you should know about tricyclic antidepressant medications.

Evaluation

The desired antidepressant effect of the drug will usually occur within 1 to 4 weeks after therapy is initiated.

If a tricyclic antidepressant is given in large doses or for a long time, the drug should be stopped by gradually reducing the dose over 4 to 8 weeks to avoid withdrawal symptoms of general listlessness, headache, and nausea.

Patient and Family Teaching

You should tell the patient and family the following:
1. The patient should take this medication exactly as ordered. It may be taken with food to avoid gastric distress. It may take up to 8 weeks before the patient begins to feel better. Therefore, it is important to take the drug in the exact amount and frequency specified, even though the patient notices no changes initially.
2. Tricyclic antidepressants should never be stopped suddenly because there could be an increase in symptoms, as well as nausea, headache, and feelings of listlessness. The patient must not stop taking the drug without talking to the nurse, physician or other health care provider.
3. Tricyclic antidepressants may cause drowsiness or make the patient feel less alert than usual. If so, the patient should avoid driving or doing other activities that require alertness. This feeling should pass after the medication is taken for a

Table 16-7

Tricyclic Antidepressants

GENERIC NAME	TRADE NAME	COMMENTS AND DOSAGE
amitriptyline	Elavil	Has a strong sedative effect, especially early in therapy. It should be taken at bedtime to decrease daytime drowsiness. Used to treat endogenous depression accompanied by anxiety. *Initial:* 25 mg PO 2 to 4 times daily. *Maintenance:* 50-100 mg/day at bedtime or in divided doses; may also give 20-30 mg IM 4 times daily.
amoxapine	Asendin	The antidepressant effect is usually seen within 2 wk after initiating therapy; used to treat a wide variety of depressions, including reactive, endogenous, and psychotic depressions. *Initial:* 50 mg PO 3 times daily; increase to 100 mg PO 3 times daily on third day. *Maintenance:* 30 mg/day or less at bedtime.
clomipramine	Anafranil	Used to treat obsessive-compulsive disorder. Give 25 mg daily and gradually increase to 100 mg over 2 wk.
desipramine	Norpramin	Has mild sedative effect; orthostatic hypotension is common during the first few weeks of therapy. Used to treat a variety of depressions, particularly endogenous type. *Initial:* 25-50 mg PO 3 times daily; give only 25-50 mg/day in adolescent and elderly patients. *Maintenance:* Up to 200 mg/day.
doxepin	Sinequan	Has marked sedative effect, particularly during initial phase of therapy. Used to treat psychotic and psychoneurotic depression with associated anxiety and somatic symptoms. The oral concentrate should be diluted in milk, fruit juice, or water before administration. *Initial:* 25 mg PO 3 times daily. *Maintenance:* 50-150 mg/day at bedtime or in divided doses.
imipramine	Tofranil	Used to treat endogenous depression; it is the only tricyclic that is also used to treat enuresis in children. *Initial:* 25 mg PO 3 to 4 times daily; or 25-50 mg IM 3 to 4 times daily; reduce to 30-40 mg/day in divided doses for adolescents and elderly patients. *Maintenance:* 50-150 mg/day PO at bedtime.
nortriptyline	Aventyl Pamelor	Used to treat endogenous depression. *Initial:* 25 mg PO 3 to 4 times daily; reduce to 30 or 50 mg/day in divided doses for adolescent or elderly patients and increase only as needed and tolerated. *Maintenance:* Up to 100 mg/day PO.
protriptyline	Vivactil	Used to treat endogenous depression, particularly when the patient is withdrawn or listless. This drug has no sedative effect and stimulates the CNS more than other tricyclics. *Initial:* 5-10 mg PO 3 to 4 times daily; reduce dose in adolescents and elderly to 5 mg 3 times daily. *Maintenance:* Not to exceed 60 mg/day.
trimipramine	Surmontil	This product has a strong sedative effect; used to treat endogenous depression accompanied by anxiety. *Initial:* 25 mg PO 3 times daily; reduce dosage to 25 mg twice daily in adolescent and elderly patients. *Maintenance:* 50-150 mg/day at bedtime. In adolescents and the elderly, increase dose to maximum of 100 mg/day only as necessary and tolerated.

short time. The patient should tell the nurse, physician, or other health care provider if drowsiness or decreased alertness persists longer than 2 weeks and interferes with usual activities.

4. Dryness of the mouth may occur when medication is first started. Chewing sugarless gum, sucking on hard candy, or rinsing the mouth frequently may help relieve the dryness.

5. Tricyclic antidepressants will increase the effects of alcohol, sleeping pills, and some medications for the relief of colds and hay fever. The patient should avoid alcohol and check with the nurse, physician, or other health care provider before taking any other medications.

6. Tricyclic antidepressants are very powerful drugs and must be kept out of the reach of children and others for whom they are not prescribed. They should not be left on dressers or low bedside tables.

7. Light-headedness, dizziness, or feelings of faintness occur in some people taking this drug, especially older people. To reduce this feeling, the patient should move slowly, especially when changing from a lying or sitting position to standing upright.

8. Tricyclic antidepressants are usually stopped several days before the patient has any surgery that requires anesthesia. The nurse, physician, or other health care provider must develop a plan to gradually stop the medication in the correct way.

9. The nurse, physician, or other health care provider should be contacted if the patient develops any new or troublesome symptoms, especially the appearance of urinary retention, constipation, blurred vision, or excessive sleepiness.

10. If the patient will be taking this medication for a long time, he should wear a Medic Alert bracelet or necklace or carry a medical identification card listing this drug.

MONOAMINE OXIDASE INHIBITORS

Action

MAO is an enzyme found in the mitochondria of cells located in nerve endings and other body tissues such as the kidney, liver, and intestines. This enzyme normally acts as a catalyst by inactivating dopamine, norepinephrine, epinephrine, and serotonin (biogenic amines) and therefore regulating the intracellular levels of these neurotransmitters. MAO inhibitors block the inactivation of the biogenic amines, resulting in an increased concentration of dopamine, epinephrine, norepinephrine, and serotonin at neuronal synapses. The antidepressant effects of MAO inhibitors are thought to be directly related to this increased concentration of biogenic amines.

Clinical Landmine

MAO Inhibitors

MAO inhibitors may cause very dangerous reactions if taken with certain foods or beverages. The patient must not eat foods such as cheese, yogurt, sour cream, raisins, bananas, avocados, bean pods, chicken livers, or pickled herring, and should avoid meat tenderizers and soy sauce. Only very small amounts of coffee, tea, cola drinks, and chocolate are permitted.

Uses

MAO inhibitors are used to relieve the symptoms of severe reactive or of endogenous depression that have not responded to tricyclic antidepressant therapy, electroconvulsive therapy, or other modes of psychotherapy.

Adverse Reactions

Adverse reactions to MAO inhibitors include postural hypotension, dysrhythmias, ataxia, drowsiness, hallucinations, headache, hyperactivity, insomnia, seizures, tremors, vertigo, anorexia, constipation, diarrhea, nausea, vomiting, fever, photosensitivity, skin rash, dysuria (painful urination), incontinence, blurred vision, dry mouth, edema, and impotence.

Overdosage produces mental confusion, restlessness, hypotension, respiratory depression, tachycardia, seizures, and shock, which may persist for 1 to 2 weeks.

Drug and Food Interactions

MAO inhibitors have many drug interactions. They may potentiate the CNS depressant effect of alcohol, anesthetics, sedatives, hypnotics, and narcotics and may

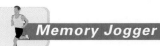

Memory Jogger

Food and Beverage Interactions

Sudden and severe hypertension can result when MAO inhibitors are used with the following foods and beverages, which are high in tyramine and other vasopressor amines: alcoholic beverages such as beer and wines (particularly sherry, hearty red wines, and Chianti), yeast extracts, meat tenderizers, soy sauce, beef or chicken liver, cured meats, dried or cured fish, sausage prepared with yeast, pickled herring, bean pods, figs, raisins, bananas, avocados, fava beans, sour cream, yogurt, and cheese. Concurrent use of MAO inhibitors and large amounts of caffeine-containing products (coffee, tea, cola, chocolate) can cause hypertension and cardiac dysrhythmias.

cause severe hypertension and hyperpyrexia. If they are used with anticonvulsants, they may cause a change in the seizure pattern of the patient, and the dosage of the anticonvulsant medication may have to be adjusted accordingly. The hypotensive effects of diuretics and antihypertensives may be enhanced when those agents are used with MAO inhibitors. The hypoglycemic effects of insulin or oral hypoglycemics may be enhanced by MAO inhibitors, and dosages may require adjustment accordingly. MAO inhibitors and tricyclic antidepressants are generally not used together because hyperpyrexia, severe convulsions, hypertensive crisis, and death may result.

Nursing Implications and Patient Teaching

Assessment

You should learn as much as possible about the health history of the patient, including the presence of any diseases that may contraindicate the use of MAO inhibitors. The patient should be asked about other medications she may currently be taking (especially tricyclic antidepressants) and the possibility of pregnancy. You should also assess the level of the patient's depression and check for suicidal ideas.

Diagnosis

What other problems does the patient have as a result of this diagnosis? Is the patient able to understand the dietary restrictions that must be followed when he is taking these medications? What assistance does the patient need in taking care of himself? The nurse should focus on things she may be able to teach the patient or learn about the patient that will be helpful to the patient in getting well.

Planning

The safe use of MAO inhibitors in pregnant patients or nursing mothers has not been established.

Implementation

MAO inhibitors are given only orally and are well absorbed by this route. The desired antidepressant effect of MAO inhibitors will usually occur within 1 to 4 weeks of drug therapy. If results are not obtained after this time, the patient will not be helped by continuing to take the drug. When improvement is noted during the first 4 weeks of drug therapy, the dosage should then be reduced gradually over a period of several weeks until an effective maintenance dosage is reached. MAO inhibitors are usually not given in the evening because of their psychomotor stimulating effect, which may produce insomnia.

The maintenance dose of MAO inhibitors can be administered in either single or divided doses. MAO inhibitors should be discontinued at least 2 weeks before elective surgery. If emergency surgery is indicated, doses of narcotics and anesthetics should be reduced. All patients treated on an outpatient basis need to be closely monitored.

Information about MAO inhibitors is provided in Table 16-8.

Evaluation

All patients taking MAO inhibitors must be monitored for symptoms of postural hypotension. If this occurs, the dosage of the drug should be reduced or the drug should be discontinued.

Patients who are agitated or who have schizophrenia may become more hyperactive. Manic-depressive patients may go into the manic phase of their illness; this may be treated by stopping the drug for a brief period of time and then starting again at a lower dosage.

The effects of MAO inhibitors continue for approximately 2 weeks after the drug is stopped. Therefore, patients who have been taking MAO inhibitors should avoid taking any drugs or eating any foods that are known to interact with MAO inhibitors for this 2-week period.

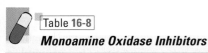

Table 16-8
Monoamine Oxidase Inhibitors

GENERIC NAME	TRADE NAME	COMMENTS AND DOSAGE
phenelzine	Nardil 🍁	*Initial:* 15 mg PO 3 times daily up to 75 mg maximum. *Maintenance:* Reduce slowly to 15 mg PO daily or every other day.
tranylcypromine	Parnate 🍁	Improvement in symptoms is usually seen 1-3 wk after therapy is begun. There is a higher incidence of hypertensive reactions with this drug than with other MAO inhibitors. Used to treat endogenous depression. *Initial:* 20-30 mg PO daily in divided doses (usually 10-20 mg in AM and 10 mg in PM). *Maintenance:* 10-20 mg PO daily.

Patient and Family Teaching

You should tell the patient and family the following:

1. The patient needs to take this medication exactly as ordered by the nurse, physician, or other health care provider. It may take up to 4 weeks before the patient begins to feel better. Therefore, it is important to take the drug in the exact amount and frequency ordered even though the patient may notice no changes.

2. MAO inhibitors can increase the effects of alcohol and other drugs such as narcotics, sleeping pills, and amphetamines. Alcohol (including beer and wine) should be avoided. The patient should check with the nurse, physician, or other health care provider before taking any other prescription or OTC medications.

3. The effect of MAO inhibitors continues for 2 weeks after the patient stops taking them. Therefore, the patient must continue to avoid eating or drinking the previously specified foods or beverages during the 2-week period.

4. The patient may experience light-headedness, dizziness, or a feeling of faintness, especially when getting up from a lying or sitting position. To reduce this feeling, the patient should move slowly when changing positions.

5. MAO inhibitors may cause drowsiness or make the patient feel less alert than usual. If so, the patient should avoid driving or other activities requiring alertness.

6. MAO inhibitors should be discontinued 2 weeks before the patient has any surgery that requires anesthesia. The nurse, physician, or other health care provider must be informed if surgery is planned so that the drug may be stopped in the correct way.

7. The nurse, physician, or other health care provider should be contacted immediately or the patient should go to the hospital emergency room if fever, severe headache, nausea, vomiting, chest pain, or rapid heartbeat develops.

8. MAO inhibitors are dangerous drugs that should be kept out of the reach of children and all others for whom they are not prescribed. These drugs must not be left sitting on a dresser or low bedside table.

9. The patient should wear a Medic Alert bracelet or necklace or carry a medical identification card listing this medication.

SELECTIVE SEROTONIN REUPTAKE INHIBITORS AND MISCELLANEOUS ANTIDEPRESSANTS

Action

Since the beginning of the 1980s, a series of new antidepressant medications have been available. Some are chemically unrelated to one another, but all act in some way to prolong serotonin in the brain. Their differences are often in terms of side effects.

Among the SSRIs, four products have become very well known. Their antidepressant action is presumed to be linked to their inhibition of CNS neuronal uptake of serotonin. These products are potent and selective inhibitors of neuronal serotonin reuptake, and they also have a weak effect on norepinephrine and dopamine neuronal uptake. Because they cause far fewer side effects than other antidepressant medications, they have become extensively used.

There are also three antidepressant products that have an effect on serotonin uptake but that are chemically unrelated to the SSRIs: bupropion, venlafaxine, and nefazodone. The neurochemical mechanism of bupropion is unknown, but it does not inhibit MAO. Its ability to block neuronal uptake of serotonin and norepinephrine is much weaker than that of the tricyclics. It does inhibit the neuronal uptake of dopamine to some extent. Venlafaxine is a potent inhibitor of neuronal serotonin and norepinephrine reuptake and a weak inhibitor of dopamine uptake. Nefazodone inhibits neuronal uptake of serotonin and norepinephrine, but the mechanism for this action is unknown.

There are three other antidepressant products that are related because they are all tetracyclic compounds. These products are maprotiline, mirtazapine, and trazodone. Tetracyclic compounds enhance central noradrenergic and serotonergic activity through an unknown mechanism. They have different amounts of antagonistic activity toward 5-HT receptors. These products inhibit the uptake of serotonin at the neuronal synaptosomes in the brain and enhance the behavioral changes caused by serotonin. The action of these drugs is more selective than that of other types of antidepressants. They have less effect on the cardiac conduction system than do tricyclic antidepressants, and they cause almost no CNS stimulation, which occurs frequently with MAO inhibitors.

Uses

These drugs are used in short-term treatment (less than 5 weeks) of outpatients with a diagnosis that is listed in the category of major depressive disorders in the fourth edition of the *Diagnostic and Statistical Manual of Mental Disorders* (DSM-IV). They have also been used extensively for long-term therapy in patients with dysthymic disorders and minor depressive episodes.

Adverse Reactions

Adverse reactions to these drugs include dizziness, tachycardia, dysrhythmias, hypertension, hypotension, rash, pruritus, constipation, weight loss, nausea and vomiting, anorexia, weight gain, diarrhea, appetite increase, dyspepsia (stomach discomfort after eating), menstrual complaints, impotence, urinary frequency, dry mouth, headache, excessive sweating, tremor, sedation, insomnia, blurred vision, agitation, confusion, hostility, and disturbed concentration.

In nearly 4% of patients taking fluoxetine, a rash develops with accompanying fever, leukocytosis, arthralgia (joint pain), edema, carpal tunnel syndrome, respiratory distress, lymphadenopathy, proteinuria, and mild transaminase elevation.

Trazodone has also produced early menses, hematuria (blood in the urine), urinary frequency, and weight changes.

Drug Interactions

If bupropion is taken with levodopa, the chance of adverse effects increases. If bupropion is used with carbamazepine, cimetidine, phenobarbital, or phenytoin, the hepatic metabolism of the drugs may be increased. Acute toxicity may develop if bupropion is given with phenelzine.

Fluoxetine increases the half-life of some drugs and may displace drugs bound to protein, such as warfarin and digitoxin, or be displaced by them. Concurrent use of trazodone and antihypertensives can cause hypotension. There are many other isolated drug interactions. Trazodone may increase the effects of alcohol, barbiturates, and other CNS depressants. The drug should be stopped as long as possible before general anesthesia because interactions are unknown.

Nursing Implications and Patient Teaching

Assessment

You should learn as much as possible about the health history of the patient, including history of hypersensitivity, presence of seizure disorder, current or prior diagnosis of bulimia or anorexia nervosa (these patients tend to have more seizures when receiving bupropion), or recent use of an MAO inhibitor. After stopping MAO inhibitor therapy, the patient should wait at least 14 days before starting bupropion.

Diagnosis

You should determine what other problems this patient may be having as a result of depression. Assessment of deficits in nutrition, safety, and knowledge are important. What other problems does this patient have specifically? For a patient who has been taking the medication, side effects such as insomnia, impotence, and taste disorders may make the underlying depression worse. Evaluate the extent of side effects and the impact on the patient's ability to function.

Planning

The incidence of seizures in patients taking bupropion is approximately four times greater than that in patients taking other antidepressant medications.

Fluoxetine has a relatively long half-life (2 to 3 days) and problems with liver or renal failure may prolong the drug's action in the body. There is growing evidence that this product may be useful in treating panic attacks, obsessive-compulsive disorders, and other psychiatric problems.

Dosage levels must be individualized based on symptoms. Patients may need to keep a diary or journal to actually realize that they are feeling better. A stable amount of the drug in the blood may not be reached until 4 to 5 weeks after starting therapy. Fluoxetine stays in the body for weeks. This may be important when drug therapy must be stopped.

Trazodone should not be used while the patient is having electroshock therapy.

Implementation

To reduce the risk of seizures while the patient is taking bupropion, the daily dosage should be kept below 450 mg, it should be given in three divided doses, and the dosage should be increased gradually.

Additional important information about these medications is summarized in Table 16-9.

Evaluation

Many patients taking bupropion experience some sort of agitation, increased restlessness, anxiety, and insomnia. If these symptoms cannot be controlled with a sedative-hypnotic, the medication should be stopped.

The desired antidepressant effect usually occurs within 1 to 2 weeks after initiating therapy. You should assess the patient's level of depression and watch for suicidal ideas.

Patient and Family Teaching

You should tell the patient and family the following:
1. The patient should take these medications exactly as ordered by the nurse, physician, or other health care provider. It is important that the patient continue to take the drug as ordered, even if she notices no changes, because it may take up to 2 weeks before the patient begins to feel better.
2. These are new medications, and there is still much to be learned about them. The drugs may produce a variety of side effects, most of them mild. They most frequently cause agitation and restlessness but may also interfere with sleep. In some individuals, these drugs can produce seizures. The nurse, physician, or other health care provider must be contacted immediately if there are any problems that are new or troublesome.
3. These drugs can cause drowsiness or make the patient feel less alert than usual. If so, the patient should avoid driving or doing other activities that require alertness. If drowsiness persists, the nurse, physician, or other health care provider should be contacted.

Table 16-9

Selective Serotonin Reuptake Inhibitors and Other Miscellaneous Antidepressants

GENERIC NAME	TRADE NAME	COMMENTS AND DOSAGE
SELECTIVE SEROTONIN REUPTAKE INHIBITORS (SSRIs)		
citalopram	Celexa	Depression, alcoholism, panic disorder, premenstrual dysphoria, social phobia. Give 20 mg every morning. Increase by 20 mg/day at weekly intervals as needed; 60 mg/day usually maximum dose.
escitalopram	Lexapro	Initially give 10 mg once daily AM or PM, with or without food. May increase to 20 mg/day after 1 wk. Reassess after 8 wk.
fluoxetine	Prozac	Full antidepressant effect may not be seen for 4 wk. Use lower dosage in patients with renal or hepatic impairment, patients with multiple diseases or medications, and the elderly. Effective in reducing symptoms of premenstrual syndrome in women, panic attacks, obsessive-compulsive disorders. *Initial:* 20 mg qd in AM. Consider dose increase after several weeks if no improvement is seen. Do not exceed maximum of 80 mg/day.
fluvoxamine	Luvox	Give 50 mg at bedtime. Increase dose by 50 mg as tolerated at 4- to 7-day intervals; titrate within range of 100-300 mg/day in divided doses.
paroxetine	Paxil	*Adults:* Initial dose 20 mg/day. Average dose 30 mg/day.
sertraline	Zoloft	*Adults:* Give 50 mg once daily initially; may increase to maximum of 200 mg/day.
MISCELLANEOUS ANTIDEPRESSANTS		
Tetracyclic Compounds		
maprotiline	—	Give 75 mg/day in single or divided doses. Some therapeutic effects seen within 3-7 days. Long half-life, so dosage should not be increased for 2 wk.
mirtazapine	Remeron	Give 15 mg at bedtime for at least 6 mo.
trazodone	Desyrel	*Initial:* 150 mg PO daily in divided doses, increasing by 50 mg/day every 3-4 days to a maximum of 400 mg/day. If drowsiness occurs, a larger dose can be given at bedtime.
Unrelated Products		
bupropion	Wellbutrin	Institute gradually to avoid producing seizures. Begin with 100 mg/day for 3 days. Wait 6 hr between dosages. May require addition of sedative-hypnotic in the first week of therapy. No single dose should be greater than 150 mg.
duloxetine	Cymbalta	Give 20-30 mg twice a day. May require prolonged duration of therapy.
venlafaxine	Effexor	Begin with 75 mg/day in divided doses and taken with food. May increase up to 225 mg/day if needed. If stopping therapy, taper off drug.

4. These medications must be kept out of the reach of children and all others for whom they are not prescribed.
5. The patient should wear a Medic Alert bracelet or necklace or carry a medical identification card listing the name of this medication.
6. The patient should avoid alcohol while taking these medications.

ANTIPSYCHOTIC DRUGS

OVERVIEW

Severe mental illness such as schizophrenia, psychotic depression, mania, or organic brain syndrome is com-

monly treated with major tranquilizers or antipsychotic drugs. These medications are used to sedate or slow the patient down, thereby reducing some of the psychotic symptoms. This allows other therapy to be used. Antipsychotic medications are usually given for long periods of time.

Antipsychotic drugs are grouped into two broad categories: (1) the phenothiazines and thioxanthenes, which are chemically and pharmacologically similar, so either type can be used; and (2) the nonphenothiazines, including haloperidol, loxapine, and molindone. All antipsychotic agents act by blocking the action of dopamine in the brain. Because they are from different chemical groups, however, they work at different sites in the brain and also produce side effects on different body systems. The two major categories will be presented separately.

PHENOTHIAZINES AND THIOXANTHENES

Action

The three major actions of phenothiazine and thioxanthene are as follows:

1. Blocking dopamine at the postsynaptic receptor sites in the brain, thus increasing the metabolism of dopamine. Phenothiazines and thioxanthenes also decrease the uptake of norepinephrine and serotonin. In the CNS, these drugs decrease the level of cyclic adenosine monophosphate (AMP), particularly in areas of the brain that control emotion and behavior. These changes are thought to produce the antipsychotic effects of the phenothiazines.
2. Reducing sensory stimulation of the reticular activating system in the brainstem, thereby producing a sedative effect.
3. Acting as an antiemetic by inhibiting action in the chemoreceptor center.

Uses

Phenothiazines and thioxanthenes are used primarily for reducing or relieving the symptoms of acute and chronic psychoses, including schizophrenia, schizoaffective disorders, and involutional psychosis. Either of these products can be used; however, thioxanthene is preferred for use in psychotic patients who are withdrawn or are exhibiting retarded behavior. Clinical evidence has shown that patients with certain types of apathetic psychosis respond well to this drug.

Adverse Reactions

Adverse reactions to phenothiazines and thioxanthenes include postural hypotension, tachycardia, confusion, drowsiness, hyperactivity, insomnia, amenorrhea, gynecomastia (enlargement of the breasts in men), hyperglycemia (high blood sugar level), hyperreflexia, tardive dyskinesia, blood cell abnormalities, contact dermatitis, photosensitivity, constipation, dry mouth, dyspnea (uncomfortable breathing), incontinence, nasal congestion, opaque deposits on the cornea and lens, and urinary retention.

Overdosage produces exaggerated CNS depression, coma, or severe hypotension, and extrapyramidal symptoms, seizures, or cardiac dysrhythmias may appear.

Drug Interactions

Phenothiazines taken concurrently with CNS depressants (alcohol, barbiturates, narcotics, and anesthetics) may increase and prolong the effects of either the CNS depressant or the phenothiazine. The effects of MAO inhibitors and tricyclic antidepressants are increased when they are taken at the same time as phenothiazines, and antacids and antidiarrheal drugs reduce the absorption rate. The effects of many other drugs and the results of laboratory tests are altered by phenothiazines and thioxanthenes.

Nursing Implications and Patient Teaching

Assessment

You should learn as much as possible about the health history of the patient, including the presence of hypersensitivity to any phenothiazines (because cross-sensitivity occurs); the history of cardiac, respiratory, or blood diseases; current use of other medications; and the possibility of pregnancy. These conditions are either contraindications or precautions to the use of phenothiazines and thioxanthenes.

The patient may have a history of emotional unrest, agitation, paranoid ideas, hallucinations (visual, auditory, or tactile), delusions, inability to think clearly, severe mood swings, and inability to cope with reality. The patient may or may not talk about his paranoid thoughts and often has difficulty paying attention and responding to things going on around him. The patient may not give appropriate answers to questions, and his behavior, dress, and general appearance may not be appropriate.

Diagnosis

What other needs does this patient have? Safety? Nutrition? Does the patient have a support system of family or friends?

Planning

Phenothiazines and thioxanthenes are not recommended for use in pregnant women or nursing mothers.

Patients with severe asthma, emphysema, or acute respiratory infections (especially children) may have slowing of respiration as a result of the CNS depressant effects of phenothiazines. Phenothiazines may also depress the cough reflex, putting a patient who is vomiting in danger of aspirating.

Implementation

Phenothiazines can be taken either orally or parenterally. The oral form is fairly well absorbed, but the absorption rate will be slowed if the drug is taken with antacids or antidiarrheal agents.

Stomach upset from the oral form of phenothiazines can be reduced or avoided by taking the drug with bland food or 8 ounces of water. Additional information about these medications is listed in Table 16-10.

Evaluation

The desired antipsychotic effects of phenothiazines may take several weeks to appear after therapy is started. The beginning dose should be the lowest recommended amount, according to the individual's tolerance and the severity of psychosis, until the psychotic symptoms are

Table **16-10**

Antipsychotic Medications

GENERIC NAME	TRADE NAME	COMMENTS AND DOSAGE
ALIPHATIC PHENOTHIAZINES		
chlorpromazine	Thorazine	A traditional phenothiazine product, popular and inexpensive. Used in psychotic disorders to control the manic phase of manic-depressive reactions, preoperatively for restlessness, to treat behavioral problems of children who are combative, or for hyperactive children with excessive motor activity. *Adults:* 30-300 mg/day PO in divided doses; or 25-50 mg IM 3 times daily; do not exceed 1000 mg/day. *Children over 6 months:* 0.55 mg/kg PO 2 to 4 times daily; or 0.55 mg/kg IM q6-8h. May also give 1 mg/kg per rectum (PR) 3 to 4 times daily.
promazine	Sparine	Used primarily in the management of psychotic disorders. Oral medication is usually preferred. *Adults:* Give 10-200 mg PO q4-6h, up to a maximum of 1000 mg/day. May also give 10-200 mg IM q4-6h. *Children over 12 yr:* 10-25 mg PO q4-6h.
triflupromazine	Vesprin	*Adults:* 100-150 mg/day PO; or 50-60 mg/day IM. *Children over 2 yr:* 2 mg/kg PO, up to 150 mg/day; or 0.2-0.25 mg/kg IM, up to 10 mg/day.
PIPERAZINE PHENOTHIAZINES		
fluphenazine	Permitil Prolixin	*Adults:* Give 0.5-10 mg/day PO in divided doses administered at 8-hr intervals initially. Normal maintenance dose is 3 mg PO daily; do not exceed 20 mg/day PO. If given IM, 1.25 mg is usual initial dose, with 2.5-10 mg IM divided and given in 6- to 8-hr intervals prn; do not exceed 10 mg/day IM. *Children:* 0.25-0.75 mg PO 1 to 4 times daily; IM dose same as for adult. *Geriatric:* 1-2.5 mg/day initially, increase as needed.
mesoridazine	Serentil 🍁	Used to treat severe emotional withdrawal, anxiety, tension, hallucinatory behavior, and blunted affect in schizophrenic patients. Reduces hyperactivity and uncooperativeness in some patients with organic brain syndrome and mental deficiencies. Also used to reduce symptoms present in alcoholism and psychoneurotic manifestations. *Adults and children over 12 yr:* 10-50 mg PO 2 to 3 times daily, up to 400 mg/day; or 25 mg IM repeated in 30-60 min if necessary, up to 200 mg/day. • *Alcoholism:* 25 mg PO twice daily initially; maintenance dose is 50-200 mg/day. • *Schizophrenia:* 50 mg PO 3 times daily; maintenance dose is 100-400 mg/day.

controlled. The dosage of phenothiazines that controls the patient's symptoms should be maintained for 2 to 3 weeks and then gradually reduced until the lowest effective maintenance dosage is reached. Phenothiazines given in large doses or for a long time should be discontinued by gradual reduction over several weeks to avoid symptoms of dyskinesia (difficulty in movements of the body), nausea, vomiting, dizziness, and trembling.

The patient should have a complete eye examination by a specialist, including inspection of the internal structures and the lens, to establish baseline data.

Patient and Family Teaching

You should tell the patient and family the following:

1. The patient should take this medication exactly as ordered. It is important that the patient continue to take the drug in the exact amount and frequency specified, even if she does not begin to feel better, because it may take several weeks before any changes occur.

2. Phenothiazines can increase the effects of alcohol, sleeping pills, and many other prescribed medications. The patient should avoid alcohol and should check with the nurse, physician, or

Table **16-10**

Antipsychotic Medications—cont'd

GENERIC NAME	TRADE NAME	COMMENTS AND DOSAGE
PIPERAZINE PHENOTHIAZINES—cont'd		
perphenazine	Trilafon	*Adults and children over 12 yr:* 2-16 mg PO 2 to 4 times daily; or 5-10 mg IM q6h, up to 15 mg/day.
prochlorperazine	Compazine	*Adults:* 5-10 mg PO 3 to 4 times daily, up to 150 mg/day; or 10-20 mg IM q4-6h, up to 200 mg/day. May also give 25 mg PR twice daily. *Children over 2 yr or 9 kg:* 0.1 mg/kg PO 4 times daily, not to exceed 10 mg/day on first day or 20 mg/day on subsequent days; or 0.132 mg/kg/day IM; or 2.5 mg PR 1 to 3 times daily, not to exceed 10 mg/day on first day or 20 mg/day on subsequent days.
thioridazine	Mellaril 🍁	Adjunct to short-term therapy in moderate-to-marked depression and anxiety. May be used in hyperactive children or children with marked behavioral problems. *Adults:* 25-100 mg PO 3 times daily initially, then 10-200 mg PO 2 to 4 times daily as maintenance; do not exceed 800 mg/day. *Children over 2 yr:* 0.25-3 mg/kg PO; or 10-25 mg PO 2 to 3 times daily.
trifluoperazine	Stelazine	Give initial dose, increasing as needed until symptoms are relieved. Then titrate dosage to lowest possible dose, based on individual response. Oral concentrate must be diluted. *Adults:* 1-5 mg PO twice daily, up to 40 mg/day; or may give 1-2 mg IM q4-6h, up to 10 mg/day. *Children over 6 yr:* 1 mg PO daily to twice daily; or may give 1 mg IM daily to twice daily.
THIOXANTHENE DERIVATIVE		
thiothixene	Navane 🍁	Monitor the patient for early signs of tardive dyskinesia and jerky movements, particularly of the hands. *Adults and children over 12 yr:* 2-5 mg PO 2 to 3 times daily initially; maintenance dose is 20-60 mg/day in divided doses. May also give 4 mg IM 2 to 4 times daily.

other health care provider before taking any other prescribed or OTC drugs.

3. Phenothiazines may cause drowsiness or make the patient feel less alert than usual, particularly when first taking the medicine. If so, the patient should avoid driving or doing other activities that require alertness. The patient should talk with the nurse, physician, or other health care provider if drowsiness or decreased alertness continues.

4. Light-headedness, dizziness, or feelings of faintness occur in some people taking phenothiazines. To reduce these feelings, the patient should move slowly when changing from a lying or sitting position.

5. Some people taking phenothiazines become more sensitive to the sun. To avoid sunburn, the patient should use a sunblock and limit exposure to the sun or sunlamps.

6. Patients taking this drug in liquid form should avoid contact of the medicine with the skin or clothes because it can cause irritation.

7. Gastric distress caused by the medication may be reduced by taking the drug with food, milk, or

8 ounces of water. The patient should not take any antacids or antidiarrheal medicine within 1 hour of taking the drug.

8. If the drug comes in a bottle with a medicine dropper, the patient should measure the prescribed dose as marked on the dropper and then dilute it in a glass of water or juice.

9. Dryness of the mouth may occur when the patient starts taking this drug. Chewing gum, sucking on hard candy, or rinsing the mouth frequently may help relieve this dryness.

10. Phenothiazines may make the patient perspire less than usual. Therefore, the patient should avoid becoming overheated in hot and humid weather or when exercising.

11. The nurse, physician, or other health care provider should be contacted immediately if urinary retention, change in vision, sore throat with fever, muscle spasms, trembling or shaking (particularly of hands), skin rash, jaundice, small uncontrollable movements of the tongue, or other new or troublesome symptoms develop.

12. This medication must be kept out of the reach of children and all others for whom it is not prescribed.

13. The patient should wear a Medic Alert bracelet or necklace and carry a medical identification card stating that he is taking a phenothiazine.

NONPHENOTHIAZINES

A variety of chemically unrelated products have come on the market over the years to help in treating psychotic patients. The mechanism of action for these products is often not precisely understood. Some of the major features of these products are briefly presented in Table 16-11.

ANTIMANICS

ACTION

Lithium is the primary drug used to treat patients in manic states. The exact mechanism of lithium is not known. The mood-stabilizing effect of the drug may be attributed to its ability to alter sodium transport at the nerve endings, inhibit cyclic AMP formation in nerve cells, and enhance the uptake of serotonin and norepinephrine by nerve cells, thus increasing the inactivation of these neurotransmitters. It has no sedative, depressant, or euphoric actions, making it unique from all other psychiatric drugs.

USES

Lithium is specifically used for patients with manic-depressive psychosis who are in an acute manic phase.

It also may be used to prevent recurrent episodes of mania in the manic-depressive patient.

ADVERSE REACTIONS

Adverse reactions to lithium include dysrhythmias, hypotension, ataxia, coma, dizziness, drowsiness, motor retardation, restlessness, slurred speech, tinnitus (ringing in the ears), pruritus, rash, abdominal pain, anorexia, diarrhea, vomiting, urinary incontinence or retention, polyuria (excretion of a large amount of urine), albuminuria, blurred vision, hyperglycemia, hypothyroidism, leukocytosis, and weight gain.

Overdosage may produce diarrhea, vomiting, muscle weakness, drowsiness, and ataxia.

Clinical Landmine

Lithium Monitoring

There is a very narrow therapeutic margin for lithium, and careful monitoring of blood levels is required to avoid toxic overdosages.

DRUG INTERACTIONS

Use of lithium together with diuretics can lead to lithium toxicity. There are many significant drug interactions with various medications.

Nursing Implications and Patient Teaching

Assessment

You should learn as much as possible about the health history of the patient, including the presence of hypersensitivity, underlying disease, the possibility of pregnancy, and other medications being used. These conditions may be contraindications or precautions to the use of lithium.

The patient may have a history of excessive talkativeness, restlessness, hyperactivity, aggressiveness, and perhaps ideas of being very important, talented, or powerful.

Diagnosis

What other problems does this patient have that might influence the effectiveness of the medication? If the patient becomes dehydrated, forgets to take medication on a regular basis, or becomes so excitable that he believes that medication is not needed, this may result in significant problems for the patient.

Planning

Lithium is not safe to use in pregnant patients and breastfeeding mothers. If a patient receiving lithium becomes pregnant, the drug should be stopped, especially

Table 16-11

Nonphenothiazine Antipsychotic Medications

DRUG	ACTION	USES	ADVERSE REACTIONS	DRUG INTERACTIONS
clozapine (Clozaril)	Increased affinity for 5-HT receptors; acts on several neurotransmitters, including antagonism of some dopamine receptors	Severely ill schizophrenics	Life-threatening agranulocytosis (very low number of white blood cells)	Increases effect of digoxin and warfarin; may decrease effects of other highly protein-bound drugs
haloperidol (Haldol)	Potently and selectively blocks dopamine at receptor sites in the brain	Used in schizophrenia and the manic phase of manic-depressive disorders	Postural hypotension; drowsiness; tardive dyskinesia (jerky, twitching movements of head, face, or neck; shaking hands; shuffling walk; stiffness of limbs); blurred vision; breast engorgement; constipation; decreased libido; dry mouth; impotence; nausea; vomiting	Potentiates CNS depressant effects of alcohol, barbiturates, narcotics, and anesthetics; may produce severe hypotension when taken with antihypertensive drugs or epinephrine
loxapine (Loxitane)	Inhibits subcortical areas of brain, producing a tranquilizing effect and decrease in aggressive behavior	Schizophrenia	Postural hypotension; tachycardia; drowsiness; hyperactivity; seizures; tardive dyskinesia; skin rash; blurred vision; opaque deposits on cornea and lens; urinary retention; constipation; dry mouth; headache; photosensitivity	Interacts with same drugs as phenothiazine
molindone (Moban)	Blocks stimuli in ascending reticular activating system; tranquilizing effect produced without relaxation of muscles	Schizophrenia	Postural hypotension; depression; drowsiness; tardive dyskinesia; blood cell changes; skin rash; urinary retention; blurred vision; dry mouth; increased libido; heavy menses	Interferes with absorption of tetracycline and phenytoin
olanzapine (Zyprexa)	Increased affinity for 5-HT receptors; acts on several neurotransmitters, including antagonism of some dopamine receptors	Schizophrenia	CNS stimulation	Carbamazepine decreases concentrations; interferes with cytochrome P-450 system

Continued

Table **16-11**

Nonphenothiazine Antipsychotic Medications—cont'd

DRUG	ACTION	USES	ADVERSE REACTIONS	DRUG INTERACTIONS
pimozide (Orap)	Increased affinity for 5-HT receptors; acts on several neurotransmitters, including antagonism of some dopamine receptors	Schizophrenia	Tardive dyskinesia after abrupt withdrawal	Anticholinergic effects potentiated; hypotensive effects seen with antihypertensives; increases dysrhythmic drug serum levels
quetiapine (Seroquel)	Increased affinity for 5-HT receptors; acts on several neurotransmitters, including antagonism of some dopamine receptors	Schizophrenia	May produce cataracts with long-term use; may increase cholesterol level	Increased levels when given with phenytoin; cimetidine decreases clearance and thus increases serum level
risperidone (Risperdal)	Increased affinity for 5-HT receptors; acts on several neurotransmitters, including antagonism of some dopamine receptors	Schizophrenia; agitation in the elderly	Lengthens the Q-T interval in some patients; elevated prolactin level; causes agitation, anxiety, headache, insomnia, constipation, dyspepsia, and rhinitis	Use with clozapine decreases clearance of risperidone
ziprasidone (Geodon)	Acts on several neurotransmitters	Schizophrenia	Lengthens the Q-T interval in some patients and may produce lethal dysrhythmias	Give 20 mg twice daily with food.

during the first trimester, because it may cause birth defects.

Elderly patients are often more sensitive to lithium toxicity. It is important to start these patients on lower doses and monitor the therapeutic and adverse effects closely while increasing dosage.

Geriatric Considerations

Lithium

Lithium is more toxic in the geriatric patient; therefore, lower lithium dosages, a lower lithium serum level, and very close monitoring are critical in this age group. The elderly are more prone to CNS toxicity, lithium-induced goiter, and clinical hypothyroidism than the average adult. Generally, excessive thirst and polyuria may be early side effects of lithium toxicity that are frequently seen in the elderly.

Implementation

You should make sure that the patient has adequate hydration (enough fluids) and that her electrolytes are balanced during lithium therapy.

Table 16-12 summarizes the important information you need to know about lithium.

Evaluation

The therapeutic level of serum lithium is relatively close to the toxic level, so the serum lithium level must be monitored on a regular basis. Blood should be drawn 12 hours after the dose of lithium is given.

Monitoring should be carried out every few days during the initial therapy and then at least every 2 months after the patient is stabilized. The therapeutic serum lithium level is 1 to 1.5 mEq/L in most laboratories. At each patient visit, you should observe for therapeutic effects and monitor the patient's mental and emotional status.

Lithium is tolerated better when the patient is in an acute manic stage than when he is in a stage where symptoms of mania have decreased. The dosage of

Modified from McKenry LM, Salerno E: *Mosby's pharmacology in nursing,* ed 21, St Louis, 2003, Mosby.

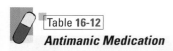

Table 16-12

Antimanic Medication

GENERIC NAME	TRADE NAME	COMMENTS AND DOSAGE
lithium	Carbolith Eskalith Lithane Lithonate Lithotabs	Lithium administered orally is rapidly absorbed in the GI tract. The desired effect of lithium may take 1 to several weeks to occur. Lithium is excreted by the kidneys, with a half-life of approximately 24 hr in a healthy adult, but in the elderly patient, half-life may be increased to 36 hr; therefore, lower dosages are indicated for this group. Lithium excretion is inhibited in the presence of low serum sodium levels. The therapeutic serum level of lithium is 1-1.5 mEq/L. Lithium is not recommended for children under 12 years of age. • *Acute mania:* 600 mg PO 3 times daily. • *Prophylaxis:* 300 mg PO 3 to 4 times daily.

lithium may have to be adjusted according to the patient's symptoms.

Patients who develop diarrhea or become ill and do not eat are at increased risk of toxicity, and their condition should be followed closely.

Patient and Family Teaching

You should tell the patient and family the following:

1. The patient should take this medication exactly as ordered. It is important that the patient continue to take the drug in the exact amount and frequency ordered, even if the patient does not begin to feel better, because it may take several weeks before any changes occur. Gastric upset caused by the medication may be reduced by taking the drug with milk or food.
2. The serum lithium levels can become toxic if the patient takes too much or becomes dehydrated from vomiting or diarrhea or does not eat. The patient should avoid activities that cause excessive sweating (strenuous exercise, sunbathing, hot tub baths) and things that produce excessive urination (consuming large amounts of caffeine in coffee, tea, or cola drinks). The nurse, physician, or other health care provider should be contacted if the patient becomes ill or does not feel well.
3. Some patients taking lithium experience side effects, but these are usually mild and disappear with time. The nurse, physician, or other health care provider should be notified of any new or troublesome symptoms, such as vomiting, nausea, shakiness, trembling, jerky movements of arms or legs, or generalized weakness.
4. The patient will need to have the level of the drug in the blood measured frequently so that the drug can be kept at the proper level and side effects may be reduced. The patient will need these blood tests every few days when beginning treatment, and then every 1 to 2 months.
5. This medication must be kept out of the reach of children and others for whom it is not prescribed.
6. The patient should wear a Medic Alert bracelet or necklace and carry a medical identification card stating that she is taking lithium.

SECTION SIX

Sedative-Hypnotic Medications

ACTION

Sedative-hypnotic medications are used in the hospital to relax patients and induce sleep before anesthesia or medical testing procedures such as electroencephalography. They are also used to treat patients with insomnia caused by mental and physical stress.

Sleep is a normal cyclic process that involves varying levels of unconsciousness from which a patient may be aroused. Normal sleep produces relaxation and relief from stress. Although individual patterns vary, each time a person sleeps, four stages occur in a cycle for varying lengths of time. Stages I and II are very light stages of sleep, during which the person may be easily aroused. Stage III is a transition to stage IV, the period of deepest sleep in which basic vital signs slow and the body totally relaxes. It is this period of sleep that makes people feel very refreshed. Approximately every 90 minutes, a period of body arousal is reached, which is often superimposed on stage I or stage II of sleep. This is called *paradoxic sleep* because, instead of relaxing, the body is more active. It is also called *REM time* because dreaming is common, as demonstrated by rapid eye movements (REM). This is an important part of sleeping, when the unconscious mind works out anxieties and tensions. When people do not have enough REM time each night, they feel anxious and unrested.

USES

At times people may be unable to sleep because of stresses or anxiety. Difficulty falling asleep is termed **initial insomnia.** The inability to stay asleep is termed **intermittent insomnia,** and **terminal insomnia** refers to early awakening with an inability to return to sleep. Terminal insomnia is often associated with depression.

If warm baths, warm drinks, appropriate temperature, and bedding changes do not help the patient relax, a medication may be prescribed on a short-term basis. A **sedative agent** is a medication that relaxes the patient and allows him or her to sleep. A **hypnotic agent** actually produces sleep in the patient. Whether a medication acts as a sedative or a hypnotic is often determined not by the drug, but by the dosage used, with smaller dosages producing sedative effects and larger dosages producing hypnotic effects.

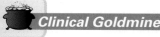
Clinical Goldmine

Sedative-Hypnotic Medications

Although most sedative-hypnotic medications increase the sleeping time, many of them produce a feeling of lethargy or a "hangover" feeling in the morning. Even a few doses of the medication may reduce the occurrence and length of REM time, making the patient feel irritable and unrested in the morning.

The ideal medication would reproduce the normal sleep pattern for the patient: the patient would sleep longer, have no side effects, and wake up feeling rested and relaxed with no risk of developing drug dependency. Unfortunately, no ideal medication exists.

Postmedication "hangover" often leads to the increased desire for more medicine so that the patient may have a refreshing sleep, with dependency or abuse resulting.

Once a patient has taken sedative-hypnotics, the normal sleep patterns may not return for several weeks. During that time, an increased period of REM will be seen, as if the body is trying to "catch up" for missed time. This may produce long, vivid, or frightening dreams.

Barbiturates are CNS depressants used for a variety of medical problems. All barbiturates act primarily on the brainstem reticular formation, reducing nerve impulses to the cerebral cortex. Barbiturates also depress the respiratory system and the activity of nerves and muscle (smooth, skeletal, and cardiac), thus producing relaxation and sleep.

Barbiturates are used for short-term treatment of anxiety, agitation, and insomnia caused by transient psychosocial stresses, and at times when rest is mandatory, such as before surgery. Large doses of short-acting barbiturates can produce surgical anesthesia (see Section Two).

The main action of benzodiazepines is CNS depression. Although the exact mechanism is not known, they are thought to act on the hypothalamus and limbic system of the brain, decreasing the vasopressor response and increasing the arousal threshold. They are used as hypnotic agents to treat insomnia. The therapeutic objective is to prevent insomnia and restore normal sleep patterns. Benzodiazepines are used in patients with acute or chronic medical problems who require restful sleep (see Section Two for more detail).

The nonbarbiturate-nonbenzodiazepine sedative-hypnotics include a variety of chemically unrelated medications. All produce some effects on REM sleep, have a potential for tolerance and habituation, and may produce rebound REM. None is as safe as the benzodiazepines. Therefore, they are not as commonly used.

ADVERSE REACTIONS

Nonbarbiturate-nonbenzodiazepine sedative-hypnotics may produce drowsiness, decreased emotional reaction, dullness, distortion of mood, impaired coordination, hypersensitivity, lethargy, headache, muscle or joint pain, and mental depression. A feeling of "hangover" commonly occurs with their use.

DRUG INTERACTIONS

Nonbarbiturate-nonbenzodiazepine sedative-hypnotics increase the sedative effects of CNS depressants, including sleeping aids, analgesics, anesthetics, tranquilizers, alcohol, and narcotics. Chloral hydrate may increase the anticoagulant effects of warfarin, whereas glutethimide and ethchlorvynol may diminish the anticoagulant effects of warfarin.

Nursing Implications and Patient Teaching

Assessment

You should learn as much as possible about the health history of the patient, including any medications the patient may be taking that may produce drug interactions,

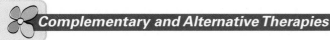

Complementary and Alternative Therapies

Insomnia

PRODUCT	COMMENTS
Valerian	May cause increased effect or toxicity with CNS depressants, sedative-hypnotics (particularly barbiturates), antidepressants, anxiolytics, antihistamines
Kava kava	Potential interactions with ethanol, CNS depressants (particularly benzodiazepines, antidepressants, sedative-hypnotics)
Passion flower	Potential interactions with antianxiety agents, antidepressants, hexobarbital, hypnotics, sedatives
Chamomile	Effects may be addictive with CNS depressants
Melatonin	Excessive dosages may cause morning sedation or drowsiness

Modified from Krinsky DL, Lavella JB, Hawkins EB, et al: *Natural therapeutics pocket guide,* ed 2, Hudson, Ohio, 2003, Lexi-Comp, Inc.

other barbiturates the patient is taking (sometimes these are present in bronchodilators or antispasmodics), response to barbiturates taken in the past, or hypersensitivity. Sedative-hypnotics are not considered safe in pregnancy. You should determine whether there are any underlying diseases that would represent contraindications to the use of sedative-hypnotics. The Complementary and Alternative Therapies box summarizes herbal preparations patients may be using to induce sleep and their potential to interact with other drugs.

Diagnosis

What are the underlying problems that require use of a sedative? Does the patient have physical or emotional concerns that could be the cause of these problems?

Planning

If sedative-hypnotics are used for more than 1 week, they may cause further disturbances in the sleep cycle and rebound insomnia. Hypothermia may occur with the use of barbiturates. Alcohol can increase the sedation produced by these drugs and depress vital brain functions.

Pediatric Considerations

Sedative-Hypnotics

- Young children are more susceptible to the CNS depressant effects of the benzodiazepines. In neonates, profound CNS depression may result because of the lower rate of drug metabolism by the immature liver.
- Paradoxic reactions have been reported in children with the use of barbiturates.

Modified from McKenry LM, Salerno E: *Mosby's pharmacology in nursing,* ed 21, St Louis, 2003, Mosby.

Geriatric Considerations

Sedative-Hypnotics

The sedative-hypnotics are particularly hazardous in elderly patients. Reductions in urinary clearance and accumulation of drug in adipose tissue may prolong the half-life of many of these drugs to a dangerous length. For example, the half-life of Dalmane can increase to 100 hours, thus increasing the potential for overdosage.

Flurazepam is increasingly effective on the second or third night of consecutive use. For one to two nights after the drug is stopped, both the amount of time before the patient falls asleep and the total awake time may still be decreased.

These are Schedule IV controlled substances. The patient may develop dependence if these drugs are used indiscriminately, and abrupt withdrawal is dangerous.

Implementation

Benzodiazepines are transformed by the liver into long-acting forms that may remain in the body for 24 hours or more and produce increasing sedation. Liver function may be impaired with long-term use. The onset of action is approximately 30 to 60 minutes; the effects last 7 to 8 hours. The drug should be given 15 to 30 minutes before bedtime. Table 16-13 summarizes important information regarding benzodiazepine sedative-hypnotics.

Use great caution when parenterally administering barbiturates to avoid intraarterial injection or extravasation because serious ischemia or gangrene could result. Barbiturates may worsen a patient's pain.

Geriatric or debilitated patients should receive lower than recommended dosages of barbiturates.

All barbiturates exhibit the same sedative-hypnotic effect, but they differ in onset time, duration, and potency. The onset and duration are determined by the

Table 16-13

Benzodiazepine Sedative-Hypnotic Medications

GENERIC NAME	TRADE NAME	COMMENTS AND DOSAGE
estazolam	ProSom	*Adults:* 1 mg at bedtime.
flurazepam	Dalmane	Flurazepam can be used for a longer time (effective for 28 nights) and has less REM rebound than some other hypnotics. Markedly suppresses stage IV, increases stage II sleep. • *Hypnotic:* 15 or 30 mg PO; 15 mg in elderly or debilitated patients.
lorazepam	Ativan	This antianxiety agent is usually used for mild or transient situational stress. It is used parenterally as a preanesthetic medication. • *Mild anxiety or insomnia:* 2-4 mg PO at bedtime; in elderly or debilitated patients use 1-2 mg/day in divided doses. • *Preanesthesia medications:* 0.05 mg/kg (maximum dose 4 mg) IM at least 2 hr before surgical procedure. • *Sedation:* 2 mg total or 0.02 mg/lb IV for adult patients younger than 50 yr of age.
quazepam	Doral	*Adults:* 15 mg initially. May reduce to 7.5 mg if response is adequate.
temazepam	Restoril	Induces sleep in 20-40 min. • *Hypnotic:* 30 mg PO before bedtime; in elderly or debilitated patients, 15 mg may be sufficient.
triazolam	Halcion	Used primarily for short-term treatment of insomnia or early morning awakening. *Adults:* 0.25-0.5 mg at bedtime; 0.125-0.25 mg in elderly.

Table 16-14

Benzodiazepine Sedative-Hypnotic Medications

DRUG	ONSET OF ACTION (min)	DURATION (hr)	SEDATIVE DOSE	HYPNOTIC DOSE
LONG ACTING				
mephobarbital (Mebaral)	60	10-16	32-200 mg PO, divided into 3-4 doses daily	100-200 mg PO daily
phenobarbital (Barbital)	60	10-16	30-120 mg PO daily, divided into 2-3 doses; 30-120 mg per rectum (PR) or IM, divided into 2-3 doses daily	50-320 mg PO daily; 100-320 mg PR or IM daily
INTERMEDIATE ACTING				
amobarbital (Amytal)	60	4-6	50-300 mg PO, divided into 2-3 doses daily	65-200 mg PO daily
aprobarbital (Alurate)	20	4-6	120-160 mg PO daily in divided doses	40-160 mg PO daily
butabarbital (Butisol)	30	6-8	40-120 mg PO daily in divided doses	50-100 mg PO daily
SHORT ACTING				
pentobarbital (Nembutal)	30	3-6	90-120 mg PO daily in divided doses	100 mg PO daily
secobarbital (Seconal)	15-30	3-6	30-90 mg PO daily divided into 2-3 doses	100 mg PO daily

lipid solubility of the particular drug. In determining dosage, it is best to begin with the lowest possible effective dose and adjust upward according to the individual patient's response. The amount prescribed should be no greater than what is needed for current treatment and less than a potentially lethal dose. Table 16-14 presents a comparison of action of the different barbiturates used for sedation and hypnosis.

When paraldehyde is given orally, it should be diluted in milk or fruit juice to mask the taste and odor. Liquids should be put in a disposable container or in a glass because plastic will absorb the odor and flavor permanently. Table 16-15 summarizes the nonbarbiturate-nonbenzodiazepine sedative-hypnotics.

Evaluation

Sedative-hypnotics should always be discontinued slowly in people who have been on long-term therapy. Tolerance is usually proportional to the total amount of the drug received. Barbiturates are controlled substances, so attempts should be made to avoid giving them to patients with a history of abuse or addiction.

Patient and Family Teaching

You should tell the patient and family the following:
1. Sedative-hypnotics are only for short-term use. Sometimes tolerance, dependence, or addiction develops with these drugs.
2. The patient should take the medication exactly as prescribed.
3. The medication should be kept out of reach of children and all others for whom it is not prescribed.
4. A hangover feeling may sometimes be experienced the day after taking the medication. The patient should avoid any driving or activities that require alertness until all drowsiness has disappeared.

Table **16-15**

Benzodiazepine Sedative-Hypnotic Medications

GENERIC NAME	TRADE NAME	COMMENTS AND DOSAGE
CHLORAL DERIVATIVES		
chloral hydrate	Aquachloral	Effective in 30-60 min and lasts 4-8 hr. Has a very disagreeable taste and causes gastric irritation; take after meals; take elixir in water, juice, or soda. • *Sedative* *Adults:* 250 mg PO 3 times daily after meals, or 325-650 mg 3 times daily per rectum (PR). *Children:* 25 mg/kg/day PO. • *Hypnotic* *Adults:* 500-1000 mg PO 15-30 min before bedtime, or 30 min before surgery. *Children:* 50 mg/kg/day; maximum dose 1 gm PO.
PIPERIDINE DERIVATIVES		
glutethimide	—	Effective in 30 min and lasts 4-8 hr. Should be stored in light-resistant containers. • *Sedative:* 25-250 mg at bedtime. • *Hypnotic:* 250 mg at bedtime.
paraldehyde	Paral Paraldehyde	Sleep induced in 10-15 min and lasts 6-8 hr. • *Sedation* *Adults:* 5-15 mL PO or PR; 5 mL IM. Children: 0.15 mL/kg PO, PR, or IM. • *Hypnosis* *Adults:* 10-30 mL PO or PR; 10 mL IM. *Children:* 0.3 mL/kg PO.
MISCELLANEOUS		
acetylcarbromal	Paxarel	*Adults:* 250-500 mg 2 to 3 times daily.
ethchlorvynol	Placidyl	Sleep induced in 15-60 min and lasts 5 hr. Do not use longer than 1 wk. • *Hypnotic:* 500-1000 mg PO at bedtime; a single dose of 100-200 mg may be given if patient awakens during the night.
propiomazine	Largon	*Adults:* Give 20 mg with 50 mg meperidine IV or IM preoperatively.
zolpidem	Ambien	*Adults:* 10 mg before bedtime.

5. It is dangerous for the patient to drink alcohol within 24 hours after taking this drug.

6. Smoking may decrease the length of time the drug helps the patient sleep.

7. The patient should avoid drinking beverages containing caffeine for at least 4 hours before taking the medication because it reduces the ability of the drug to produce sleep.

8. Some people experience side effects while taking this drug, so the nurse, physician, or other health care provider should be notified if any new or uncomfortable symptoms appear, such as rash, fever, unusual bleeding, bruising, sore throat, jaundice, or abdominal pain.

9. The patient may develop excessive dreaming when the drug is stopped; this should lessen each night.

10. Tablets and capsules should be kept in a dry, tightly closed container. Elixirs should be kept in a tightly closed brown glass bottle.

11. If using this drug primarily to relax and go to sleep, the patient should investigate alternative methods of relaxation to help reduce the need for medication.

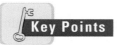

Key Points

- CNS medications include analgesics, antimigraine agents, seizure medications, antiemetics, antivertigo medications, antiparkinsonian agents, antipsychotics, and sedative-hypnotics.
- It is important to understand how nerves transmit information from the brain through chemical neurotransmitters and how these medications interact with the body.
- Neurotransmitters fit into receptors in various parts of the body to act on them, and many CNS drugs act on more than one type of receptor.
- Each agent acts differently.
- It is extremely important for you to administer dosages carefully because serious adverse reactions are possible if dosages are exceeded.

Go to the free CD-ROM for an Audio Glossary, animations, video clips, and Review Questions for the NCLEX-PN® Examination.

evolve Be sure to visit the companion Evolve website at http://evolve.elsevier.com/Edmunds/LPN/ for WebLinks, a link to the top 200 drugs by prescription, and sign-up pages for newsletter drug updates.

CASE STUDY

Mrs. Jane Michner, a 65-year-old widow, was admitted 2 weeks ago with a fractured hip. She has a 6-year history of Parkinson's disease. Her hip is healing well, but she is having difficulty learning to walk with crutches. This has made her very depressed, and she is concerned about how she will manage when she returns home. She has also developed symptoms of a urinary tract infection, a problem she has had repeatedly. She is currently receiving:

Ascorbic acid (vitamin C): 1 gm PO 4 times daily

Levodopa (Larodopa): 1 gm PO 3 times daily with meals

Nitrofurantoin (Macrodantin): 100 mg PO 3 times daily

1. Why is Mrs. Michner taking ascorbic acid?
2. What special information do you need to give Mrs. Michner about her antiparkinsonian medications?
3. Several days after admission, Mrs. Michner developed a maculopapular eruption of the skin all over her trunk. What is the likely cause of this problem?
4. What medications might Mrs. Michner take to treat the urinary tract infection?
5. The doctor starts Mrs. Michner on imipramine HCl (Tofranil) 20 mg PO twice daily. Why was this drug ordered? What does the patient need to know about it?
6. Does Mrs. Michner have any contraindications to the use of imipramine HCl?

DRUG CALCULATION REVIEW

1. The physician orders valproic acid (Depakote) at 15 mg/kg/day PO. The patient weighs 150 lbs today. What will be the daily dose in milligrams of this antiseizure medication for this patient?

2. Order: Dilantin 200 mg by gastrostomy tube twice a day

   Supply: Dilantin 125 mg/5 mL

Question: How many milliliters of Dilantin is needed for each dose?

3. Order: Lorazepam 0.5 mg IV push stat

   Supply: Lorazepam 2 mg/mL

   Question: How many milliliters of lorazepam is needed?

CRITICAL THINKING ?

1. Describe the properties of antimigraine products that differentiate them from other nonnarcotic analgesics.

2. With antianxiety agents, how would you distinguish signs of overdosage from adverse reactions? What patient data would you need to obtain to make this distinction?

3. What nonpharmacologic suggestions could you make to your patients to assist them with management of their insomnia? Why are antihistamines often used in place of sedative-hypnotics for elderly patients?

4. Antiemetics, among other CNS-acting medications, should not be taken with any other drugs or substances that act on the central nervous system because of the increased risk of sedative effects. What would you assess for in a hospitalized patient admitted to your unit for observation for oversedation?

17 Medications for Pain Management

After reading and studying this chapter, you should be able to do the following:

- List medications commonly used for the treatment of moderate to severe pain.
- Evaluate different forms of narcotic agonists and narcotic agonist-antagonists in their ability to control pain.
- Explain why there are so many rules about how narcotics and related analgesic drugs may be given.
- Compare and contrast drug tolerance and drug addiction.
- List behavior that would make you believe a patient is addicted to the drug.

Key Terms

Be sure to check out the bonus material on the free CD-ROM, including selected audio pronunciations.

Acute pain (p. 313)
Addiction (p. 314)
Chronic pain (p. 313)
Dependence (p. 314)
Hydration (hī-DRĀ-shŭn, p. 321)
Miosis (mī-Ō-sĭs, p. 314)
Narcotic (năr-KŎT-ĭk, p. 312)
Opioids (Ō-pē-ōydz, p. 312)
Pain (p. 313)
Tolerance (p. 314)
Withdrawal symptoms (p. 314)

OVERVIEW

A wide range of drugs are used in controlling pain. The most common drugs for mild pain relief include over-the-counter analgesics such as aspirin and acetaminophen. (These drugs are described in Chapter 22 because they have actions other than pain reduction). Many of the drugs used for treating severe pain are narcotics. (A **narcotic** is any substance that produces stupor associated with analgesia, and specifically refers to **opioids,** which are used to treat severe pain.) Natural opioids come from opium, which comes from unripe seed capsules of the poppy plant. Opium contains many chemicals, including morphine and codeine. (Heroin is diacetylmorphine, which chemically breaks down into morphine.) There are also nonnarcotic analgesics that produce intermediate pain relief for conditions not severe enough to require a narcotic.

In addition to natural opioids, man-made or synthetic opioids have been developed. It was hoped that many of these new drugs would not be as addictive as morphine—but this was not so. However, these new drugs are useful for pain management and to reverse the effects of opioids. Many of these new drugs are made by changing morphine chemically. Morphine is the "mother" of the synthetic opioid analgesics, hydrocodone, hydromorphone, and oxycodone. Other classes of synthetic opioids are made of different chemicals but have actions similar to morphine.

Analgesics used in pain management are classified according to their mechanism of action. Opioids are classified as agonist, partial agonist, or agonist-antagonist medications. The term *agonist* means "to do"; the term *antagonist* means "to block." An agonist drug binds with the receptor(s) to activate and produce the maximum response of the individual receptor. A partial agonist produces a partial response of this type. An opioid agonist-antagonist drug produces mixed effects, acting as an agonist at one type of receptor and as a competitive antagonist at another type of receptor.

The mechanism of action for opioids is determined by where they bind to specific opioid receptors inside and outside the central nervous system (CNS). The primary opioid receptors concentrated in the CNS are mu, kappa, delta, and sigma receptors. Although analgesia is associated with the first three receptors, most action occurs at the mu and kappa receptors (Table 17-1). The sigma receptors seem to produce mostly unwanted effects.

Morphine is the main opioid drug to which all other pain management drugs are compared (Table 17-2). It is used a great deal in acute care and in hospice settings for dying patients who have severe pain. Codeine, hydrocodone, and oxycodone are often used in combination with acetaminophen in the office or clinic setting. Hydromorphone is very strong and is only used for treating severe pain not relieved by morphine.

Opioid agonist-antagonist drugs are also used. Agonist-antagonists may be preferred over agonist opioids for use in patients in the community because their risk for abuse is less. Tramadol is an agonist-antagonist in common use in office practice. However, pentazocine has limited use because of its CNS toxicity.

Table 17-1

Selected Opioid Receptor Responses

RECEPTOR	MEDICATION EXAMPLES	RESPONSE
Mu	*Strong agonist:* morphine; hydromorphone *Partial agonist:* buprenorphine *Weak agonist:* meperidine *Antagonist:* naloxone, opioid agonist-antagonist	Supraspinal analgesia, euphoria, respiratory depression, sedation, constipation, urinary retention, drug dependence Reversal of opioid effects; acute withdrawal induced in opioid dependency
Kappa	*Agonist:* pentazocine, morphine, nalbuphine, butorphanol *Little or no activity:* levorphanol, methadone, meperidine *Antagonist:* naloxone, buprenorphine	Spinal analgesia, sedation Reversal of opioid effects; acute withdrawal induced in opioid dependency

From McKenry LM, Salerno E: *Mosby's pharmacology in nursing,* ed 21, St Louis, 2003, Mosby, p. 269.

Table 17-2

Equivalent Doses of Opioid Analgesics Compared to Morphine 10 mg IM

ANALGESIC	ORAL DOSE (mg)	SUBCUTANEOUS DOSE	TRANSDERMAL DOSE
morphine	60	10	
morphine (MS Contin)	60	NA	
hydromorphone	7.5	1.3	
fentanyl (Duragesic patch)	NA	NA	100 mcg/hr = morphine 10 mg IM q4h
codeine	200	130	
hydrocodone	5-10	NA	
oxycodone	5-10	NA	
propoxyphene	65	NA	
tramadol	ND		
meperidine	300	75	
methadone	20	10	
pentazocine	180	30-60	

Modified from Brunton L, Lazo L, Parker K, editors: *Goodman and Gilman's pharmacological basis of therapeutics,* ed 11, New York, 2005, McGraw-Hill.
NA, Not applicable; *ND,* not determined.

In order to limit the abuse of these drugs, the federal government had created many rules that describe who may prescribe narcotics. As a nurse, you will have to learn and follow these rules. You may have responsibility to keep the narcotics in a safe place and account for their use in the hospital or nursing home setting.

This chapter is divided into three sections. Section One deals with narcotic agonist analgesics. Section Two presents narcotic agonist-antagonist analgesics. Nonnarcotic (centrally acting) analgesics are presented in Section Three.

PAIN AS A PROCESS

Pain is defined by the International Association for the Study of Pain (IASP) as an unpleasant sensation or emotion that produces or might produce tissue damage. Pain is always subjective; that is, pain is something the patient feels and that cannot be felt or measured by someone else.

Researchers believe that four things are required fo pain to occur:

1. An unpleasant stimulus affects nerve endings and sets off electrical activity.
2. The nerve endings carry the unpleasant stimulu along the nerves through electrical signals to the spinal cord, using different types of nerve fibers Different types of fiber carry different types o pain signals.
3. The signals go to the brain.
4. A feeling of pain develops that includes behav ioral, psychologic, and emotional factors.

Acute pain is usually related to an injury, sucl as recent surgery, trauma, or infection, and end within an expected time. **Chronic pain** is any pain that continues beyond the usual course of a acute injury process. Persons with cancer-related pain or chronic disorders (for example, arthritis migraine) are the majority of people with chroni pain.

TOLERANCE, DEPENDENCE, AND ADDICTION

All opioid drugs cause tolerance and dependence. This is not the same as abuse. **Tolerance** is a drug-related problem that is seen when the same amount of drug produces less effect over time. More drug is needed to have the same effect. **Dependence** is a state in which the body shows withdrawal symptoms when the drug is stopped or a reversing drug or antagonist is given. **Withdrawal symptoms** are changes in the body or mind, such as nausea or anxiety, that occur when a drug is stopped or reduced after regular use. Tapering off (slowly taking less of the drug) can prevent withdrawal symptoms. Psychologic dependence, or **addiction,** is the desperate need to have and use a drug for a nonmedical reason. Tolerance and dependence are the result of regular use of an opioid for a certain length of time and are not a problem. Addiction is a problem; however, a patient in pain should not be denied pain relief because of fear of addiction.

SECTION ONE

Narcotic Agonist Analgesics

ACTION

Drugs called narcotic agonist analgesics are thought to prevent painful feelings in the central nervous system in the substantia gelatinosa [gray matter] of the spinal cord, brain stem, reticular formation, thalamus, and limbic system.) The nerves that act with the opiates (have opiate receptors) in each of these areas interact with the nerves of the autonomic nervous system that carry the pain messages (have neurotransmitters), to produce changes in the person's reaction to pain. (See Chapter 16 for additional information on receptors and neurotransmitters in the CNS.) The narcotic action of the drug is shown through pain relief (analgesia), sleepiness, euphoria, unclear thinking, slow breathing, **miosis** (the pupil of the eye constricts or gets smaller), peristalsis (slowing of the action of smooth muscle in the bowel) causing constipation, reduced cough reflex, and hypotension (low blood pressure).

USES

Narcotic agonist analgesics are used to treat moderate to severe acute pain. They may be used to relieve pain from acute heart, lung, liver, or kidney disease or pain in the veins of the legs; for presurgery medications; in severe diarrhea and cramping; for people who are addicted to narcotics (methadone only); for constant cough (codeine); for difficulty breathing caused by heart failure or fluid in the lungs; in pain felt after surgery; and in labor.

ADVERSE REACTIONS

Adverse reactions to narcotic agonist analgesics drugs include bradycardia (slow heartbeat), hypotension, anorexia (lack of appetite), constipation, confusion, dry mouth, euphoria (excessive happiness), fainting, vomiting, pruritus (itching), skin rash, skin itch, slow breathing, and shortness of breath. Overdosage may cause bradypnea (very slow breathing, with a rate less than 12 breaths/minute); irregular, shallow breathing; sedation; coma; miosis; cyanosis (blue color to the skin); gradual drop in blood pressure; oliguria (reduced ability to form and pass urine); clammy skin; and hypothermia (abnormally low body temperature). Chronic overdosage symptoms seen in drug abusers include very small pupils, constipation, mood changes, reduced level of alertness, skin infections, pruritus, needle scars, and abscesses. Respiratory rate and sleepiness are the variables most closely watched for signs of overdosage.

DRUG INTERACTIONS

The CNS depressant effects of narcotic agonist analgesics may be increased by the use of other narcotic agonist analgesics, alcohol, antianxiety agents, barbiturates, anesthetics, nonbarbiturate sedative-hypnotics, phenothiazines, skeletal muscle relaxants, and tricyclic antidepressants. Narcotics act with many other medications to increase or decrease their effects. You should find out if the patient who is using narcotics takes any other medicines.

Nursing Implications and Patient Teaching

Assessment

It is important to determine the cause of the pain in order to end it whenever possible. Some organizations have called for pain assessment to be the fifth vital sign, but this is not universally accepted. Do not simply treat pain without understanding the source of the particular pain. Even in a patient with terminal cancer, evaluate each new pain for a specific cause that may be

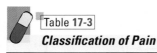

Table 17-3
Classification of Pain

CATEGORY	CHARACTERISTICS	EXAMPLE
Nociceptive	Somatic Well localized Dull, aching, or throbbing	Laceration, fracture, cellulitis, arthritis
Visceral	Poorly localized Continual aching Referred to dermatomal sites that are distant from the source of the pain	Subscapular pain arising from diaphragmatic irritation; right upper quadrant pain arising from stretching of liver capsule
Neuropathic	Shooting or stabbing pain superimposed over a background of aching and burning	Postherpetic neuralgia, postthoracotomy neuralgia, poststroke pain, trigeminal neuralgia, diabetic polyneuropathy

From McKenry LM, Salerno E: *Mosby's pharmacology in nursing*, ed 21, St Louis, 2003, Mosby, p. 269.

specifically treated. For example, bone pain can be ended by radiation. Table 17-3 lists the classifications of pain and their characteristics.

You should ask the patient about what she is feeling and the history of the pain, including when it started, where it is, what it is like, how often she has it, and what makes it worse or relieves it. Accept that patients have pain when they say they have it, and, it is the intensity level they say it is. In addition to what patients tell you, you may see tense muscles; changes in their breathing, blood pressure, and pulse; sweating; and pupil reaction. Also, they may be restless, crying, or moaning.

You should also learn as much as you can about other parts of the health history, such as whether the patient has a history of allergic or adverse reaction to morphine or related drugs, whether he seems to be able to deal with pain, and whether there is any reason to think he might abuse narcotics.

The Agency for Health Care Policy and Research (AHCPR) clinical practice guidelines include the following principles of pain assessment (A-A-B-C-D-E-E):

Ask about pain regularly. Medication is to be given regularly and is more effective if you do not wait until the patient is in severe pain and begging for medication. There is acceptance that addiction is generally not a concern, especially for patients with chronic pain or terminal illness.

Assess pain systematically. Use pain intensity scales (Figures 17-1 and 17-2).

Believe the patient and family in their reports of pain and what relieves it.

Choose pain-control options appropriate for the patient, family, and setting. The health care provider who makes this decision should be aware of the wishes of the family and individual.

Deliver interventions in a timely, logical, and coordinated fashion.

Empower patients and their families.

Enable them to control their course to the greatest extent possible.

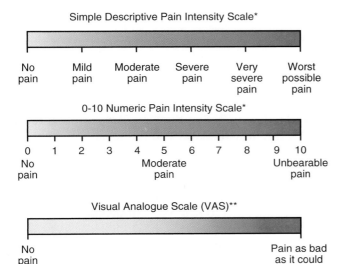

FIGURE **17-1** Pain measurement scales.

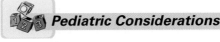

Pediatric Considerations

Pain Measurement

Pain measurement scales exist to help evaluate how much pain the patient is feeling. Children experience pain in the same way as adults. Sometimes they have more difficulty communicating their pain, so providers need to be alert. A pain scale using smiling or frowning faces may help assess their pain (see Figure 17-2).

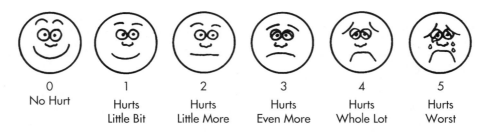

0 — No Hurt
1 — Hurts Little Bit
2 — Hurts Little More
3 — Hurts Even More
4 — Hurts Whole Lot
5 — Hurts Worst

Brief word instructions: Point to each face using the words to describe the pain intensity. Ask the child to choose face that best describes own pain and record the appropriate number.

FIGURE **17-2** Wong-Baker FACES Pain Rating Scale.

Diagnosis

Are there reasons the patient should not use these medications? Risk factors for their use? Are you aware of other things that might pose a problem for a patient taking these medications? Report any problems discovered to the registered nurse or physician.

Planning

Whenever possible, pain treatment should begin with simple analgesics and nonnarcotic analgesics and supportive pain measures first. These measures are described later.

Remember that pain relief is best if the drug is given before the patient is in intense pain.

The main problem in using opioids, especially when the patient is at home and not in a hospital, is the risk of physical and psychologic addiction or dependence for the patient. Be careful when opioids are given to the elderly, to pregnant women, to weak persons, to patients in shock or drunk with alcohol, and to children or newborns.

Clinical Landmine

Narcotic Agonist Analgesics

Pain is often a key symptom that helps identify the patient's problem. Narcotic agonist analgesics remove pain, so it is sometimes hard to determine what is wrong with the patient. Diagnosis will be difficult if the patient's condition is caused by a problem in the stomach or abdomen. Narcotic agonist analgesics should not be used in these situations. Narcotic agonist analgesics, as well as any CNS depressants, should not be used in persons with increased pressure in their eyes (intraocular pressure), head injury, or loss of consciousness.

Nonpharmacologic treatment of pain can be used alone or in combination with medications. This type of treatment includes patient education, management of anxiety and depression, cognitive-behavioral therapy,

and appropriate exercise and activity. Complimentary and alternative medicine therapies may be helpful, although there is little scientific evidence to support the use of chiropractic manipulation, homeopathy, and spiritual healing. Heat, ice, massage, topical analgesics, acupuncture and transcutaneous electrical nerve stimulation (TENS) may provide relief alone or in combination with analgesic medications. Guided imagery and distraction are especially good in pediatric patients.

Geriatric Considerations

Opioids

Elderly patients are more susceptible to the CNS and constipation side effects of opioids. Usually these patients should be placed on a bowel regimen when opioids are started. Elderly patients should be given a lower dose of opioids. Avoid propoxyphene, tramadol, and methadone, or use these drugs with caution, in elderly patients.

Implementation

Because these drugs are often abused, there are many rules to follow in giving these medications. You must learn and follow the laws that tell what you must do when giving these narcotic agonist analgesics. The Controlled Substances Act of 1970 (see Chapter 3) classed the narcotic agonist analgesics by how easily people can get addicted to them and how often they are abused. The rules are strict to help prevent people from easily abusing these drugs.

Once the narcotic agonist analgesic is metabolized by the body, the patient may feel even more pain. This is why these patients often need regular doses of medication. The drugs should also be given 2 hours before a baby is delivered or before surgery to prevent respiratory depression (severe slowing of breathing) in the newborn baby or the surgery patient.

The cough reflex is reduced by these drugs; this may be a problem in patients with lung disease. The drugs may also produce a faster heart rate in patients who have a particular heart rhythm problem. These drugs may also make convulsions worse in people who have seizures. The amount of pain felt by the patient will help you determine the dose of the narcotic and how it should be given. Narcotics may be given orally or rectally, by injection into the muscle, the subcutaneous tissue, or directly into the vein, or by epidural or intrathecal administration.

Continuous infusion of opioids into the bloodstream may be required when the patient has pain from terminal cancer or has some other chronic condition that causes severe pain. This method is also often used for short-term treatment of severe pain after surgery. The medication is delivered through an infusion pump using a microdrop infusion set. This pump allows the patient to receive a predetermined IV bolus (a preset quantity of drug injected into a vein at one time) of an analgesic (usually morphine) by using the syringe pump mechanism. Figure 17-3, *A*, shows a patient controlled analgesia (PCA) unit used in a hospital setting. Using this equipment, the patient can control when she gets pain medication. The health care provider orders the dose of medication and how often the patient can get a dose. The pump is then set or calibrated to deliver the ordered dose whenever the patient pushes the button (see Figure 17-3, *B*). The equipment can be locked from 5 to 20 minutes after a dose is given. The lockout mechanism prevents the patient from getting an accidental overdose or excessive dosing by the patient. The pump also records the number of times the button is pushed and the total amount of all medication given. The pump may be programmed for continuous administration, patient-activated delivery, or clinician-activated delivery. The pump also records all bolus attempts, successful and unsuccessful, made by the patient. This helps the provider determine if the patient feels she needs more medicine than she is getting.

The specific dose information for the narcotic agonist analgesics is listed in Table 17-4.

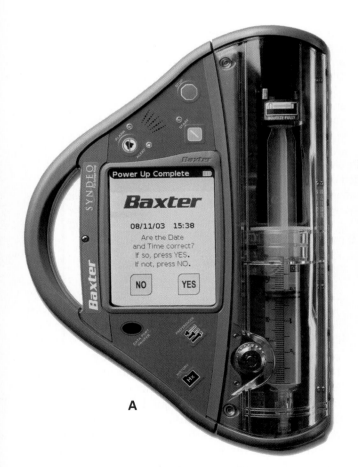

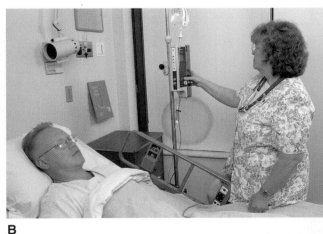

FIGURE **17-3 A,** Syndeo® PCA Syringe Pump, designed for patient- or clinician-activated medication delivery. **B,** The nurse sets the pump to deliver an ordered dose, which the patient can administer by pushing buttons on the hand-held device at the bedside. (*A,* Copyright Baxter Healthcare Corporation, Deerfield Creek, IL.)

Table **17-4**

Narcotic Agonist Analgesics

GENERIC NAME	TRADE NAME	COMMENTS AND DOSAGE
alfentanil HCl	Alfenta	Individualize dosage in maintenance of anesthesia.

codeine	Codeine Phosphate
	Codeine Sulfate
		Schedule II drug.
		• *Pain relief*
		  Adults: 15-60 mg PO, IM, or subcutaneously q4h prn.
		  Infants and children: 0.5 mg/kg PO, IM, or subcutaneously q4h prn.
		• *Antitussive*
		  Adults: 5-10 mg PO 4-6 times daily.
		  Infants and children: 0.175-0.25 mg/kg PO 4-6 times daily.

fentanyl	Duragesic
	
	Actiq
	Fentanyl Oralet
	
	Sublimaze
		Transdermal system: 25- to 100-mg patch q72h. (Available in 25, 50, 75, and 100 mg.)
		Transmucosal system: Lozenges, 100-400 mcg; suck 20-40 min before needed. Dispose of unused medication as required by law.
		Schedule II drug; potent, short-acting narcotic. The respiratory depressant effects of fentanyl are particularly dangerous; have resuscitation equipment nearby.
		• *Preoperative*
		  Adults: 0.05-0.1 mg IM.
		  Children 2-12 yr: 0.02-0.03 mg/20-25 lb IM.

hydromorphone	Dilaudid	Potent synthetic compound that maximizes analgesic effects and minimizes some of the common side effects of morphine; Dilaudid has 7-10 times the analgesic action of morphine. *Adults:* 2-4 mg IM or subcutaneously q4-6h; 2 mg PO q4-6h; one suppository twice daily.
levomethadyl acetate HCl	Orlaam	Used in managing opioid dependence. Give 20-40 mg 3 times weekly, increase by 5-10 mg to maintenance of 60-90 mg 3 times weekly.
levorphanol	Levo-Dromoran	Used to relieve moderate to severe pain; often used preoperatively to reduce apprehension and to prolong analgesia. It has a relatively longer onset of action than other narcotic agonist analgesics. *Adults:* 2-3 mg PO or subcutaneously. May also be given by slow IV injection.
meperidine	Demerol	Schedule II drug; synthetic narcotic analgesic with less potency than morphine; each dose of syrup should be taken in one-half glass of water, because if undiluted, it can exert a topical anesthetic effect on mucous membranes. *Adults:* 50-150 mg IM, subcutaneously, or PO q3-4h. *Children:* 0.5-0.8 mg/lb IM, subcutaneously, or PO q3-4h.

Evaluation

Usually, oral narcotic agonist analgesics begin to take effect in 15 to 30 minutes. The time needed for opioids injected into the tissue to take effect may vary a lot. This is because of differences in the ability of these drugs to dissolve in the tissue, which causes differences in how fast the body can absorb them. Opioids given by mouth are much less effective than those given by injection. However, oral narcotic agonist analgesics produce pain relief for a longer time. Intravenous (IV) opioids may be given in small doses by the patient or nurse through IV tubing following institutional policies.

The dose of the narcotic agonist analgesic depends on the severity of the pain experienced by the patient, the patient's response to the pain and the medication, and the nature of the illness. In the past, many patients had pain because the dose of medication was not high enough. In the last 10 years, higher doses have been recommended for treating patients with cancer or chronic pain. The new guides suggest much higher doses at more frequent intervals and for longer times than previous guides. The doses for such patients are much higher than presurgery doses or doses for acute pain.

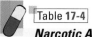

Table 17-4

Narcotic Agonist Analgesics—cont'd

GENERIC NAME	TRADE NAME	COMMENTS AND DOSAGE
methadone	Dolophine	Schedule II drug; synthetic narcotic analgesic used primarily in the detoxification, treatment, and maintenance of heroin addicts or for severe pain. When the drug is used for severe pain, it is administered IM. The drug is highly addictive. When used for heroin addicts for more than 3 wk, methadone moves from a treatment phase to a maintenance phase. • *Pain relief* *Adults:* 2.5-10 mg IM, subcutaneously, or PO q3-4h.
morphine	Duramorph MS Contin Oramorph SR MSIR	Schedule II drug; the primary narcotic analgesic used for relief of severe pain. It is the narcotic analgesic against which all others are compared. It also produces sedation and euphoria when pain is present. Traditionally used for preoperative sedation and postoperative analgesia. Morphine is more effective against dull, continuous pain than sharp, spasmodic pain. IV medication should be given slowly over a 4- to 5-min period. Protect drug from light and freezing. *Adults:* Administer 5-20 mg subcutaneously or IM q4h as indicated; IV administration doses range from 2 to 15 mg/5 mL injected over a 5-min period. *Children:* 0.1-0.2 mg/kg per dose subcutaneously; maximum dose not to exceed 15 mg.
opium combinations	Opium Tincture Paregoric	Schedule II drug. Paregoric is equivalent to 0.04% morphine. Opium tincture is equivalent to 1% morphine. Avoid confusing these two medications. Paregoric is used for cramps, diarrhea, and teething pain in infants (as a topical application to gums). • *Diarrhea* *Adults:* Tincture 0.6-1.5 mL PO 4 times daily; camphorated tincture 5-10 mL PO 4 times daily. *Children:* Camphorated tincture 0.25-0.5 mL/kg prn.
oxycodone	OxyContin Roxicodone	*Adults:* 5 mg or 5 mL q6h prn.

oxycodone
  hydrocodone
  combinations
	Lorcet
	Oxycodone
	Percocet
	Percodan
	Tylox
	Vicodin
		These agents are similar in action and structure but are not identical; they are opium alkaloids and are morphine-like in action. Used for moderate to severe acute pain.
		Adults: 1-2 tablets q4-6h prn for pain.

oxymorphone	Numorphan	*Adults:* 0.5 mg IV; or subcutaneously/IM, give 1-1.5 mg q4-6h.
remifentanil	Ultiva	Individualize dosage as analgesia adjunct.
sufentanil	Sufenta	Individualize dosage as analgesia adjunct.

The patient who is receiving any type of narcotic should be checked at regular, frequent intervals. Because narcotic agonist analgesics may decrease the cough and sigh reflexes, patients who have had surgery, especially those who have smoked for a long time, may develop areas where the lungs do not inflate well or may have fluid in them (atelectasis) and pneumonia.

You should also assess each patient's behavior while he is taking the drug. For example, the patient may be unable to stop taking the drug, may make frequent requests for the drug, or may use more than one health care provider or office. These behaviors may be sign of dependence or addiction.

Narcotic agonist analgesics are metabolized by the liver, and the leftover chemicals leave the body through the kidneys; 90% of the drug is passed with the urine i first 24 hours.

Patient and Family Teaching

You should tell the patient and family the following:
   1. The patient should take this medication as o dered by the nurse, physician, or other healt care provider and not change the dosag

Although this product could cause addiction, it is most effective when taken before the patient has severe pain.

2. If the patient is not feeling a lot of pain, other methods for getting rid of pain should be used whenever possible.
3. The patient should not take any other medications without telling the nurse, physician, or other health care provider. Alcohol increases the effect of the medication, and taking both of them together may cause a problem.
4. Some patients have side effects from this drug, such as dizziness, light-headedness, nausea, drowsiness, sweating, flushing (red color in the face and neck), or stopping of the cough reflex. The patient or family should report any new or troubling symptoms to the nurse, physician, or other health care provider.
5. The patient taking this medicine should not operate heavy machinery, drive, or perform tasks that require her to be alert.
6. The patient should urinate often and make sure he is not constipated by increasing fluid intake and adding extra fiber into his diet.

7. The patient should get up slowly from lying or sitting positions to decrease feelings of light-headedness and should avoid standing in one position for long periods.
8. When taking the first doses of opioids, the patient should lie down for a short period to prevent nausea.
9. The patient should take the medication exactly as prescribed, and should make an effort to wait for longer periods of time between doses if the medication is taken for a long time. The patient should write down the time when the medication was last taken to prevent taking too much medication by accident.
10. This medication must be kept out of the reach of children and all others for whom it is not prescribed. All extra medication should be thrown away when there is no longer any need for it; it should not be kept for another time.

SECTION TWO

Narcotic Agonist-Antagonist Analgesics

ACTION

Narcotic agonist-antagonist analgesics are strong drugs that act through the CNS, possibly at the limbic system. They act with other chemicals at specific nerve sites. Drugs in this category have different sites of action, but they usually act like morphine in producing analgesia, euphoria, and respiratory and physical depression. Some drugs may compete with other narcotics. Thus they may produce withdrawal symptoms in patients who are dependent on narcotics, but they are also less likely to be abused than pure narcotic agonists.

USES

Narcotic agonist-antagonist analgesics are used mostly for the relief of moderate to severe pain. They are also used in the injectable form for presurgery analgesia and for pregnant women during active labor. These drugs may be better than narcotics for use in patients outside the hospital because their risk for abuse is lower.

Narcotic-analgesic combination drugs include other chemicals that also work on the pain centers of the CNS. These drugs may contain acetaminophen, aspirin, and caffeine, combined with narcotics such as codeine, oxycodone, or hydrocodone. Some agents also contain a form of barbiturate, which is added for its sedative (calming) effects. Narcotics and barbiturates are legally defined as controlled substances, so there are many rules about how they must be used.

Combination drugs are used for the relief of moderate to severe pain of an acute origin, such as postsurgical or dental pain when a tooth is pulled. They are often ordered when the patient leaves a hospital or are ordered when the patient is not in a hospital. These drugs are addictive and should be used for only a brief time. Table 17-5 lists common combination products used for analgesia.

ADVERSE REACTIONS

Adverse reactions to narcotic agonist-antagonist analgesics include bradycardia, hypertension (high blood pressure) or hypotension, tachycardia (rapid heartbeat), changes in mood, blurred vision, confusion, dizziness, headache, weakness, nervousness, nystagmus (rhythmic movement of the eyes), syncope (light-headedness and fainting), tingling, tinnitus (ringing in the ears),

Table 17-5
Narcotic-Analgesic Combination Products

TRADE NAME	CHEMICAL COMPONENTS
Acetaminophen with Codeine	Codeine, acetaminophen
ASA with Codeine Compound	Codeine, aspirin (acetylsalicylic acid [ASA])
Empirin with Codeine	Codeine, aspirin
Fiorinal with Codeine	Codeine, aspirin, caffeine, butalbital
Percocet	Oxycodone, acetaminophen
Percodan	Oxycodone, oxycodone terephthalate, aspirin
Phenaphen-650 with Codeine	Codeine, acetaminophen
Tylox	Oxycodone, acetaminophen
Vicodin	Hydrocodone bitartrate, acetaminophen

tremor, unusual dreams, pruritus, rash, hardening of the soft tissue from swelling, stinging on injection, ulcers, anorexia, abdominal cramps, constipation, diarrhea, dry mouth, dyspepsia (stomach discomfort after eating), nausea, vomiting, low production of white blood cells, dyspnea (uncomfortable breathing), flushing, speech difficulty, and either the urge to urinate or difficulty urinating. Overdosage may produce sleepiness and respiratory depression.

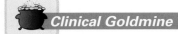

Clinical Goldmine

Narcan

Because there is a very real danger of overdosage of narcotics, it is important to know about a drug called naloxone (Narcan). This drug is a narcotic antagonist that may be used to reverse symptoms of overdoses of narcotics (whether by accident or on purpose). Narcan is shorter acting than narcotics. If it is given, you must watch for an increase in the narcotic symptoms (rebound) when the Narcan wears off.

DRUG INTERACTIONS

Alcohol and drugs that slow the actions of the body (depressants) should be used with caution with these products because of the risk for increased CNS depression.

Nursing Implications and Patient Teaching

Assessment

You should learn as much as possible about the health history of the patient, including the presence of lung, liver, or kidney disease; pregnancy or breastfeeding; recent heart attack; or clues that they might have emotional problems or might have problems with drug

dependency or drug misuse. These conditions may b contraindications or precautions to the use of narcoti agonist-antagonist analgesics.

The patient's feelings of the pain and the amount c pain she can handle should be determined. A history c the pain, including when it started, where it is locatec what it feels like, how bad it is, and things that make worse or make it better should be obtained. You may se that the patient has tensed muscles, low breathing changes in blood pressure or pulse, sweating, change in reaction of the pupils, or restlessness, crying, c moaning.

Diagnosis

Are there any other problems in addition to the medic diagnosis that will affect the patient's response to thes drugs? Is the patient frightened? Are there concern about blood loss, ability to breathe, safety, and whethe the tissues have enough fluid (**hydration**)? Any prob lems discovered should be reported to the registere nurse or physician.

Planning

Narcotic agonist-antagonist analgesics should be use with caution in patients who have emotional problem or in those who have a history of drug abuse. Becaus both physical and emotional dependence may occu these drugs should be given to such patients only whe they can be carefully watched, and given only in limite amounts.

Narcotic agonist-antagonists should not be given t patients with head injury, because you need to be abl to monitor how the patient acts without the confusin effects of the medication. It has not been establishe whether it is safe to use these drugs in children or i pregnant women (other than during labor). Becaus these drugs tend to cause slowed breathing, they shoul be used very carefully in patients with breathing prob lems (especially asthma), obstructive breathing cond tions, and cyanosis.

Narcotic agonist-antagonists may produce withdrawal symptoms in patients who have developed dependence on narcotics. These products may also cause seizures, especially in patients with known seizure disorders.

Patients who take combination drug products may have adverse effects from or develop problems because of any of the drugs used in the medications.

Implementation

All of these narcotic agonist-antagonist analgesics are available in injectable form, but only pentazocine is available in oral form. These medications should be given by intramuscular (IM) injection, because subcutaneous injection may damage tissues.

When frequent injections are needed, each dose should be given in a different site. The injection sites should be changed every time to avoid damaging the tissues. (Refer back to Figure 10-15, which shows a typical injection rotation plan).

For acute pain, one to two tablets or capsules of narcotics combined with other medications are given every 4 to 6 hours. These drugs are not to be given to children.

Table 17-6 presents a review of narcotic agonist-antagonist analgesics.

Evaluation

You should monitor the patient to determine whether he is getting relief from his pain and whether he is developing any problems as a result of the medicine. If the patient starts seeing things that are not there (hallucinations), or becomes confused or semicomatose, the medication should be stopped.

You should also watch the patient's behavior. For example, the patient may be unable to stop taking the drug, may want the drug all the time, or may try to get the drug from different physicians or hospitals.

Patient and Family Teaching

You should tell the patient and family the following:
1. The patient should take this medication as ordered by the nurse, physician, or other health care provider and not change the dosage. Even though this product has a risk for addiction, it is most effective when taken before the patient has severe pain.
2. As the patient begins to feel better, other methods for pain relief should be used whenever possible.

Table 17-6

Narcotic Agonist-Antagonist Analgesics

GENERIC NAME	TRADE NAME	COMMENTS AND DOSAGE
buprenorphine	Buprenex	Onset of action in 15 min, peak at 60 min, duration 6 hr. Give 0.3 mg IM or slow IV q6h.
butorphanol	Stadol	Onset of action in 10 min after IM injection and almost immediately after IV injection. The respiratory depressant effect is similar to that of morphine, is dose related, and is easily reversed with naloxone. *Intramuscular:* 1-4 mg, repeated q3-4h prn; do not give doses greater than 4 mg. *Intravenous:* 0.5-2 mg, repeated q3-4h prn.
dezocine	Dalgan	Onset of action in 15-30 min; duration 2-4 hours. Give 5-20 mg IM.
nalbuphine	Nubain	Onset in 15 min, duration 3-6 hr. This product tends to be more expensive than other agonist-antagonist products. *Adults:* 10 mg subcutaneously, IM, or IV, repeated q3-6h prn; do not give more than 20 mg in 1 dose or more than 160 mg/day.
pentazocine	Talwin	Onset in 15 min, duration 3 hr. Schedule IV drug; synthetic opioid used for moderate to severe pain or as a preoperative or preanesthetic medication. Although it may be given subcutaneously, it is better to give deep IM and rotate sites, because subcutaneous injection may produce severe tissue damage at injection site. Do not mix this product with other chemicals during injection. • *Pain relief:* *Adults:* 30 mg IM, subcutaneously, or IV q3-4h; do not exceed doses of 60 mg IM or 30 mg IV. Total daily dose should not exceed 360 mg. For chronic administration, 50-mg oral tablets are recommended q3-4h.

3. Some patients have side effects from these drugs, such as drowsiness, nausea, vomiting, dizziness, blurred vision, sweating, dry mouth, headache, and confusion. The patient should report any new or troubling symptoms to the nurse, physician, or other health care provider.

4. The patient should avoid working with heavy machinery, driving, or tasks that require alertness after taking this medication.

5. This medicine must be kept out of the reach of children and others for whom it is not prescribed.

SECTION THREE
Nonnarcotic Centrally Acting Analgesics

ACTION AND USES

Nonnarcotic analgesics are drugs that act at the level of the brain (centrally acting) to control mild or moderate pain. Although propoxyphene and ethoheptazine are chemically similar to narcotic analgesics, they are not as strong and do not have the abuse risk of narcotics. Methotrimeprazine has strong CNS depressant activity and is related to the phenothiazine drugs. This drug is used most commonly when a patient will be receiving anesthetic. These products are used mostly to relieve mild to moderate pain. They are also used in combination with other products for pain alone or when pain and fever are both present.

Nonnarcotic analgesic combination drugs are used mainly to control pain. They include agents such as acetaminophen, aspirin, caffeine, antacids, and butalbital. Caffeine, a plant extract, has mild brain, lung, and heart stimulant effects, as well as some diuretic activity. It has no analgesic properties, but it is used to treat some types of headaches. Combination products are used when additional actions are desired along with mild or moderate analgesia (Table 17-7).

ADVERSE REACTIONS

Adverse reactions to nonnarcotic analgesics include postural hypotension (low blood pressure when a person suddenly stands up), disorientation, dizziness, euphoria, headache, light-headedness, minor visual disturbances, sleepiness, slurring of speech, weakness, skin rashes, pain in stomach or abdomen, constipation, dry mouth, nausea, vomiting, difficulty urinating, chills, stuffy nose, and pain at the injection site. Overdosage usually produces extreme sleepiness, although the patient may have slowed breathing and be in a coma. Cyanosis and low oxygen levels are also present because of the slow breathing rate, hypotension, and weak heart function. Hepatotoxicity (damage to the liver) may also occur in alcoholics who use the drug acetaminophen.

DRUG INTERACTIONS

Nonnarcotic analgesics have CNS depressant effects that add to those of other depressants, including alcohol. Each product interacts with other drugs, although these products have fewer chemical interactions than narcotics.

Nursing Implications and Patient Teaching

Assessment

You should learn as much as possible about the patient's health history, including whether the patient has any respiratory or hepatic disease, or is pregnant or breastfeeding. In addition, you should look for clues that the patient has emotional problems or has had problems

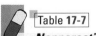
Table **17-7**
Nonnarcotic Analgesic Combination Products

	TRADE NAME	CHEMICAL COMPONENTS
	Anacin	Aspirin, caffeine
	Bromo-Seltzer	Acetaminophen, sodium bicarbonate, citric acid
	Equagesic	Aspirin, meprobamate
	Excedrin	Aspirin, acetaminophen, caffeine
	Fiorinal	Aspirin, caffeine, butalbital
	Vanquish	Aspirin, acetaminophen, caffeine, antacids

with drug dependency or drug misuse. These conditions may be contraindications or precautions to use of nonnarcotic analgesics.

You should determine the patient's feelings about the pain and its history, including when it started, where it is located, what it feels like and how severe it is, and things that make it worse or make it better. You may also see that the patient has tensed muscles, changes in breathing, sweating, change in pupils, restlessness, crying, or moaning, as well as changes in blood pressure and pulse rate. How well the patient can accept pain should be determined. Use a pain scale to grade the intensity of the patient's pain.

Diagnosis

What other problems does the patient have that might interfere with the action of this medication? Are there concerns about moving around, sensory awareness, or level of alertness?

Planning

You should not give nonnarcotic analgesics, including phenothiazines, to patients who are allergic to the products they contain. Always ask the patient about whether he has any allergies before giving a medication. Methotrimeprazine should not be given at the same time as an antihypertensive medication or some antidepressants (monoamine oxidase inhibitors), or to patients who are very ill with drug overdosages, are in a coma, have very low blood pressure, have had a heart attack, or have severe kidney or liver disease.

Methotrimeprazine is rarely given more than a few times and should not be given for longer than 30 days, unless narcotics cannot be given and unless you can obtain periodic blood counts and liver function studies.

Nonnarcotic Analgesics

Elderly and weakened patients may react more strongly to many nonnarcotic analgesics. These patients should not do anything that requires them to be alert while taking these drugs because the medication may slow down their ability to respond quickly.

Implementation

Propoxyphene comes in a capsule, and methotrimeprazine comes as an injection. Table 17-8 lists important drug information about major nonnarcotic agents.

Evaluation

After methotrimeprazine is given, hypotension, fainting, dizziness, or sleepiness may occur. Patients should be watched carefully while taking this product, especially for the first 6 hours after the first dose.

You should check the patient regularly and frequently to determine her response to the drug and look for symptoms of overdosage. Patients who get too much medication may die within the first hour, so it is important to watch the patient carefully. Patients who have emotional problems, who have abused drugs in the past, or who may not take their medicine properly should not be given these medications.

Dependence may develop when propoxyphene products are taken in high doses over a long time. These drugs should be treated with the same caution as narcotics.

You should watch how the patient behaves. For example, the patient may be unable to stop taking the

Table 17-8

Nonnarcotic Centrally Acting Analgesics

GENERIC NAME	TRADE NAME	COMMENTS AND DOSAGE
clonidine	Duraclon	Give 30 mcg/hr for continuous epidural infusion.
methotrimeprazine	Levoprome	This product is a phenothiazine derivative with potent CNS depressant activity. Give deep IM injection into large muscles, with rotation of injection sites. • *Pain:* 10-20 mg deep IM q4-6h prn. Although up to 40 mg may be given, start with 10-mg doses until patient response is assessed. Reduce dose in elderly patients to 5 mg.
propoxyphene	Darvon-N	Schedule IV drug; a centrally acting opioid, structurally related to methadone. It is used primarily as a weak analgesic but has physical and psychologic addictive properties. *Adults:* 65-100 mg PO q4h prn.
tramadol	Ultram	Give 50-100 mg PO q4-6 hr. Do not exceed 400 mg/day.

drug, may keep asking for the drug, or may use several different health care providers or hospitals.

Because of the risk of hepatotoxicity in former alcoholics using acetaminophen, watch for any sign of alcohol abuse.

Patient and Family Teaching

You should tell the patient and family the following:

1. The patient should take this medication as ordered by the nurse, physician, or other health care provider and not change the dosage. Although these drugs have a risk for addiction, they are most effective when taken before the patient has severe pain.
2. As the patient begins to feel better, other methods for reducing pain should be used whenever possible.
3. Some patients have side effects from these drugs, such as dizziness, sleepiness, nausea, and vomiting. The patient may also note a feeling of lightheadedness, especially when getting up from lying down so the patient should stand up slowly to stop this feeling. The patient should tell the nurse, physician, or other health care provider about any new or troublesome symptoms.
4. The patient should not use any heavy machinery, drive, or perform tasks for which he needs to be alert while taking this medication.
5. This medication must be kept out of the reach of children and others for whom it is not prescribed.

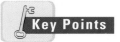

Key Points

- Pain is something we all feel.
- For many years, patients suffered with pain because there was a fear that they would become addicted to narcotics. New guidelines have tried to change this.
- Morphine is the standard against which all other narcotics are judged.
- There are now many new synthetic narcotics available to help reduce pain.
- You have a special job in learning and following the many rules for giving narcotics and in preventing abuse of these drugs.

Go to the free CD-ROM for an Audio Glossary, animations, video clips, and Review Questions for the NCLEX-PN® Examination.

evolve   Be sure to visit the companion Evolve website at http://evolve.elsevier.com/Edmunds/LPN/ for WebLinks, a link to the top 200 drugs by prescription, and sign-up pages for newsletter drug updates.

CASE STUDY

Mr. Rim, a hard-working Korean immigrant, works in an inner-city convenience store. He has recently hurt his back lifting heavy boxes.

1. What would be the most appropriate form of initial pain control?
2. The pain continues and now Mr. Rim experiences pain shooting from his lower back down his left leg. X-ray studies reveal a ruptured vertebral disk and he undergoes surgery. What type of analgesia is likely to be ordered after surgery?

3. Mr. Rim does not want to take any pain medication. He believes that he should only have pain medication if his pain is so bad that he cannot tolerate it. What would you tell him?
4. Is there any reason why Mr. Rim is likely to become addicted to this medicine because of his ethnic background?
5. What type of behavior might lead you to believe that a patient has become addicted to pain medicine?

DRUG CALCULATION REVIEW

1. Order: Morphine sulfate gr¼ intramuscular every 4 hours as needed for pain

   Supply: Morphine sulfate 10 mg/mL

   Question: How many milliliters of morphine sulfate is needed for each dose?

2. Order: Dilaudid 0.5 mg/hr IV continuous drip

   Supply: Dilaudid 20 mg in 200 mL 0.9% normal saline

   Question: How many milliliters per hour should the IV infusion device be set for?

3. Order: Narcan 0.4 mg IV for respiratory rate (RR) <8 breaths/min

   Supply: Narcan 0.2 mg/mL

   Question: How many milliliters of Narcan should be given if the RR is <8 breaths/min?

CRITICAL THINKING ?

1. Why are increased caution and lower doses of narcotic analgesics recommended for use in elderly patients?

2. Your postoperative abdominal surgery patient has been requesting increasingly frequent pain medication. Her medication has been ordered every 4 hours, but she is now requesting it every 2-2½ hours. What would be the most appropriate nursing action for this patient?

3. A nursing entry on a patient's chart recorded, "Quiet evening." Also recorded was that the same nurse had administered "ASA 625 mg PO for headache" to the patient. What information is missing?

4. Mr. Taylor has just returned to your surgical unit from the postanesthesia care unit, following left total knee joint replacement surgery. When would be the best time to administer pain medication to Mr. Taylor?

5. Mr. Robbins was started on a narcotic agonist analgesic immediately after his surgery. Several days after the surgery, he seems to be requesting medication more often than you had anticipated. Mr. Robbins is not addicted to his medication, but both he and his family are concerned about that possibility. Draw up a teaching plan for a narcotic agonist analgesic.

18 Gastrointestinal Medications

Objectives

After reading and studying this chapter, you should be able to do the following:

1. Identify common uses for antacids and histamine H_2-receptor antagonists.
2. Compare and contrast the actions of anticholinergic and antispasmodic medications on the gastrointestinal (GI) tract.
3. Compare the actions and adverse reactions of the five major classifications of laxatives.
4. Identify indications for the use of at least two common antidiarrheals, antiflatulents, digestive enzymes, and emetics.
5. Describe indications for disulfiram use and what is meant by "disulfiram reaction."

Key Terms

Be sure to check out the bonus material on the free CD-ROM, including selected audio pronunciations.

antacids (ănt-ĂS-ĭdz, p. 329)
antidiarrheals (ăn-tĭ-dī-ă-RĒ-ălz, p. 334)
antiflatulents (ăn-tĭ-FLĂ-tū-lĕnts, p. 342)
digestive enzymes (dī-JĔS-tĭv ĕn-ZĪMZ, p. 344)
disulfiram reaction (dī-SŬL-fĭ-răm, p. 345)
emetics (ĕm-ĔT-ĭks, p. 346)
histamine H_2-receptor antagonists
 (HĬS-tă-mēn, ăn-TĂG-ō-nĭsts, p. 329)
laxatives (LĂK-să-tĭvz, p. 338)
motility (mō-TĬL-ĭ-tē, p. 334)

OVERVIEW

This chapter discusses medications used to treat the many diseases and disorders that affect the gastrointestinal (GI) tract. Many of these drugs are available over the counter (OTC); many others are used, often in combination, to relieve the symptoms of common GI tract problems.

There are three major types of GI medications. The first major type includes products designed to help restore or maintain the lining that protects the GI tract. These drugs include antacids, which act to neutralize or reduce the acidity of the gastric contents, and the his-tamine H_2-receptor antagonists, which reduce gastric acid secretion by limiting the action of histamine at the H_2 receptors in the stomach. A third type of drug, the proton pump inhibitors, reduce gastric acid through blocking the proton pump. These medications are described in Section One.

A second type of medication affects the general motility, or movement, of the GI tract. These medications include the anticholinergics and antispasmodics, which not only reduce gastric motility but also decrease the amount of acid secreted by the stomach, and the antidiarrheals, which reduce diarrhea by slowing the intestinal peristalsis. These drugs are discussed in Section Two.

The third major group of GI drugs is the laxative agents. These preparations also affect motility, but their action is primarily in the colon. They promote bowel emptying in a variety of ways. They may increase intestinal bulk, lubricate the intestinal walls, soften the fecal mass by retaining water, or produce increased peristalsis through local tissue irritation or by direct action on the intestine. These drugs are discussed in Section Three.

Section Four presents miscellaneous medications. These preparations include antiflatulents, which are used to reduce gas and bloating; digestive enzymes, which are used in deficiency states to break down fats, starches, and proteins in the digestive process; emetics, which are used to produce vomiting, primarily in poisoning or overdose; and medications used to treat gallstones and alcoholism. Antiemetic preparations are discussed in Chapter 16 along with antivertigo agents.

DIGESTIVE SYSTEM

The digestive system is composed of the mouth, esophagus, stomach, intestines, and accessory structures (Figure 18-1). This system performs the mechanical and chemical process of digestion, absorbs nutrients, and eliminates waste.

Digestion begins in the mouth with chewing and mixing of food with enzyme-rich saliva secreted by salivary glands. The passages and spaces from the mouth to the anus are called the alimentary canal, in which the complex compounds created in the mouth are reduced to soluble, absorbable substances; the usable

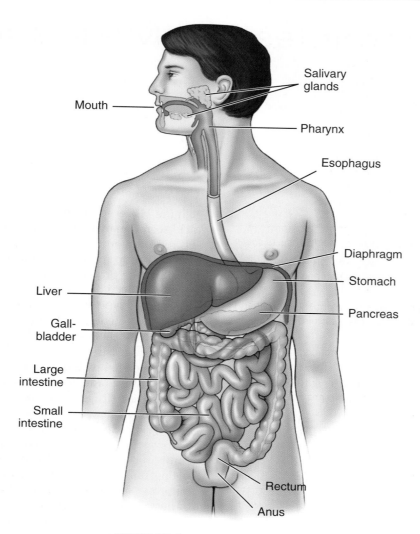

FIGURE **18-1** The digestive system.

food substances are absorbed; and the indigestible and waste material is eliminated. The digestive glands secrete enzymes and other chemicals essential to the breakdown of food substances and their absorption into the bloodstream. The salivary glands, gallbladder, liver, and pancreas are included as accessory glands.

Almost all oral medications use the digestive system as a means to reach target organs or tissues. Many of the side effects, such as diarrhea, nausea, or constipation, are results of the direct action of medications on the alimentary tract itself. Medications, as well as all swallowed materials, are acted on by the digestive tract, and are metabolized and excreted.

The digestive tract must work without being destroyed by the strong acid it makes to digest food. Several protective factors work together to protect the GI tract mucosa from injury. The gastric mucosal barrier resists backward diffusion of hydrogen and thus has the ability to have a high concentration of hydrochloric acid (HCl) within the gastric lumen unless something breaks this barrier. Endogenous prostaglandins (those produced in the GI tract) are thought to protect the cells

against injurious agents and are produced in great numbers in the mucosa of the stomach and duodenum. They are known to produce both mucus and bicarbonate and to maintain mucosal blood flow. Mucus helps protect the mucosa. It is secreted by surface epithelial cells and forms a gel that covers the mucosal surface and physically protects the mucosa from abrasion. It also resists the passage of large molecules such as pepsin. Bicarbonate is produced in small amounts by surface epithelial cells and moves up from the mucosa to create a thin layer of alkalinity between the mucus and the epithelial surface. Other protective factors include mucosal blood flow, epithelial healing or renewal, and epidermal growth factor that is secreted in saliva and by the duodenal mucosa.

There is a lot of variability in the body's ability to absorb medications from the GI tract over the course of a lifetime. Changes in GI blood flow, amount of surface available, and motility are found in very young and more elderly patients. Thus dosages of some medications may need to be changed when the patient is very young or very old.

SECTION ONE

Antacids, H$_2$-Receptor Antagonists, Proton Pump Inhibitors

OVERVIEW

The lining of the stomach is usually strong enough to resist the powerful digestive juices and acids that bathe it. When stress or disease produces excess secretion of gastric acids, or when there is destruction of the protective mucosal lining because of alcohol, chemicals, or disease, gastric distress is produced. If the protective lining is not repaired or the gastric acid level reduced, duodenal, gastric, or peptic ulcers are produced, which lead to increased pain and bleeding. Antacid therapy, histamine H$_2$-receptor antagonists, and proton pump inhibitors reduce gastric acidity and promote healing. More than one medication may be used at the same time to help in healing. Two unique medications, sucralfate and misoprostol, are designed to assist in the protection of GI mucosa from the effects of nonsteroidal antiinflammatory drugs (NSAIDs).

ACTION

Antacids are OTC agents that neutralize hydrochloric acid and increase gastric pH, thus inhibiting pepsin (a gastric enzyme). Antacids work in a variety of ways. Some antacids cause hydrogen ion absorption, or buffering of the acid; tightening of the gastric mucosa; and increased tone of the cardiac sphincter. Formation of gas that may be burped is another way in which antacids work.

Histamine H$_2$-receptor antagonists are unique because they promote healing of ulcers and act with antacids to produce more alkaline conditions in the GI tract. Histamine H$_2$-receptor antagonist drugs can bind to the H$_2$ receptor, thereby displacing histamine from receptor binding sites and preventing stimulation of the secretory cells. Thus they block histamine, inhibit the secretion of gastric acid, and are rapidly absorbed; they reach their peak of effectiveness in 45 to 90 minutes.

Another class of drugs that works to heal gastric ulcers is the proton pump inhibitors. These drugs irreversibly stop the acid secretory pump embedded within the gastric parietal cell membrane by altering the activity of H$^+$,K$^+$-ATPase, the enzyme inhibiting hydrogen ion transport into the gastric lumen, and thus decrease acid secretion. Because proton pump inhibitors act on the basolateral membrane of the parietal cells, they do not affect gastric emptying, basal or stimulated pepsin output, or secretion of intrinsic factor. These drugs do not seem to affect the level of adenosine triphosphatase (ATPase) of other organ systems.

USES

Antacids are used with other drugs to treat peptic ulcer disease, gastritis, gastric ulcer, peptic esophagitis, hiatal hernia, gastric hyperacidity, and esophageal reflux.

Histamine H$_2$ blockers are generally considered first-line therapy to relieve symptoms and prevent complications of peptic ulcer disease when used over 6 to 8 weeks. (It is common for the patient to have a relapse after the medication is stopped.) They are also used in the prophylaxis and treatment of peptic esophagitis, benign gastric ulcers, duodenal ulcers, stress ulcers, and Zollinger-Ellison syndrome. The H$_2$ blockers are similar in effectiveness and side effects. Many peptic ulcers may be caused by *Helicobacter pylori*. This organism may be controlled and the ulcer healed by use of antibiotics plus ranitidine products.

Proton pump inhibitors are used in the short-term treatment of active duodenal ulcers, usually after adequate courses of H$_2$-receptor antagonists have not been successful. Longer therapy is not indicated. Severe erosive esophagitis and poorly responsive gastroesophageal reflux disease (GERD) are indications for these types of medications as well. Long-term treatment with proton pump inhibitors is needed for pathologic hypersecretory conditions.

There are other important drugs that also assist in the healing of ulcers that do not fit into these three categories. Sucralfate is an aluminum salt of sulfated sucrose and a polysaccharide with antipeptic activity. It aids in the healing of ulcers by forming a protective layer at the ulcer site, providing a barrier to hydrogen ion diffusion, but does not alter gastric pH. It also works to stop pepsin's action and adsorbs bile salts. Misoprostol is a synthetic prostaglandin analogue with both an antisecretory and a mucosal protective action. It is indicated for use in patients who have gastric distress or ulceration secondary to the use of NSAIDs.

ADVERSE REACTIONS

Some adverse reactions occur only with a certain category of antacids; others are common to most. Antacids may produce malaise (weakness), anorexia (lack of appetite), bowel obstruction, constipation, diarrhea, frequent burping, thirst, and muscle weakness. In cases of extreme hypermagnesemia, cardiotoxicity with bradyarrhythmia, asystole, and hypotension may be seen. The most severe reactions include coma, decreased reflexes, and respiratory depression.

With histamine H$_2$-receptor antagonists, side effects are unusual, but the patient may have mild and self-limiting problems such as dizziness, headaches, somnolence, mild and brief diarrhea, some hematology changes, rash, impotence, mild gynecomastia (enlargement of the breasts in men), muscle pain, and fever. With proton pump inhibitors, reactions include headache, diarrhea, abdominal pain, and nausea. Rare reactions include rash, vomiting, and dizziness.

DRUG INTERACTIONS

Antacids prevent the absorption of tetracycline. Enteric coatings of various medications dissolve more quickly in the presence of antacids, leaving the upper GI tract more sensitive to irritation. Some antacids have been known to either bind with or alter the absorption rate of digitalis products, anticoagulants, iron, phenothiazines, antiinflammatory agents, antihypertensives, antiarthritic agents, hydantoin, and possibly propranolol. Aluminum-magnesium hydroxide gel may increase absorption of aspirin. Dicumarol is absorbed 50% faster when taken at the same time as antacids.

 Clinical Landmine

Cimetidine

Cimetidine inhibits the cytochrome P-450 system and interacts with many other medications.

Antacids may increase the absorption of cimetidine, a histamine antagonist agent. Cimetidine may increase the effects of anticoagulants, hydantoin, beta-adrenergic blocking agents, lidocaine, benzodiazepine derivatives, and theophylline. Decreased white blood cell counts have been reported in cimetidine-treated patients who also received other drugs and treatments known to produce neutropenia. Apnea, confusion, and muscle twitching may be produced when cimetidine is administered with morphine. Serum digoxin levels may be reduced when digoxin and cimetidine are administered together. Cigarette smoking may neutralize the action of cimetidine. Ranitidine does not appear to interact with warfarin-type anticoagulants, theophylline, or diazepam, although it does produce false-positive urine protein tests.

Proton pump inhibitors also inhibit the cytochrome P-450 system and may interfere with the metabolism of other drugs using the P-450 system. They may also increase concentration of oral anticoagulants, diazepam, and phenytoin, making overdosage a possibility.

Nursing Implications and Patient Teaching

Assessment

You should learn all you can about the patient's health history, including GI symptoms, the presence of disease (especially renal failure), the presence of allergy, and whether any medications that might cause drug interactions are currently being taken by the patient.

Diagnosis

In addition to the medical diagnosis, what is the source of the patient's problem? Does the patient drink too much coffee or alcohol or use cigarettes extensively—all of which are harmful to the gastric mucosa? Is the patient under stress from financial, family, or job-related difficulties? Does the patient experience gastric distress because of other medications (such as NSAIDs) or disease processes? Look beyond the symptoms to find the cause of increased gastric acid production. This may assist the patient in focusing on the true source of the problem.

Planning

The patient's fluid intake should be increased, and you should carefully monitor the patient who is taking antacids that cause constipation, such as those containing calcium or aluminum. These drugs may be alternated with antacids that have cathartic-like actions, such as those containing magnesium.

Implementation

Antacids are available in several different forms. Liquids or solutions are the preferred choice whenever possible, because they neutralize acid more rapidly. Suspensions, gels, chewable tablets, effervescent tablets, and powders are also available. Tablets should be considered the last alternative even though they may be the patient's first choice. The gastric emptying time of the peptic ulcer patient may vary, so it is wise to individualize the antacid schedule. The neutralizing abilities of antacids vary, requiring different quantities of medication, depending on the product. You should discuss flavor preferences with the patient. Many patients discontinue antacid therapy because they dislike the flavor. Products come in many flavors, and various drugs may be tried if compliance becomes a problem.

Antacids with a laxative effect should be taken at bedtime to allow adequate rest before the bowel is stimulated.

The sodium content of various antacids must be carefully assessed before giving them to patients who are on restricted sodium intake. This would include pregnant women and patients with congestive heart failure (CHF) or other cardiac conditions, hypertension (high blood pressure), edema (fluid buildup in the body tissues), or renal failure.

Histamine H$_2$-receptor antagonists may be given intravenously (IV) or orally (PO). Oral preparations

Geriatric Considerations

Antiulcer Therapies

- Gastrointestinal problems are very common in elderly patients. Every complaint should be properly considered before drug therapy is started.
- In the elderly, melena (a black stool that contains digested blood) is more common than pain as an indication of ulcer disease.
- Acid secretion reaches its peak during sleep between the hours of 10 PM and 2 AM. Therefore H_2-receptor antagonists given once a day should be taken at bedtime.
- Cigarette smoking, which increases the amount of acid produced in the stomach, may decrease the effect of H_2 blockers. Patients should be advised to stop smoking, if possible, or at least to not smoke after the last dose of medication is taken.
- Confusion and dizziness with the use of H_2 blockers are more commonly reported by elderly persons than by younger adults. Mental status changes have been seen with cimetidine (Tagamet), especially in elderly persons who have damaged liver or renal function or who are severely ill. Acute mental changes in elderly patients may show a need to lower the drug dose or to stop the medication.
- Antacids neutralize gastric acid; food also serves as a buffer for gastric acid. Thus antacids are most beneficial if given between meals and at bedtime.
- When H_2-receptor antagonists are ordered with antacids, the medications should be scheduled at least 1 hour apart, with the antacid taken first.

Modified from McKenry LM, Salerno E: *Mosby's pharmacology in nursing*, ed 21, St Louis, 2003, Mosby.

should be given with meals and at bedtime. IV injections should be diluted and injected over 1 to 2 minutes or given by infusion, and are usually given to patients with hypersecretion of gastric acid or intractable pain from ulcers. These medications should be given for 2 to 6 weeks, until endoscopy tests reveal healing. This drug may mask underlying malignancy.

Table 18-1 presents a summary of antacids and histamine H_2-receptor antagonists.

Evaluation

You should watch to see if the patient seems to have less GI distress or if he develops any adverse reactions.

Patient and Family Teaching

You should tell the patient and family the following:

1. The patient should take the medication exactly as ordered. Antacids are generally taken 1 hour after meals. If the patient is being treated for peptic ulcer, the gastric emptying time (usually between 1 and 3 hours) will determine when she should take the antacid. The patient should not switch to another antacid or take new drugs without consulting the nurse, physician, or other health care provider.
2. Antacids may cause diarrhea or constipation. The patient should report any major problems with these symptoms to the nurse, physician, or other health care provider. A good fluid intake should be maintained, and the amount of fluids and fiber in the diet should be increased if constipation becomes a problem.
3. The chewable tablets should be chewed thoroughly before swallowing and followed with a full glass of water.
4. Liquid preparations should be shaken well before taking them to ensure accurate dosage.
5. The nurse, physician, or other health care provider should be asked about whether the antacids will affect any other medications the patient may need to take. Spacing of other medication at different times may limit drug interactions.
6. Liquid medications should be stored in a cool place but not allowed to freeze; refrigeration makes them taste better.
7. Antacids lose their effectiveness over time; the patient should not use old medication.
8. If the nurse, physician, or other health care provider prescribes an aluminum-containing antacid, the patient's diet must contain adequate amounts of dietary phosphorus (up to 1.5 gm/day). Phosphorus is found in the protein of meat, almonds, beans, barley, bran, cheese, cocoa, chocolate, eggs, lentils, liver, milk, oatmeal, peanuts, peas, walnuts, whole wheat, rye, asparagus, beef, carrots, cabbage, celery, cauliflower, chard, chicken, clams, corn, cream, cucumbers, eggplant, fish, figs, prunes, pineapples, pumpkins, raisins, and string beans.
9. The patient with a peptic ulcer will need to make several visits to the nurse, physician, or other health care provider for examination and laboratory tests; this is done to assess the healing process.
10. Peptic and duodenal ulcers tend to recur, so it is important to determine what causes the problem and to try to correct it. The medication is only part of the therapy. Controlling stress, avoiding irregular eating and stressful living habits, and eliminating other diseases and infections are also important.
11. Antacids are often taken with histamine H_2-receptor antagonists. The patient should keep medications at home, at school, or at the office so they can be used as soon as there is any gastric distress.
12. Antacids dissolve the enteric coating on tablets. Thus antacids should not be taken within 1 hour of a medication with an enteric coating.

13. Patients taking proton pump inhibitors must swallow the tablets whole. The patient must not crush or chew tablets.

14. Proton pump inhibitors should be taken before meals.

15. Proton pump inhibitors and H₂ blockers should not be used at the same time. Now that H₂ blockers may be purchased OTC in half-strength doses, patients should be reminded of this each time proton pump inhibitors are prescribed.

Table 18-1

Antacids, Histamine H₂-Receptor Antagonists, and Proton Pump Inhibitors

GENERIC NAME	TRADE NAME	COMMENTS AND DOSAGE
ANTACIDS		
aluminum carbonate gel	Basaljel	Give 1-2 tablets or capsules, or 2 teaspoonsful of suspension in water or fruit juice q2h; may use up to 12 times daily.
aluminum hydroxide gel	Alu-Cap Amphojel Dialume	Helps delay stomach emptying and binds bile salts. Drug of choice in peptic ulcer disease. *Oral:* 5-10 mL q2-4h, followed by a sip of water if desired. *Tablets:* 2 tablets (300 mg or 600 mg) 5 to 6 times daily; chew thoroughly and follow with water.
calcium carbonate	Dicarbosil Tums	Very effective; promotes prolonged and powerful neutralizing effect greater than aluminum hydroxide. It is primarily suited for short-term therapy and is given in small doses. The constipating effects may be minimized by alternating it with doses of a magnesium-containing antacid such as magnesium carbonate. Give 2-4 gm (30-40 gr) qh. Tums should be taken 1 or 2 tablets at a time, chewed or dissolved slowly in the mouth between the cheek and gum.
dihydroxyaluminum sodium carbonate	Calcium Rich Rolaids Tablets	Give 1-2 tablets, chewed, prn.
magaldrate	Losopan Riopan	Combination of magnesium and aluminum hydroxide. Effectiveness depends on GI pH. Give 1-2 tablets or 1-2 teaspoonsful between meals and at bedtime; not to be taken for more than 2 wk or more than 20 tablets in 24 hr.
magnesium hydroxide	Milk of Magnesia	Helpful because cathartic effect counteracts constipation of aluminum hydroxide. Osmotic diarrhea may occur when given alone. *Adults:* 1-3 teaspoonsful with water up to 4 times daily.
magnesium oxide	Mag-Ox Maox Uro-Mag	Acts more slowly than sodium bicarbonate but has a more prolonged action and increased neutralizing ability. As with other magnesium antacids, osmotic diarrhea may develop, but it may be alleviated if alternated with aluminum or calcium salts. Give 250 mg PO as required.
sodium bicarbonate	Bell/ans	Give 0.3-2 gm 1 to 4 times/day.
sodium citrate	Citra pH	Give 30 mL daily.
ANTACID COMBINATIONS		
aluminum hydroxide and magnesium hydroxide	Maalox	Combined to provide a nonconstipating, noncathartic antacid for relief of hyperactivity of peptic ulcer. Give 2 tablets or 2 teaspoonsful q4h prn; suspension may be followed by a sip of water.
aluminum hydroxide, magnesium hydroxide, and simethicone	Gelusil Mylanta	Products use simethicone to reduce gas formation, and they come in many flavors and a variety of combinations. *Suspension:* 1-2 teaspoonsful 4 times daily between meals and at bedtime. *Tablets:* 1-2 tablets (chewed well) 4 times daily between meals and at bedtime. Do not exceed 24 teaspoonsful or 24 tablets in a 24-hr period or use the maximum dosage for longer than 2 wk.

Table **18-1**

Antacids, Histamine H₂-Receptor Antagonists, and Proton Pump Inhibitors—cont'd

GENERIC NAME	TRADE NAME	COMMENTS AND DOSAGE
ANTACID COMBINATIONS—cont'd		
calcium carbonate and glycine	Titralac Tablets	Form an insoluble antacid-protective compound for the relief of hyperacidity. Give 1 teaspoonful or 2 tablets qh after meals; tablets can be chewed, swallowed, or allowed to dissolve slowly in the mouth; do not exceed 19 tablets or 8 teaspoonsful in 24 hr.
HISTAMINE H₂-RECEPTOR ANTAGONISTS		
cimetidine	Tagamet	Widely used in prophylaxis and treatment of ulcers. Has more drug interactions than other preparations and a much wider range of actions than other preparations. • *Duodenal ulcer:* 300 mg PO 4 times daily with meals and at bedtime, or 300 mg q6h IV. Should be taken with antacids.
famotidine	Pepcid	Give 20-40 mg daily at bedtime.
nizatidine	Axid	Give 150-300 mg daily at bedtime.
ranitidine	Zantac	Similar in action to cimetidine but has fewer drug interactions. Headaches are frequent; extrapyramidal symptoms may be noted. • *Duodenal ulcer:* 150 mg PO twice daily. Do not give more than 150 mg/24 hr if creatinine clearance is below 50 mL/min.
AGENTS TO TREAT *H. PYLORI*		
bismuth subsalicylate, metronidazole, and tetracycline	Helidac	Each dose includes 4 pills: 2 pink, round, chewable, 262.4-mg tablets (bismuth subsalicylate); 1 white, 200-mg tablet (metronidazole); and 1 pale, orange and white, 500-mg capsule (tetracycline). Take each dose 4 times daily with meals and at bedtime. Chew and swallow the pink tablets; swallow the others whole. Drink plenty of water with medication, especially at night.
ranitidine bismuth citrate	Tritec	Give 400 mg twice daily for 4 wk together with clarithromycin 500 mg 3 times daily for the first 2 wk. May be taken with or without food.
MISCELLANEOUS PRODUCTS		
misoprostol	Cytotec	*Adults:* Take 200 mcg 4 times daily with meals and at bedtime. If this dose cannot be tolerated, take 100 mcg. Use throughout the course of NSAID therapy.
sucralfate	Carafate	• *Duodenal ulcer:* 1 gm 4 times daily on an empty stomach 1 hr before meals and at bedtime. Take antacids as needed for pain relief, but not within ½ hr before or after this medication. Continue for 4-8 wk. May take 1 gm twice daily for maintenance.
PROTON PUMP INHIBITORS		
esomeprazole	Nexium	Give one 20- or 40-mg delayed-release capsule 1 hr before eating.
lansoprazole	Prevacid 🍁	Take 15 mg once daily before meals for 4 wk. May also use 30 mg with 500 mg clarithromycin and 1 gm amoxicillin twice daily for 14 days; or 30 mg with 1 gm amoxicillin 3 times daily for 14 days for those intolerant to clarithromycin.
omeprazole	Losec 🍁 Prilosec	Take 20 mg daily before eating for 4-8 wk; most ulcers heal within 4 wk, but some require an additional 4 wk. Do not open, chew, or crush capsule.
pantoprazole	Protonix	Give 40-mg delayed-release capsule once daily for 8 wk. Also available as an IV infusion.
rabeprazole	Aciphex	Give one 20-mg delayed-release tablet every morning for 4-8 wk.

Anticholinergics, Antispasmodics, and Antidiarrheals

OVERVIEW

Motility is the spontaneous but unconscious or involuntary movement of food through the GI tract. Much of the discomfort of GI disease is caused by increased intestinal peristalsis (muscle contraction). Abdominal cramping, bloating, and pain may be related either to acute minor illnesses associated with diarrhea and increased gas, or to chronic diseases such as ulcers or colitis. Also, many drugs have both diarrhea and increased bowel motility as common adverse reactions.

The medications used to treat these problems are classed as anticholinergics, antispasmodics, or antidiarrheals. Their actions are somewhat different, although they are often used interchangeably.

ACTION

The anticholinergic-antispasmodic preparations are parasympatholytic drugs (natural and synthetic) that act with antacids in prolonging the therapeutic benefits of both drug categories. Anticholinergics reduce GI tract spasm and intestinal motility, acid production, and gastric motility and thus reduce the associated pain. Gastric emptying time is slowed, and neutralization is increased. Pancreatic secretions of fluid, electrolytes, and enzymes are also stopped. However, the adverse reactions resulting from the high dosages necessary to obtain these effects make the use of such dosages questionable. GI motility stimulants are also available and are particularly helpful in the elderly patient with GERD because they do not have cholinergic activity.

Antidiarrheals reduce the fluid content of the stool and decrease peristalsis and motility of the intestinal tract. They increase smooth muscle tone and diminish digestive secretions. The bismuth salts absorb toxins and provide a protective coating for the intestinal mucosa.

USES

Anticholinergic-antispasmodic agents are used primarily to treat peptic ulcer, pylorospasm, biliary colic, hypermotility, hyperacidity, irritable colon, and acute pancreatitis.

Antidiarrheals are used to treat nonspecific diarrhea or diarrhea caused by antibiotics.

ADVERSE REACTIONS

Adverse reactions are common in anticholinergic therapy because high dosages are usually required. The most common adverse reactions include rapid, weak pulse; blurring of vision; dysphagia (difficulty swallowing); difficulty talking; dilation of pupils; drowsiness; excitation; photophobia (sensitivity to light); confusion; restlessness; staggering; talkativeness; rash primarily over the face, neck, and upper trunk (especially in children); flushing of skin; constipation; dry mouth; great thirst; urinary urgency; and difficulty emptying the bladder. Anticholinergics containing phenobarbital may produce convulsions, delirium, excitement, musculoskeletal pain, and various dermatologic and allergic responses. Antidiarrheals may cause tachycardia (rapid heartbeat), dizziness, drowsiness, fatigue, headache, sedation, pruritus (itching), urticaria (hives), abdominal distention, constipation, dry mouth, nausea, vomiting, urinary retention, and physical dependence.

DRUG INTERACTIONS

Anticholinergics containing phenobarbital may decrease the effects of anticoagulants, requiring higher doses of the anticoagulant. Anticholinergics have many drug interactions; see Chapter 16 for a more specific discussion. The newer GI stimulants may cause serious dysrhythmias (irregular heartbeats) when given with other drugs that inhibit the cytochrome P-450 3A4 system and must be used with caution.

Nursing Implications and Patient Teaching

Assessment

You should learn all you can about the patient's health history, including the presence of allergy, underlying diseases, current use of medications, previous GI history, and history of bowel function (regularity, consistency, and frequency). The patient with diarrhea may have frequent loose, watery stools, often with mild, cramping abdominal pain before bowel movements.

Diagnosis

Determine if the patient has other problems relating to hydration or nutrition. Is the patient eating enough fiber? Are other medications or foods producing constipation? Does the patient need education to help in managing GI symptoms?

Planning

Preparations with phenobarbital may be habit forming, so they should not be given to patients with a history of addiction. Initial doses should be small. These drugs should be used with caution in patients who have hepatic dysfunction or prostatic hypertrophy or who are at risk for glaucoma.

Opiates, loperamide, and diphenoxylate may cause psychologic or physical dependence if used in high dosages or for long periods. The nonspecific antidiarrheal agents provide symptomatic relief until the cause of the diarrhea can be determined and specific therapy can be instituted. These agents should not be used in patients with diarrhea caused by poisoning until the toxin has been removed from the GI tract.

Implementation

Anticholinergics may be given orally or parenterally (when oral dosages cannot be retained or when immediate relief is needed). It is usually better to begin the oral dosage as soon as possible. All of the antidiarrheal agents are given orally; individual dosages are determined by need. Dietary changes are usually part of the treatment plan. The patient's diet is restricted to clear liquids for 24 hours, and then foods are gradually added as tolerated.

Table 18-2 gives a summary of anticholinergic, antispasmodic, and antidiarrheal medications. Synthetic forms of these anticholinergic drugs are more expensive than the natural forms (belladonna, atropine, and scopolamine).

Table **18-2**

Anticholinergic, Antispasmodic, and Antidiarrheal Medications

GENERIC NAME	TRADE NAME	COMMENTS AND DOSAGE
ANTICHOLINERGICS		
Belladonna Alkaloid		
atropine sulfate	Anaspaz	Among the most effective of the anticholinergic drugs with minimal side effects. Give 0.4-0.6 mg PO or subcutaneously q4-6h. *Children:* 0.1-0.4 mg, depending on size.
belladonna tincture	Cystospaz	*Adults:* 0.6-1.0 ml 3 to 4 times daily. *Children:* 0.03 ml/kg 3 times daily.
L-hyoscyamine	Levsin	Reduces hypermotility and hyperacidity; several contraindications for use. *Adults:* 0.125-0.25 mg PO or subcutaneously q4h; use 1-2 mL drops q4h prn; use 0.375 mg in sustained-release tablets q12h. In severe cases, use 2 timecaps q12h or 1 timecap q8h. *Children:* Calculate dosage based on weight.
scopolamine	Scopace	Similar to atropine in peripheral action, but parenteral dosages cause CNS depression, resulting in drowsiness, euphoria (excessive happiness), relief of fear, sleep, relaxation, and amnesia. *Adults:* 0.3-0.6 mg subcutaneously or IM, 0.4-0.8 mg PO q4-6h. *Children:* 0.006 mg/kg PO or SQ.
Quaternary Anticholinergics		
anisotropine	Valpin	Reduces motility and hyperacidity. *Adults:* 50 mg (1 tablet) PO 3 times daily.
clidinium	Quarzan	*Adults:* 2.5-5 mg PO 3 to 4 times daily before meals and at bedtime.
glycopyrrolate	Robinul	Used orally as adjunctive treatment in peptic ulcer disease. Give 1-2 tablets 2 to 3 times daily.
isopropamide iodine	Darbid	Synthetic anticholinergic that suppresses gastric secretions and reduces hypermotility for 10-12 hr. *Adults:* 5-10 mg q12h; may use more frequently if symptoms are severe.
mepenzolate	Cantil	Decreases gastric acid and pepsin secretion while slowing contractions of the colon. *Adults:* 25-50 mg PO with meals and at bedtime.
methantheline	Banthine	This drug is similar in action to atropine. *Adults:* 50 mg initially, then 100 mg q6h. *Children:* 6 mg/kg daily in 4 divided doses.
methscopolamine	Pamine	Synthetic substitute for atropine as an antispasmodic. *Adults:* 2.5 mg 30 min before eating and 2.5-5 mg at bedtime.

Continued

Table 18-2

Anticholinergic, Antispasmodic, and Antidiarrheal Medications—cont'd

GENERIC NAME	TRADE NAME	COMMENTS AND DOSAGE
ANTICHOLINERGICS—cont'd		
Quaternary Anticholinergics—cont'd		
propantheline	Pro-Banthine	An analogue to methantheline, this drug is more effective than methantheline in the reduction of volume and acidity of the stomach's secretions. *PO:* 15 mg with meals and 30 mg at bedtime, adjusted according to therapeutic response. *IM or IV:* 30 mg q6h prn; maintenance is usually 15 mg.
tridihexethyl	Pathilon	Synthetic anticholinergic effective in relaxing pain by reducing spasms of the GI tract. Also used in irritable bowel syndrome. *PO:* 25-50 mg 3 to 4 times daily, or 75 mg sequels q12h. *IM, IV, or subcutaneously:* 10-20 mg q6h; switch to oral preparation as soon as possible.
ANTISPASMODICS		
dicyclomine	Antispas Bentyl Di-Spaz	Synthetic antispasmodic controls spasms of the GI tract; also used in irritable bowel syndrome. *Adults:* 10-20 mg PO 3 to 4 times daily; or 20 mg IM q4-6h. *Children:* 10 mg PO 3 to 4 times daily. *Infants:* 5 mg syrup diluted with an equal volume of water, 3 to 4 times daily for colic.
ANTICHOLINERGIC COMBINATION DRUG		
hyoscyamine, atropine, scopolamine, and phenobarbital	Donnatal	This medication is one of many combination products combining anticholinergic and sedative drugs. Because of the phenobarbital, these products may be habit forming. Give 3-8 capsules or tablets in equally divided doses 3 to 4 times daily. *Elixir:* 15-40 mL/day in equally divided doses. *Extentabs:* 2 tablets q12h.
GASTROINTESTINAL STIMULANT		
metoclopramide	Reglan	• *Nocturnal heartburn related to GERD:* Give 10 mg 30 min before each meal and at bedtime for 2-8 wk. May increase to 15 mg if needed.
ANTIDIARRHEALS		
attapulgite	Donnagel	Because of the presence of the belladonna alkaloids, caution must be used in patients with glaucoma or bladder neck obstruction.
bismuth subsalicylate	Bismatrol Pepto-Bismol	Contains salicylates; ask patient about aspirin sensitivity. Has risk of producing Reye's syndrome in children. May cause temporary darkening of the stool and tongue. *Adults:* 30 mL or 2 tablets PO every 30 min to 1 hr until symptoms are relieved or until a maximum of 8 doses has been given. *Children:* Calculate dosage by weight. Give with oral rehydration solution in children with severe diarrhea.
difenoxin with atropine	Motofen	*Adults:* 2 tablets, then 1 after each loose stool to a maximum of 8 tablets in 24 hr.
diphenoxylate and atropine sulfate	Lomotil Logen	These are Schedule V controlled substances. The addition of atropine sulfate helps prevent abuse. *Adults:* 2 tablets or 2 teaspoonsful 4 times daily until diarrhea is controlled. *Children:* Calculate dosage by weight.
kaolin and pectin	Kaopectate Parapectolin	These are nonprescription products widely used in self-treatment of diarrhea; their clinical effectiveness has not been established. *Adults:* 2 tablespoonsful at once and 1 or 2 tablespoonsful after each bowel movement. *Children:* Calculate dosage by weight.

Table 18-2

Anticholinergic, Antispasmodic, and Antidiarrheal Medications—cont'd

GENERIC NAME	TRADE NAME	COMMENTS AND DOSAGE
ANTIDIARRHEALS—cont'd		
lactobacillus	Bacid Lactinex	Nonprescription product specifically used to treat diarrhea caused by antibiotics. It reestablishes normal intestinal flora and may be used prophylactically in patients with a history of antibiotic-induced diarrhea. *Adults:* 2 capsules or 4 tablets of Bacid, or use 1 packet of granules of Lactinex, 2 to 4 times daily, preferably with milk.
loperamide	Imodium Kaopectate II	More potent and has a longer duration of action with less CNS depression than diphenoxylate; now available OTC. *Adults:* Initially give 4 mg PO, then 2 mg after each unformed stool; maximum of 16 mg PO daily.
mesalamine	Asacol Rowasa	Give 800 mg 3 times daily for 6 wk in ulcerative colitis.
olsalazine	Dipentum	Give 1 gm/day PO in 2 divided doses for ulcerative colitis.
opium tincture (paregoric, tincture of opium)		This is a Schedule III controlled substance. It is given orally mixed with water. A white, milky fluid forms when they are mixed together. • *Tincture of opium* *Adults:* Give 0.6 mL PO 4 times daily. • *Camphorated opium tincture (paregoric)* *Adults:* 5-10 mL PO 4 times daily until diarrhea subsides. *Children:* 0.25-0.5 mL/kg PO 4 times daily until diarrhea subsides.
sulfasalazine	Azulfidine	Use for mild to moderate ulcerative colitis. Give 3-4 gm in evenly divided doses.

Evaluation

Long periods of diarrhea can cause dehydration and electrolyte imbalance. You should encourage the patient to increase fluid intake to replace the fluid lost in the stool.

Patients who are also taking diphenoxylate and atropine sulfate (Lomotil) or laxatives and narcotics should be watched for signs of CNS depression. CNS side effects are rare with synthetic anticholinergic therapy, which is one of the advantages of the synthetic products.

Antidiarrheals should not be used on a long-term basis. You should watch for diarrhea to decrease and to see if any adverse effects develop.

Long-term anticholinergic therapy may mask or alter the symptoms of GI disease, so it may be difficult to tell if GI disease has occurred again.

Patient and Family Teaching

You should tell the patient and family the following:

1. The patient should take this medication exactly as ordered by the nurse, physician, or other health care provider.
2. This medication should be kept out of the reach of children and all others for whom it has not been prescribed.
3. Many people experience mild side effects with these medications. The patient should alert the nurse, physician, or other health care provider if any new or troublesome problems occur, especially diarrhea, so that the problems may be evaluated.
4. High environmental temperatures may make the patient feel unusually hot and fatigued. The patient should avoid becoming overheated while taking this drug.
5. The antidiarrheal agents are used to relieve symptoms and to prevent dehydration until the underlying cause can be found and treated.
6. The patient with diarrhea should be restricted to clear liquids (tea, gelatin, broth, carbonated beverages) for 24 hours; the patient can then begin adding bland foods and continue to add more solid foods if diarrhea does not reappear.
7. Diarrhea that persists for more than 48 hours should not be self-treated. The patient should return to the nurse, physician, or other health care provider for further evaluation and diagnosis.
8. Some antidiarrheal medications contain habit-forming drugs; therefore, they should be used only at the dosage recommended and for the length of time prescribed.

OVERVIEW

Laxatives are drugs that help draw fluid into the intestine to promote fecal softening, speed the passage of feces through the colon, and aid in the elimination of stool from the rectum. They are classified in five major categories, based on their mechanism of action. These categories are bulk-forming agents, fecal softeners, hyperosmolar or saline solutions, lubricants, and stimulant or irritant laxatives.

Laxatives are one of the major groups of drugs used by patients as self-treatment for constipation, with use increasing as patients age. Laxatives have a high rate of overuse, and they destroy the body's natural emptying rhythm when they are used excessively. Laxatives are used in bowel training of individuals who have lost neurogenic control of the bowel, and are commonly used in preparing patients for x-ray, obstetric, or surgical procedures.

ACTION

Bulk-forming laxatives absorb water and expand, increasing both the bulk and the moisture content of the stool. The increased bulk stimulates peristalsis, and the absorbed water softens the stool. These agents do not have systemic effects.

Fecal softeners soften stool by lowering the surface tension, which allows the fecal mass to be softened by intestinal fluids. They also inhibit fluid and electrolyte reabsorption by the intestine.

Hyperosmolar laxatives such as lactulose and glycerin produce an osmotic effect in the colon by distending the bowel with fluid accumulation and promoting peristalsis and bowel movement. Saline laxatives also produce an osmotic effect by drawing water into the intestinal lumen of the small intestine and colon.

Lubricant laxatives create a barrier between the feces and the colon wall that prevents the colon from reabsorbing fecal fluid, thus softening the stool. The lubricant effect also eases the passage of feces through the intestine.

Stimulant or irritant laxatives increase peristalsis by several mechanisms, depending on the agent. These mechanisms include primary stimulation of colon nerves (senna preparations), stimulation of sensory nerves in the intestinal mucosa (bisacodyl), or direct stimulation of smooth muscle and inhibition of water and electrolyte reabsorption from the intestinal lumen (castor oil).

USES

Bulk-forming laxatives are used in simple constipation and in atonic constipation, when the colon loses muscle tone as a result of overuse of other cathartics. Bulk-forming laxatives are also very useful in postpartum, elderly, and weakened patients. They have been used to treat diverticulosis and irritable bowel syndrome.

Fecal softeners help relieve constipation produced by a delay in rectal emptying. They are also useful when it is important to reduce straining at stool, such as in patients with hernia or cardiovascular disease, postpartum patients, or patients after rectal surgery.

Saline laxatives are used to cleanse the bowel in preparation for endoscopic or colonoscopic examination, x-ray studies, or surgery. They are used to hasten evacuation of worms after the administration of anthelmintics, and after the ingestion of poisons to help get rid of toxic material quickly. Lactulose and glycerin are most commonly used to treat simple constipation.

Lubricant laxatives are used to soften stool in conditions where straining at stool should be avoided, such as in patients with myocardial infarction, aneurysm, stroke, or hernia or after abdominal or rectal surgery. They are also used to prevent discomfort and tearing or laceration of hemorrhoids or fissures.

Stimulant or irritant laxatives are used to treat constipation resulting from prolonged bed rest or poor dietary habits or constipation induced by other drugs. They are also used to cleanse the bowel in preparation for endoscopic/colonoscopic examination, x-ray studies, or surgery.

ADVERSE REACTIONS

Bulk-forming laxatives may produce abdominal cramps, diarrhea, strictures (narrowing), and obstructions (blockages) when taken without sufficient liquid. Nausea and vomiting are also common. Hypersensitivity may be demonstrated by development of asthma, dermatitis, rhinitis, and urticaria.

Fecal softeners may cause mild cramping or diarrhea.

Hyperosmolar or saline laxatives may produce abdominal cramping, nausea, and fluid and electrolyte disturbance if used daily or in patients with renal impairment. Hypermagnesemia may occur in patients with chronic renal insufficiency and is aggravated by increased intake of magnesium in hyperosmolar laxatives.

In patients with cardiac disease or CHF, the increased sodium intake in the sodium-containing saline cathartics can start or worsen the condition.

Lubricant laxatives may produce abdominal cramps, vomiting, decreased absorption of nutrients and fat-soluble vitamins, diarrhea, and nausea. Lipid pneumonia caused by aspiration and deficiency syndromes resulting from low absorption of the fat-soluble vitamins may occur with long-term or excessive use.

Stimulant or irritant laxatives may produce muscle weakness (following excessive use of laxatives), dermatitis, pruritus, abdominal cramps, diarrhea, nausea, vomiting, alkalosis, and electrolyte imbalance (with excessive use).

Long-term or excessive use of stimulant laxatives may result in irritable bowel syndrome or a severe, prolonged diarrhea. These conditions may lead to hyponatremia and hypokalemia (decreased sodium and potassium in the blood) and dehydration. Cathartic colon, a syndrome resembling ulcerative colitis both radiologically and pathologically, may develop after chronic misuse.

DRUG INTERACTIONS

Antibiotics, anticoagulants, digitalis preparations, and salicylates may have reduced effectiveness if used at the same time as bulk-forming agents because of binding and hindrance of absorption. A 2-hour interval between doses of these medications is required.

Fecal softeners should never be used along with mineral oil or other laxatives. The systemic absorption of other agents is enhanced, causing an increased laxative effect and greater risk of toxic effects, especially to the liver. Hyperosmolar saline laxatives should not be taken within 1 to 3 hours of tetracyclines, because they may form nonabsorbable complexes. Lubricant laxatives may reduce the effectiveness of anticoagulants, contraceptives, digitalis, and fat-soluble vitamins if taken together.

Antacids or milk should not be taken with bisacodyl tablets because they cause the enteric coating to dissolve too rapidly, resulting in gastric irritation. Some laxatives cause rapid transit through the bowel, and so current use of many medications that require time to dissolve may be adversely affected.

Nursing Implications and Patient Teaching

Assessment

You should learn all you can about the patient's health history, including underlying disease, allergies, edema, or CHF; use of a sodium-restricted diet; and other drugs being taken. The patient should be evaluated for potential abuse. Constipation that persists should always be evaluated for serious organic causes. Changes in bowel habits, especially waking up at night to defecate, should always be investigated.

The patient may complain of increased hardness of stool or of difficulty in passing stool. Decreased frequency of stools, mild abdominal discomfort and distention, and occasionally mild anorexia may be present. Confused geriatric patients may show only increased restlessness when they are constipated.

Laxatives should not be given to patients with abdominal pain, nausea, vomiting, other signs of appendicitis, or acute surgical abdominal conditions. Other contraindications include fecal impaction, intestinal ulcerations, stenosis or obstruction, disabling adhesions, or dysphagia.

Diagnosis

What are the factors that have caused constipation? Does the patient have other problems in terms of hydration, lack of nutritional fiber, or eating disorders that underlie the development of constipation?

 Geriatric Considerations

Laxatives

Elderly patients often use and abuse laxatives, even though studies have indicated that 80% to 90% of persons over 60 years old have at least one bowel movement daily.

To reduce the potential for chronic laxative use and dependency, the elderly patient should be taught nondrug measures to prevent constipation, such as increasing fluid intake to 6 to 8 glasses of water each day if permitted and tolerated. Also recommended is a regular exercise routine, such as a daily walk or active and passive exercise for bedridden patients.

You should get a dietary and laxative history from the patient. Consistent intake of a low-fiber diet or a regular intake of foods that tend to harden stools, such as processed cheese, hard-boiled eggs, liver, cottage cheese, high-sugar-content foods, and rice, may result in constipation.

High-fiber or high-residue diets, along with adequate fluid intake, serve to speed up food travel time in the GI tract and have a mild laxative effect.

High-fiber foods include orange juice with pulp or a fresh orange, bran or whole-grain cereals, whole-grain or bran breads, leafy vegetables, and fresh fruits. Although prunes, bananas, figs, and dates are high in dietary fiber, prunes also contain a laxative substance that stimulates intestinal motility.

Modified from McKenry LM, Salerno E: *Mosby's pharmacology in nursing,* ed 21, St Louis, 2003, Mosby.

Planning

Many bulk-forming products contain significant amounts of dextrose, galactose, and sucrose and should be avoided in patients with diabetes mellitus. Allergic reactions (urticaria, rhinitis, and asthma) may occur as a result of the plant gums present in these agents. This should be considered in patients with a history of allergic reactions, especially to plants.

Bulk-forming agents may become dry, thick, and hardened in the throat or within the intestine if they are swallowed without sufficient water. They can cause esophageal or intestinal obstruction or impaction if this occurs. The drugs should never be chewed or swallowed without one or more full glasses of water. Before giving medication for constipation, you should ensure that the patient is well hydrated (has enough fluids).

Products with sodium salt should be avoided in patients with edema, pregnancy, CHF, and sodium-restricted diets. Potassium salt should be avoided in patients with renal impairment. Because laxatives are available without prescription, it is especially important to teach the patient about these serious side effects.

You should begin educating the patient by explaining the usefulness of exercise, diet, and liquids to reduce constipation. The patient should be taught to eat bulk-forming foods, fruits, vegetables, and whole-grain cereals and encouraged to perform more physical activities if she is able to do so. Proper bowel habits should be discussed and encouraged, and increased fluid intake should be stressed.

Overdosage or overuse of stimulant laxatives may cause excessive fluid loss and electrolyte imbalance, particularly hypokalemia. Overuse of any laxative can lead to atonic constipation and create dependence on the laxative.

Implementation

All bulk-forming and stimulant laxatives are given orally, with one or more glasses of liquid. Most other laxatives are available for oral administration or as enemas.

You should plan medication administration to allow the drug's effects to occur at a time that will not interfere with the patient's rest or digestion. Administration of lubricant laxatives should be timed so that they are not given within 2 hours of meals or medication.

Bisacodyl enteric-coated tablets must be swallowed whole, never chewed or crushed, and never taken with milk or antacids.

A summary of laxative products is given in Table 18-3. The need for mixtures of laxatives has not been documented. The actions of various laxatives show that combinations are unnecessary and may produce harmful or undesirable effects. They also tend to be more expensive than drugs sold individually. A partial listing of some of the available drug mixtures that patients may ask you about is provided in Table 18-4, but it is not recommended that combination drugs be used.

Evaluation

Laxatives should be used only for short periods of time and should not require any patient monitoring. If for any reason they are used on a long-term basis, ask the patient about bowel habits, diet, and exercise, and monitor for adverse reactions. Many of the stimulant laxatives discolor alkaline urine red-pink and acidic urine yellow-brown. They may give a reddish color to feces.

Patient and Family Teaching

You should tell the patient and family the following:

1. Bulk-forming laxatives require large amounts of fluid to work properly; they should never be chewed or swallowed without water. The patient must take at least one full glass of liquid with each dose.
2. Laxatives should be taken exactly as specified by the nurse, physician, or other health care provider and are indicated for short-term use only. Overuse of laxatives robs the bowel of its ability to perform well on its own.
3. Some agents are high in sodium or glucose. The content should be checked if the patient's diet is restricted or he is a diabetic.
4. Laxatives should be used only as additional therapy with good, regular bowel habits, daily exercise, and the use of high-bulk foods and fruits in the diet to help maintain regularity.
5. Bulk-forming laxatives should not be taken within 2 hours of any other medications.
6. Allergic reactions may occur in response to any of these products. If rash, itching, nasal congestion, or wheezing occurs, the patient should stop taking the medication immediately and contact the nurse, physician, or other health care provider.
7. The laxative effect of bulk-forming laxatives may occur within 12 hours or may take up to 3 days to appear. Fecal softeners act within 24 to 48 hours. Lactulose may require 24 to 48 hours to produce a normal bowel movement. Saline laxatives produce results within 2 to 8 hours and should not be taken at bedtime. The fastest effect of hyperosmolar products is obtained when the drug is taken on an empty stomach with a full glass of water. Mineral oil should not be taken within 2 hours of taking food or other medication. The stimulant laxatives act within 6 to 10 hours, except castor oil, which acts within 1 to 3 hours. The stimulant laxatives include many of the chewing gum and chocolate types and are the kind most often abused.
8. Fecal softeners should be used only in addition to good, regular bowel habits, daily exercise, and the use of high bulk or fiber in the diet to help maintain regularity. They do not treat preexisting constipation but do prevent constipation from developing.

Table 18-3

Laxatives

GENERIC NAME	TRADE NAME	COMMENTS AND DOSAGE
BULK-FORMING LAXATIVES		
methylcellulose	Citrucel Unifiber	Produces a laxative effect in 12-72 hr. All doses should be taken with 1 full glass or more of liquid. *Adults:* 5-20 mL liquid PO 3 times daily with a full glass of water; or 1-3 capsules or tablets may be taken PO 4 times daily with meals and at bedtime.
psyllium seed	Fiberall Metamucil	This product is indigestible and is not absorbed, and does not interfere with absorption of nutrients. These laxatives are least likely to cause laxative abuse. *Adults:* 1-2 teaspoonsful PO in full glass of water 1 to 3 times daily; follow with second glass of water.
FECAL SOFTENERS OR WETTING AGENTS		
docusate	Colace Modane	Give 50-200 mg PO daily.
HYPEROSMOLAR OR SALINE LAXATIVES OR ENEMAS		
glycerin	Sani-Supp	*Suppository:* Use 1 and retain for 15 min.
lactulose	Cephulac Cholac	Available by prescription only. Give as needed.
magnesium (magnesium citrate, milk of magnesia)	Philips Milk of Magnesia	*Adults:* 15-30 mL PO daily; may be increased to 60 ml PO daily if necessary. *Magnesium citrate:* 5-10 oz PO at bedtime. *Milk of magnesia:* 30-60 mL PO, usually at bedtime.
sodium salts	Fleet Enema Phospho- Soda	Approximately 10% of the sodium in these products may be absorbed. *Oral:* 20 mL PO mixed with half a glass of water; follow with another full glass of water; should be taken as soon as patient gets up in the morning. *Enema:* 4 oz per rectum (PR) for adults; 2½ oz for children over 2 yr.
LUBRICANT LAXATIVES		
castor oil	Purge Emulsoil	Used orally and also given rectally as an enema for retention and softening. It should be given at least 2 hr after meals. *Adults:* 5-30 mL PO at bedtime. *Children over 6 yr:* 5-15 mL PO; give 4 oz PR as enema.
STIMULANT OR IRRITANT LAXATIVES		
bisacodyl	Dulcolax Correctol Feen-a-Mint	Enteric-coated tablets must be swallowed whole; do not chew or crush. Do not take within 1 hr of antacids or milk. Drink at least 1 full glass of water with each dose. Suppository should be inserted at time bowel movement is desired; acts within 15-60 min. Enema is administered rectally at time evacuation is desired. *Adults:* 10-15 mg PO in evening or before breakfast. Approximately 30 mg PO may be safely used in preparation for special procedures.
Cascara sagrada	Cascara aromatic	The fluid extract contains 18% alcohol. Sold under various brand names; some tablets are sugar coated, others are uncoated. They may discolor alkaline urine red-pink, and acidic urine yellow-brown. *Adults:* Aromatic: 5 mL daily with full glass of water; plain: 1 mL PO daily with glass of water; tablet: one 325-mg tablet at bedtime.
senna	Senokot Ex-Lax Agoral	May cause yellow or yellow-green cast to feces; red-pink discoloration of alkaline urine; yellow-brown color in acid urine. Give 1-8 tablets/day PO.

Table 18-4
Laxative Combination Products

TRADE NAME	CHEMICAL COMBINATION
Haley's MO	Milk of magnesia, mineral oil
Peri-Colace	Casanthranol, docusate sodium
Senokot-S	Senna, docusate sodium

9. The patient should take milk or fruit juice with fecal softeners to mask the bitter taste. The flavor of the hyperosmolar laxatives may be improved by taking the medication with fruit juice or a citrus-flavored carbonated beverage. Fruit juices or carbonated drinks may help disguise the oily taste of lubricant laxatives.

10. The nurse, physician, or other health care provider should give the patient a list of foods high in bulk or fiber that can assist in maintaining bowel regularity.

11. Saline laxatives should not be taken daily on a prolonged basis or used in children under 6 years of age.

12. Large doses of lubricant laxatives may cause a leakage of oil from the rectum. The use of pads to protect clothing may be necessary if tight sphincter control is not present.

SECTION FOUR
Miscellaneous Gastrointestinal Drugs

OVERVIEW

Many diseases and symptoms affect the GI tract; there are also many drugs used in their treatment. Antiflatulents such as simethicone break up GI gas bubbles through a defoaming action so that they may be more easily expelled by belching or as flatus. Pancreatic digestive enzymes are used as replacement therapy for individuals with pancreatic enzyme insufficiency. Emetics are used mostly in emergency situations to produce vomiting by direct action on the vomiting center. Chenodiol acts on the liver to increase breakdown of radiolucent cholesterol gallstones. Disulfiram is used in alcoholic patients to produce a severe sensitivity to alcohol. Each of these drugs will be briefly described.

Table 18-5 summarizes the important miscellaneous GI medications.

ANTIFLATULENTS

ACTION

Simethicone is an **antiflatulent** that breaks up and prevents mucus-surrounded pockets of gas from forming in the intestine. Mucus surrounding the gas bubbles is broken down, and the gas bubbles all come together, freeing the gas. Gastric pain is then reduced. Charcoal is occasionally used as an antiflatulent but is used primarily in the treatment of drug overdosage to absorb chemicals.

USES

Antiflatulents are used to treat problems that produce bloating, flatulence, or postoperative gas pains. They may also be used for chronic air swallowing, functional dyspepsia (stomach discomfort after eating), peptic ulcer, spastic or irritable colon, and diverticulitis. The patient may complain of being bloated or distended, of feeling "full" or gaseous, or of frequent belching. Gas pains may also be noted, especially after surgery. You should determine if the flatulence is caused by food and whether changing the diet may decrease the symptoms. Antiflatulents are often used along with antacid therapy. This medication is intended for short-term use only. More rigorous evaluation should be undertaken if symptoms do not disappear with therapy.

GALLSTONE-SOLUBILIZING AGENTS

ACTION

Gallstone-solubilizing agents act on the liver to suppress cholesterol and cholic acid synthesis. Biliary cholesterol desaturation is enhanced, and breakup or dissolution of radiolucent cholesterol gallstones (those that allow x-rays to pass through and thus show up as dark images) eventually occurs. There is no effect on calcified or radiopaque gallstones (those that absorb x-rays and thus show up as white images) or radiolucent bile pigment stones.

USES

Gallstone-solubilizing agents are useful in selected patients with radiolucent stones in gallbladders that opacify well (show up when dye is used). These patients are poor surgical risks because of disease or advanced age. Success is likely to be higher with small stones that float.

Table 18-5

Miscellaneous Gastrointestinal Medications

GENERIC NAME	TRADE NAME	COMMENTS AND DOSAGE
ANTIFLATULENTS		
activated charcoal	CharcoCaps	520-975 mg after meals or at first sign of discomfort; repeat prn.
simethicone	Mylanta Gas Relief Mylicon	Available in both drops and tablet form. Chew tablets thoroughly before swallowing. Shake drops well before using. Give 40-80 mg tablets after each meal and at bedtime, or use 40 mg (0.6 mL) drops 4 times daily after meals and at bedtime.
GALLSTONE DISSOLUTION		
chenodiol	Chenix	Recommended dosage range is 13-16 mg/kg/day in 2 divided doses taken morning and evening. Increase dosage by 250 mg/day each week until the recommended or tolerated dose is obtained. Dosages less than 10 mg/kg are usually ineffective and may in fact contribute to increased risk of cholecystectomy. Give 3-7 tablets/day based on patient's weight.
monoctanoin	Moctanin	Given by physician as a direct perfusion into biliary tract.
ursodiol	Actigall	Give 8-10 mg/kg/day in 2 or 3 divided doses.
DIGESTIVE ENZYMES		
pancreatin	Creon Digepepsin Hi-Vegi-Lip	This product tends to be cheaper than pancrelipase, although it is not as effective. Give 325 mg to 1 gm with meals.
pancrelipase	Cotazym Cotazym-S Ku-Zyme HP Pancrease Viokase	Pancrelipase is a prescription drug combination of the pancreatic enzymes used in replacement therapy. It works more effectively than pancreatin. It provides a catalyst effect in the hydrolyzation of fats, proteins, and starch. The amount of dietary fat is the key to dosage. For every 17 gm of fat, 300 mg of pancrelipase should be taken. Use 1-3 capsules or tablets (or 1-2 packets) just before each meal or snack.
ANTIALCOHOLIC PRODUCT		
disulfiram	Antabuse	The adult dosage is approximately 500 mg daily for 1-2 wk, followed by 125-500 mg daily for maintenance. It may take up to 3 wk for the drug to reach full effectiveness, and drug is still effective for approximately 2 wk after therapy is discontinued. The average maintenance dosage is 250 mg daily. Maintenance therapy is needed until the patient is fully recovered socially and a basis for permanent self-control has been established. This may take months or even years.
EMETICS		
apomorphine		*Adults:* 5 mg subcutaneously.
ipecac	Syrup of Ipecac	*Children:* 0.1 mg/kg subcutaneously. Do not repeat. Do not confuse with fluid extract ipecac, which is 14 times more concentrated. *Older than 1 yr:* 1 tablespoonful (15 mL), followed by 2-3 glasses of water (200-300 mL). *Younger than 1 yr:* 2 teaspoonsful, followed by 1-2 glasses of water. Dose may be repeated once after 20 min if vomiting does not occur.

ADVERSE REACTIONS

Adverse reactions to gallstone-solubilizing agents may include dose-related diarrhea, anorexia, constipation, cramps, dyspepsia, epigastric distress, flatulence, heartburn, nausea, nonspecific abdominal pain, and vomiting. Laboratory test results may be altered; nonspecific decreases in white cell count may also develop.

DRUG INTERACTIONS

Biliary cholesterol secretion and gallstones may be increased by estrogens, clofibrate, and oral contraceptives. Therefore, those drugs may counteract the effectiveness of gallstone-solubilizing agents. Bile acid–sequestering agents such as cholestyramine and colestipol may reduce the absorption of gallstone-solubilizing agents.

Aluminum-based antacids may absorb bile acids and also reduce the absorption of gallstone-solubilizing agents.

These medications should not be used in patients with known liver or other gallbladder disease. If the gallbladder fails to show up after two consecutive single doses of dye, or if radiopaque or radiolucent bile pigment stones are seen, these medications should not be used. These products may produce hepatotoxicity (damage to the liver), ranging from mild toxicity to fatal hepatic failure. They should be used only in patients without previous hepatic problems, and careful monitoring of the patient's liver function is required. There is also the chance that chenodiol therapy might contribute to the development of colon cancers in individuals who are predisposed to develop them.

If diarrhea develops, reducing the dosage usually eliminates the symptoms. The patient is often able to resume higher dosages without diarrhea occurring again.

Evaluation of patient compliance is important. The patient must be reliable in keeping appointments, reporting problems, and having periodic health evaluations.

Memory Jogger

Gallstone Recurrence

Stone recurrence can be expected within 5 years in 50% of all patients using gallstone-solubilizing agents. Low-cholesterol, low-carbohydrate diets with increased dietary bran may help reduce biliary cholesterol. Weight reduction may help postpone stone recurrence.

DIGESTIVE ENZYMES

ACTION

Pancreatic **digestive enzymes** promote digestion by acting as replacement therapy when the body's natural pancreatic enzymes are lacking, not secreted, or not properly absorbed. They are made from pork pancreas. Healthy patients may find intestinal gas is decreased when they take the medication.

USES

Digestive enzymes are often indicated for individuals with poor digestion, for predigestive purposes, and as replacement therapy. They may be used to relieve the symptoms of cystic fibrosis, cancer of the pancreas, or chronic inflammation of the pancreas causing malabsorption syndromes. Patients who have had GI bypass

surgery may also be helped. Obstruction of the pancreatic or common bile duct by a tumor may produce a need for these enzymes.

ADVERSE REACTIONS

If a proper dietary balance of fat, protein, and starch is not maintained, temporary indigestion may develop. Nausea, abdominal cramps, and diarrhea have been reported in patients taking high doses. Inhalation of the powder may provoke asthma.

DRUG INTERACTIONS

Antacids containing calcium carbonate or magnesium hydroxide may cancel out the therapeutic effect of digestive enzymes. In addition, serum iron levels produced by iron supplements may be decreased by these enzymes.

Nursing Implications and Patient Teaching

The patient may complain of sudden, intense pain in the gastric region; hiccups; belching of gas; vomiting; constipation; pain radiating to the back; weakness; diarrhea; indigestion; ravenous appetite without weight gain; and chronic cough and infections.

Those individuals hypersensitive to pork protein should avoid this therapy. The patient should avoid breathing the powdered form of the enzymes or allowing it to come into contact with the skin, because it may produce irritation.

Digestive enzymes are given with meals or snacks. They are available in tablet or capsule form, which is swallowed, not chewed. They also come in a powder, or the capsules may be opened and sprinkled on food for those who have difficulty swallowing tablets. Medication granules are not to be taken without food, because this will destroy the enzymes.

The correct dosage to take can be determined after several weeks of therapy. Different flavors are available.

You should monitor the patient for the therapeutic effect and the absence of adverse reactions. Question the patient about the appearance of stools because this may help evaluate the degree of malabsorption present.

Patient and Family Teaching

You should tell the patient and family the following:
1. The patient should take this medication exactly as ordered. The capsules or tablets should be swallowed at mealtime, or the capsules of powder can be opened and sprinkled on the food if the patient has difficulty swallowing pills.
2. The granules should always be taken with meals or snacks. The body will destroy the granules and not receive any benefit from them if the patient does not take food with them.
3. The patient must be careful not to breath in the powder or touch it with the hands when opening

the powder and pouring it. Direct exposure to the powder produces a strong irritation.

4. The patient should eat a well-balanced diet, with adequate amounts of fat, starch, and protein. She should develop and maintain a normal eating routine; this will help prevent indigestion.

5. The patient can try the various flavors of medication until he finds the ones that he prefers.

6. The patient should report any discomfort or troublesome symptoms to the nurse, physician, or other health care provider.

DISULFIRAM

ACTION

Disulfiram produces a severe sensitivity to alcohol that results in a very unpleasant reaction. This **disulfiram reaction** includes severe nausea, vomiting, and diarrhea, as well as many other adverse reactions, when even small amounts of alcohol are swallowed. This drug causes excessive amounts of acetaldehyde to develop by stopping the normal liver enzyme activity after the conversion of alcohol to acetaldehyde. Increased levels of acetaldehyde produce the disulfiram reaction. The reaction is present until the alcohol is completely metabolized. The intensity of the reaction is variable, but it is usually related to the amount of disulfiram and alcohol swallowed.

Clinical Landmine

Disulfiram Reaction

A disulfiram reaction may include the following symptoms: flushing and warming of the face, severe throbbing headache, shortness of breath, chest pain, nausea, vomiting, sweating, weakness, hyperventilation, tachycardia, syncope (light-headedness and fainting), and confusion. Severe reactions could include dysrhythmias, respiratory distress, cardiovascular collapse, myocardial infarction, acute CHF, convulsions, and death.

USES

Disulfiram is used only for the management of alcoholism. It is used to discourage alcohol intake, which in turn forces the patient to be sober. This drug is used in addition to psychiatric therapy or alcohol counseling and in patients who are motivated and fully cooperative.

ADVERSE REACTIONS

Disulfiram may produce drowsiness, fatigue, headache, optic neuritis (with impaired vision, decreased color perception, and blindness), psychotic reactions, restlessness, acneiform eruptions, dry mouth, elevation of serum liver enzyme levels, hepatotoxicity, metallic or garlic-like aftertaste, and impotence.

DRUG INTERACTIONS

Use of disulfiram with even small amounts of alcohol produces a severe reaction. When used together, disulfiram increases the effects of anticoagulants, phenytoins, and barbiturates, and may increase the side effects of isoniazid. Use with metronidazole and marijuana has an additive effect and may produce psychotic episodes. Exaggerated clinical effects of diazepam and chlordiazepoxide are produced when these drugs are taken at the same time as disulfiram. Use with paraldehyde may produce the disulfiram-alcohol reaction.

Some medications, such as metronidazole, produce similar reaction when taken with alcohol. Patients must be warned of these *disulfiram-like reactions*.

Nursing Implications and Patient Teaching

Disulfiram should not be used if the patient has swallowed alcohol in any form within the last 12 hours. This includes the use of cough mixtures, tonics, vanilla, vinegar, some sauces, aftershave lotions, back-rubbing solutions, some creams, or other products containing alcohol. Do not use disulfiram if there has been recent ingestion of paraldehyde or metronidazole. Do not use in the presence of severe myocardial disease or coronary occlusion, psychoses, or hypersensitivity (allergy) to disulfiram. Do not use disulfiram in pediatric patients.

Disulfiram should be used with extreme caution in patients with any of the following conditions: diabetes mellitus, epilepsy, cerebral damage, hypothyroidism, chronic and acute nephritis, hepatic cirrhosis or insufficiency, conditions requiring multiple drug usage, coronary artery disease, and hypertension. In these patients, there is the possibility of an accidental disulfiram reaction.

The patient should give permission for disulfiram therapy. The patient and a responsible family member need to understand the consequences of this therapy. Disulfiram reactions may occur for up to 2 weeks after a single dose of disulfiram. The longer a patient takes this drug, the more sensitive she will become to alcohol. The disulfiram reaction may be provoked by even small amounts of alcohol. The patient should be cautioned against hidden forms of alcohol (tonics, cough syrup, aftershave lotions).

Disulfiram users should wear a Medic Alert bracelet or necklace or carry a medical identification card indicating that they use this drug and describing the symptoms most likely to occur in the disulfiram reaction. Cards to give to patients taking this drug may be obtained from the drug company.

The patient should be actively involved in support and counseling to reduce psychologic dependence and should be monitored for compliance and for development of adverse effects.

EMETICS

ACTION

Emetics are drugs used in emergency situations to cause vomiting so as to remove poisons from the stomach before the poisons can be absorbed. Emetics have largely replaced gastric lavage as the treatment of choice in management of poisoning or drug overdosage. Except in situations for which they are contraindicated, emetics are superior to lavage for rapid elimination of poisons before extensive absorption of gastric contents can occur. There are only two emetics commonly used in current clinical practice: apomorphine and syrup of ipecac. Apomorphine is given by injection and acts directly on the CNS. Syrup of ipecac acts primarily as a gastric irritant to produce vomiting. After ingestion, it stimulates the chemoreceptor trigger zone in the brain to induce vomiting.

USES

Ipecac is used when toxic substances are swallowed, to empty the stomach before the toxins can be absorbed.

ADVERSE REACTIONS

Ipecac is not absorbed and has no systemic effect unless vomiting does not occur within 30 minutes. If the drug is absorbed or an excessive dose is swallowed, it may cause cardiac dysrhythmias, atrial fibrillation, or other cardiotoxic effects. For this reason, gastric lavage is necessary if vomiting does not occur within 30 minutes.

DRUG INTERACTIONS

Ipecac should not be given with activated charcoal, because the charcoal will adsorb the ipecac, neutralizing the emetic effect.

Nursing Implications and Patient Teaching

Vomiting should never be provoked after a patient swallows corrosive or caustic substances such as lye; vomiting in that situation will only cause additional injury to the esophagus.

Emetics should never be used in unconscious patients; in those who are convulsing, severely inebriated, or in shock; or in those who have loss of the gag reflex.

Always make certain you are giving *ipecac syrup*, not just ipecac, to avoid confusion with the fluid extract, which is 14 times more concentrated.

You should learn all you can about the patient's history from the patient or anyone who can give details about what was swallowed, when, and what has happened since that time. A local poison control center should be consulted if there is uncertainty about how to proceed. If two doses of ipecac do not produce vomiting within 30 minutes, referral and gastric lavage are necessary.

It is wise for patients to keep 1-oz bottles of syrup of ipecac readily available in their homes in case of a poisoning emergency.

COMPLEMENTARY AND ALTERNATIVE THERAPIES

The Complementary and Alternative Therapies box describes herbal preparations commonly used by patients and potential drug interactions with other medications.

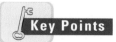

Key Points

- Many medications are used to treat the variety of diseases or disorders affecting the GI tract.
- The major medications covered in this chapter are antacids, which neutralize or reduce stomach acidity; histamine H_2-receptor antagonists, which stop the action of histamine at receptor cells in the stomach; anticholinergics and antispasmodics, which reduce gastric motility and decrease acid secretions; antidiarrheals, which reduce diarrhea; laxatives, which promote emptying of the bowel; antiflatulents, which reduce gas and bloating; digestive enzymes, which break down fats, starches, and proteins; and emetics, which produce vomiting.
- Many of these medications are used by the patient as self-medications. Therefore, it is important that you teach the patient or family about serious adverse reactions to watch for and any special administration considerations, such as fluid intake or foods to avoid.

Go to the free CD-ROM for an Audio Glossary, animations, video clips, and Review Questions for the NCLEX-PN® Examination.

evolve Be sure to visit the companion Evolve website at http://evolve.elsevier.com/Edmunds/LPN/ for WebLinks, a link to the top 200 drugs by prescription, and sign-up pages for newsletter drug updates.

Complementary and Alternative Therapies

Gastrointestinal Problems

CONDITION	PRODUCT	COMMENTS
Constipation	Cascara Senna	Use may decrease absorption of oral medications; potential interaction with antiarrhythmics, digoxin, phenytoin, laxatives, lithium, theophylline
	Milk thistle	No toxicity or serious side effects noted
	Psyllium	
Diarrhea	Grapefruit seed extract	Avoid concurrent administration of terfenadine, astemizole, cisapride; use other medications metabolized by the cytochrome P-450 (CYP) 3A4 subsystem with caution
	Olive leaf	No reported toxicities
	Green tea Bilberry	Potential interaction with anticoagulants, aspirin, NSAIDs, antiplatelet agents
Gallbladder/gallstones	Milk thistle Artichoke Goldenseal	No reported toxicities with any of these products
Indigestion/heartburn	Bromelain	Potential interactions with anticoagulants, aspirin, NSAIDs, antiplatelet agents
	Ginger	Potential interactions with anticoagulants, aspirin, NSAIDs, antiplatelet agents, cardiac glycosides
	Cayenne	Potential interaction with anticoagulants, aspirin, NSAIDs, antiplatelet agents; potential interference with monoamine oxidase inhibitors, antihypertensives
	Artichoke Chamomile Peppermint	No known interactions with the rest of these products
Irritable bowel	Cat's claw	Potential interaction with anticoagulants, aspirin, NSAIDs, antiplatelet agents
	Grapefruit seed extract	Avoid concurrent administration of terfenadine, astemizole, cisapride; use other medications metabolized by the CYP 3A4 subsystem with caution
	Evening primrose	Potential interaction with anticoagulants, aspirin, NSAIDs, antiplatelet agents
	Peppermint	No known interactions
Nausea/vomiting	Chamomile	No known interactions
	Ginger	Potential interactions with anticoagulants, aspirin, NSAIDs, antiplatelet agents, cardiac glycosides
Ulcer	Licorice	Potential interaction with nitrofurantoin
	Mastic	No known interactions
	Marshmallow	Potential interactions with insulin, oral hypoglycemic agents

Modified from Krinsky DL, Lavella JB, Hawkins EB, et al: *Natural therapeutics pocket guide*, ed 2, Hudson, Ohio, 2003, Lexi-Comp, Inc.

CASE STUDY

Mr. Frost is a 73-year-old man who is being treated for CHF that developed after an acute myocardial infarction. His stay in the hospital has been upsetting for him, and both his eating and bowel habits have changed. He usually reports a bowel movement every morning but has been unable to pass stool for the last 3 days. He is currently sitting on a commode and straining. The doctor orders:

Metamucil: 1 rounded tsp 1 to 2 times/day
Lanoxin: 0.25 mg PO daily
Hydrochlorothiazide: 50 mg daily

1. Why is the Metamucil ordered?
2. If the Metamucil does not work, what type of laxative might be effective?
3. What type of laxative would not be indicated for this patient?
4. Why is the Lanoxin ordered?
5. What is the purpose of the hydrochlorothiazide?
6. Are there any things to be concerned about in a patient taking hydrochlorothiazide?
7. What dietary modifications might assist Mr. Frost in returning to normal bowel activity?

DRUG CALCULATION REVIEW

1. Order: Pepcid 20 mg by gastrostomy tube (per GT) twice a day
   Supply: Pepcid 40 mg/5 mL
   Question: How many milliliters of Pepcid are needed with each dose?
2. Order: Anzemet 1.8 mg/kg 30 min before chemotherapy

   Supply: Anzemet 20 mg/mL
   Question: How many milligrams of Anzemet should be given to a patient weighing 143 lbs?
3. Order: Sucralfate 1.5 gm per GT 4 times per day
   Supply: Sucralfate 1 gm/10 mL
   Question: How many milliliters of sucralfate is needed with each dose?

CRITICAL THINKING

1. Ms. McKelvey has been taking OTC antacids for her stomach ulcer. Now, however, the clinic physician has prescribed the addition of a histamine H_2-receptor antagonist. When the physician leaves the room, Ms. McKelvey tells you that she is unhappy about this, because she has prided herself on keeping her "medical costs" down by using only home remedies and OTC drugs. "If they're both for ulcers," she says, "then what's the difference? Why can't I just double my dose of the antacid?" Describe the differences between these two drugs in their actions and uses in a way that makes it easy for Ms. McKelvey to understand.

2. Explain why adverse reactions are more frequent with anticholinergics than with antidiarrheals.

3. Mrs. Harris, age 82, has been admitted to the hospital for treatment of severe diarrhea. She is placed on antidiarrheal therapy and admitted to your unit for inpatient treatment and observation. Identify signs of dehydration and electrolyte imbalance, as well as any adverse reactions that might be associated with antidiarrheal therapy, particularly in the elderly patient.

4. On the second day of treatment, Mrs. Harris does show signs of both dehydration and electrolyte imbalance, as you had anticipated. Draw up a treatment plan for this patient.

5. Mr. Weigand has been using fecal softeners on an almost daily basis "for quite a while," he says, but is still having trouble with constipation. The physician has examined Mr. Weigand and tells him that he needs to be switched to a lubricant type of laxative instead of the softeners. Mr. Weigand is uncomfortable with this and asks you why he cannot use his "old stand-by."

6. Mrs. Magid has been prescribed a digestive enzyme. What are the possible indications for this drug? What kind of patient teaching would be necessary to give Mrs. Magid about this drug? How can she minimize adverse reactions?

7. Why would digestive enzymes be prescribed for a child with cystic fibrosis?

8. What is a "disulfiram reaction?" Why is disulfiram prescribed? Explain why patient compliance is so important with this drug.

19 Hematologic Products

After reading and studying this chapter, you should be able to do the following:

1. Identify drugs that act in the formation, repair, or function of red blood cells.
2. Describe the influence of anticoagulants on blood clotting.
3. Identify at least three adverse reactions associated with hematologic products.
4. Develop a teaching plan for patients taking anticoagulants on a long-term basis.

■ Key Terms

Be sure to check out the bonus material on the free CD-ROM, including selected audio pronunciations.

anticoagulants (ăn-tī-kō-ĂG-ū-lĕnts, p. 349)
fibrin (FĪ-brĭn, p. 349)
fibrinogen (fĭ-BRĬN-ō-jĕn, p. 349)
thrombi (THRŎM-bī, p. 349)
thromboplastin (thrŏm-bō-PLĂS-tĭn, p. 349)

OVERVIEW

Hematologic products act in the formation, repair, or function of red blood cells. There are four major groups of medications that have hematologic effects. They include the anticoagulants (heparin and coumarin) and the heparin antagonist protamine sulfate. Thrombolytic agents and antiplatelet factors also have a major influence on blood clotting. Related vitamins and minerals that are needed for red blood cell development are iron, vitamin K, vitamin B$_{12}$, and folic acid; these are presented in Chapter 24.

ANTICOAGULANTS

One of the body's protective functions is to clot blood in response to tissue injury. Any damage to the cells starts a series of chemical reactions to protect the body (Figure 19-1). Cellular damage results in the formation of **thromboplastin,** which then acts on prothrombin to form thrombin. Calcium must be present for this reaction to occur. Thrombin then acts on **fibrinogen** (a protein found in the blood plasma) to produce **fibrin,** a netlike substance in the blood that traps red and white blood cells and platelets and forms the matrix, or skeleton, of the clot. Vitamin K must be present to produce prothrombin and other clotting factors that are made in the liver. All **anticoagulants** prevent the formation of blood clots, or thrombi, by interfering with this complex clotting mechanism of blood and increasing the time it takes for blood to clot. In cases of overdosage, protamine sulfate is given to counteract the effect of heparin. In response to some bleeding disorders, vitamin K may be given either orally or parenterally to manufacture prothrombin and serve as an anticoagulant antagonist (see Chapter 24).

ACTION

There are two major categories of anticoagulants. The first category, the coumarin and indandione derivatives, limits formation of blood coagulation factors II, VII, IX, and X in the liver by interfering with vitamin K. These drugs do not destroy existing blood clots; however, they may limit the extension of existing blood clots or thrombi.

The second category, heparin sodium, acts at multiple sites in the normal coagulation system to stop reactions that lead to the clotting of blood and the formation of fibrin clots. It increases the action of antithrombin III (heparin cofactor) on several other coagulation factors, primarily activated factor X (Xa), to slow new clot development. Heparin does not dissolve existing clots either, although thrombolytic agents do. Low-molecular-weight heparin is a special formulation used in special circumstances, such as to prevent deep vein thrombosis after surgery.

USES

As part of the circulatory system, the arterial vessels carry oxygenated blood throughout the body. If these small arteries become plugged with **thrombi** (clots made of fibrin, platelets, and cholesterol), the oxygen cannot get to the tissues and death may result. Abnormal

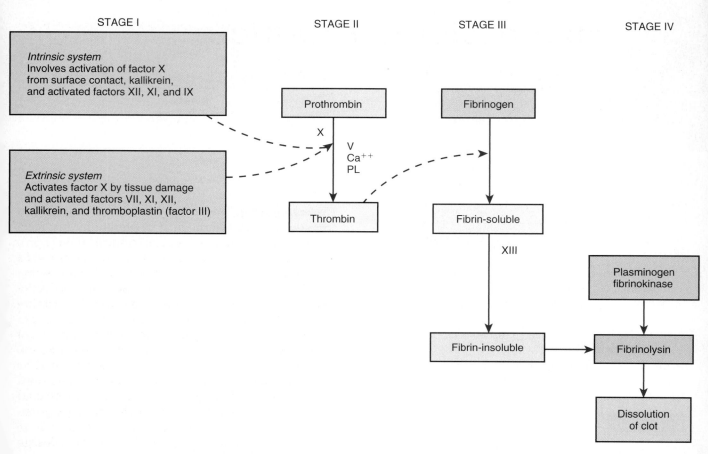

FIGURE **19-1** Blood coagulation and clot resolution. *PL,* Phospholipid.

blood clotting may produce a thrombus in the coronary artery, which nourishes the heart muscle. Emboli (small pieces of a blood clot) may break off from a site of thrombophlebitis (inflammation and blood clot in a vein) in the lower extremities and travel through the bloodstream to block vessels in areas of the heart, brain, or lung (see Figure 15-7). This blockage can cause stroke or death. Drugs that can slow or reduce clotting, then, are very helpful.

Anticoagulant therapy is used to prevent new clot formation or to stop existing clots from growing in size. Anticoagulant therapy is used prophylactically during and after many types of surgery, especially surgery involving the heart or circulation. It is also used in patients with heart valve disease, in patients with some dysrhythmias (irregular heartbeats), and in patients receiving hemodialysis. Any patient on bed rest for a long time is at risk for development of blood clots, especially patients with a history of clotting problems or recent orthopedic, thoracic, or abdominal surgery.

Heparin is the anticoagulant of choice when an immediate effect is needed. For long-term therapy, a coumarin or indandione derivative is used. The U.S. Food and Drug Administration (FDA) has classified coumarin preparations as "possibly" effective as part of the therapy for treatment of transient cerebral

ischemic attacks (TIA). Indandione derivatives (phenindione) are used to treat pulmonary emboli and as prophylaxis to treat deep vein thrombosis, myocardial infarction, rheumatic heart disease with valve damage, and atrial dysrhythmias. Low-intensity coumarin therapy (prothrombin time [PT] ratio between 1.2 and 1.5) greatly decreases the risk of stroke from nonrheumatic atrial fibrillation and has few side effects.

ADVERSE REACTIONS

Warfarin may produce alopecia (hair loss), rash, urticaria (hives), cramping, diarrhea, intestinal obstruction, nausea, paralytic ileus, vomiting, excessive uterine bleeding, hemorrhage with excessive dosage, leukopenia, and fever.

Heparin sodium may produce hypertension (high blood pressure); headache; hematoma, irritation, and pain at the injection site; conjunctivitis; tearing of eyes; rhinitis; frequent or persistent erection; hemorrhage; thrombocytopenia; shortness of breath; wheezing; chills; fever; alopecia; and hypersensitivity (allergic) reaction.

Early signs of overdosage or internal bleeding include bleeding from gums while brushing teeth, excessive bleeding or oozing from cuts, unexplained bruising or nosebleeds, and unusually heavy or unexpected menses in women.

DRUG INTERACTIONS

Other anticoagulants (coumarin or indandione derivatives), methimazole, and propylthiouracil increase the anticoagulant effect of heparin.

Antihistamines, digitalis, nicotine, and tetracycline decrease the anticoagulant effect of heparin.

Acetylsalicylic acid (ASA), coumarin-derivative anticoagulants, dextran, nonsteroidal antiinflammatory drugs (NSAIDs), and other selected drugs increase the risk of bleeding and hemorrhage in a patient receiving heparin.

ASA, corticotropin, ethacrynic acid, glucocorticoids, and NSAIDs increase the risk of gastrointestinal (GI) bleeding and hemorrhage in a patient receiving heparin.

Allopurinol, ASA, anabolic steroids, antibiotics, androgens, many sedatives, some antacids, dextran, disulfiram, drugs affecting blood elements, glucagon, heparin, narcotics (with prolonged use), phenylbutazone, propylthiouracil, quinidine, quinine, salicylates, thyroid drugs, and vitamin E increase the PT response of patients receiving coumarin.

Adrenocorticosteroids, antacids, antihistamines, barbiturates, contraceptives (oral), estrogens, griseofulvin, haloperidol, meprobamate, primidone, rifampin, thiazide diuretics, and vitamin K decrease the PT response of a patient on coumarin.

Anticoagulant effects may be increased with acute alcohol intoxication and decreased with chronic alcohol abuse. Oral hypoglycemics taken with anticoagulants may increase the effect of either the hypoglycemic or anticoagulant.

Alkylating agents, antimetabolites, corticosteroids, ethacrynic acid, indomethacin, quinidine, and salicylates increase the risk of bleeding in a patient taking coumarin.

Nursing Implications and Patient Teaching

Patients requiring rapid anticoagulation are commonly hospitalized. Coagulation and PT tests are ordered when the patient is started on anticoagulants. Heparin is usually started for an immediate effect and gradually replaced by oral anticoagulants. Thereafter, the physician or other health care provider orders coagulation and PT tests at regular intervals. When the oral anticoagulant shows proper effect and the prothrombin activity is in the therapeutic range, heparin therapy may be stopped and the oral anticoagulant therapy continued.

Several issues are being debated with regard to heparin therapy; one is the method used to calculate the dose of heparin. Standard heparin dosing protocols use a 5000-unit intravenous (IV) bolus followed by a continuous infusion of 800 to 1000 units/hr. The dose is adjusted based on the activated partial thromboplastin time (APTT) results, determined from blood drawn 6 hours after the start of the heparin infusion and regularly thereafter. Standard dosing can cause inadequate dosing or excessive anticoagulation.

Weight-based dosing and adjusted dosing are alternative methods for determining the dosing of heparin. Weight-based dosing uses the patient's body weight in kilograms, infusing 80 units/kg as an IV bolus. The maintenance infusion is 18 units/kg/hr through an infusion pump. There are indications that weight-based dosing is safer, achieves therapeutic levels in less time than with standard dosing, and results in fewer bleeding complications and a lower rate of thromboembolic recurrences.

In adjusted dosing, the standard heparin IV dose is used initially, but subsequent dose adjustments are based on raising the APTT 2 to 5 seconds above the normal level. Certain conditions—liver disease, advanced age, sepsis, disseminated intravascular coagulation (DIC), and severe trauma—cause the regular antithrombin II activity to decline, thus increasing the risk of thrombosis. Using adjusted-dose heparin rather than fixed-dose heparin may result in fewer thromboembolic events because of more precise control of anticoagulation.

The standard tests for determining the general effect of heparin on clotting are the Lee-White method, the whole blood activated partial thromboplastin time (WBAPTT), and the APTT. The most commonly used test is the APTT. The dosage of heparin is considered adequate when the whole blood clotting time is approximately $2\frac{1}{2}$ to 3 times the control value.

Traditionally, PTs were used to determine the dosage for coumarin preparations. Initially, PT tests were done daily until the results stabilized in the therapeutic range ($1\frac{1}{2}$ to $2\frac{1}{2}$ times the normal control value). After stabilization, the tests were performed at 1- to 4-week intervals, depending on patient status.

The validity of PT determinations is dependent on the thromboplastin reagent used to perform the test. In 1983, the World Health Organization recommended a system called the International Normalization Ratio (INR) to standardize PT reporting so that all laboratory reports would be the same. The INR is based on the PT ratio that would be obtained if a standard reference thromboplastin were used. Thromboplastin sensitivity is given by the drug maker using the International Sensitivity Index (ISI). PT numbers are changed to INR measurements by a standard math equation. Laboratories commonly report both numbers (PT/INR) when PT is ordered.

The goal of prolonging the PT to 1.5 to 2.5 times the normal has largely been replaced by specific INR goal recommendations for each clinical indication. The typical INR goal is 2.0 to 3.0, except in mechanical cardiac valve replacement, in which a higher INR is necessary to prevent clot formation.

Assessment

You should learn as much as possible about the patient's health history, including the presence of hypersensitivity, underlying systemic disease, the current nature of he problem, and use of other medications. You should nquire about conditions that would contraindicate use of some anticoagulants, such as alcoholism, blood dyscrasias, bleeding tendencies of the GI, genitourinary, or espiratory tracts, or malignant hypertension. Patients vith congestive heart failure may be more sensitive to oumarin anticoagulants and indandione derivatives.

Heparin is derived from animal tissue and should be used with caution in any patient with a history of allergy. This drug should be used cautiously in patients vith hepatic or renal disease or hypertension, during nenses, after delivery, or in patients with indwelling catheters. A higher incidence of bleeding may be seen in vomen over the age of 60. Make sure that female patients taking a coumarin or indandione derivative are not pregnant or breastfeeding. These drugs are usually not given to children.

Geriatric Considerations

Anticoagulants

The elderly may be more sensitive to the effects of anticoagulants, and a lower maintenance dose is usually recommended for the geriatric patient, along with very close supervision and monitoring.

The primary adverse effects of excessive drug usage are prolonged bleeding from the gums when brushing teeth or from small shaving cuts, excessive or easy skin bruising, blood in urine or stools, and unexplained nosebleeds. There may be early signs of overdose that indicate the need for medical intervention.

Be aware that giving other drugs at the same time that may cause gastric irritation increases the risk for GI bleeding. Drugs such as NSAIDs (for example, ibuprofen, indomethacin) that are commonly prescribed for the elderly patient often cause GI effects.

Modified from McKenry LM, Salerno E: *Mosby's pharmacology in nursing*, ed 1, St Louis, 2003, Mosby.

Diagnosis

There are many medical and surgical contraindications o the use of anticoagulant drugs, particularly in patients who have recently had surgery, trauma, or obstetric complications. Review the patient's problems nd make certain that none of these contraindications exist.

Planning

The dosages listed for heparin are given in United States Pharmacopeia (USP) heparin units. Heparin is not effective if given orally and should be given by IV injection, IV infusion, or deep subcutaneous (intrafat) injection. Heparin should not be given intramuscularly (IM) because these injections produce hematomas, irritation,

and pain at the injection site. Use a small (25-gauge) needle and a tuberculin syringe for the subcutaneous intrafat injection.

Implementation

Anticoagulant drugs should not be used if there are not good laboratory facilities available or if the patient is not compliant in taking medications or keeping appointments for laboratory and health assessment. Coumarin derivatives should not be used in a patient undergoing diagnostic or therapeutic procedures with risk for uncontrolled bleeding.

The sites of intrafat injections of heparin should be rotated to avoid formation of hematomas. (See Figure 10-15 for rotation site suggestions.) Because of the adverse effects if inaccurate doses are given, once the heparin is drawn into the syringe, you should double-check the dosage with another nurse. There are several things to remember about heparin injection that make the process unique. First, you should not attempt to pull back on the plunger or aspirate blood before injection. Second, you must be extra careful to not move the needle while the heparin is being injected. Third, injection sites should not be massaged before or after injection. Patients receiving heparin are not good candidates for IM injections of other medications, because hematomas and bleeding into nearby areas may occur.

If the heparin solution is discolored or contains a precipitate (solid at the bottom), it must not be used. Heparin is strongly acidic and is chemically incompatible with many other medications in solution, so it must not be piggybacked with other drugs into an infusion line. Never mix any drug with heparin in a syringe when bolus therapy is given.

If intermittent IV therapy is being given, blood for partial thromboplastin time determination should be drawn one-half hour before the next scheduled heparin dose. Blood for partial thromboplastin times can be drawn anytime after 8 hours of continuous IV heparin therapy. However, blood should not be drawn from the tubing of the heparin infusion line or from the vein being used for infusion. Blood should always be drawn from the arm not being used for heparin infusion.

If heparin is being given at the same time as a coumarin or an indandione derivative, blood should not be drawn for PTs within 5 hours of IV heparin administration, or 24 hours if heparin is given subcutaneously. IV heparin infusions should be checked frequently, even if pumps are in good working order, to make sure that the proper dosage is being given.

If anticoagulant therapy is started with heparin and continued with a coumarin or an indandione derivative, it is recommended that both drugs be given until the PT or INR results indicate an adequate response to the coumarin or indandione derivative.

A summary of anticoagulants is provided in Table 19-1.

Table **19-1**

Anticoagulants and Other Drugs Affecting the Blood

GENERIC NAME	TRADE NAME	COMMENTS AND DOSAGE
ANTICOAGULANTS		
Coumarin and Indandione Derivatives		
anisindione	Miradon	Give 300 mg the first day, 200 mg the second day, 100 mg the third day, and 25-250 mg daily thereafter, as indicated by PT or INR levels. Store tablets at 59-99° F.
dicumarol	Dicumarol	Give 200-300 mg the first day, then 25-200 mg on subsequent days as indicated by PT or INR levels. Store tablets at <70° F.
warfarin (sodium)	Coumadin	Individualize dosage. Usual initiation dose is 2-5 mg/day with dosage adjustments based on the results of INR and/or PT ratio determinations. Store tablets at 59-86° F and protect from air and light.
Heparin		
heparin	Heparin	Dosage is adjusted according to patient's coagulation time. *Adults:* *Deep subcutaneous:* 10,000-20,000 USP units initially. Then 8000-10,000 USP units q8h. *IV:* 10,000 USP units initially, then 5000-10,000 USP units q4-6h. Give either undiluted or diluted with 50-100 mL of isotonic NaCl. *IV infusion:* Give 20,000-40,000 USP units in 1000 mL of isotonic NaCl solution over 24 hr. Loading dose of 5000 USP units may be given by IV injection. Also available as a lock flush solution. *Children:* *IV:* 50 USP units/kg initially, then 50-100 USP units/kg q4h. *IV infusion:* 50 USP units/kg as a bolus initially, then 100 USP units/kg added and absorbed q4h.
Glycosaminoglycans		
danaparoid	Orgaran	Give 750 anti-Xa units twice daily administered by subcutaneous injection beginning 1-4 hr preoperatively and then not earlier than 2 hr after surgery. Continue as needed for approximately 10 days postoperatively. Dosages are not equivalent to heparin dosages. Clotting times are unreliable in monitoring effect. Obtain CBC with platelets and stools for occult blood.
Low-Molecular-Weight Heparins		
ardeparin sodium	Normiflo	Give 50 units/kg q12h by subcutaneous injection. Begin treatment the evening of the day of surgery or the following morning and continue for about 14 days or until patient is fully ambulatory.
dalteparin sodium	Fragmin	Give 2500 International Units subcutaneously only, starting 1-2 hr before abdominal surgery.
enoxaparin	Lovenox 🍁	Low-molecular-weight heparin used to prevent deep vein thrombosis after hip replacement. Give 30 mg subcutaneously twice daily for 7-10 days. Begin immediately after surgery.
tinzaparin	Innohep	Give 175 anti-Xa International Units/kg of body weight subcutaneously once daily for about 6 days until the patient is adequately anticoagulated with warfarin. Draw blood for PT/INR just before giving scheduled dose of tinzaparin for patients also receiving warfarin.
HEPARIN ANTAGONIST		
protamine sulfate	Protamine Sulfate	The onset of action for protamine sulfate is 0.5-1 min. The duration of action is 2 hr. *Adults and children:* 1 mg of protamine sulfate for every 90 USP units of beef lung heparin or for every 115 USP units of porcine intestinal mucosa heparin to be neutralized. Administer IV at a slow rate over 1-3 min (limit is 50 mg given in 10 min). Additional doses may be given if need is indicated by coagulation studies.

Continued

Table **19-1**

Anticoagulants and Other Drugs Affecting the Blood—cont'd

GENERIC NAME	TRADE NAME	COMMENTS AND DOSAGE
THROMBOLYTIC AGENTS		
Tissue Plasmogen Activators		
alteplase, recombinant	Activase	For lysis of coronary artery thrombi. Best results if given IV within 6 hr of onset of symptoms of MI. Give 6-10 mg IV bolus over the first 1-2 min, 20 mg over the second hour, and 20 mg over the third hour. May be slightly more effective but costs 10 times more than the other products.
reteplase	Retavase	Give as IV bolus only.
tenecteplase	TNKase	Give no more than 50 mg by IV administration only. Do not exceed recommended volume per 5 sec when giving as IV bolus.
Other Thrombolytic Agents		
anistreplase	Eminase	For lysis of thrombi obstructing coronary arteries. Give 30 units by IV injection over 2-5 min.
streptokinase	Streptase	Used in acute evolving transmural MI, deep vein thrombosis, arterial thrombosis and embolism, and occluded AV cannula. Patients may have severe, uncontrolled hypertension or severe allergic reactions. Dosage is calculated and administered by physician.
urokinase	Abbokinase	Used to dissolve clots from pulmonary emboli or a coronary artery thrombosis, or to clear IV catheters obstructed by clotted blood or fibrin. Physician gives priming dose and follows with a constant infusion pump dosage calculated and administered by physician.
ANTIPLATELET AGENTS		
abciximab	ReoPro	Give IV bolus of 0.25 mg/kg administered 10-60 min before the start of PTCA, followed by a continuous IV infusion of 10 mcg/min for 12 hr.
acetylsalicylic acid	ASA	Give 600 mg PO stat with first indication of MI. Do not give ASA in addition to coumarin anticoagulants.
anagrelide	Agrylin	Used in treating essential thrombocythemia to reduce elevated platelet count and the risk of thrombosis. Give 0.5 mg 4 times daily or 1 mg twice daily for about 1 wk and then adjust to lowest effective dosage required to reduce and maintain platelet count <600,000/μL.

 Clinical Landmine

Internal Bleeding

Signs suggesting internal bleeding include abdominal pain or swelling, back pain, bloody or tarry stools, bloody or cloudy urine, constipation (resulting from paralytic ileus or intestinal obstruction), coughing up blood, dizziness, severe or continuous headaches, and vomiting blood or "coffee-ground" substance.

Evaluation

f heparin is given by continuous IV infusion, the coagulation time should be determined every 4 hours in the early stages of treatment.

You should watch for signs of overdosage of anticogulants and internal bleeding as therapy progresses.

This might include bleeding gums when the patient brushes her teeth, blood in the urine, or coughing up blood.

Patient and Family Teaching

You should tell the patient and family the following:
1. The patient should take the oral medication only as directed. If a dose is missed, it should be taken as soon as possible, but not if it is almost time for the next dose. The doses should not be doubled. The patient should keep a record of all missed doses.
2. The patient will need regular INR time or coagulation blood tests and regular visits to the physician to ensure that blood clotting stays within special and narrow limits. The dosage may require changes from time to time, based on results of laboratory tests.

Table 19-1

Anticoagulants and Other Drugs Affecting the Blood—cont'd

GENERIC NAME	TRADE NAME	COMMENTS AND DOSAGE
ANTIPLATELET AGENTS—cont'd		
cilostazol	Pletal	For intermittent claudication, give 1100 mg twice daily taken about 30 min before or 2 hr after breakfast and dinner. May need a smaller dose if concurrent administration of some CYP3A4 drugs.
clopidogrel	Plavix	Give 75 mg daily with or without food. No adjustment necessary for elderly patients or those with renal disease.
dipyridamole	Persantine	Give 75-100 mg 4 times daily as adjunct to warfarin therapy.
ticlopidine	Ticlid	Reconstitute drug and give IV at rate of 0.4 mcg/kg/min for 30 min and then continue at 0.1 mcg/kg/min. Specific dosage based on weight.
OTHER MISCELLANEOUS PRODUCTS		
antihemophilic factor	Hemofil M/E Koate-HP Monoclate P	Used in treating patients with hemophilia A. Individualize dosage based on needs of patient.
antiinhibitor coagulant complex	Autoplex T/E Feiba VH	Individualize dosage based on needs of patient.
antithrombin III	ATnativ	Used in treating patients with hereditary antithrombin III deficiency. Individualize dosage based on needs of patient.
eptifibatide	Integrilin	Give IV bolus of 1890 mcg/kg as soon as possible after diagnosis of acute coronary syndrome, followed by continuous infusion of 2 mcg/kg/min until hospital discharge or CABG surgery.
hydroxyurea	Droxia	Antisickling agent. The initial dose of hydroxyurea is 15 mg/kg/day as a single dose. The patient's CBC must be monitored every 2 wk.
pentoxifylline	Trental	Used in intermittent claudication from chronic occlusive arterial disease and in cerebrovascular insufficiency. Give 400 mg 3 times daily with meals. Decrease dosage if GI side effects develop.
tirofiban	Aggrastat	Used with heparin in the treatment of acute coronary syndrome, including patients who are to be managed medically and those with PTCA. Can be administered in the same IV catheter as heparin. Give for 48-108 hr, including during surgical procedure and after. Medication must be diluted and administered according to the patient's weight.

AV, Atrioventricular; *CABG,* coronary artery bypass grafting; *CBC,* complete blood cell count; *MI,* myocardial infarction; *NaCl,* sodium chloride; *PTCA,* percutaneous transluminal coronary angioplasty.

3. The patient should not take other medications without checking with the nurse, physician, or other health care provider; this includes aspirin or any over-the-counter (OTC) medicines.

4. The patient should wear a Medic Alert bracelet or necklace or carry a medical information card explaining that he is taking an anticoagulant.

5. The patient should inform all nurses, physicians, or other health care providers, dentists, or podiatrists whom she sees for care that she is taking an anticoagulant.

6. The patient should use caution in brushing teeth, trimming nails, and shaving. (An electric razor should be used when possible.)

7. Pressure should be used to stop bleeding from accidental cuts or scrapes; if bleeding persists after 10 minutes, the nurse, physician, or other health care provider should be contacted.

8. The patient should not engage in contact sports or other activities that could lead to injuries.

9. The patient should eat a normal, balanced diet, but should avoid eating excessive amounts of foods high in vitamin K (tomatoes, onions, dark leafy greens, bananas, or fish).

10. The patient should avoid alcohol.

11. The patient should know the possible side effects of anticoagulants: active bleeding or signs of bleeding such as tarry stools, blood in the urine, bleeding gums, nosebleeds, dizziness, coughing up blood, abdominal or joint pains, unexplained bruising, or unusually heavy or unexpected menstrual periods in women.

12. After anticoagulation therapy has been stopped, the patient should use caution until the body recovers its blood-clotting abilities.

PROTAMINE SULFATE

ACTION

Protamine sulfate is a strongly basic (alkaline) protein that acts as a heparin antagonist to neutralize (reverse) the actions of heparin. However, it may also serve as an anticoagulant when used as the sole medication. It forms a stable salt in the presence of heparin, which is strongly acidic. This cancels out the anticoagulant activity of both drugs. When protamine sulfate is used with heparin, these results occur almost immediately and may persist for 2 hours or more.

USES

Protamine sulfate is used to treat heparin overdosage. It may also be used after surgical procedures to neutralize the effects of heparin given during extracorporeal circulation on a heart-lung machine.

ADVERSE REACTIONS

Adverse reactions to protamine sulfate include bradycardia (slow heartbeat), dyspnea (uncomfortable breathing), lassitude (weariness), sudden drop in blood pressure, transitory flushing (red color in the face and neck), and a feeling of warmth. Overdosage may produce anticoagulant effects.

Nursing Implications and Patient Teaching

Assessment

Because of the anticoagulant activity of protamine sulfate, overdoses of this drug when used as a heparin antagonist may produce additional anticoagulation.

Diagnosis

Does the patient have any other problems that might result from excessive anticoagulation? Is the patient taking other medications or using a diet that would interfere with anticoagulation?

Planning

Protamine sulfate may be inactivated by blood. Thus, there may be a rebound effect when a large dose is used to neutralize heparin. This requires an increased dose of protamine sulfate. Hyperheparinemia or bleeding may be seen in some patients 30 minutes to 18 hours after open heart surgery, even when adequate amounts of protamine sulfate have been given.

Implementation

Protamine sulfate should be given only by a physician. You would usually assemble the medications but allow the physician to draw up the dose. It should be given slowly by IV injection over 1 to 3 minutes in doses not exceeding 50 mg of protamine sulfate activity (5 mL)

during any 10-minute period. It is rare that more than 100 mg is given at a time.

Severe hypotension and anaphylactic-like reactions may be provoked if it is given too rapidly. This drug contains no preservatives, so the unused portion of the medication in the ampule should be discarded.

Evaluation

You should closely monitor the patient for signs of further anticoagulant activity and have equipment readily available to treat shock.

Patient and Family Teaching

The family and patient should know that this is a standard drug used to neutralize heparin. See Table 19-1 for information on protamine sulfate and other hematologic products.

THROMBOLYTIC AGENTS

ACTION

Thrombolytics convert plasminogen to the enzyme plasmin, which degrades or breaks down fibrin clots, fibrinogen, and other plasma proteins. These products are used for lysis (dissolving) of thrombi.

USES

Thrombolytic agents are used in acute myocardial infarction for lysis of thrombi blocking coronary arteries, in acute pulmonary emboli for lysis of clot when the patient is hemodynamically unstable, and in acute ischemic stroke and acute arterial occlusion. Use of thrombolytics reduces the extent of cellular damage from blockage.

ADVERSE REACTIONS

Bleeding is the most obvious adverse effect. Dysrhythmias, hypotension (low blood pressure), polyneuropathy, cholesterol embolism, pulmonary embolism, and hypersensitivity are all possible effects.

DRUG INTERACTIONS

Administering these products along with other anticoagulants may increase the potential for bleeding.

Nursing Implications and Patient Teaching

Assessment

These medications are given by the physician in life-threatening situations of vascular block because of thrombosis. They are most helpful if administered within the first hour after the thrombosis.

You should learn as much as you can about the health history of the patient. Through talking to the patient or other primary witnesses, attempt to determine the exact time sequence of events and what happened before the patient was seen. Determine whether any other medications have been taken. For example, because aspirin helps reduce platelet adhesion, patients who are suspected of having a myocardial infarction are urged to take a 600-mg aspirin (ASA) tablet. Obtain the history of any recent surgery.

Diagnosis

What other factors in addition to the medical diagnosis are important? Does this patient have risk factors for bleeding, myocardial infarction, stroke, or pulmonary emboli? This patient is probably very frightened and anxious. He may also be worrying about finances, career, and family if he believes he is seriously ill.

Planning

These medications come as a powder that requires reconstitution. Are all of the equipment and materials that the physician will require for infusion present?

Implementation

Carefully monitor the vital signs of the patient receiving thrombolytic therapy. Report these findings frequently to the physician or other health care provider.

Evaluation

Observe the patient carefully for bleeding. Bleeding may be superficial, coming from the infusion site. Other more significant bleeding indicates overdosage and is shown by hematuria (blood in the urine), hematemesis (blood in the vomitus), signs of abdominal tension, and internal bleeding.

Patient and Family Teaching

Explain the basis of thrombolytic therapy to the patient and family as necessary. Make sure the physician speaks with them about what is being done.

ANTIPLATELET AGENTS

ACTION

Through a variety of mechanisms, these products act to limit or inhibit platelet aggregation (clumping) and thus reduce thrombus formation.

USES

ASA reduces the incidence of myocardial infarction–related deaths in men older than 50 years of age. ASA is the drug of choice in ischemic stroke; it plays no role in hemorrhagic stroke.

Dipyridamole (Persantine), ticlopidine (Ticlid), and clopidogrel (Plavix) are used for myocardial infarction prophylaxis for men and as additional or adjunct therapy with thrombolytics in preventing infarction or

stroke. Abciximab (ReoPro), anagrelide (Agrylin), and a variety of other specialty products may be used during cardiac catheterization or other cardiovascular procedures.

ADVERSE REACTIONS

Bleeding is the most frequently seen adverse event. Diarrhea, nausea, dyspepsia (stomach discomfort after eating), rash, GI pain, neutropenia, purpura (bruising), vomiting, flatulence, pruritus (itching), dizziness, and anorexia (lack of appetite) are also seen.

DRUG INTERACTIONS

Variable interactions with antacids, cimetidine, digoxin, and theophylline are possible.

Nursing Implications and Patient Teaching

Assessment

These drugs are used in critically ill patients to help limit damage from thrombosis or occlusion. You will be involved in monitoring vital signs and assisting with the monitoring of the patient's cardiovascular status.

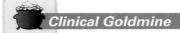 **Clinical Goldmine**

Myocardial Infarction

ASA is often given as soon as it is suspected that the patient may be having a myocardial infarction.

Diagnosis

Evaluate for changes in level of consciousness, renal function, and respiration. Be alert for any signs of bleeding.

Planning

Have all materials available for monitoring the patient's vital signs and for giving medications.

Implementation

Assist in recording the medications given and the patient's response. Assist in the ordering and collection of any blood work required to monitor therapy.

Evaluation

Changes in vital signs and levels of consciousness provide important feedback about the status of the blood circulation.

Patient and Family Teaching

Assist in calming the patient, explaining the situation to the family, and providing information. Some of these medications may be given orally over time to help maintain a good circulation.

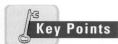

Key Points

- Hematologic products act in the formation, repair, or function of red blood cells.
- There are four major groups of hematologic products. They are the anticoagulants, the heparin antagonist protamine sulfate, thrombolytics and antiplatelet factors, and the vitamins and minerals needed for red blood cell development (discussed in Chapter 24).
- Patient and family teaching is especially important for the patient undergoing long-term therapy.

Go to the free CD-ROM for an Audio Glossary, animations, video clips, and Review Questions for the NCLEX-PN® Examination.

evolve Be sure to visit the companion Evolve website at http://evolve.elsevier.com/Edmunds/LPN/ for WebLinks, a link to the top 200 drugs by prescription, and sign-up pages for newsletter drug updates.

CASE STUDY

Mrs. Lily, 34 years old, arrives at the office late for her appointment. She is limping and says her right calf is very sore. It is swollen, red, and very painful to touch. Mrs. Lily is a heavy smoker, takes oral birth control pills, and was recently involved in a car accident in which her right leg was badly bruised. The doctor admits her to the hospital with the following orders:
- Bed rest
- Right leg elevated and wrapped with warm, moist compresses
- Heparin IV q6h
1. If Mrs. Lily has thrombophlebitis, what is the probable cause?
2. What risk factors does she have now for other adverse reactions?
3. What blood test is useful in determining how much heparin should be given?
4. The dosage of heparin is considered adequate when the whole blood clotting time is approximately _____ the control value.
5. Low-intensity coumarin therapy (prothrombin time ratio between 1.2 and 1.5) greatly decreases the risk of stroke from what condition?
6. The doctor also orders Coumadin during Mrs. Lily's stay in the hospital. Why?
7. On admission, Mrs. Lily was found to have a hematocrit of 32% and a hemoglobin of 11 gm/dL. The doctor believes that this is because of blood loss during several pregnancies and heavy periods. What will be the likely course of treatment?

DRUG CALCULATION REVIEW

1. Order: Heparin 7500 units subcutaneously twice a day

    Supply: Heparin 20,000 units/mL

    Question: How many milliliters of heparin should be given with each dose? (Round to the nearest hundredth.)

2. Order: Give 500 mL of dextran 40 over 24 hr

    Question: How many milliliters per hour should the IV infusion device be set for? (Round to the nearest whole number.)

3. The physician orders enoxaparin (Lovenox) 30 mg subcutaneously twice daily for 7 to 10 days for prevention of deep vein thrombosis after hip replacement surgery. Available are prefilled syringes of 150 mg/1 mL concentration. How many milliliters will you expect to administer to this patient with each dose?

CRITICAL THINKING ?

1. Briefly point out the major differences in the three major groups of hematologic agents with regard to actions and uses.

2. Mrs. Gardner is being treated for a deep vein thrombosis (DVT). She is concerned about her treatment regimen, pointing out differences in the treatment her sister received for the same thing. As you listen to Mrs. Gardner's worries, you realize she keeps referring to her "embolism." Explain to Mrs. Gardner the difference between a thrombus and an embolism and why this difference may affect methods of treatment.

3. Mr. Pierce is brought to your unit and placed on anticoagulant therapy. Explain the rationale for needing to know why this patient is being put on anticoagulation therapy. Why would you need laboratory values to validate accurate dosage?

4. Describe the possible problems that can arise if anticoagulants are used in conjunction with some other specific drugs.

5. In the emergency department, Ms. Zukerman needs an immediate anticoagulant effect. Which is the drug of choice? Why?

6. Ms. Zukerman receives the appropriate medication, as indicated by Question 5, but now she exhibits signs of overdosage. What are the signs and symptoms of overdosage with this drug? Describe the needed interventions, both nursing and pharmacologic.

7. Which coagulation value is most accurate in monitoring the effect of Ms. Zukerman's therapy and why?

8. Ms. Zukerman's condition is stabilized now, but she is experiencing pain at injection sites. How can you respond?

9. Mrs. Martinez has just started taking Coumadin 2.5 mg every day. She is also "cutting down" on her caloric intake, at her doctor's recommendation, to help control her type 2 diabetes. She seems confused at her follow-up visit, however, and asks you, "If I'm supposed to lose weight, why can't I have salads? I thought they were low in sugar and calories, and I should eat a lot of vegetables on a diet." What does Mrs. Martinez need to know about Coumadin therapy?

10. Mr. Harris wants to know if his "Coumadin is working. I had some blood taken yesterday, and my doctor told me my platelets were OK. I thought the Coumadin was supposed to make me take longer to clot. Does this mean I need to take more?" What would you explain to Mr. Harris?

20 Hormones and Steroids

Objectives

After reading and studying this chapter, you should be able to do the following:

1. Describe the use of antidiabetic medications.
2. Identify preparations that act on the uterus.
3. Compare and contrast the action of adrenal and pituitary hormones.
4. Describe at least five adverse reactions that may result from the use of glucocortical and mineralocortical steroids.
5. Compare the actions of various male and female hormones.
6. List the indications for the use of thyroid preparations.

Key Terms

Be sure to check out the bonus material on the free CD-ROM, including selected audio pronunciations.

abortifacients (ă-BŎR-tĭ-FĀ-shĕnts, p. 372)
androgens (ĂN-drō-jĕnz, p. 382)
corticosteroids (KŎR-tĭ-kō STĔR-ŏydz, p. 375)
diabetes mellitus (dī-ă-BĒ-tēz mĕ-LĪ-tĭs, p. 362)
estrogen (ĔS-trō-jĕn, p. 382)
glucometers (GLŪ-kō-mēt-ĕrz, p. 365)
hormones (HŎR-mōnz, p. 360)
hyperglycemia (hī-pĕr-glī-SĒ-mē-ă, p. 364)
hyperthyroidism (hī-pĕr-THĪ-rŏyd-ĭzm, p. 393)
hypoglycemia (hī-pō-glī-SĒ-mē-ă, p. 364)
hypothyroidism (hī-pō-THĪ-rŏyd-ĭzm, p. 393)
insulin (ĬN-sū-lĭn, p. 362)
insulin-dependent diabetes mellitus (IDDM) (p. 363)
lipodystrophy (lĭp-ō-DĬS-trō-fē, p. 363)
myxedema (mĭk-sĕ-DĒ-mă, p. 394)
non–insulin-dependent diabetes mellitus (NIDDM) (p. 363)
oral hypoglycemics (hī-pō-glī-SĔM-ĭks, p. 369)
oxytocic agents (ŏk-sē-TŌ-sĭk, p. 372)
progesterone (prō-JĔS-tĕr-ōn, p. 382)
sex hormones (p. 375)
Somogyi effect (SŌM-ō-jē, p. 368)
steroids (STĔR-ŏydz, p. 360)
systemic acidosis (sĭs-TĔM-ĭk ăs-ĭ-DŌ-sĭs, p. 364)
tocolytics (tō-kō-LĪT-ĭks, p. 373)
type 1 diabetes (p. 363)
type 2 diabetes (p. 363)
uterine relaxants (Ū-tĕr-ĭn rē-LĂK-sănts, p. 372)

OVERVIEW

This chapter discusses the different hormones and steroids used in medical therapy. Unlike many other categories of medications, these are natural or synthetic preparations that replace, increase, or decrease natural chemicals already present within the patient. At times, the body may produce too much of a hormone (for example, in hyperthyroidism), and medication is given to reduce the hormone (such as methimazole, which limits the production of thyroid hormones). In diabetes mellitus, medication is given to replace the hormone insulin when not enough is produced by the pancreas.

Hormones are chemicals that are made in an organ or gland and are carried through the bloodstream to another part of the body. Once it arrives, the hormone stimulates that part of the body to increase its activity or secretion. **Steroids** are a specific chemical group of hormones that have powerful effects on cell sensitization, healing, and development. They are all part of a complex message system of the body, linking together various organs and systems. Lack of one basic hormone will stimulate, or signal, the glands to produce more hormone. When the right amount of the hormone is reached, the signal is turned off, and the gland slows production of the hormone. This is called a feedback mechanism and is important in creating stability of the body. If some part of the system does not work properly, failure in one organ system may then cause changes in other hormonal systems.

This chapter is divided into five basic sections. Section One describes insulin and the oral hypoglycemic agents used to treat diabetes mellitus. The various drugs that act on the uterus are presented in Section Two. Section Three describes the pituitary and adrenocortical hormones, the major steroids that act throughout the body. Section Four presents the male and female hormones and the different hormones in oral contraceptives. The various drugs used to treat the overproduction and underproduction of thyroid hormones are described in Section Five.

ENDOCRINE SYSTEM

The regulation and coordination of body activities happens in two ways: (1) through nerve impulses carried by the nervous system and (2) through chemical substances or hormones carried by the blood and lymph. The organs that secrete hormones are called endocrine glands, or glands of internal secretion. All together, these glands make up the endocrine system (Figure 20-1). This system includes the pituitary gland, thyroid gland, parathyroid glands, adrenal glands, pancreas, duodenum, testes, ovaries, and placenta. Sometimes the thymus gland and the pineal body are listed as part of the endocrine system. Endocrine glands are ductless; their secretions go directly into the blood or lymph and are then carried to all parts of the body. In this respect they are different from exocrine glands (glands of external secretion) such as salivary or sweat glands, whose products go through ducts that open onto a surface.

Of special importance are the hormones that affect the reproductive system. The gonads, accessory structures, and genitals of males and females are involved in reproduction and control sexual function and behavior (Figures 20-2 and 20-3). How these reproductive organs develop and function is under the control of hormones.

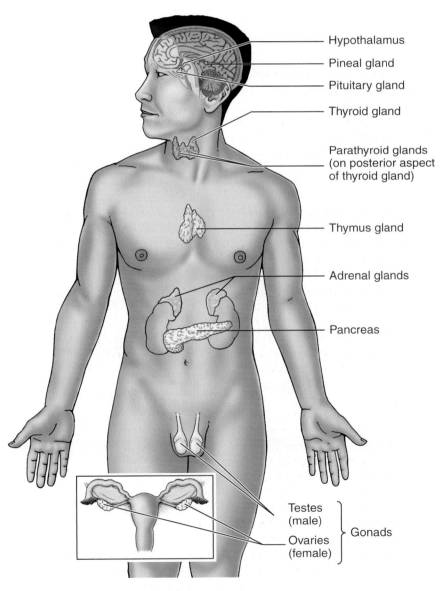

FIGURE **20-1** The endocrine system.

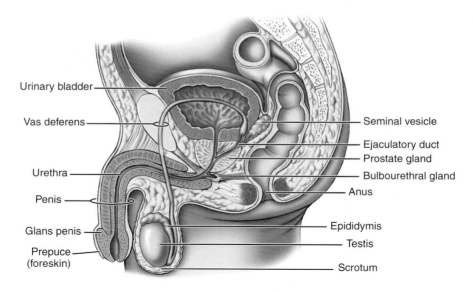

FIGURE **20-2** The male reproductive system.

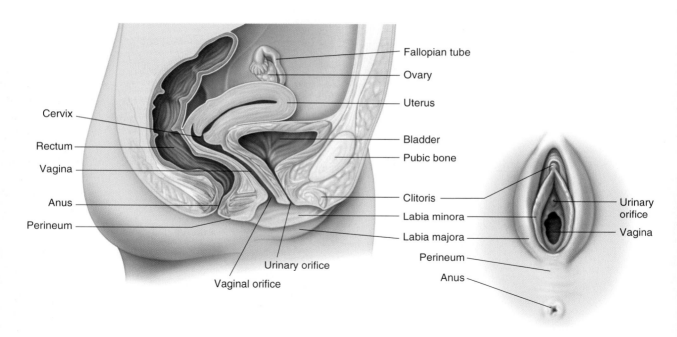

FIGURE **20-3** The female reproductive system.

SECTION ONE

Antidiabetic Drugs

OVERVIEW

Diabetes mellitus is a chronic disorder of carbohydrate (glucose) metabolism as well as abnormal fat and protein metabolism. With time, these abnormalities result in microvascular, macrovascular, and neurologic complications. Diabetes mellitus can be described as a catabolic state (a state in which the body breaks down complex compounds into simple substances) that is caused by a relative or absolute lack of insulin, insulin resistance, and impaired or insufficient target cell receptors. **Insulin** is the hormone necessary for the metabolism and use of glucose in the body and is produced by the beta cells of the pancreas. Insulin helps glucose move into fat and striated muscle cells by turning on a carrier system. The patient with diabetes mellitus has a pancreas that fails to produce enough insulin for the needs of the body.

When there is not enough insulin, glucose is not available for metabolism in the cell, and so it circulates unused and at high levels in the blood. The lack of insulin forces the liver to convert protein and fat to use for energy, increasing the amounts of fatty acids. Some of these fatty acids will convert to cholesterol; over time, this increases the development of atherosclerosis. Acutely, a lack of insulin can increase the production of free fatty acids and increase ketogenesis. Along with an increase in glucagon and other hormones, a decrease in pH can occur, resulting in ketoacidosis. If left untreated, ketoacidosis can result in death.

The two major types of diabetes are **type 1 diabetes,** formerly known as **insulin-dependent diabetes mellitus (IDDM)** or juvenile diabetes, and **type 2 diabetes,** formerly known as **non–insulin-dependent diabetes mellitus (NIDDM)** or latent-onset diabetes. Patients with type 2 diabetes usually have a pancreas that functions a little and that can be encouraged by medication to produce more insulin. Patients with type 1 diabetes usually have little or no production of insulin by the pancreas. These patients must take insulin to control the symptoms of diabetes mellitus. Insulin may also be necessary for some cases of type 2 diabetes, although diet, weight reduction, and oral hypoglycemic agents are usually effective in controlling symptoms.

Antidiabetic agents are used along with diet, exercise, and lifestyle changes to control blood glucose levels. These agents include insulin and five classes of oral agents.

INSULIN

ACTION

Insulin's primary effect is to lower blood glucose levels by helping glucose move into target tissues. Once insulin binds to and stimulates an insulin receptor, a series of reactions take place in the cell, making it easier for glucose to pass into the cell. In addition to its role in glucose control, insulin is also very important in fat metabolism. Adequate amounts of insulin inhibit lipoprotein lipase, thereby preventing the release of fatty acids into the blood. Insulin also promotes glucose transport and storage of glucose as triglycerides in fat cells. Thus, insulin is an anabolic hormone (one that converts simple substances into more complex compounds) that helps maintain stores of fatty acids, glycogen, and protein.

USES

Patients with type 1 diabetes do not produce enough insulin and must receive insulin to survive and prevent ketosis. This disorder is thought to be caused by an autoimmune T-lymphocyte attack on the beta cells of the pancreas, leading to destruction of the insulin-producing cells in the individual who has a genetic risk of diabetes.

In type 2 diabetes, tissues are insensitive to insulin and beta cell response to glucose is altered. This results in a lack of the circulating insulin that is needed by the body. Unlike in type 1 diabetes, ketosis is not likely to occur because some insulin is present. A nonketotic state with high osmotic pressure may occur in patients with infection or other underlying disease. Lack of tissue sensitivity to insulin, particularly in the muscles and liver, leads to hyperglycemia and insulin resistance. Therefore, higher levels of insulin are necessary to overcome the resistance.

The Diabetes Control and Complications Trial (DCCT) and the Kumamoto study clearly showed that intensively treated type 1 and 2 patients with diabetes had a delay in the onset and the progress of diabetic complications. The American Diabetes Association (ADA) consensus statement recommends treatment to produce glucose levels as close to normal as possible.

The best glucose control in type 1 diabetes can be reached with multiple insulin injections. Multiple injection programs have replaced the standard one-per-morning injection of intermediate-acting insulin or one-per-morning injection of mixed short- and intermediate-acting insulin. Open-loop insulin pumps or continuous subcutaneous insulin delivery devices now allow insulin to be delivered in much the same way as it would be in the nondiabetic patient. Over the last several years, various devices have also been developed to simplify insulin injection. However, the standard insulin syringe and vial of insulin are still used by most patients.

Insulin has been produced from various animal sources and by recombinant technology. Animal-source insulins are produced from the pancreas glands of cows and pigs. Synthetic human insulin is prepared using a nonpathogenic strain of *Escherichia coli* bacteria or *Saccharomyces cerevisiae* fungus. As of 1999, only pure pork insulin and synthetic insulin have been produced. The advantage of using synthetic human insulin or purified pork insulin is a decrease in the production of antibodies in the diabetic patient. In addition, there is a lower risk of developing **lipodystrophy,** or shrinkage and loss of the fatty tissue when insulin is given in the same spot too frequently. Human insulin is also now less expensive than animal-source insulin. However, substituting human insulin is not required when successful treatment has already been achieved with pork insulin.

Lispro, a rapid onset short-acting insulin, was introduced in the 1990s. This insulin analogue has a more rapid onset and shorter duration of action than regular insulin and provides an insulin with action more like that produced by the body.

Patients with type 2 diabetes may require insulin because of oral antidiabetic agent failure or to give an additional glucose-lowering effect when oral agents alone are not adequate. Insulin is also used in patients with type 2 diabetes if the patient has oral agent allergies or liver or renal dysfunction or is pregnant or contemplating pregnancy. Most patients with type 2 diabetes can be successfully treated with oral antidiabetic medications for years.

ADVERSE REACTIONS

Adverse reactions to insulin include lipodystrophy; local itching, swelling, or erythema (redness or irritation) at the injection site; and symptoms of insulin allergy or resistance. The most important adverse reaction is **hypoglycemia** (serum glucose levels <60 mg/dL), which is caused by taking too much insulin. Symptoms of hypoglycemia include sudden onset of nervousness; hunger; malaise (weakness); cold, clammy, skin; lethargy (sleepiness); no urine glucose or acetone; pallor (paleness); diaphoresis (sweating); change in level of consciousness (awareness and ability to respond); and shallow respirations.

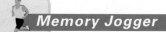

Memory Jogger

Hypoglycemia

Hypoglycemia may develop, especially with insulin overdosage, increased work or exercise, skipping a meal or eating the meal later than usual, or an illness associated with vomiting, diarrhea, or delayed digestion. Meals must be timed with respect to the activity of the insulin (i.e., onset, peak, and duration).

If the patient does not take enough insulin or does not take it on a regular schedule, **hyperglycemia** (fasting blood glucose levels >150 mg/dL) may develop. Signs of hyperglycemia include glycosuria and ketonuria (abnormal amounts of glucose and ketone bodies in the urine), Kussmaul's respiration (deep, rapid sighing breaths), tachycardia (rapid heartbeat), and acetone breath (fruity odor to the breath).

DRUG INTERACTIONS

Insulin needs may be increased by insulin antagonists such as oral contraceptives, corticosteroids, epinephrine, and preparations used for thyroid hormone replacement therapy. Thiazide diuretics may elevate glucose levels. A variety of other drugs, alcohol, and anabolic steroids may increase the hypoglycemic effects of insulin. Insulin promotes the movement of potassium into cells and lowers the serum potassium levels. Propranolol can mask the signs and symptoms of hypoglycemia.

Nursing Implications and Patient Teaching

Assessment

A patient whose diabetes mellitus was not previously diagnosed or is poorly controlled or out of control may have a history of polyuria (excretion of a large amount of urine), polydipsia (excessive thirst), polyphagia (excessive uncontrolled eating), weight loss, blurred vision, and fatigue. In severe cases of hyperglycemia, the patient may develop **systemic acidosis**, a condition in which the basic fluid and electrolyte balance of the body is disturbed and the blood pH is decreased. Symptoms of systemic acidosis include nausea, vomiting, and changes in level of consciousness.

You should ask the patient about signs of pregnancy, infection, and kidney, liver, or thyroid disease, because these conditions will alter the requirement for insulin. The patient should be asked about any earlier sensitization (allergy to a foreign protein) to beef or pork and whether the patient is taking other drugs that may interact with insulin.

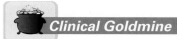

Clinical Goldmine

Patients Taking Insulin

In patients taking insulin, you should look for a history of hypoglycemia: sudden onset of nervousness; hunger; malaise; cold, clammy sweat; lethargy; serum glucose levels less than 60 mg/dL; no urine glucose or acetone; pallor; diaphoresis; change in level of consciousness; and shallow respirations. These symptoms are relieved by having the patient eat or drink a source of fast-acting sugar. You may also see signs of hyperglycemia: elevated fasting blood glucose levels (greater than 150 mg/dL), glycosuria, ketonuria, Kussmaul's respiration, tachycardia, and acetone breath.

Diagnosis

What other needs does the patient have? Weight loss, nutrition, knowledge? What other diseases does this patient have that might influence the therapy for diabetes?

Planning

The successful management of diabetes mellitus depends on the patient understanding about her disease. Control and maintenance require that the patient know about the nature of the disease, her diet and the need for weight control, and the importance of hygiene and exercise. The patient must understand how to do blood and urine testing, and how to correctly draw up and inject insulin. She must know the signs and symptoms of hypoglycemia and hyperglycemia and the appropriate actions to take for each, as well as procedures to follow on days when she is ill.

The patient should be shown the proper injection technique, including drawing up, injection, and storage of insulin. You should ask the patient to demonstrate to you that he knows how to give the injection.

The patient should be taught about rotation of injection sites to prevent lipodystrophy. Although use of human insulin has reduced the incidence of lipodystrophy, all patients should be encouraged to rotate injection sites regularly to help with absorption (see Figure 10-15).

It may be preferable to have patients use prefilled insulin cartridges and syringes that automatically dispense standard dosages if their vision is bad or they have difficulty understanding. Routine follow-up and evaluation of injection technique is important. The patient should be asked to give you a demonstration of the technique periodically as she makes return visits to the clinic or office.

Clinical Landmine

Errors in Insulin Administration

Errors in insulin administration are common among diabetic patients. Review the patient's technique regularly.

Patients must also be taught how to test their blood glucose level using a **glucometer** (hand-held testing machine). Have the patient practice pricking his finger or skin, placing the blood drop in the machine, and accurately interpreting the results according to the requirements of the equipment being used. You should provide a booklet or chart in which the patient can record his findings. Information on times when the blood should be tested for glucose should be given to the patient as part of written instructions. Times to test blood glucose may vary based on the type of medication taken and the degree of control required.

Individuals with cerebral vascular disease, coronary disease, or advanced complications may be at higher risk of hypoglycemia and may not benefit from tight glucose control. In general, the goal for the fasting blood sugar (FBS) is less than 120 mg/dL.

The goal for the bedtime glucose level is 100 to 140 mg/dL. Treatment adjustment should occur if the glucose is less than 100 mg/dL or greater than 160 mg/dL. The goal is to keep the hemoglobin (Hb) A_{1c} level around 7%, which is equivalent to a blood glucose level of 150 mg/dL. The blood glucose level goes up by about 30 points for every 1% increase of the Hb A_{1c} (for example, 8% = 180 mg/dL; 9% = 210 mg/dL).

Clinical Landmine

Insulin Dosage Adjustment

Dosage adjustment should occur if the FBS is less than 80 mg/dL or greater than 140 mg/dL.

Insulin allergy (transient local itching, swelling, and erythema at the injection site) commonly develops when therapy is started, particularly with beef and pork insulin. Use of Humulin insulin has decreased this problem. Insulin resistance (requirements of more than 200 units of insulin per day) is rare and may be caused by infection, inflammatory diseases, obesity, or stress. You should closely monitor the patient with insulin resistance who is being treated with a concentrated insulin injection to make sure that hypoglycemia is avoided. Long-acting insulins are not adequate in the treatment and management of acidosis and emergencies.

Administration of insulin by an aerosol inhaler is under investigation. This would allow some diabetic patients to give up injections.

Implementation

Techniques for calculation of insulin dosage, preparation of injection, mixing of insulin types, injection sites, and injection technique are all presented in Chapter 10. Refer to this material to review this information.

Insulin is a protein and therefore is inactivated by gastrointestinal (GI) enzymes. Thus insulin is generally given subcutaneously and timed so that it is available in the body when the glucose level rises after eating. The time of administration also depends on the type of insulin preparation. Only regular insulin can be administered intravenously (IV), as is done during ketoacidosis or diabetic coma.

All insulin chemically begins as regular insulin. Various substances such as protamine or zinc may be added to delay insulin absorption or turn it into a suspension. The different insulin preparations, with different onsets, peaks, and durations of action, are required so that patients can individualize their treatment. Premixed insulin products are also available as combinations of neutral protamine Hagedorn (NPH) and regular insulin in ratios of 70/30, 30/70, and 50/50. Information about these products is summarized in Tables 20-1 and 20-2.

Insulin dose depends on the patient's response. The dosage should be gradually increased or decreased (titrated) to get the best response with the lowest dosage. Generally, the minimal goal of therapy is to avoid extremes of ketoacidosis and hypoglycemia.

The individual presenting with ketones in the blood must be started on insulin. The goal of therapy is to maintain blood glucose levels as follows: fasting, 90-130 mg/dL; 1 hour after eating (postprandial), <18

Table 20-1

Comparison of Action of Insulin Preparations

SPECIES	ONSET	PEAK	DURATION	PRODUCT
SHORT ACTING/RAPID ONSET				
Human	15 min	30-90 min	≤5 hr	Lilly Humalog
SHORT ACTING (REGULAR)				
Animal	½-2 hr	3-4 hr	6-8 hr	Lilly Iletin II Regular Novo Nordisk Purified Pork Regular
Human	½-1 hr	2-3 hr	4-6 hr	Lilly Humulin R Novo Nordisk Novolin R Velosulin BR
INTERMEDIATE ACTING (LENTE "L")				
Animal	4-6 hr	8-14 hr	20-24 hr	Lilly Iletin II Lente Novo Nordisk Purified Pork Lente
Human	3-4 hr	4-12 hr	16-20 hr	Lilly Humulin L Novo Nordisk Novolin L
INTERMEDIATE ACTING (NPH "N")				
Animal	4-6 hr	8-14 hr	20-24 hr	Lilly Iletin II NPH Novo Nordisk Purified Pork NPH
Human	2-4 hr	4-10 hr	14-18 hr	Lilly Humulin N Novo Nordisk Novolin N
LONG ACTING				
Human	6-10 hr	Minimal	0-30 hr	Lilly Humulin U
Human	4-8 hr	4-24 hr	36 hr	Protamine Zinc (PZ)
Human	4-8 hr	10-30 hr	>36 hr	Extended Zinc (Ultralente)
Recombinant human analogue	1 hr	None	24 hr	Glargine (Lantus)

CATEGORY	DESCRIPTION OF ACTIVITY	PRODUCT
COMBINATION PRODUCTS		
Humulin 30/70 (NPH, 30 units; regular 70, units)	Provides rapid activity onset within ½ hr with duration of up to 24 hr	Lilly, Novo Nordisk
Humulin 50/50 (NPH, 50 units; regular, 50 units)	Provides rapid activity onset within ½ hr with duration of approximately 24 hr	Lilly, Novo Nordisk
Humulin 70/30 (NPH, 70 units; regular, 30 units)	Provides rapid activity onset within ½ hr with duration of up to 24 hr; maximal effect is within 4-8 hr	Lilly, Novo Nordisk

Table 20-2

Insulin Dosage Regimens

REGIMEN	TYPE OF INSULIN USED	TIME ADMINISTERED WITH EXPECTED TIME-ACTION CURVE*	ADVANTAGES	DISADVANTAGES
I. Single dose	Intermediate insulin (I)	(curve) 7 AM (I), Noon, 6 PM, Midnight, 7 AM	One injection should cover noon and PM meal; hypoglycemia during sleep is not a problem	No fasting, breakfast, or nighttime coverage of hyperglycemia
II. Split-mixed dose	Intermediate insulin (I) and regular insulin (R)	(curve) 7 AM (I + R), Noon, 6 PM, Midnight, 7 AM	Two injections provide coverage over 24-hr period	Two injections required; "locks" patient into set meal pattern
III. Split-mixed dose	Intermediate insulin (I) and regular insulin (R)	(curve) 7 AM (I + R), Noon, 7 PM (R), 9 PM (I), Midnight, 7 AM	Three injections provide coverage over 24 hr, particularly over early AM hours	Three injections required; evening intermediate insulin dose may potentiate early morning hypoglycemia
IV. Multiple dose	Regular insulin (R) and intermediate (I) insulin	(curve) 7 AM (R), Noon (R), 7 PM (R), 9 PM (I), Midnight, 7 AM	Allows more flexibility in meal times and amount of food intake	Four injections required; requires before-meal blood glucose checks; requires establishing and following individualized regimen; tighter control may predispose to hypoglycemia
V. Multiple-dose (insulin delivery via the pump is similar to this regimen)	Regular insulin (R) and longest acting insulin (LA)	(curve) 7 AM (R) + (LA), Noon (R), 7 PM (R), Midnight, 7 AM	Provides insulin delivery pattern that more closely simulates normal endogenous insulin pattern; allows for some flexibility in food-intake pattern	Requires three or four injections plus blood glucose checks before meals and on retiring; requires establishing and following individualized algorithm; tight control may predispose to hypoglycemia
VI. Long acting	Glargine (constant small surge from 7 PM through the night to 7 PM the next day)	(curve) 7 AM, Noon, 7 PM, Midnight, 7 AM, 7 PM	Provides a pattern that closely simulates normal endogenous insulin production	Cannot be mixed with other types of insulin

*Solid lines indicate short-acting insulin; dashed lines indicate long-acting insulin.

mg/dL; and 2 hours postprandial, <150 mg/dL. There are a variety of recommendations for how insulin might be given daily to achieve these goals:

1. Give daily doses of short-acting or ultra-short-acting insulin before meals based on carbohydrate counting: 1 unit of insulin per 10-15 gm of carbohydrate content initially (adjust ratio up or down as needed for each patient). Give a split dose of long-acting insulin (ultralente) before breakfast and before dinner, with the dose (= [0.5 × patient's weight in kg] ÷ 2) divided evenly between these two times.

2. Give daily doses of short-acting or ultra-short-acting insulin before meals based on carbohydrate counting: 1 unit of insulin per 10-15 gm of carbohydrate content initially (adjust ratio up or down as needed for each patient). Give a single dose of insulin glargine (Lantus) at nighttime (dose = [0.5 × patient's weight in kg] ÷ 2).

3. Combine short-acting or ultra-short-acting and intermediate-acting (NPH) insulin as follows:
   - Before a meal, give short-acting or ultra-short-acting insulin based upon carbohydrate counting as described earlier
   - Calculate total daily dose of NPH (= [0.5 × patient's weight in kg] ÷ 2)
   - Give one half of NPH dose at nighttime
   - Divide the remaining half of the NPH dose evenly among the three meals and give before each meal with short-acting or ultra-short-acting insulin

The insulin vial in use may be stored outside of the refrigerator for 1 month, provided it does not get extremely hot or cold. An extra supply of insulin should be stored in the refrigerator. Insulin should be warmed to room temperature for use because the injection of cold insulin may irritate the tissues. The expiration date on the bottle should be checked regularly to make sure the insulin is not too old to use safely.

Rapid-acting insulin is used during treatment of ketoacidosis and in other acute situations (infection, surgery) when the patient's food intake is variable. It is also used in combination with longer acting insulins to achieve greater control. Regular insulin may be used in divided dose therapy. The dosage is determined by the level of blood glucose. Long-acting insulin is used primarily for patients whose blood sugar level is constantly high at night.

For insulin suspensions, the vial is gently rolled and tipped from end to end before the insulin is drawn up so that any particles that may have settled out are returned to suspension. Vigorous shaking may result in air bubbles that can make it difficult to accurately draw the insulin. Shaking also breaks down protein molecules in the insulin.

Most diabetic patients can control their symptoms with 40 to 60 units of insulin per day. Occasionally a patient develops resistance to the insulin or becomes so unresponsive to insulin that several hundred or even thousands of units of insulin may be necessary. Patients who require dosages in excess of 300 to 500 units often have impaired insulin receptors. Concentrated insulin injection allows a higher dosage to be given in a smaller amount of fluid. Each milliliter of the concentrated insulin contains 500 units of purified pork, rather than the 100 units in the normal products. Glargine is an insulin product that provides a basal level of insulin for 24 hours.

Evaluation

The patient's response to the insulin dose is seen by testing the blood. The nurse, physician, or other health care provider should inform the patient about how frequently she should return for checkups, what blood levels are being found at these visits, and what the desired levels should be. The patient must be encouraged to take responsibility for managing her own disease.

The plan of insulin therapy is to keep blood glucose levels within specific limits and to prevent symptoms of hyperglycemia and hypoglycemia. Patients with home glucometers should be told when to check their blood glucose level, depending on the type of insulin they are taking. Urine ketones should be measured during acute illness or periods of increased glycosuria and in ketosis-prone diabetic patients. The records the patient keeps will provide information regarding control between office visits and should be taken to each visit with the health care provider.

If hypoglycemia occurs, the patient should be taught to eat some form of carbohydrate immediately. The family should also be involved in patient teaching about therapy for hypoglycemia. If the patient is unconscious, honey or Karo syrup may be put under the tongue or on the buccal mucosa in the mouth. Additional carbohydrates, such as bread, crackers, or milk, should be provided for the next 2 hours, or a sandwich should be eaten if a snack or meal would not be regularly eaten within an hour. Glucagon may be administered by a family member or a care provider.

The **Somogyi effect** (rebound elevation of glucose levels brought on by hypoglycemia) can lead to overtreatment of the patient with insulin when less insulin is actually needed. Patients older than 60 years of age are often sensitive to hypoglycemia. They should be observed for confusion and abnormal behavior because repeated episodes of hypoglycemia may cause brain damage.

Patient and Family Teaching

You should tell the patient and family the following:

1. The patient should keep on a diet (regular meals, snacks, and caloric requirements) and maintain an ideal body weight to promote glycemic control and prevent hypoglycemia.

2. The patient must know the signs and symptoms of hypoglycemia (too little sugar) and hyperglycemia (too much sugar), their causes, prevention, and treatment. The patient should notify the nurse, physician, or other health care provider if any of the symptoms occur.

3. Pork or beef insulin can cause an increase (hypertrophy) or a decrease (atrophy) in the size of fatty tissue when injected into the same site frequently. A plan for rotation of insulin injection sites should be developed, followed, and recorded.

4. The patient must use the proper syringe and the correct type, strength, and dose of insulin to avoid dosage errors.

5. The patient should avoid drinking alcohol because it can intensify the hypoglycemia produced by insulin, causing blood glucose levels to fall too low.

6. The patient's blood glucose levels can be measured by daily blood testing. The patient should be taught the proper technique for testing, recording, and interpreting the results. This will help the patient and the nurse, physician, or other health care provider manage the disease successfully.

7. Insulin requirements increase when the patient is under stress or becomes ill, especially with an infection. The patient must faithfully test the urine or blood when ill and must not stop taking insulin. The patient may take a liquid diet if he has an upset stomach, nausea, or vomiting. The nurse, physician, or other health care provider should be contacted for information on how to adjust the insulin dosage.

8. The patient must be prepared for emergency situations by:
   a. Carrying a medical identification card.
   b. Wearing a Medic Alert bracelet or necklace.
   c. Carrying a readily available source of sugar at all times.

9. When traveling, patients should carry an extra supply of insulin, syringes, and needles in a separate container that they keep with them in case they cannot get to their luggage. Patients will need to make adjustments for time zone changes to avoid hypoglycemia.

10. The patient should be alert for hypoglycemia when driving, operating machinery, or engaging in activities that require alertness.

ORAL HYPOGLYCEMICS

ACTION

The primary action of the **oral hypoglycemics** is to stimulate insulin release by the beta cells of the pancreas. Therefore, the patient must have some functioning beta cells if these drugs are to work. These products also increase the peripheral use of insulin and influence other fat and carbohydrate processes.

USES

The number of oral antidiabetic agents has dramatically increased since the 1980s. There are now five classes of oral agents. They can be used in monotherapy (therapy with one drug) or combined oral agent therapy, or can be combined with insulin to achieve the optimal (best) glucose control in patients with type 2 diabetes. The first available class of oral agents was the sulfonylureas. Sulfonylureas lower serum glucose levels by increasing beta cell insulin production and, to a lesser extent, by decreasing insulin resistance. In the early 1980s, a second generation of sulfonylureas became available and over time these have replaced the first-generation sulfonylureas. Second-generation sulfonylureas are approximately 1000 times more potent than first-generation agents. Unlike first-generation oral agents, which bind to ionic and nonionic sites, second-generation agents bind only to nonionic sites. This type of binding usually results in fewer interactions with other medications. The major side effect of sulfonylureas is hypoglycemia. These drugs can be used as monotherapy or in combination with insulin, acarbose, or metformin.

The second class of oral agents that became available was the biguanides. The only drug in this class that is now available in the United States is metformin. Metformin use is associated with a very small risk for lactic acidosis, usually in patients who may also have some renal dysfunction. This class of medication lowers glucose levels by decreasing glucose production in the liver, decreasing insulin resistance, and slowing the absorption of glucose from the intestines. As monotherapy, metformin generally does not cause hypoglycemia. Metformin can be used in combination with insulin, sulfonylureas, repaglinide, or acarbose.

Alpha-glucosidase inhibitors became available in the 1990s. Acarbose, currently the only drug available in this class, lowers glucose by slowing the breakdown of polysaccharides into simple sugars. As monotherapy, it cannot cause hypoglycemia. It can be used with sulfonylureas, insulin, or metformin.

The newest oral agent class, the meglitinides, was released in 1998. The drug repaglinide, although chemically unrelated to the sulfonylureas, works by stimulating the release of insulin from the beta cells of the pancreas. Its use can result in hypoglycemia. It can be used as monotherapy or in combination with metformin.

Research is under way for a new class of oral antidiabetic agents to be known as DPP-4 inhibitors. Several new drugs in this class are in clinical trials.

ADVERSE REACTIONS

Hypoglycemia is the most common adverse reaction. Allergic reactions manifested by urticaria (hives), ras pruritus (itching), and erythema may occur at the beginning of therapy and generally temporary. More common reactions to sulfonylureas include heartburn, nausea, vomiting, abdominal pain, and diarrhea caused by increased gastric acid secretion. Occasionally, sulfonylureas cause hepatotoxicity (damage to the liver) and cholestatic jaundice, with symptoms of jaundice (yellow color of skin, eyes, and mucous membranes), dark urine, and light-colored stools. Leukopenia, agranulocytosis, thrombocytopenia, hemolytic anemia, aplastic anemia, and pancytopenia have also been reported. There are rare reports of disulfiram-like reactions when alcohol is taken with tolbutamide. Lactic acidosis may rarely occur with metformin, and the risk is increased with the use of alcohol. Nausea, vomiting, diarrhea, flatulence, and anorexia are the most common adverse reactions with metformin; these problems tend to improve over time.

Clinical Landmine

Alcohol Consumption

Alcohol consumption with oral hypoglycemics may result in a violent disulfiram-like reaction.

DRUG INTERACTIONS

The hyperglycemic effects of the sulfonylureas and metformin are potentiated (made worse) by oral anticoagulants and various other drugs. Sulfonamide-type antibacterial agents and salicylates displace the sulfonylureas from protein-binding sites, which leads to high blood levels of the active drug. Barbiturates, sedatives, and hypnotics may have a prolonged effect when taken at the same time as the sulfonylureas because of a decreased rate of elimination from the body. Thiazide diuretics oppose the secretion of insulin from the beta cells and decrease the effectiveness of sulfonylureas. Many of these drugs, when used along with oral contraceptives that contain ethinyl estradiol and norethindrone, may decrease contraceptive effectiveness.

Nursing Implications and Patient Teaching

Assessment

You should try to learn as much as possible about the patient's health history, including what other drugs the patient is taking that may interact with the oral products, and if the patient is pregnant or has renal insufficiency, impaired liver function, or a history of ketoacidosis. Ask if the patient has any sensitivity (allergy) to sulfa drugs, because they may have cross-sensitivity to sulfonylureas (a patient who is sensitive to one type of sulfa drug may be sensitive to all types).

Diagnosis

Does patient have any other problems that would interfere with drug therapy? Problems with weight, nutrition, vision, finances? How compliant do you believe this patient will be with diet, exercise, medication, and testing requirements?

Planning

No transition period is necessary when a patient is switched from one oral hypoglycemic to another. Plan the teaching that will be necessary as you work with this patient.

Implementation

These products are administered orally. The duration of the hypoglycemic effect is the main difference between the various products. The duration of action, serum half-life, dosage range, and approximate doses per day are given in Table 20-3.

Evaluation

The patient's blood glucose levels should be monitored, and the patient should be watched for signs and symptoms of hypoglycemia.

Rashes may develop when sulfonylurea therapy begins, but they generally last only a short time. If they persist, the medication should be stopped. Cholestatic jaundice has been reported in a small number of patients on oral hypoglycemic therapy. Any liver damage that has developed generally goes away when the drug is stopped. Watch for any signs of blood dyscrasias, GI intolerance, or allergic reactions.

Patient and Family Teaching

You should teach the patient and family about diabetes, diet, and exercise, much as you would if the patient were starting to take insulin. Teach patients specifically about nutrition, blood testing, and general precautions to follow. In addition, you should tell the patient and family the following:

1. The patient taking oral hypoglycemic agents should report jaundice, dark urine, light-colored stools, fever, sore throat, fatigue, or any unusual bleeding or bruising to the nurse, physician, or other health care provider.
2. Allergic skin reactions may develop when oral hypoglycemic therapy begins. Red, raised rashes are generally brief and will disappear with continued drug therapy.
3. The patient should avoid drinking alcohol when taking these products because lactic acidosis or a disulfiram-like reaction, with severe nausea and vomiting, dizziness, headache, diaphoresis, and flushing (red color in the face and neck), may develop.

Table 20-3

Oral Treatment of Type 2 Diabetes

GENERIC NAME	TRADE NAME	DOSING RANGE	COMMENTS
SULFONYLUREAS			
glimepiride	Amaryl 1-, 2-, 4-mg tablets	0.5-8 mg daily	After reaching 2 mg/day, increase by no more than 2 mg at 1- to 2-wk intervals.
glipizide extended release	Glucotrol XL 5-, 10-mg tablets	5-20 mg daily	Premeal dosing not necessary.
glipizide	Glucotrol 5-, 10-mg tablets	2.5-40 mg	Divide daily doses >15 mg; take 30 min before meals.
glyburide	DiaBeta Micronase 1.25-, 2.5-, 5-mg tablets	1.25-20 mg	Can divide daily doses >10 mg; doses >10 mg may not further lower glucose levels.
micronized glyburide	Glynase Prestab 1.5-, 3-, 6-mg tablets	0.75-12 mg	Small particle size facilitates rapid absorption; can divide doses >6 mg.
BIGUANIDES			
metformin	Glucophage 500-, 850-mg tablets	500-2500 mg	Take with meals to decrease GI symptoms; avoid in liver and kidney disease; hold dose for contrast studies; lactic acidosis potential; called an *insulin sensitizer.*
ALPHA-GLUCOSIDASE INHIBITORS			
acarbose	Precose 25-, 50-, 100-mg tablets	25 mg daily to 100 mg 3 times daily	Take with the first bite of the meal; adjust dose at 4- to 8-wk intervals based on glucose level 1 hr postmeal; increase to 100 mg 3 times daily only if weight >60 kg; avoid in liver and intestinal disorders; treat hypoglycemia with glucose or lactose.
miglitol	Glyset	25 mg 3 times daily	Give medication with first bite of each meal. May be used as monotherapy or in combination therapy with a sulfonylurea.

Continued

Table 20-3

Oral Treatment of Type 2 Diabetes—cont'd

GENERIC NAME	TRADE NAME	DOSING RANGE	COMMENTS
THIAZOLIDINEDIONES			
rosiglitazone	Avandia	4 mg daily or 2 mg twice daily	May increase dosage to 8 mg daily. May be used as monotherapy or with existing dosages of sulfonylurea or metformin.
pioglitazone	Actos	15-45 mg daily	Give once daily without regard to meals. May be used with sulfonylurea, metformin, or insulin.
MEGLITINIDES			
repaglinide	Prandin 0.05-, 1-, 2-mg tablets	0.5-4 mg before meal to maximum daily dose of 16 mg	*Dosing:* up to 30 min before a meal; if meal is added or skipped, add or skip dose; if not previously treated or if hemoglobin A_{1c} <8%, start with 0.5 mg; if previously treated or A_{1c} ≥8%, begin at 1-2 mg before meals; the dose should be doubled, up to 4 mg before meals, until glucose goal is achieved.
nateglinide	Starlix	120 mg 3 times daily with meals	May be used as monotherapy or with metformin.

SECTION TWO

Selected Drugs Used with Pregnancy and Delivery

OVERVIEW

Medications used throughout the end of pregnancy and during delivery are a special category of drugs that is beyond the focus of this text. However, any drug used for the mother also affects the fetus, so paying special attention to drug use is required during the immediate delivery period. Therefore, a few of these products are selected for discussion. Excluding anesthetics, most drugs used during the antepartum (before), intrapartum (during), and postpartum (after birth) periods are given primarily for their effect on the uterus. These include tocolytics, oxytocics, uterine relaxants, and abortifacients. These products are used primarily to slow labor at the time of delivery or to help expel the fetus from the uterus to terminate pregnancy.

ACTION

Abortifacients stimulate uterine contractions and cause the uterus to empty. **Oxytocic agents** and ergot preparations cause the uterus to contract, helping labor move on to delivery. Oxytocin acts directly on the smooth muscles of the uterus, especially when the mother is at or near full term, to produce firm, regular contractions. They also act on the blood vessels to produce vasoconstriction (narrowing), and on the mammary gland cells in the postpartum phase to stimulate the flow of milk. Because these drugs are given so frequently, most of the information presented here is about oxytocics.

In contrast to abortifacients, oxytocin, and the ergots, the **uterine relaxants** act on the beta-adrenergic receptors to stop uterine smooth muscle contractions. **Tocolytics** are agents used to stop preterm labor. They generally act through uterine relaxation.

USES

Abortifacients are used early in pregnancy to end pregnancy by emptying the uterus. Oxytocics are used for a number of purposes:

- To stimulate or induce labor at term when there are medical problems threatening the life of the mother or fetus
- To assist in the delivery of the shoulder of the infant
- To assist in the release of the placenta
- To control postpartum bleeding or lack of muscle tone in the uterus
- To relieve breast swelling or engorgement caused by lack of lactation
- To stimulate uterine contraction after a cesarean section birth or other uterine surgery
- To treat incomplete abortion

The ergots are used to prevent or control hemorrhage after the delivery of the placenta and in the postpartum period.

Uterine relaxants and tocolytics are used when a mother goes into preterm labor and the goal is to delay delivery. Women who show signs of preterm delivery may be treated with a subcutaneous injection and then sent home on an oral maintenance dose. Magnesium sulfate, a common anticonvulsant, has some success as a tocolytic; however, it is not a first-line agent. It has also been used with ritodrine therapy, although with questionable efficacy and an increase in adverse reactions.

ADVERSE REACTIONS

Abortifacients may produce severe cramping and pain. Tocolytics often produce visual disturbances, malaise, nausea, and confusion. Oxytocin may produce dysrhythmias (irregular heartbeats), edema (fluid buildup in the body tissues), fetal and neonatal bradycardia (slow heartbeat), anxiety, redness of skin during administration, nausea and vomiting, anaphylaxis (shock), postpartum hemorrhage, cyanosis (blue color to the skin), and dyspnea (uncomfortable breathing).

In the appropriate dosage and in the absence of contraindications, the ergots are fairly safe. The most common adverse reactions are nausea and vomiting. Other, more unusual reactions include allergic reactions, bradycardia, hypotension (low blood pressure), hypertension (high blood pressure), or cerebral-spinal symptoms and spasms.

Excessive doses of oxytocics during labor can produce uterine hypertonicity (extreme muscle tension), spasm, and tetanic contractions and ruptures of the uterus. Smaller overdoses in labor yield a sustained, forceful contraction without rest. Overdosage with ergots during labor yields a similar reaction, with cardiovascular and GI symptoms progressing to more dangerous problems.

DRUG INTERACTIONS

Vasoconstrictors and local anesthetics increase the effects of oxytocics.

Nursing Implications and Patient Teaching

Assessment

It is important to determine the exact due date for delivery. The patient may be past the anticipated due date for the baby or have a history of engorged breasts. A history of incomplete abortion, cesarean section births, or excessive postpartum bleeding may require use of oxytocics or ergots. Finally, a patient may also want to terminate an unwanted pregnancy early in gestation.

Diagnosis

What additional problems might this patient have? Is there unreasonable anxiety or fear associated with the delivery? Does the mother have concerns about the health of the child? Have previous experiences been positive? What other medical conditions might make this delivery more risky?

Planning

The uterine contractions produced by oxytocics should be about the same as those of spontaneous, normal labor.

There are numerous precautions or contraindications to the use of oxytocics. These medications must be given by qualified nurses under the direct supervision of physicians or other health care providers. Inappropriate use of either oxytocic or ergot preparations has caused fetal and maternal death or injury, subarachnoid hemorrhage, and uterine rupture.

Implementation

Oxytocin is the drug of choice to cause or induce labor in many areas of the country. However, prostaglandins are now preferred in some regions. These are usually given by IV infusion pump.

Ergonovine is now the drug of choice to control postpartum bleeding. It can be given sublingually, intramuscularly (IM), or IV in emergency situations. Methylergonovine is the synthetic homologue of ergonovine and has been found to produce fewer vasoconstrictive or hypertensive side effects than ergonovine. It is noted that IV administration of either of these ergot preparations increases the danger of side effects.

A summary of drugs acting on the uterus is provided in Table 20-4.

Table 20-4

Drugs Acting on the Uterus

GENERIC NAME	TRADE NAME	COMMENTS AND DOSAGE
OXYTOCICS		
ergonovine	Ergotrate	Used to prevent or control postpartum hemorrhage secondary to uterine atony or subinvolution. Note similarity in names between ergotamine (used for migraines) and ergonovine; they are not the same, although they may be listed the same in some books. Protect the ampule from light, store in a cool place, and discard after 60 days. *Sublingual* (appropriate in nonemergency situations and for prophylaxis after leaving the labor and delivery suite): 200-400 mcg (0.2-0.4 mg) 2 to 4 times daily for 48 hr postpartum. *IM* (postpartum to facilitate uterine contraction and decrease bleeding): 0.2 mg.
methylergonovine	Methergine	Synthetic ergonovine produces stronger and more prolonged contractions. Protect vials from heat and light, and discard colored vials. Onset of action from IV is immediate; after IM, it is 2-5 min, and with PO it is 5-10 min. *IV:* 0.2 mg over a period of not less than 1 min with continuous blood pressure monitoring. *IM:* 0.2 mg not more often than every 2-4 hr or not more than a total of 5 doses. *PO:* 0.2 mg 3 or 4 times daily for a maximum of 1 wk
oxytocin	Pitocin Syntocinon	Used to induce or stimulate labor at term and secondarily in the stimulation of milk flow. It is the drug of choice in many areas of the country for medical induction of labor. Syntocinon is a synthetic derivative without the cardiovascular or vasopressor effects. The nasal form is useful for initial milk letdown. Never administer intravenously in undiluted form or in high concentrations. *To induce labor:* 10 units in 1 L D_5W or isotonic saline as an IV infusion. Initially give 1-2 milliunits/min. If no response within 15 min, gradually increase to a maximum of 20 milliunits/min. The total induction dose ranges from 600 to 12,000 milliunits, with the average being 4000 milliunits. *For postpartum bleeding:* 3-10 units IM after delivery of the placenta; or 10-40 units in 1 L isotonic saline IV at a rate to control the bleeding.
UTERINE RELAXANTS		
ritodrine HCl	Yutopar	Begin with 0.1 mg/min IV; increase based on patient response and follow with 10-20 mg q2-6h PO.
ABORTIFACIENTS		
carboprost	Hemabate	Initially, 250 mcg IM; then 250-500 mcg prn.
dinoprostone	Prostin E_2	1 suppository high into vagina; repeat prn.
mifepristone	Mifeprex	Patient takes three 200-mg tablets after reading and signing consent form. If abortion does not occur within 3 days, the patient is seen and must take 400 mcg misoprostol. Patient returns for examination 14 days later.
TOCOLYTICS		
magnesium sulfate	Magnesium Sulfate	Give 4-5 gm IM of a 50% solution q4h prn; or 4 gm of a 10%-20% solution not to exceed 1.5 mL/min of a 10% solution IV. Drug has a narrow therapeutic range of 4-7 mEq/L. Also used for treatment of preeclampsia and eclampsia conditions.
terbutaline sulfate	Brethine Bricanyl	Initiate IV administration at 10 mcg/min; titrate upward to a maximum dose of 80 mcg/min. Maintain IV dosage at the minimum effective dose for 4 hr. Oral doses of 2.5 mg q4-6h have been used as maintenance therapy until term.

Table 20-4
Drugs Acting on the Uterus—cont'd

GENERIC NAME	TRADE NAME	COMMENTS AND DOSAGE
AGENTS FOR CERVICAL RIPENING		
dinoprostone	Cervidil Prepidil	Use in pregnant women at or near term with a medical or obstetric need for labor induction. *10-mg gel insert:* Wash hands after handling product. Bring to room temperature just before administration. Physician should use aseptic technique to insert endocervical catheter and introduce gel into cervical canal. Patient should remain in supine position for 15-30 min to help retain fluid. May repeat after 6 hr if no response. Give IV oxytocin 6-12 hr after gel insertion as needed.

D₅W, 5% dextrose in water.

Evaluation

If oxytocin is used during induction of labor, the patient should be monitored for degree of contractions and the development of adverse reactions. The blood pressure and pulse should be checked frequently, and there should be continuous monitoring of the fetal heart rate. You should monitor the dilation of the cervix and the progression of contractions. Drastic increases in the frequency, force, and duration of contractions and in resting uterine tone may require the drug to be stopped. The contractions should not be over 50 mm Hg, the frequency should be no longer than every 2 minutes, and the duration should be no longer than 90 seconds. Both the mother and fetus should be monitored with internal monitoring equipment (fetal scalp electrode [FSE] and intrauterine pressure catheter [IUPC]).

You should watch for the symptoms of ergotism: vomiting; diarrhea; unquenchable thirst; tingling, itching, and coldness of the skin; a rapid, weak pulse; confusion; and unconsciousness.

Ergonovine might stimulate cramping. If this becomes too uncomfortable, either decrease the dosage or treat the symptoms.

The most common side effects of ergonovine are nausea and vomiting. These symptoms can sometimes be stopped if the patient is given a phenothiazine antiemetic.

If overdosage of an oxytocic occurs, producing a continuous contraction, the drug must be stopped immediately. It may be necessary to give a general anesthetic to relax the uterus, particularly if the fetus is threatened.

Patient and Family Teaching

You should tell the patient and family the following:
1. Oxytocics or ergots are given to augment the body's natural action during and after labor and delivery.
2. The patient will be watched continually throughout this treatment.
3. Contractions should not be more intense than normal contractions.
4. Ergonovine might stimulate cramping; if this becomes intense, the patient should inform the nurse or physician.

Pituitary and Adrenocortical Hormones

OVERVIEW

The pituitary, or "master" gland, lies in the sella turcica in the sphenoid bone in the skull and is connected to the brain by a slender stalk. This area is almost directly between the eyes in the middle of the brain. The anterior (front) portion of the pituitary, or the adenohypophysis, and the posterior (back) portion of the pituitary, or the neurohypophysis, produce hormones that control growth, metabolism, electrolyte balance, water retention or loss, and the reproductive cycle.

The adrenal cortex manufactures the **corticosteroid** and a small amount of the **sex hormones.** These hormones are substances that influence many organs, structures, and life processes of the body. The corticosteroid are composed of the glucocorticoids and the mineralocorticoids, and the sex hormones include the androgen and estrogens.

PITUITARY HORMONES

ANTERIOR PITUITARY HORMONES

Actions and Uses

The major anterior pituitary hormones include two gonadotropins: follicle-stimulating hormone (FSH) and luteinizing hormone (LH). They are called *gonadotropins* because they influence the gonads, which are the organs of reproduction. They influence the production of sex hormones, the development of secondary sex characteristics, and the pattern and regularity of the reproductive cycle. An additional anterior pituitary hormone, prolactin, stimulates the production of breast milk after childbirth.

There are a number of sources for gonadotropins that are used clinically. Human chorionic gonadotropin is taken from human placentas and contains FSH and LH. A purified form of FSH and LH, known as menotropins, is taken from the urine of postmenopausal women. These hormones may be given to produce ovulation in women with ovulatory failure, to stimulate production of sperm in men, or to assist in treatment when the testes have failed to descend into the scrotum. Clomiphene is a synthetic nonsteroidal compound that is also used to promote ovulation.

Somatotropic hormone (STH or somatotropin) and adrenocorticotropic hormone (ACTH or corticotropin) are also produced by the anterior pituitary. Somatotropin comes from human pituitary glands removed at autopsy. This hormone regulates growth during childhood and is given to children who have failed to grow because of a growth hormone deficiency. ACTH stimulates the adrenal cortex to produce and secrete hormones, primarily glucocorticoids. ACTH is used in diagnostic testing and in the treatment of some acute neurologic problems.

Adverse Reactions

Because all of these medications are hormones, their primary adverse reactions include systemic or local hormonal reactions. Menotropins may produce ovarian enlargement, blood inside the peritoneal cavity, and febrile reactions; when it is used to increase fertility, multiple births may be produced. Clomiphene may produce abdominal discomfort, ovarian enlargement, blurred vision, nervousness, and nausea and vomiting; vasomotor flushes (hot flashes) much like those seen in menopause may also occur. Chorionic gonadotropin may cause headache, irritability, restlessness, fatigue, and edema. Precocious puberty (onset of sexual development at an early age) may result from its use in treatment for undescended testes.

Somatotropin may provoke antibody stimulation in some individuals, resulting in failure of the drug to produce any growth. ACTH is involved with numerous adverse reactions because it stimulates the adrenal gland. A summary of the most commonly used types of ACTH is provided in Table 20-5.

POSTERIOR PITUITARY HORMONES

Action and Uses

The posterior pituitary gland produces the antidiuretic hormone (ADH) vasopressin, as well as oxytocin, a hormone that stimulates the uterus. Vasopressin regulates the reabsorption of water by the kidneys. This hormone is specifically released whenever the brain senses that the urine is becoming concentrated because the patient has had severe diarrhea or vomiting or has become dehydrated through some other condition.

Vasopressin may be given when the body loses water when it should not do so, as in diabetes insipidus, or when the pituitary fails to secrete vasopressin because of disease or surgical removal. Vasopressin is also used in

Table 20-5

Common Anterior Pituitary Hormones

GENERIC NAME	TRADE NAME	COMMENTS AND DOSAGE
corticotropin (ACTH)	ACTH Acthar	Very rapid absorption and use necessitates administration q6h to maintain desired production; use 20-100 units IM or subcutaneously.
corticotropin repository	ACTH-80 HP Acthar Gel	Slowly absorbed and can be administered in a single daily IM dose. *Adults:* 40-80 units IM q24-72h.
corticotropin zinc hydroxide	Cortrophin-Zinc	*Adults:* 40 units IM or subcutaneously q12-24h.
cosyntropin	Cortrosyn	Synthetic subunit of ACTH but exhibits all the pharmacologic properties of natural ACTH. Cosyntropin 0.25 mg is equivalent in action to 25 units natural ACTH and is less likely to produce allergies. • *Adrenocortical insufficiency testing:* 0.25-0.75 mg IM or IV; children younger than age 2 may respond to a dose of 0.125 mg.

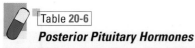

Table 20-6
Posterior Pituitary Hormones

GENERIC NAME	TRADE NAME	COMMENTS AND DOSAGE
desmopressin	DDAVP Stimate	Synthetic antidiuretic inhalant. Drug of choice in patients with mild to moderate diabetes insipidus. Offers prolonged antidiuretic activity without vasopressor or oxytocic side effects. Give 2.5-10 mcg in the evening. Note the effect and increase nightly by 2.5 mcg until satisfactory sleep duration is attained.
vasopressin	Pitressin Vasopressin tannate	Water-insoluble derivative of vasopressin that has a longer duration of action and is of use in long-term treatment of diabetes insipidus in children and some adults. *Adults:* 5-10 units (0.25-0.5 mL) IM or subcutaneously, 2 to 4 times daily; maximum 60 units.

some GI problems and in the treatment of nighttime bed-wetting. Pituitary extract is also given to increase smooth muscle contraction of the digestive tract and blood vessels. Information on vasopressin and desmopressin (DDAVP, the synthetic form) is provided in Table 20-6.

Oxytocin acts directly on the smooth musculature of the uterus to produce firm, regular contractions as described in Section Two of this chapter.

ACTH usually is reserved for testing and replacement therapy. ACTH stimulates the adrenal cortex to secrete cortisol, corticosterone, aldosterone, and several other weaker substances.

Adverse Reactions

Adverse reactions to small doses of vasopressin include abdominal cramps, anaphylaxis, bronchial constriction, circumoral pallor, diarrhea, flatus (gas in the intestine), intestinal hyperactivity, nausea, "pounding" headaches, sweating, tremors, urticaria, uterine cramps, vertigo (feeling of dizziness and spinning), and vomiting. Vasopressin given in larger doses may produce death.

ACTH use, particularly over a sustained period of time, is associated with substantial adverse effects of the cardiovascular, endocrine, GI, musculoskeletal, and ophthalmic systems. The patient must be monitored closely while using these products. Suddenly stopping the medication may worsen symptoms.

Drug Interactions

Oral antidiabetic agents, urea, and fludrocortisone increase the effects of vasopressin, and large doses of epinephrine, heparin, and alcohol decrease the effect. The antidiuretic effect of desmopressin is decreased by lithium, large doses of epinephrine, demeclocycline, heparin, and alcohol. The antidiuretic effect of desmopressin may be increased by chlorpropamide, urea, and fludrocortisone.

ACTH interacts with aspirin, anticholinesterases, diuretics, barbiturates, and hydantoins.

Nursing Implications and Patient Teaching

Assessment

You should learn all you can about the patient's health history to determine medication use and the presence of other diseases or conditions that would influence whether it is safe to use pituitary hormones.

Diagnosis

Patients needing anterior pituitary hormones often have many symptoms that must be dealt with while the primary problems are resolved. These patients often have emotional, financial, and physical problems. Diagnosing problems that bother the patient and helping take care of them will be important in meeting the long-term treatment goals for each individual.

Planning

There are no oral forms of pituitary hormones. They are given intramuscularly, subcutaneously, intravenously, or intranasally. Patients taking posterior pituitary products must be monitored closely. Additional doses may be required in times of stress.

Implementation

The dosages of desmopressin are individualized so that the patient has an adequate daily rhythm of water metabolism and adequate duration of sleep. Generally, the administration should be at the same time as polyuria or polydipsia and before sleep.

Even though vasopressin is given in an injection, the patient should drink one to two glasses of water at the time of administration to reduce the incidence of adverse effects.

Evaluation

You should monitor the patient taking ADH for a decrease in the frequency and the amount of urination, monitor the specific gravity of the urine, and watch for water intoxication or signs of dehydration.

Patient and Family Teaching

You should tell the patient and family the following:

1. The patient and family should meet regularly with the nurse, physician, or other health care provider. No medications should be stopped, or the dosage altered, without that person's knowledge and approval.
2. Patients taking ADH should measure fluid intake and the amount and specific gravity of their urine. They should keep accurate records that should be reviewed by the nurse, physician, or other health care provider.
3. The patient should be aware of the symptoms of water intoxication: drowsiness, listlessness, headache, and convulsions. The drug should be stopped and the nurse, physician, or other health care provider should be contacted at once if any of these symptoms develop. Signs of dehydration—failure to urinate, dry skin and mouth, complaint of thirst, and furrowed tongue—should also be reported.

ADRENOCORTICAL HORMONES

ACTION

The adrenal cortex manufactures glucocorticoids, mineralocorticoids, and small amounts of sex hormones. Hydrocortisone and cortisone are two of the many glucocorticoids produced by the adrenal glands. These hormones regulate glucose, fat, and protein metabolism and control the antiinflammatory response and the immune response system. The mineralocorticoids consist of aldosterone and desoxycorticosterone. These hormones work with others to maintain the fluid and electrolyte balance in the body. They conserve sodium and increase the elimination of potassium. They are used in replacement therapy for adrenal insufficiency.

USES

Glucocorticoids may be given in normal or physiologic doses for replacement of missing hormones in adrenal insufficiency (Addison's disease). They are more commonly given in pharmacologic doses to reduce inflammatory, allergic, or immunologic responses, and with antineoplastics to treat hematologic and malignant diseases. Examples of when glucocorticoids might be used are acute emergencies, allergic states, collagen diseases,

connective tissue disease, diagnostic testing of adrenocortical hyperfunction, edematous states, hematologic and neoplastic diseases, ophthalmologic diseases, respiratory diseases, and miscellaneous conditions such as acute Bell's palsy, chronic kidney disease, ulcerative colitis, and thromboembolic disease.

Local steroids might be used for intraarticular (into joints), soft tissue, or intrabursal (into bursae) problems, or for intralesional (into lesions) or subcutaneous dermatologic problems. Steroids might also be used topically for acute and chronic dermatoses, rectal problems, and some eye or ear problems.

ADVERSE REACTIONS

The side effects of systemic corticosteroids in pharmacologic doses are predictable exaggerations of the actions of the corticosteroids that are normally produced by the adrenal glands, or the results of reduced function of the hypothalamic-pituitary-adrenal axis. These are not benign drugs. Some adverse reactions are quite common; others are more unusual. Adverse reactions that might develop are listed in Table 20-7.

DRUG INTERACTIONS

Corticosteroids increase the effects of barbiturates, sedatives, narcotics, and anticoagulants. They decrease the effects of insulin and oral hypoglycemics, coumarin anticoagulants, isoniazid, aspirin, and broad-spectrum antibiotics. Drugs that increase the effects of steroids are indomethacin, aspirin, and oral contraceptives, especially estrogen. Drugs that decrease the effects of steroids include ephedrine, barbiturates, phenytoin, antihistamines, chloral hydrate, rifampin, and propranolol. Some drugs produce exaggerated side effects when given with steroids. These include alcohol; aspirin and antiinflammatory drugs; amphotericin B; thiazides and other potassium-wasting diuretics; stimulants such as adrenalin, amphetamines, and ephedrine; anticholinergics; and cardiac glycosides. Steroids also interfere with numerous laboratory tests.

Nursing Implications and Patient Teaching

Assessment

There are many contraindications and precautions to the use of these drugs. You should learn all you can about the patient's health history to determine if she has other diseases, is already taking other medications that might interact with corticosteroids, and if she might have an infection or be pregnant. You should also document the usual daily pattern of water metabolism and sleep duration.

Table 20-7

Adverse Reactions Associated with Corticosteroids

BIOLOGIC SYSTEM	POTENTIAL ADVERSE REACTIONS
Endocrine	Atrophy of adrenal cortex* (can occur after 10 days); anterior pituitary suppression; diabetes* (catabolism of fat, protein, glycogen, resulting in hyperglycemia); fluid/electrolyte imbalance* (from overlapping mineralocorticoid effect); hypokalemia; muscle cramps; irregular heart rate; redisposition of lipids* (moon face, buffalo hump, truncal obesity, striae, hirsutism, acne); and androgenic effects from sex hormones
Gastrointestinal	Gastritis,* peptic ulcer* (unrelated to local irritation of oral tablets); esophagitis; and pancreatitis
Immune	Absence of signs of infection*; uninhibited invasion and proliferation of virus, bacteria, fungus; and inhibition of fibroplasia with delayed wound healing
Musculoskeletal	Muscle wasting* (catabolism of protein) and osteoporosis
Neurologic	Mood changes (euphoria, insomnia, nervousness, irritability); mood swings (psychotic episodes, depression, exaggerated sense of well-being); and EEG changes
Ophthalmologic	Induces or aggravates glaucoma by decreasing aqueous outflow; cataracts; optic nerve damage; increased susceptibility to viral or fungal infection; and corneal perforation (when used in conditions that cause cornea to thin)
Vascular	Thrombosis, thromboembolism, thrombophlebitis, hypercholesterolemia, and atherosclerosis; these problems are especially prominent with cortisone
Miscellaneous	Hypertension; collagen tissue breakdown can activate latent TB by liberating organisms from deposits in pulmonary tissue; hypersensitivity reactions

EEG, Electroencephalogram; *TB,* tuberculosis.
*Most common potential adverse effects.

Diagnosis

Once a patient has started on glucocorticoids, there is a constant need to look for adverse effects, both physical and psychologic. You must be constantly aware of new symptoms that may represent pathology or disease.

Planning

Steroids come in many forms. Corticosteroids may be administered by the following routes: oral, inhalation, intranasal, intravenous, intramuscular, subcutaneous, intrabursal, intradermal, intrasynovial, intralesional, soft tissue injection, topical, and per rectum. Only corticosteroid preparations with specific labels should be used for ophthalmologic or otic administration.

Steroids that are used topically affect only a small part of the body. Steroids that are injected or taken by mouth affect the whole body—they have effects throughout the body's systems. Although glucocorticoids are highly potent drugs, short-term use of even very large doses is not likely to cause long-term problems. However, intermediate and long-term administration (longer than 6 days of systemic treatment) places the patient at high risk for a large number of serious adverse effects, and how much risk and how much benefit the patient will receive must be carefully considered. These medications stop production of steroids by the body, so if the medication is suddenly stopped, the body may be unable to function. The immediate and long-term effects of these drugs vary greatly and depend on the disease, the route of administration, dosage, duration, and frequency and time of administration.

Generic forms of the drugs are much less expensive than brand-name drugs. Generally, prednisone is considered to be the drug of choice to reduce inflammation and depress the immune system. It is recommended that antacids be taken with or between doses to help reduce the chance of peptic ulcer. Systemic corticosteroids are given orally, except in emergency circumstances or when the patient is unable to take oral medication. The onset of action is 2 to 8 hours, and the effect last for 24 hours. Oral corticosteroids are almost completely absorbed in the GI tract.

When corticosteroids are given orally to patients with functioning adrenal glands, the total dose should be taken first thing in the morning. This is the time when the adrenal glands are normally secreting the most hormones, so the corticosteroid dose will not cause problems with the body's feedback loop.

For conditions requiring a local injection, a single injection yields sufficient antiinflammatory effects to reduce symptoms in many cases. The slowly absorbed forms (acetate, diacetate, tebutate) of corticosteroid generally give relief for 1 to 2 weeks.

Implementation

Dosages vary a lot; the dose must be determined for each patient and each problem depending on the diagnosis, severity, prognosis, and estimated length of the disease. Patient response and tolerance must also be considered when deciding on dosage. Individuals may respond better to one form than another, but this is unpredictable. The general rule, regardless of route of administration, is to prescribe as high a dose as necessary initially to get a favorable response, then decrease the amount gradually to the lowest level that will maintain the therapeutic effect but not produce complications.

In systemic administration, dosage regimens are of two types: (1) physiologic, for replacement of glucocorticoids in adrenal insufficiency, and (2) pharmacologic, to reduce symptoms.

Corticosteroids cannot be stopped without tapering, or slowly reducing, the dose over time. Stopping the drug suddenly leads to steroid withdrawal syndrome, with symptoms of anorexia, nausea and vomiting, lethargy, headache, fever, joint pain, skin peeling, myalgia (widespread muscle pain), weight loss, and hypotension. Abruptly stopping the drug may also result in a rebound of symptoms of the condition being treated.

When corticosteroids are administered for longer than 1 to 2 weeks at pharmacologic doses, pituitary release of ACTH is stopped, and this causes secondary adrenocortical insufficiency. Patients undergoing physiologic, emotional, or psychologic stress may need additional support through larger amounts of steroids. This suppression of ACTH may last up to 2 years after the patient stops taking the drug.

During tapering to maintenance doses or to stop the drug, the patient must be watched carefully and taught the signs of adrenal insufficiency (malaise, hypotension, and anorexia [lack of appetite] are common, but many other symptoms may also occur). If these symptoms occur, or if the patient's disease flares up, the steroid dose is increased until symptoms go away. Tapering then begins again on a more gradual plan. After shorter steroid courses (1 to 2 weeks), the dosage is reduced by 0% each day. The same scheduled dose intervals are kept.

Table 20-8 provides a summary of adrenocortical hormones.

Evaluation

All patients receiving systemic corticosteroids should be watched carefully, and the dosage should be adjusted to reflect reduced or increased symptoms, the patient's response, and any periods of stress in the patient's life (injury, infection, surgery, and emotional crisis). Patients should be monitored for 1 or 2 years after high-dosage or long-term treatment. While receiving steroids, patients are usually given prescriptions that cannot be refilled to prevent unmonitored steroid use.

Corticosteroids hide infection and increase the patient's risk for infection. Corneal fungal infections are particularly likely to develop with extensive ophthalmologic corticosteroid use. Corticosteroids are particularly dangerous to use in patients with a history of tuberculosis, because the disease can be reactivated. Active psychologic disorders may be made worse, or hidden disorders may be made active, with long-term use because steroids affect mood. Long-term use may also produce osteoporosis, leading to vertebral collapse.

Although steroids are often used illegally in sports because they affect muscle size and strength, you can see how dangerous it would be to take steroids for a long time because of all the damage they can do to the body.

Patient and Family Teaching

You should tell the patient and family the following:

1. The patient will need to visit the nurse, physician, or other health care provider frequently to monitor progress during and after steroid therapy.
2. Nicotine raises the blood level of naturally produced cortisone; therefore, heavy smoking may add to the expected action.
3. Alcohol may enhance the tendency of steroids to cause ulcers. The patient should avoid alcohol during the course of therapy.
4. Steroids may decrease resistance to infection and the ability to tolerate stress, injury, or surgery (including dental surgery). The patient should inform the nurse, physician, or other health care provider or dentist or surgeon that a steroid is being taken.
5. The patient may need an increased dosage of steroids during times of injury, illness, or emotional or psychologic stress for up to 2 years after long-term treatment with steroids.
6. The patient and family should know the signs and symptoms of adrenal insufficiency. Malaise, weakness, hypotension, anorexia, nausea and vomiting, aching of bones and muscles, headache, increased temperature, and diarrhea are common, but many other symptoms may also develop. The nurse, physician, or other health care provider should be contacted immediately if any of these problems develop.
7. The patient must not stop taking the steroids suddenly. The body will slowly grow to depend on them and will not be able to survive well without them.
8. The patient should wear a Medic Alert bracelet or necklace or carry a medical identification card indicating that he is taking a corticosteroid during and after treatment.

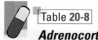

Table 20-8

Adrenocortical Hormones

GENERIC NAME	TRADE NAME	COMMENTS AND DOSAGE
GLUCOCORTICOIDS		
Short Acting		
cortisone	Cortone	*Initially:* 25-300 mg/day PO, 20-300 mg/day IM. • *Physiologic replacement:* 0.5-0.75 mg/kg/day PO; 0.25-0.75 mg/kg/day IM.
hydrocortisone	Cortef	*Initially:* 20-240 mg/day PO; dosage may be as low as 0.1 mg 3 times/wk.
hydrocortisone acetate	Hydrocortisone Acetate	For intralesional, intraarticular, or soft tissue injection only. Do not give IV. Give 5-37.5 mg depending on site.
hydrocortisone sodium succinate	Solu-Cortef	Give 100-500 mg IV or IM and repeat at 2-, 4-, or 6-hour intervals depending on patient response.
Intermediate Acting		
methylprednisolone	Depo-Medrol	40-120 mg IM.
prednisolone	Delta-Cortef	*Initially:* 5-60 mg/day PO.
prednisone	Meticorten	*Initially:* 5-60 mg/day PO.
triamcinolone	Aristocort	*Initially:* Aristocort.
triamcinolone diacetate	Aristocort Forte	40 mg/wk IM.
Long Acting		
betamethasone	Celestone	0.6-8.4 mg/day PO, IM, or IV.
dexamethasone	Decadron	*Initially:* 0.75-9 mg/day PO.
MINERALOCORTICOIDS		
fludrocortisone acetate	Florinef Acetate	Give 100-500 mg IV or IM and repeat at 2-, 4-, or 6-hour intervals depending on patient response.

9. The patient should not receive any immunizations without consulting the nurse, physician, or other health care provider first.
10. The patient should take oral medication with food to minimize stomach upset.
11. The patient may need to eat a diet rich in potassium and low in sodium. The nurse, physician, or other health care provider should give the patient a list of foods to eat and foods to avoid.
12. The patient should keep the tablets in tightly sealed, brown bottles away from heat.
13. The patient should tell the nurse, physician, or other health care provider if she becomes pregnant or begins to take medications from another health care provider, especially aspirin, diuretics, digitalis preparations, insulin, oral hypoglycemics, phenobarbital, rifampin, phenytoin, and somatotropin.
14. If the patient misses a dose:
    a. If the patient is on an alternate-day schedule, the dose should be taken as soon as possible, and the regular schedule should be followed. If the patient does not remember until the evening, the missed dose should be taken the next morning, the day after that should be skipped, and a new schedule should be started.
    b. If the patient is on a daily-dose schedule, the dose should be taken as soon as possible. If the patient does not remember until the next day, only the normal dose should be taken and the normal schedule should be followed.
    c. If the patient is on divided doses (taking medication more than once a day), the dose should be taken as soon as possible and the normal schedule should be followed. If the patient forgets to take his or her medication until it is time for the next dose, that dose should be doubled and then the patient should go back on the regular schedule.

15. Patients should call the nurse, physician, or other health care provider if they have rapid weight gain, black or tarry stools, unusual bleeding or bruising, or signs of hypokalemia (decreased potassium in the blood), including anorexia, lethargy, confusion, nausea, and muscle weakness.

16. It will be important to have frequent appointments to monitor therapy while the patient is taking this drug.

Sex Hormones

OVERVIEW

The sex hormones are produced under the influence of the anterior pituitary gland. The male hormone testosterone and its related hormones are called androgens; the female hormones are estrogen and progesterone. **Androgens** help to develop and maintain the male sex organs at puberty, and develop secondary sex characteristics in men: facial hair, deep voice, body hair, body fat distribution, and muscle development. They promote the anabolic or tissue-building processes in the body. Anabolic steroids are synthetic drugs with the same use and actions as androgens. These medications may be given as replacement therapy for testosterone deficiency. Androgen therapy may also be given to women as part of the treatment for estrogen-dependent inoperative metastatic breast carcinoma in patients who are past menopause. Androgens are also used to reduce postpartum breast pain and engorgement. Some postmenopausal women also use low-dose androgen therapy to treat a relative androgen deficiency. This helps reverse some of the masculinizing symptoms of menopause.

In addition to the two naturally occurring female hormones, estrogen and progesterone, there are also a number of synthetic estrogen and progesterone preparations. **Estrogen** is secreted by the ovarian follicle and the adrenal cortex. Estrogens help develop and maintain the female reproductive system and the primary and secondary sex characteristics in women. They also are part of the feedback system to the pituitary, providing signals for the release of the gonadotropins. Estrogens play a role in the fluid and electrolyte balance in the tissues, especially in relation to calcium. They are active in most of the tissue and muscular processes involved in for pregnancy and labor.

Progesterone is produced by the corpus luteum in the ovary, by the placenta, and in small amounts by the adrenal cortex. Progesterone is essential for the development of the placenta, and helps to maintain pregnancy once it occurs. It also helps to prevent pregnancy by inhibiting the pituitary gonadotropins that cause the ovarian follicle to mature in order to produce ovulation.

Estrogen, progesterone, and combinations of the two hormones are very effective as oral contraceptives. They prevent ovulation and cause a state that mimics pregnancy in the female.

ANDROGENS

ACTION

The main action of the androgens is to develop secondary male sex characteristics. Androgens are anabolic, increasing the building of tissue. Androgens are also antineoplastic when used to treat certain breast cancers in women. Erythropoiesis, or an increase in red blood cell formation, occurs with the administration of androgens.

USES

Androgens are used in hypogonadism, hypopituitarism, dwarfism, eunuchism, cryptorchidism, oligospermia, and general androgen deficiency in males. They are used to restore a positive nitrogen balance in patients with chronic, debilitating illness or trauma; in treatment of anemia secondary to renal failure and in other blood dyscrasias in which increased erythropoiesis is needed; for palliative therapy (therapy to treat symptoms in terminal cases) for advanced breast cancer in postmenopausal women; and for treatment of endometriosis in younger women. Androgens are also used to suppress milk production. They are commonly misused by body builders and athletes who wish to have bigger and stronger muscles.

ADVERSE REACTIONS

Adverse reactions to androgens include edema caused by sodium retention (usually only with large doses), acne, hirsutism (excessive body hair), male pattern baldness, cholestatic hepatitis with jaundice, buccal irritation, diarrhea, nausea, and vomiting. In women, androgens may produce clitoral enlargement and masculinization. In men androgens may cause a decrease in sperm count, excessive sexual stimulation, gynecomastia (enlargement of the breasts), impotence, and urinary retention. In children, use of androgens may produce precocious puberty. Children may also develop short stature because of premature bone epiphyseal closure.

DRUG INTERACTIONS

Anabolic steroids may increase the effects of anticoagulants, antidiabetic agents, and other drugs. Corticosteroids given at the same time as androgens increase the possibility of edema. Barbiturates decrease the therapeutic effects of androgens because of increased breakdown in the liver. Androgens may affect the results of many laboratory tests.

Nursing Implications and Patient Teaching

Assessment

You should learn as much as you can about the health history of the patient, including the presence of carcinoma; cardiac, renal, or liver dysfunction; other drugs the patient may be taking; and the possibility of pregnancy.

The male patient may have a history of impotence, reduced libido (sex drive), weight loss, male climacteric, or castration. There may be a history of traumatic castration or failure to develop secondary sex characteristics by 15 to 17 years of age.

Diagnosis

These patients often have other problems that you should diagnose and address. In addition to their medical problems, they often have great concern about their sexuality, body image, and self-esteem.

Planning

When androgens are given for hypogonadism, careful descriptions of secondary sex characteristics and measurements should be recorded for a baseline to monitor the therapeutic effects.

If cholestatic jaundice develops or liver function decreases, the drug should be stopped. Stomatitis (inflammation of the mouth) may result from buccal administration.

Implementation

Androgens can be given by mouth, buccally, and sublingually, depending on the specific drug and the reason for therapy. Dosages vary from 2 to 10 mg daily for replacement therapy. Higher divided doses are given for antineoplastic therapy.

Patients must be taught not to swallow the pill and not to eat, drink, or smoke or chew tobacco until the buccal tablet is absorbed.

Table 20-9 provides a summary of androgen products.

Evaluation

The therapeutic response may be slow, requiring 3 or more months to affect symptoms. You should monitor for the development of secondary sex characteristics and improvement in sexual functioning.

Patient and Family Teaching

You should tell the patient and family the following:
1. The patient should take this medication as instructed by the nurse, physician, or other health care provider.
2. Response to the drug may take several weeks or months.
3. The patient should eat a diet high in calories, protein, vitamins, and minerals unless otherwise instructed by the nurse, physician, or other health care provider.
4. The patient should report any new or troublesome symptoms that may develop. Men should report fluid retention, especially in the feet and hands; enlargement of breasts; shortness of breath; excessive physical or sexual stimulation; prolonged or painful erection of the penis; impotence; urinary retention; and jaundice. Women should report jaundice; fluid retention, especially in the feet and hands; shortness of breath; changes in vaginal bleeding; increased sex drive; and masculinization of appearance (signs of masculinization in women usually are reversed when the drug is discontinued).
5. If medicine is taken under the tongue (sublingually) or buccally (putting medicine in cheek), the patient should rinse the mouth and brush the teeth after taking medicine.

FEMALE SEX HORMONES

ESTROGENS

Action

Exogenous estrogens (those produced outside the body) aid in the development of both primary and secondary sex characteristics, including growth and development of the uterine musculature and endothelium, vaginal epithelium, and fallopian tubes; development of breasts; increased cervical mucus and decreased vaginal pH; increased uterine motility; growth of axillary and pubic hair; decreased long bone growth in prepubertal and pubertal girls; and decreased calcium loss from bones. Estrogens suppress the release of gonadotropins (FSH and LH) from the pituitary or hypothalamus through a feedback mechanism. Estrogens are anabolic and cause retention of salt, water, and nitrogen, an increase in serum lipoproteins and triglycerides, and a decrease in cholesterol. They suppress ovulation when given in adequate doses.

Uses

Estrogens are used for hormone replacement therapy in menopause or other conditions in which the natural estrogens are decreased, such as ovarian failure

Table 20-9

Androgens

GENERIC NAME	TRADE NAME	COMMENTS AND DOSAGE
danazol	Danocrine	Synthetic androgen is used to treat endometriosis, fibrocystic breast disease, and hereditary angioedema through suppression of pituitary gonadotropins and subsequent reduction in menstruation. • *Endometriosis:* 400 mg PO twice daily for 3-6 mo; may continue for 9 mo. Use only for those who cannot tolerate other drugs or who fail to respond; begin therapy during menstruation to rule out pregnancy. • *Fibrocystic breast disease:* 50-200 mg PO twice daily for 4-6 mo; begin during menstruation; use only when pain is severe.
fluoxymesterone	Halotestin	GI disturbances are more frequent with this product than with other oral androgens. • *Hypogonadism:* 2-10 mg/day PO. • *Breast cancer:* 15-30 mg/day PO in divided doses.
methyltestosterone	Android Testred Virilon	Patient should not drink, eat, or smoke or chew tobacco until tablet is absorbed buccally. Check mouth each visit for signs of local irritation. • *Male eunuchism:* 10-40 mg/day PO; 5-20 mg buccal. • *Androgen deficiency:* 10-40 mg/day PO; 5-20 mg buccal. • *Undescended testicle after puberty:* 30 mg/day PO; 15 mg buccal. • *Female breast cancer:* 200 mg/day PO; 100 mg buccal.
testosterone	Delatestryl	• *Male eunuchism:* Give 50-200 mg every 2-4 wk. • *Androgen deficiency:* Give 50-200 mg every 2-4 wk. • *Undescended testicle after puberty:* Give 50-200 mg every 2-4 wk. • *Female breast cancer:* Give 50-200 mg every 2-4 wk.
testosterone cypionate (in oil)	Depo-Testosterone	Give 200-mg injection every 2-4 wk.
testosterone pellets	Testopel	150- to 450-mg pellets given subcutaneously every 3-6 mo. Each pellet contains 75 mg of testosterone. Number of pellets to be implanted gradually increases as parenteral injection dosage decreases.
testosterone transdermal system	Androderm	Use 5 mg/day or 2 systems initially. Apply system at night to a clean, dry area of skin on the back, abdomen, upper arms, or thighs. Do NOT apply to scrotum. Wear patches for 24 hours. Test blood levels and titrate up or down through use of additional patch.
testosterone transdermal system	Testoderm	For primary or secondary hypogonadism. Start therapy with a 6-mg/day system applied daily. Place the patch on a clean, dry scrotal area. Wear 22-23 hr daily. After 3-4 wk of use, check blood levels 2-4 hr after applying patch. Patient should achieve adequate blood levels in 6-8 wk or shift to another form of therapy.
ANDROGEN HORMONE INHIBITOR		
finasteride	Propecia Proscar	Used in benign prostatic hyperplasia and prostatic carcinoma. Give 5 mg once daily. May require 6 mo of therapy or more. Also used in treating male pattern alopecia.

primary amenorrhea, and oophorectomy. They are used in infertility work-ups and for palliative therapy in prostatic cancer and in breast cancer that occurs at least 5 years after menopause. After many years of controversy, it has now been demonstrated conclusively that estrogens are effective for prevention of postmenopausal osteoporosis when used with other measures, but they do increase the risk for stroke, heart attack, and breast cancer. Estrogen-progestin combinations also seem to provide a decreased incidence of uterine cancer.

Adverse Reactions

Adverse reactions to estrogens include edema, hypertension, thrombophlebitis, depression, migraine headaches, skin rash, decreased glucose tolerance, intolerance to contact lenses, abdominal cramps, diarrhea, nausea, vomiting, breast tenderness and enlargement, changes in vaginal bleeding, worsening of estrogen-dependent malignancies, increase in size of uterine fibroids, vaginal candidiasis, and changes in weight and libido.

Drug Interactions

Rifampin and barbiturates may reduce the effects of estrogen. Estrogens may reduce the effects of oral anticoagulants, tricyclic antidepressants, anticonvulsants, and antidiabetic agents. They may potentiate antiinflammatory or glycosuric effects of hydrocortisone and the effect of meperidine. Estrogens alter the results of many diagnostic tests.

PROGESTINS

Action

Progestins cause the uterine endometrium to shed during menses after tissue growth stimulated by estrogen. They maintain the endometrium and vaginal epithelium and decrease uterine motility during pregnancy. Acting with estrogen, they cause the breasts to secrete milk and become more vascular. Some progestins have estrogenic or androgenic effects. Progestins suppress pituitary gonadotropins through a feedback mechanism. They can suppress ovulation, control uterine bleeding caused by hormonal imbalance, increase sodium excretion, and cause a negative nitrogen balance.

Uses

Progestins are used for contraception; control of excessive uterine bleeding caused by hormonal imbalance; treatment of secondary amenorrhea, dysmenorrhea, and premenstrual tension; and control of pain in endometriosis. They may be used in the diagnosis and treatment of infertility. They are also used as palliative therapy for endometrial cancer. When used for contraception, progestin-only preparations are known as "mini-pills."

Adverse Reactions

Adverse reactions to progestins include fluid retention; thromboembolic events, including pulmonary embolism; dizziness; headache; mental depression; rashes; decrease in glucose tolerance; weight gain or loss; cholestatic jaundice; diarrhea; nausea; vomiting; amenorrhea; breast tenderness or enlargement; decreased libido; galactorrhea; increased vaginal discharge; spotting; and withdrawal bleeding (bleeding that occurs when the drug is stopped). Overdosage produces changes in menses, nausea, vomiting, and withdrawal bleeding.

Drug Interactions

Progestins alter the results of several laboratory tests.

Nursing Implications and Patient Teaching

Assessment

For patients of prepubertal age, you should ask about primary amenorrhea and sexual infantilism. For women of childbearing age, ask about the possibility of pregnancy, history of ovarian failure, need for contraception, and dysmenorrhea. For patients of perimenopausal age, obtain a history of hot flashes, menstrual irregularities, dyspareunia, vaginal discharge, vulvar pruritus, urinary frequency, and history of oophorectomy or hysterectomy.

There is an increased dose-related risk of thromboembolic disease, especially in premenopausal women. Progestins should not be used during pregnancy, especially the first 3 months, because of the risk of congenital anomalies and of vaginal adenosis or vaginal or cervical cancer in female offspring when they reach childbearing age. There is an increased risk of gallbladder disease with long-term use. Postmenopausal estrogen therapy is associated with an increase in the risk of endometrial cancer of 5 to 15 times the normal risk; the level of risk is related to the length of treatment. Administration of estrogen may result in hypercalcemia in patients with breast or bone cancer.

Diagnosis

Based on the assessment, you must be prepared to diagnose and deal with other emotional or physical problems arising from estrogen or progestin use. As women go through their reproductive years, they have different concerns and physical problems. Determine age-related factors that may be of concern to the patient. Individualize therapy as much as possible.

Planning

Estrogen therapy affects many body systems. When estrogens are used before puberty, short stature and decreased growth can result. Use in adult women can increase the risk for migraine headaches, hypertension, diabetes, and certain benign and malignant tumors. Because estrogens are metabolized in the liver and excreted through the kidneys, renal or hepatic dysfunction can alter their actions. Fibroid tumors of the uterus may increase in size. Because fluid is retained, symptoms of hypertension, asthma, epilepsy, migraine, and heart or kidney dysfunction may be increased. Topical estrogens are readily absorbed and may have systemic effects.

Progestins are especially valuable in women who cannot take estrogen. Progestins often cause menstrual cycle changes, and patients must understand this before taking these drugs if they are to have a successful experience. These medications can be used for contraception in women who are breastfeeding.

Implementation

Estrogens can be given orally, intramuscularly, or topically. For control of menopausal symptoms, ovarian failure, or postoophorectomy symptoms, they are usually given in cycles of one tablet daily for 3 weeks, followed by 1 week off the drug. Usually, the lowest effective dose is given for the shortest period of time. High dose or long-term therapy should be tapered gradually.

Table 20-10

Estrogens and Progestins

GENERIC NAME	TRADE NAME	COMMENTS AND DOSAGE
ESTROGENS		
conjugated estrogens	Premarin	Contain 50%-65% sodium estrone sulfate and 20%-35% sodium equilin sulfate; these are naturally occurring and extracted from the urine of pregnant mares. Store in closed containers. Give 0.3-7.5 mg PO daily; medication should be given for 3 wk on a daily basis, with 1 wk off the medication.
esterified estrogens	Estratab Menest	These products contain 75%-85% sodium estrone sulfate and 6%-15% sodium equilin sulfate. Store medication in a tightly closed container. • *Vasomotor menopausal (natural or surgical) symptoms:* 1.25-3.75 mg PO daily. Adjust to lowest dose that controls symptoms.
estradiol	Climara Delestrogen Estrace Estraderm	• *Vasomotor menopausal symptoms, senile vaginitis, kraurosis vulvae, or replacement therapy in hypogonadism or female castration, ovarian failure:* 1-2 mg PO daily cycled 3 wk on and 1 wk off. Use lowest therapeutic dosage. Transdermal system: 0.05-mg patch 2 times/wk, increasing dose until symptoms resolve. May use 3-wk cycle on patch, 1 wk off.
estrogen vaginal creams	Estrace Estring Ogen Premarin	These preparations are used vaginally and on the vulva to treat atrophic epithelial changes related to low estrogen levels. Can be absorbed systemically and produce side effects. Most effective when used at bedtime. Contain various synthetic estrogens. Give 2-4 gm daily. Use applicator that is included, or rub on topically. Use lowest dose for shortest time that will control symptoms.
estrone	Kestrone 5	Give 0.1-1 mg IM weekly as replacement or to halt abnormal uterine bleeding as a result of hormonal imbalance.
estropipate or piperazine estrone	Ogen	This drug is composed of crystalline estrone and piperazine for stability. • *Prevention of postmenopausal osteoporosis, senile vaginitis, or vasomotor menopausal symptoms:* Cycle 3 wk on, 1 wk off with 0.625-5 mg daily. Use lowest dose that controls symptoms.
ethinyl estradiol	Estinyl	This is the most active synthetic estrogen known. • *Vasomotor menopausal symptoms:* 0.02-0.05 mg PO daily cycled 3 wk on, 1 wk off. Use decreasing doses as menopause progresses. Use lowest effective dose.
ESTROGEN AND PROGESTIN COMBINATION		
premphase	Prempro	• *Moderate to severe vasomotor symptoms associated with menopause, prevention of osteoporosis:* 0.625-mg/2.5-mg tablet once daily. • *Atrophic vaginitis:* Use vaginal cream 2-4 gm daily for 1-2 wk and then reduce dosage to 1 gm 1-3 times/wk.

Natural progestins are poorly absorbed orally; therefore, oral progestins are synthetic products. Tablets are given daily. Progestins are quickly metabolized in the liver, but daily doses are effective.

Table 20-10 presents a summary of estrogens and progestins.

Evaluation

The nurse should watch for adverse effects. Patients on replacement therapy should be monitored regularly. The nurse should watch for thrombophlebitis and edema in women and monitor men for changes that make them more feminine and impotent.

Timing and description of any vaginal bleeding should be noted to determine if response is therapeutic or adverse.

Patient and Family Teaching

You should tell the patient and family the following:
1. Estrogenic drugs, by law, must be dispensed with a patient package insert titled "What You Should Know About Estrogens." When the patient

Table 20-10

Estrogens and Progestins—cont'd

GENERIC NAME	TRADE NAME	COMMENTS AND DOSAGE
SELECTIVE ESTROGEN RECEPTOR MODULATION		
raloxifene	Evista	• *Osteoporosis prevention:* Give 60 mg daily.
PROGESTINS		
hydroxyprogester one in oil	Hylutin	• *Primary and secondary amenorrhea, dysfunctional uterine bleeding, metrorrhagia:* 375 mg IM.
medroxyprogeste rone acetate	Amen Curretab Cycrin Provera	Duration of action is long and somewhat variable. • *Secondary amenorrhea, abnormal uterine bleeding caused by hormonal imbalance:* 5-10 mg PO daily for 5-10 days, beginning on 16th or 21st day of menstrual cycle. Maximum therapeutic effect will be noted with 10 mg/day for 10 days beginning on 16th day of cycle. Withdrawal bleeding should occur 3-7 days after last dose.
megestrol acetate	Megace	Used for appetite enhancement in AIDS patients and for palliative treatment of advanced carcinoma of the breast or endometrium.
norethindrone	Micronor Nor-QD Ovrette	This medication represents the only ingredient in some "mini-pill" contraceptives. Take with meals to reduce nausea. Store in a closed container. • *Amenorrhea or uterine bleeding caused by hormonal imbalance:* 5-20 mg daily on 5th to 25th day of the menstrual cycle. • *Endometriosis:* 10 mg daily for 2 wk, increasing 5 mg at 2-wk intervals until a total dose of 30 mg is reached. Continue 6-9 mo or until breakthrough bleeding occurs. Then it can be stopped temporarily.
norethindrone acetate	Aygestin	This medication is twice as strong as norethindrone. It is mildly androgenic. Take with meals to reduce nausea. Store in a closed container. • *Uterine bleeding caused by hormonal imbalance:* 2.5-10 mg daily on 5th to 25th day of the menstrual cycle. • *Endometriosis:* 5 mg for 2 wk, increasing 2.5 mg at 2-wk intervals until a dose of 15 mg/day is reached. Continue 6-9 mo or until breakthrough bleeding occurs. Then it can be stopped temporarily. The object of therapy is to prevent menstruation.
progesterone	Crinone	• *For amenorrhea, abnormal uterine bleeding, AIDS wasting:* 5-10 mg daily for 6-8 days by IM injection.

AIDS, Acquired immunodeficiency syndrome.

receives a prescription, she should look for this package insert and read it thoroughly.

2. Some patients experience side effects when taking this medication. If any of the following symptoms develop, the patient should stop taking the medication and contact the nurse, physician, or other health care provider immediately: chest pain, abdominal or leg pain or swelling, sudden severe headaches, visual changes, sudden loss of coordination, sudden shortness of breath, or slurred speech.

3. The patient should discontinue the drug immediately if she believes she is pregnant.

4. Less dangerous symptoms that require care or consultation with a health care provider include changes in vaginal bleeding or discharge, skin rash, breast lumps, jaundice, hypertension, abdominal pain, and mental depression.

5. Nausea and breast tenderness may occur early in therapy but should lessen after 1 to 3 weeks; taking oral medicines with food may reduce nausea

6. Less common side effects are changes in libido photosensitivity, chloasma (facial skin changes often seen in pregnancy), and vomiting.

7. Use of estrogens for replacement is associated with an increased risk of developing endometria

cancer. The patient should report any vaginal bleeding after menopause to the nurse, physician, or other health care provider.

8. If surgery is anticipated, the surgeon should be notified so that doses may be changed or briefly stopped.

9. Patients of all ages should be monitored regularly while on any estrogen preparation.

10. The patient should take the pills exactly as directed and keep them out of the reach of children or anyone for whom they are not prescribed.

11. When used for a short period to treat dysfunctional bleeding, progestins should first stop the bleeding and then cause the endometrial lining to shed when the drug is stopped (withdrawal bleeding). Improvement of heavy bleeding should occur in 24 to 48 hours.

12. Breakthrough or withdrawal bleeding can occur, especially in long-term use for contraception. The patient should report abnormal or unexplained vaginal bleeding to the nurse, physician, or other health care provider.

13. The patient should not take progestins if there is a history of breast or genital cancer, except as palliative treatment in advanced disease.

14. Diabetic patients should tell the health care provider if they begin developing positive urine tests so that antidiabetic medication can be adjusted.

15. Many herbal products are marketed to provide hormone replacement therapy. These products are not regulated, standardized, or tested, and caution should be used in their use.

ORAL CONTRACEPTIVES

ACTION

Most oral contraceptives are combination drugs that contain both an estrogen and a progestin. The principal action is to prevent ovulation by inhibiting FSH and LH. The progestin-only "mini-pill" prevents ovulation by the same mechanism but is more variable in suppressing the gonadotropins. The progestins in both types of oral contraceptive pills have several other contraceptive effects: creating thick cervical mucus hostile to sperm, slowing ovum transport by decreasing motility of the fallopian tubes, and blocking implantation.

USES

Oral contraceptives are used to prevent pregnancy when a highly effective method is needed and heterosexual activity is regular.

ADVERSE REACTIONS

Information on adverse reactions to oral contraceptives is provided in the previous sections on estrogen and progestin. Most adverse reactions are caused by hormonal imbalance. The types of hormonal imbalance and the symptoms they cause include the following:

- *Estrogen excess* may produce nausea, dizziness, edema, cyclic weight gain, bloating, increase in fibroid size, uterine cramps, irritability, increased fat deposition, poor contact lens fit, vascular-type headache, hypertension, suppression of lactation, cystic breast changes, breast tenderness, thrombophlebitis, cerebrovascular infarction, myocardial infarction, and hepatic adenoma.

- *Progestin excess* may cause increased appetite and weight gain (noncyclic), tiredness, malaise, depression and decrease in libido, acne, alopecia (hair loss), cholestatic jaundice, decreased length of menstrual flow, hypertension, headaches during the "resting" phase of the cycle (the time that the patient is off the drug), breast tenderness, decreased carbohydrate tolerance, dilated leg veins, and pelvic congestion syndrome.

- *Androgen excess* may produce increased appetite and weight gain, hirsutism, acne, oily skin, rash, increased libido, cholestatic jaundice, and pruritus.

- *Estrogen deficiency* may cause irritability, nervousness, hot flashes, vasomotor symptoms, uterine prolapse, pelvic relaxation symptoms, early and midcycle spotting, decreased amount of menstrual flow, no withdrawal bleeding, decreased libido, dry vaginal mucosa, atrophic vaginitis and dyspareunia, headaches, and depression.

- *Progestin deficiency* may produce late breakthrough bleeding and spotting, heavy menstrual flow and clots, delayed onset of menses, dysmenorrhea, and weight loss.

Emergency Contraception

Anytime a woman has unprotected intercourse and does not want to become pregnant, she may use a kit containing two tablets or take two multiple-tablet doses of selected combined oral contraceptive pills. Treatment must be started within 72 hours of intercourse, with two doses taken 12 hours apart. Emergency contraceptive pills work primarily by blocking or delaying ovulation, or by changing the way sperm or ova are transported, thereby preventing conception. The risk of pregnancy is decreased by 75%. The pills often produce nausea and irregular menstrual bleeding.

DRUG INTERACTIONS

There may be an increase in breakthrough bleeding and a decrease in contraceptive effectiveness in patients taking antitubercular medication, many antibiotics, barbiturates, and anticonvulsants.

Oral contraceptives may decrease the effectiveness of anticoagulants, antihypertensives, anticonvulsants, tricyclic antidepressants, oral hypoglycemics, and vitamins. When oral contraceptives are given with troleandomycin, the effect may be additive in causing jaundice. Oral contraceptives may alter many laboratory test results.

 Clinical Goldmine

Obtaining a History

You should ask the patient for a detailed menstrual history and history of any thromboembolic events, migraine headaches, and liver or kidney problems.

Nursing Implications and Patient Teaching

Assessment

To determine the most appropriate type of contraception for a patient, you should learn as much about the patient's history as possible, including a thorough menstrual, contraceptive, and reproductive history. This must include any current diseases, the patient's drug history, and whether or not the patient smokes. You must make certain the patient is not breastfeeding or pregnant, assess the patient's sexual activity and knowledge of contraceptive methods, and discover whether there are any contraindications for drug use (Box 20-1).

Diagnosis

Does the patient have other knowledge deficits or financial, nutritional, or social problems that would interfere with her taking this medication? For example, women who smoke and use oral contraceptives are at much greater risk for venospasm and thromboembolic events. These women should not be placed on oral birth control (OBC) if they are older than 35 years or should

 Clinical Landmine

Adverse Effects of Smoking

Patients should be questioned about smoking while taking the pill. Patients who smoke while taking oral contraceptives, especially if they are older then 35 years, are at increased risk of adverse effects.

Box 20-1 | *Contraindications for Oral Contraceptives*

ABSOLUTE CONTRAINDICATIONS

History or presence of thromboembolic disorders, cerebrovascular accident, coronary artery disease, hepatic adenoma, malignancy of breast or reproductive system, known impairment of liver function, and pregnancy.

STRONG RELATIVE CONTRAINDICATIONS

Severe headaches (particularly vascular or migraine),* hypertension (with resting diastolic blood pressure of 90 mm Hg or greater on three or more separate visits or an accurate measurement of 110 mm Hg or more on a single visit),* diabetes,* prediabetes or a strong family history of diabetes, gallbladder disease, including cholecystectomy,* previous cholestasis during pregnancy, congenital hyperbilirubinemia (Gilbert's disease), mononucleosis (acute phase), sickle cell disease (SS) or sickle C disease (SC),* undiagnosed, abnormal vaginal bleeding,† elective surgery (planned in next 4 weeks or major surgery requiring immobilization),* long leg casts or major injury to lower leg, patient over 40 years of age,* patient over 35 years of age with a history of heavy smoking,* and impaired liver function within the past year.

OTHER RELATIVE CONTRAINDICATIONS

Termination of term pregnancy within past 10 to 14 days,* weight gain of 10 pounds or more while on the pill,* failure to have established regular menstrual cycles,* profile suggestive of anovulation and infertility problems (late onset of menses and very irregular, painless menses),* presence of or history of cardiac or renal disease,* conditions likely to make patient unreliable at following dosage instructions (mental retardation, major psychiatric problems, alcoholism, history of repeatedly taking pills incorrectly),* lactation (oral contraceptives may be started as weaning begins and may be an aid in decreasing the flow of milk).*

May start the pill for women with these problems, but observe carefully for worsening or improvement of the problem: depression,* hypertension (with resting diastolic blood pressure of 90 to 99 mm Hg at a single visit),* presence of or history of chloasma or alopecia related to pregnancy,* asthma,* epilepsy,* uterine fibromyoma,* acne, varicose veins,* history of hepatitis (but liver function tests are normal now and have been for at least 1 year).

---

*These are contraindications to estrogen-containing pills, but may not be contraindications to progestin-only pills or may be less of a contraindication to progestin-only pills than to combined pills.
†Some believe this to be an absolute contraindication.

be helped to discontinue smoking. For women using emergency contraception, do they understand other more effective ways to prevent pregnancy?

Planning

Although breakthrough bleeding may be a side effect, nonfunctional causes should be investigated. Bleeding irregularities are more common with progestin-only pills.

There is some risk of infertility after oral contraceptives are stopped, especially in women who have had irregular or scanty periods before taking pills.

Research suggests that many women forget to take pills, resulting in many unintentional pregnancies. Discuss with the patient how the pill will fit into her life style in such a way that she will remember to take it.

Implementation

To be effective, oral contraceptives must be taken at about the same time each day. This is particularly true with progestin-only pills. Taking medication with meals will reduce the nausea common in the first cycles.

All oral combination contraceptives are to be taken for 21 days. Usually, therapy is started either the fifth day after or the Sunday after menstruation starts. Another method of contraception should be used for the first 7 to 10 days of the first cycle. Pills are packaged in a 1-month packet with the days named or numbered. Some preparations contain 28 pills to be taken daily, 7 of which contain an inert substance or iron. Others require the patient to go 7 days without pills before starting another 28-day cycle. During the "resting" phase of the cycle, vaginal bleeding should occur.

Combination pills vary in the type and amount of estrogen and progestin they contain (Box 20-2). All have at least one estrogen and one progestin. Two estrogens, ethinyl estradiol and mestranol, may be used in the different pills. Mestranol is half as strong as ethinyl estradiol. Several progestins are used in with them. Some progestins are estrogenic, antiestrogenic, or androgenic in effect. A dose of 50 micrograms or less of estrogen is used to start therapy. Less than this dose may cause breakthrough bleeding, but doses of less than 50 micrograms are increasingly being prescribed. New combinations are introduced frequently. For the progestin-only pills, the medication is taken daily on a continuous basis.

Table 20-11 provides a summary of oral contraceptives.

Evaluation

You should monitor for adverse effects, which may vary in severity. They may be a result of the different strengths of estrogen and progestin. Side effects may be

---

| Box 20-2 | *Content of Oral Combination (Estrogen and Progestin) Contraceptive Pills* |

MESTRANOL AND NORETHINDRONE
Genora 1/50
Nelova 1/50
Norethin 1/50
Norinyl 1+50
Ortho-Novum 1/50

ESTRADIOL AND NORETHINDRONE
Brevicon
Genora 1/35; 0.5/35
Modicon
NEE 1/35
Nelova 1/35E; 0.5/35E
Norcept-E 1/35
Norethin 1/35E
Norinyl 1+35
Ortho-Novum 1/35
Ovcon-50; Ovcon-35

ESTRADIOL AND NORETHINDRONE BIPHASIC OR TRIPHASIC PILLS
Nelova 10/11 (Norethindrone dose increases in phase 2)
Ortho-Novum 10/11 (Norethindrone dose increases in phase 2)
Ortho-Novum 7/7/7 (Norethindrone dose increases in phases 2 and 3)

Tri-Levlen (Norethindrone dose increases in phases 2 and 3)
Tri-Norinyl (Norethindrone dose increases in phases 2 and 3)
Triphasil (Norethindrone dose increases in phases 2 and 3)

ESTRADIOL AND NORETHINDRONE ACETATE
Loestrin 21 1.5/30; Fe 1.5/30; 21 1/20; Fe 1/20
Norlestrin 1/50; Fe 1/50; 21 2.5/50; Fe 2.5/50

ESTRADIOL AND ETHYNODIOL DIACETATE
Demulen 1/35; 1/50

ESTRADIOL AND LEVONORGESTREL
Levlen
Nordette

ESTRADIOL AND NORGESTREL
Lo/Ovral
Ovral

ESTRADIOL AND DESOGESTREL
Ortho-Cept

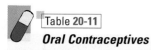

Table 20-11

Oral Contraceptives

GENERIC NAME	TRADE NAME	COMMENTS AND DOSAGE
estrogen and progestin combinations	• *Monophasic* Demulen Loestrin Lo/Ovral Lunelle Modicon Nelova Nordette Norinyl Ortho-Cept Ortho-Novum Ovcon Ovral • *Biphasic* Jenest-28 Mircette Necon Nelova 10/11 Ortho-Novum 10/11 • *Triphasic* Estro Step Estro Step 21 Fe Ortho Novum 7/7/7 Ortho-Tri-Cyclin Tri-Levlen Tri-Norinyl Triphasil Trivora-28	The patient should take 1 pill each day for 21 days, beginning with the regimen the nurse, physician, or other health care provider suggests, either starting the Sunday after a period begins or starting 5 days after the onset of the period. If there are 7 inert pills, they should be taken after the 21-day cycle. If not, the patient should start a new pack 7 days after finishing the 21-day cycle. If 1 pill is missed, the forgotten one should be taken and a backup contraceptive method used. If 2 pills are missed, two should be taken for 2 consecutive days and another method used until the end of the cycle. If 3 are missed, a new pack should be started on the 8th day or the first Sunday after the last pill was taken. Another birth control method must be used for 7-14 days, depending on the dosage.
progestin only (mini-pills)	Micronor Nor-QD Ovrette	Pills must be taken at the same time each day to be most effective. Only the most reliable patients should use these pills. Slightly less effective than combination products in preventing pregnancy. Incidence of pregnancy is highest in the first 6 mo of use. Breakthrough bleeding is more common than with combination pills; therefore, undiagnosed genital bleeding is an important contraindication, especially in older women. The patient should take 1 pill at the same time every day continually. Do not stop during menses.

OTHER CONTRACEPTIVE FORMS

emergency contraception	Plan B
	Preven
	  Emergency
	  Contraceptive
	  Kit
		Initiate treatment within 72 hr of intercourse, with 2 doses taken 12 hr apart. (Patients may also use 2 multiple-tablet doses of combined oral contraceptive medications such as Ovral, Lo/Ovral, Levlen, Nordette, Tri-Levlen, and Triphasil according to the instructions given in the package insert.)

levonorgestrel implants	Norplant	Medication implanted in a set of 6 flexible closed capsules made of Silastic, each containing the progestin levonorgestrel. This is an implantable system effective in contraception for up to 5 yr and completely reversible. Contraindicated in patients with abnormal bleeding, thrombophlebitis, pregnancy, liver disease, and carcinoma of the breast. Implant subdermally in the midportion of the upper arm about 8-10 cm above the elbow crease during the first 7 days after the onset of menses. Breakthrough bleeding is a common occurrence.

Continue

Table 20-11
Oral Contraceptives—cont'd

GENERIC NAME	TRADE NAME	COMMENTS AND DOSAGE
OTHER CONTRACEPTIVE FORMS—cont'd		
levonorgestrel intrauterine system	Mirena	For women who have had at least 1 child, this system is implanted in the uterus. It provides contraception for up to 5 yr.
medroxyprogesterone acetate	Depo-Provera	Long-term injectable contraceptive. Give 150 mg every 3 mo after the onset of normal menses. Give in gluteal or deltoid muscle. Make certain that the patient is not pregnant.
progesterone intrauterine insert	Progestasert	A T-shaped unit containing a reservoir of 38 mg progesterone with barium sulfate dispersed in a silicone fluid is inserted into the uterine cavity. Contraceptive effectiveness is maintained for 1 yr, and then the unit must be replaced. Bleeding and cramps may occur during the first few weeks after insertion, sometimes requiring removal.

avoided by changing to a different combination of estrogen and progestin pill. Some spotting can be tolerated in younger women.

You should evaluate the patient's compliance in taking medications. Patients who have trouble remembering to take other medications are not good candidates for oral contraceptives.

Patient and Family Teaching

You should tell the patient and family the following:

1. The patient must take the pills exactly as prescribed. If a pill is missed, the patient should follow the directions given by the nurse, physician, or other health care provider. Usually the patient takes two pills the next day or discards one tablet and takes one tablet the next day. The risk for bleeding or conception increases with two or more pills missed. The patient may need to use a backup method of contraception for a period of time. Another method should also be used in the first 3 weeks of the first cycle and if vomiting for several days occurs because of illness.

2. Certain side effects should be reported to the nurse, physician, or other health care provider immediately: pain in the chest, groin, or legs; sudden, severe headaches; sudden slurring of speech; sudden loss of coordination; sudden visual changes; and sudden shortness of breath. Other symptoms may require attention but are not emergencies: changes in vaginal bleeding, hypertension, breast lumps, jaundice, vaginal discharge, stomach or side pains, and mental depression. Other side effects may be present but are not serious: nausea, anorexia, acne, stomach cramps, edema of ankles and feet, breast swelling and tenderness, tiredness, brown spots on the skin, changes in libido, changes in weight, hirsutism, some hair loss on the scalp, and sensitivity to the sun.

3. The patient must return for scheduled checkups.

4. The patient should immediately stop taking the pill if she thinks she is pregnant or if she misses two periods. The patient must not take oral contraceptives while breastfeeding.

5. The patient should keep one extra month's supply of pills on hand so there is no chance of running out and breaking the cycle.

6. The patient should not smoke while taking the pill.

7. All other medications the patient is taking should be reported to the nurse, physician, or other health care provider because of possible drug interactions. This is particularly true for antibiotics, which may make the pill less effective and thus allow the woman to get pregnant.

8. For women younger than 40 years of age, the risk of death from complications from the pill is less than the risk of death from complications of pregnancy. (Patients should not be so frightened of taking the pill that they fail to recognize that it is safer statistically to take the pill than to be pregnant.)

9. For patients using the Norplant or the Progestasert systems, special instructions are needed. Patient should watch for signs of infection or excessive bleeding after insertion. Difficulties should be reported to the nurse, physician, or other health care provider immediately.

Each visit to the health care provider should include a history of possible side effects or adverse reactions since the previous visit, a review of whether the patient is taking the pill correctly, and a reminder of signs and symptoms to report.

Thyroid Hormones

OVERVIEW

The thyroid gland, located in the neck in front of the trachea, produces the hormones thyroxine (T_4) and triiodothyronine (T_3), which influence almost every organ and tissue of the body. Although their exact mechanism of action is unknown, their primary action is to control the metabolic rate of the tissues.

The anterior pituitary gland secretes thyroid-stimulating hormone (TSH), which tells the thyroid gland to release the hormones that it has stored. When the level of circulating thyroid hormones is high, TSH from the anterior pituitary gland is withheld; when the circulating level falls, this information is also signaled and TSH is once again released. This type of arrangement is called a *feedback mechanism,* because physiologic action influences the organ sending the signals.

Two general types of diseases can influence the hormone-producing activity of the thyroid gland. A decrease in the amount of thyroid hormones that are manufactured or secreted is called **hypothyroidism.** Symptoms include fatigue, malaise, lethargy, moderate weight gain (around 10 pounds) with minimal appetite, cold intolerance, menorrhagia, dry skin, coarse hair, hoarseness, impaired memory, and constipation. An increase in the amount of thyroid hormones that are manufactured and secreted is called **hyperthyroidism.** Symptoms include weight loss, decreased or absent menstruation, rapid or pounding heart, heat intolerance, nervousness, irritability, diarrhea, sweaty skin, insomnia (inability to sleep), fever, or chest pain.

Synthetic hormones, natural hormones, or a combination product may be given to increase the level of thyroid hormone in hypothyroid conditions or given as replacement therapy when the thyroid gland has been surgically removed. In hyperthyroid conditions, other preparations are given that slow the rate of thyroid production. Both thyroid supplements and antithyroid medications will be described.

THYROID SUPPLEMENTS OR REPLACEMENTS

ACTION

The main action of the thyroid hormones is to increase metabolic rate. This results in an increase in tissue oxygen consumption, body temperature, heart and respiratory rate, cardiac output, and carbohydrate, lipid, and protein metabolism. In addition, thyroid hormones influence growth and development of the skeletal system, especially ossification in the epiphyses of long bones (the growth center).

USES

Thyroid hormones are used in replacement therapy to manage hypothyroidism, myxedema, cretinism, or nontoxic goiter caused by deficiency of thyroid hormones, atrophy, congenital defects, and the effects of surgery, antithyroid products, or radiation. They are also used to treat chronic thyroid infections and tumors that depend on thyrotropic hormone.

ADVERSE REACTIONS

Adverse reactions to thyroid replacements include dysrhythmias, hypertension, tachycardia, hand tremors, headache, insomnia, nervousness, diarrhea, vomiting, weight loss, menstrual irregularities, rash, glycosuria, hyperglycemia, increased prothrombin time, and increased serum cholesterol levels. Overdosage produces signs of hyperthyroidism.

DRUG INTERACTIONS

Thyroid preparations may increase the patient's need for antidiabetic agents. Anticoagulant effects may be exaggerated by thyroid replacement because of increased hypoprothrombinemia. Corticosteroid needs are increased for patients taking thyroid preparations because of increased tissue demands. Effects of tricyclic antidepressants are increased by thyroid hormones. Many other isolated medications may be affected.

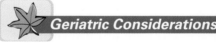
Geriatric Considerations

Thyroid Hormones

Because elderly patients are usually more sensitive to and have more adverse reactions to thyroid hormones than patients in other age groups, it is recommended that thyroid replacement doses be individualized. In some patients, the dose should be 25% lower than the usual adult dose.

Hypothyroidism, the second most common endocrine disease in the elderly population, is often misdiagnosed. Only one third of geriatric patients exhibit the typical signs and symptoms of cold intolerance and weight gain. Most often, the symptoms are nonspecific, such as failing to thrive, stumbling and falling episodes, weight loss, and incontinence. If neurologic change has occurred, the patient may be misdiagnosed as having dementia, depression, or a psychotic episode.

Modified from McKenry LM, Salerno E: *Mosby's pharmacology in nursing,* e 21, St Louis, 2003, Mosby.

Nursing Implications and Patient Teaching

Assessment

You should try to learn as much as possible about the patient's health history, including other drugs being taken that may produce drug interactions and the possibility that the patient has diabetes mellitus, cardiovascular disease, adrenocortical insufficiency, or pregnancy; these conditions are precautions to the use of thyroid supplements. The patient may also have a history of hypothyroidism.

On examination, you may find skin changes associated with **myxedema,** the most severe form of hypothyroidism. These changes include nonpitting edema, doughy skin, puffy face, large tongue, decreased body hair, and cool, dry skin. The thyroid gland may be normal in size, enlarged, or not palpable, depending on the cause of hypothyroidism. Neurologic signs include slow thinking, muscle weakness, slowed relaxation phase of the deep tendon reflexes, dull facial expression, and carpal tunnel syndrome. Cardiac signs include bradycardia and decreased blood pressure.

Laboratory findings in thyroid disease may include reduced free T_4 index and elevated serum TSH; other tests may be abnormal.

Diagnosis

Because thyroid disease may be insidious (hard to notice because of small changes) in onset, the patient may have many symptoms that require therapy at the time of diagnosis. Patients may have become depressed, have gained weight, or have problems with body image and self-esteem that should be addressed. Patients may find it hard to wait for the length of time it takes for thyroid medications to return them to normal functioning and resolve some of these problems.

Planning

Patients older than 50 years of age are often very sensitive to thyroid hormones. It is important to begin the patient on a small dose and observe for signs and symptoms of cardiovascular disease before increasing the dosage.

Implementation

Begin all treatment with small doses and increase gradually. A cut in dosage followed by a slower increase in the dose may be necessary when side effects occur. Therapy should be withdrawn for 2 to 6 days and then restarted at a lower dosage if this happens.

The patient's age, the presence of cardiac disease, and the severity of symptoms should be considered when beginning therapy. Titration of dosage (gradual adjustment of dose up or down) to gain the best response with the lowest dosage is the goal. The usual maintenance dosage in the treatment of hypothyroidism is 0.5 to 2 gm as a single daily dose before breakfast.

T_4 is the treatment of choice for hypothyroidism because of its purity and long duration of action. Because T_4 has a slow onset of action, therapeutic effects may not occur for 3 to 4 weeks. T_3, which has a rapid onset, may be given if rapid correction of hypothyroidism is necessary. The equivalent strengths of the various thyroid products vary, and care must be used in changing from one product to another. Patients should take the medication at the same time every day, preferably before breakfast. If medication is taken late in the day, insomnia may result.

Table 20-12 presents a summary of thyroid supplements or replacements.

Evaluation

Response to therapy is not immediate. Most patients begin to feel better within 2 weeks, and the therapeutic results are often seen in 3 months.

You should teach patients the signs and symptoms of hypothyroidism and hyperthyroidism so that they can determine if they are receiving too much or too little medicine.

If symptoms of overdosage occur, the medication should be stopped for several days and therapy should be started again at a lower dosage.

Periodic blood tests should be done before starting thyroid hormone therapy and once the patient is on a maintenance dose.

Patient and Family Teaching

You should tell the patient and family the following:

1. The patient should take the medication exactly as directed by the nurse, physician, or other health care provider. The medication should be taken at the same time every day, preferably before breakfast. If it is taken too late in the day, the patient may have difficulty going to sleep.
2. Response to this medication is not immediate; symptoms should improve within 2 weeks. The patient should not increase the dosage unless instructed to do so by the nurse, physician, or other health care provider. Taking the medication regularly as ordered is very important.
3. If the patient is also being treated for diabetes mellitus, any changes in blood or urine sugar and acetone test results should be reported to the health care provider.
4. If the patient is receiving anticoagulant therapy, bleeding or excessive bruising should be reported to the health care provider.
5. The patient should check with the health care provider before taking any other medications; this will decrease the chance of drugs interacting.
6. The patient should report signs and symptoms of overdosage (hyperthyroidism) or underdosage (hypothyroidism) to the health care provider promptly (these signs and symptoms are summarized earlier).

Table 20-12

Thyroid Supplements or Replacements

GENERIC NAME	TRADE NAME	COMMENTS AND DOSAGE
levothyroxine	Levothroid Synthroid Levo-T Eltroxin	Synthetic preparation; drug of choice because effect is predictable. *Initial therapy:* 0.05-0.1 mg PO daily with increases in dosage of 0.05-0.1 mg at 2-wk intervals until therapeutic effect is achieved. *Maintenance:* 0.1-0.2 mg/day PO.
liothyronine (T_3)	Cytomel Triostat	A synthetic hormone; has rapid effect and short duration of action, which allow fast dosage adjustment and quick reversibility of overdosage. The therapeutic effects are achieved in 24-72 hr and persist up to 72 hr after withdrawal of drug. • *Mild hypothyroidism:* Initiate therapy at 25 mcg daily and increase by 12.5-25 mcg every 1-2 wk until effects are achieved. Maintenance dosage is usually 25-100 mcg/day.
liotrix	Thyrolar	Liotrix is a combination of synthetic levothyroxine sodium (T_4) and liothyronine sodium (T_3) in a 4:1 ratio. Predictable therapeutic effect is an advantage. Initiate therapy with one ½ tablet and increase by one ½ tablet at 1- to 2-wk intervals.
thyroid, desiccated	Armour-USP S-P-T Thyrar USP	Desiccated thyroid contains T_4 and T_3 thyroid hormones in their natural state. Because these drugs are composed of desiccated animal thyroid glands, the hormonal content is variable and T_3 and T_4 levels fluctuate; therefore, avoid varying brands. • *Myxedema without hypothyroidism:* Initiate therapy at 30 mg/day with increases of 60 mg/mo until therapeutic effects are achieved. Maintenance is usually 60-180 mg/day.

ANTITHYROID PRODUCTS

ACTION

These are the main drugs used to treat hyperthyroidism. The main action of antithyroid products is to stop the new production of thyroid hormones. These agents do not inactivate or inhibit the thyroid hormones (T_3 and T_4) that are already stored or are circulating in the blood.

USES

Antithyroid products are used to treat hyperthyroidism or to improve hyperthyroidism in preparation for surgery or radioactive iodine therapy.

ADVERSE REACTIONS

Adverse reactions to antithyroid products include drowsiness, headaches, neuritis, paresthesias (numbness and tingling), vertigo, epigastric distress, jaundice, nausea, vomiting, skin rash, urticaria, myalgia, edema, alopecia, and lymphadenopathy. Hypothyroidism may occur as a result of prolonged therapy. Agranulocytosis (very low number of white blood cells) is a rare but serious occurrence. In addition, other more serious problems may develop.

DRUG INTERACTIONS

The effects of anticoagulants are increased or potentiated by propylthiouracil. Caution should be taken in giving antithyroid drugs to patients who are receiving additional drugs known to cause agranulocytosis (e.g., hydantoin).

Nursing Implications and Patient Teaching

Assessment

You should try to learn as much as possible about the patient's health history, including hypersensitivity (allergy) to antithyroid drugs, other medications being taken that could cause drug interactions, and pregnancy or breastfeeding.

The patient may have a history of hyperthyroidism, including nervousness or tremor, weight loss with increased appetite, heat intolerance and excessive sweating, mood swings, and muscle weakness. On physical examination, the nurse may find exophthalmos (bulging eyes); thyroid enlargement; tachycardia; increased blood pressure; tremor; warm, moist, smooth skin; and proximal muscle weakness. Weight loss and the signs of chronic heart failure may be the most obvious signs of hyperthyroidism in the elderly.

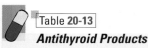

Table 20-13
Antithyroid Products

GENERIC NAME	TRADE NAME	COMMENTS AND DOSAGE
iodine products	Lugol's Iodine	Give 2-6 drops solution 3 times daily. Used before surgery.
	Thyro-Block	Give 130-mg potassium iodine tablets.
methimazole	Tapazole	Does not inhibit peripheral conversion of thyroxine to T_3. It is more potent than PTU, and doses are one tenth those of PTU. It acts more rapidly but less consistently than PTU. Initial dosage is 15-60 mg PO daily; maintenance is usually 5-15 mg daily.
propylthiouracil	Propylthiouracil	PTU interferes with synthesis of thyroxine and blocks peripheral conversion of thyroxine to T_3. It may cause hypoprothrombinemia and bleeding. Give 100-150 mg PO 3 times daily at 8-hr intervals. Initial dose is 300 mg PO daily at 8-hr intervals, with adjustments in dosage made after 2 wk depending on free T_4 levels and symptoms. Continue therapy 6-18 mo before tapering.

PTU, Propylthiouracil.

Laboratory findings may show elevated free T_4 index, increased T_3, or decreased TSH.

Diagnosis

Because thyroid disease may be slow in onset, the patient may have many symptoms that require therapy at the time of diagnosis. Patients may be restless or anxious, have eating and sleeping problems, or have problems with concentration and memory that must be addressed. Patients may find it hard to wait for the length of time it takes for thyroid medications to return them to normal functioning and resolve some of these problems.

Planning

Antithyroid drugs usually remove symptoms of hyperthyroidism if taken correctly for 1 to 2 years. Patient compliance with therapy should be encouraged to help them return to normal thyroid levels.

Implementation

The therapeutic objective is to correct the hypermetabolic state with a minimum of side effects and without producing hypothyroidism. Clinical response to the antithyroid drugs usually takes 1 to 2 weeks, because the drugs do not affect the release of thyroid hormone. Response depends on stopping the production of thyroid

Complementary and Alternative Therapies

Hyperglycemia, Hyperthyroidism, or Hypothyroidism

CONDITION	PRODUCT	COMMENTS
Hyperglycemia/ diabetes	Gymnema	Potential interactions with insulin, oral hypoglycemics
	Bitter melon	Potential interaction with anticoagulants, aspirin, NSAIDs, antiplatelet agents
	Evening primrose	
Hyperthyroidism	Milk thistle	No known interactions
	Passion flower	Potential interactions with antianxiety agents, antidepressants, hexobarbital, hypnotics, sedatives
	Valerian	Potential interactions with CNS depressants, sedative-hypnotics (barbiturates), antidepressants, anxiolytics, antihistamines
Hypothyroidism	Bitter melon	Potential interactions with insulin, oral hypoglycemics
	Garcinia	

Modified from Krinsky DL, Lavella JB, Hawkins EB, et al: *Natural therapeutics pocket guide*, ed 2, Hudson, Ohio, 2003, Lexi-Comp, Inc.
CNS, Central nervous system; *NSAIDs*, nonsteroidal antiinflammatory drugs.

hormone in the thyroid gland. This in turn depends on the amount of hormone production materials present in the gland, and the rate of conversion of these materials into the thyroid hormones. Generally, therapy is maintained for 12 to 24 months and then reduced to see if the hyperthyroidism starts again. Titration to gain the best therapeutic response with the lowest dosage is the objective. Table 20-13 provides a summary of antithyroid products.

Evaluation

Laboratory blood tests should be completed before beginning antithyroid therapy and periodically once the patient is on a regular maintenance dosage. Before therapy is started, a white blood cell count (WBC) with differential is done; this should be repeated if there is any sign of infection. Serum T_4 and TSH levels are monitored initially and after every 2 weeks of therapy until a euthyroid state (normal function of the thyroid gland) is achieved, usually in 3 to 5 months. Once the patient has been euthyroid for 6 to 12 months, a decision may be made to reduce the dosage and see whether the hyperthyroidism is under control. If hyperthyroidism seems to be absent, therapy is stopped.

Patient and Family Teaching

You should tell the patient and family the following:
1. The patient should take this medication exactly as directed by the nurse, physician, or other health care provider.
2. Because clinical response usually takes from 1 to 2 weeks to achieve, the dosage should not be increased until the results at the present dosage level can be evaluated.
3. Some patients experience side effects from this drug, such as fever, sore throat, malaise, unusual bleeding or bruising, headache, skin rash, and enlargement of cervical lymph nodes; these symptoms should be reported to the nurse, physician, or other health care provider.
4. Bed rest, adequate diet, and avoidance of occupational and domestic stress are also useful modalities of therapy.

COMPLEMENTARY AND ALTERNATIVE THERAPIES

Some herbal preparations may be used by patients for the treatment of hyperglycemia, hyperthyroidism, or hypothyroidism. These products may interact with other medications, as indicated in the Complementary and Alternative Therapies box.

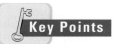
Key Points

- A variety of hormones and steroids are used in medical therapy.
- Unlike many other medications, hormones and steroids are natural or manufactured preparations that replace, increase, or decrease the effects of substances already produced in the body.
- Hormones and steroids are part of a complex message system linking together various organs and biologic systems. Increases or decreases of hormones send signals to other organ systems about whether to increase or decrease production of other substances.
- Important hormones or steroids covered in this chapter are insulin and oral hypoglycemics, agents that act on the uterus, pituitary and adrenocortical hormones, sex hormones, oral contraceptives, and thyroid preparations.
- It is important for you to have a basic understanding of how these preparations work in the body, a familiarity with the major adverse effects that can occur, and a lesson plan with the important points to cover when teaching the patient and family.

Go to the free CD-ROM for an Audio Glossary, animations, video clips, and Review Questions for the NCLEX-PN® Examination.

evolve Be sure to visit the companion Evolve website at http://evolve.elsevier.com/Edmunds/LPN/ for WebLinks, a link to the top 200 drugs by prescription, and sign-up pages for newsletter drug updates.

CASE STUDY

Lucy Bradford is a 33-year-old type 2 diabetic. She developed diabetes after a pregnancy 3 years ago, and she has been able to keep her blood glucose level under control with diet until recently. Her blood sugar has been around 136 mg/dL. Over the past few months, the glucose level has begun to vary a great deal, sometimes reaching as high as 180 mg/dL. She has no other health problems or previous surgeries but has smoked 1 pack of cigarettes a day for 12 years. She takes oral contraceptives. She reports developing a red itchy rash after taking sulfa as a child. Today the doctor decided she needed to start on some oral antidiabetic medication and ordered glyburide 5 mg/day PO.

1. What would you tell Lucy about the medication she is going to start taking?
2. Is this a low, medium, or high dose of glyburide?
3. What blood sugar level would be an appropriate goal for Lucy?
4. What blood test monitors the effectiveness of blood sugar control over a 6- to 8-week period?
5. From your knowledge of Lucy's condition and what you know about glyburide, how do you anticipate Lucy will react to the glyburide?
6. All sulfonylureas have the same mechanism of action. What differs is: _____.
7. The physician decides to switch Lucy to _____, which has a similar mechanism of action to the sulfonylureas. Why would this drug be a good substitute?
8. Lucy comes back several months later. Her glycohemoglobin A_{1c} is less than 7%. Is this a problem?
9. Diet and exercise are the foundation of any diabetes management plan. Develop a teaching plan

for communicating these important things to Lucy:
a. A more ideal body weight reduces insulin resistance and can significantly impact glucose control.
b. The total number of calories that are adequate to promote a reasonable weight and good nutrition should be established.
c. Generally, dividing the total number of calories into three smaller meals and 2 to 3 snacks minimizes postprandial glucose spikes. Spreading out calories may also control increased hunger associated with skipped meals.
d. Generally 10% to 20% of the total daily calories are from protein, 20% of calories are from saturated and polyunsaturated fat, and 60% to 70% of calories are from monounsaturated fats and from carbohydrates.
e. Exercise helps achieve and maintain an ideal body weight, resulting in decreased insulin resistance. Exercise also improves insulin sensitivity. For reasons not well understood, the exercising muscle requires little insulin but can mobilize moderate amounts of glucose.
10. Lucy's potential for hyperglycemia is increased because: _____.
11. Lucy does not want to have another child. She has been taking a biphasic oral contraceptive pill. Are there any contraindications to diabetics taking oral contraceptive pills?
12. Does Lucy have any other risk factors that would limit oral contraceptive use?

DRUG CALCULATION REVIEW

1. The physician orders an injection of dexamethasone (Decadron) 6 mg IM for a patient with bronchial asthma. In stock is dexamethasone 4 mg/1 mL in a 5-mL multidose vial. How many milliliters of this medication will you prepare?

2. Order: Synthroid 125 mcg by mouth (PO) daily
   Supply: Synthroid 0.25 mg per tablet
   Question: How many tablets of Synthroid should be given?

3. Order: Solu-Medrol 60 mg IV push stat
   Supply: Solu-Medrol 125 mg/mL
   Question: How many milliliters of Solu-Medrol should be given? (Round to the nearest tenth.)

CRITICAL THINKING ?

1. Identify the major similarities in the treatment of type 1 and type 2 diabetes.

2. Seven-year-old Jessica has recently been diagnosed with type 1 diabetes. Which insulin preparation(s) is Jessica most likely to receive? Why?

3. What would indicate that a patient understands his androgen therapy regimen?

4. Ms. Marra, who is 26, has begun an initial course of oral contraceptives. What would indicate her understanding of and likelihood of compliance with her OBC regimen?

5. Mr. Moore is starting a thyroid replacement regimen. As you are preparing to instruct him regarding his medication regimen, he makes the comment,

"Sounds to me like these pills will have me feeling fine in no time." How would you address this?

6. What information would you want to include in your education of a patient who takes oral contraceptives and has been prescribed furosemide?

7. Immunosuppression is one of the serious effects of steroid therapy. If your patient with chronic obstructive pulmonary disease (COPD) has been maintained on prednisone 40 mg PO daily for 6 months, how would you instruct her to monitor herself for signs and symptoms of infection?

8. Why should your patient taking oral steroids also be receiving a histamine H_2-receptor antagonist such as ranitidine or cimetidine?

21 Immunologic Medications

Objectives

After reading and studying this chapter, you should be able to do the following:

1. Define common terms used in immunology.
2. Explain the differences between the three different types of immunity.
3. Outline typical immunization plans for children and adults.
4. List the major adverse reactions of common immunologic drugs.
5. Identify at least three drugs used for in vivo testing.

Key Terms

Be sure to check out the bonus material on the free CD-ROM, including selected audio pronunciations.

antigen-antibody response (ĂN-tĭ-jĕn ĂN-tĭ-bŏ-dē, p. 400)
antiserums (ĂN-tĭ-sĭ-rŭmz, p. 401)
artificially acquired active immunity (ĭ-MŪ-nĭ-tē, p. 400)
immunity (ĭ-MŪ-nĭ-tē, p. 400)
naturally acquired active immunity (p. 400)
passive immunity (p. 401)
toxoid (TŎKS-ŏyd, p. 401)
vaccines (văk-SĒNZ, p. 400)

OVERVIEW

Immunologic agents are biologic preparations such as vaccines, toxoids, and other serologic agents used primarily to prevent or modify disease in an otherwise healthy person. Depending on the formulation of the biologic agents, they provide active or passive immunity to specific diseases. These different mechanisms are discussed in general, with specific product information presented later in Table 21-1.

IMMUNE SYSTEM

The immune system is part of the lymphatic system, which is made up of the lymph vessels, lymph nodes, and other lymph organs (Figure 21-1). This system removes foreign substances from the blood and lymph,

combats disease, maintains tissue fluid balance, and absorbs fats. It moves lymph from its source, the body tissues, to the point where it reenters the bloodstream. The structures of the lymphatic system are of two kinds: those that are concerned with the transport of lymph (lymph capillaries, lymph vessels, and lymph ducts) and those that are composed mostly of lymphatic tissue but serve other specific functions (lymph nodes, spleen, tonsils, and thymus—together these structures are called *lymph organs*).

The lymphatic system produces the T cells that help provide immunity and moves them throughout the lymphatic system.

ACTION

A bacterium, virus, or foreign protein that invades the body is called an *antigen.* The body senses the foreign antigen and responds by making antibodies. *Antibodies* are special proteins made by the lymphatic tissue and the reticuloendothelial system that are designed to help neutralize, or resist the effects of, the invading proteins. In this **antigen-antibody response,** a specific antigen causes the body to produce an antibody that reacts specifically with that antigen. Some antibodies keep circulating for the life of the person, providing constant active immunity to certain antigens. Other antibodies are active for only a short period of time, providing passive immunity.

The antigen-antibody response results in **immunity,** or resistance to invading proteins and diseases. One way that a person can develop immunity is by having a disease and recovering from it. An example is when a child develops chickenpox, and the body develops antibodies to the chickenpox virus. These antibodies travel around in the bloodstream for the rest of the person's lifetime, providing **naturally acquired active immunity.**

The lymphoid tissue and the reticuloendothelial system tissues will also produce antibodies to a live but weakened antigen (known as a live, attenuated antigen), or an antigen that has been killed. Thus laboratories can produce **vaccines** that contain either attenuated or killed antigens, so that people can be immunized to prevent them from getting some diseases. This is called **artificially acquired active immunity.** Whether

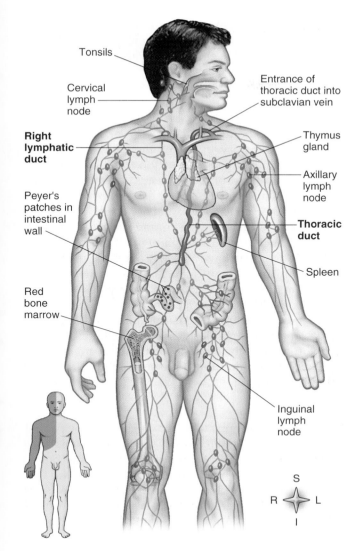

FIGURE **21-1** The lymphatic system. *I,* Inferior; *L,* left; *R,* right; *S,* superior.

cannot distinguish between the toxin and the toxoid. The most common example is the use of tetanus toxoid to protect patients from *Clostridium tetani.*

Once a person has had an antigen-antibody response, the antibodies are stored in the body. Immune globulins are specific types of protein antibodies that are stored in blood serum and plasma. Concentrated immune globulins are also called **antiserums,** and may be collected from human or animal sources. A common example is the hepatitis B immune globulin. These antibodies can be injected into a person who does not have immunity to the antigen. These antibodies then circulate to immediately protect this person, but the protection lasts for only a short time. This form of protection is called artificially acquired **passive immunity.** This type of temporary immunity can also occur when antibodies pass from the mother to the fetus through the placenta or to the nursing infant through breast milk. This is known as naturally acquired passive immunity.

Infants and children can be immunized against diphtheria, tetanus, pertussis, hepatitis B, *Haemophilus influenzae* type B, polio, measles, mumps, rubella, and varicella. These primary immunizations dramatically reduce the incidence of disease in a community and lower mortality and morbidity rates from these diseases, which used to kill so many young children. Although most children in the United States have gotten these immunizations by the time they enter school, the United States lags behind many other countries in the percentage of children immunized at an early age. Thus these diseases continue to be widespread and to do damage. We now know that some of these early immunizations lose their ability to provide long-term immunity. Thus some adults who were vaccinated when they were children may develop pertussis or other diseases to which they believed they were immune.

Immunization Schedule

The American Academy of Pediatrics, the Advisory Committee on Immunization Practices, and the American Academy of Family Physicians collaborate on immunization guidelines that are updated each January.

USES

Vaccines and toxoids are the biologic agents used in the routine schedule of active immunizations for adults and children. Specific biologic agents are reserved for use in people who live in areas where specific diseases (for example, yellow fever, cholera, typhoid) are endemic (common in the community) and there is a high risk of infection. Other vaccines (for example, pneumococcal

a weak or dead antigen is given depends on the disease and on what the research has shown is the best way to protect patients. Rubeola (measles) vaccine is an example of a vaccine made from live, attenuated measles antigen. A person who is vaccinated against measles develops a very mild case of measles. The immune system then produces antibodies that protect the person from getting a full infection with measles. Some diseases may require periodic booster injections of vaccine to keep the antibody level high enough to protect the patient from disease.

Some disease-causing proteins that come from invading bacteria are called *toxins.* Toxins act like antigens to stimulate the immune system to produce antitoxins, which act to neutralize the toxins in the same way that antibodies neutralize antigens. When a toxin is attenuated, or weakened, it is called a **toxoid.** A toxoid can be used to produce immunity because the body vaccine, influenza vaccine) are recommended for people at high risk for specific diseases such as pneumonia or flu.

An additional group of biologic agents (for example, purified protein derivative [PPD], histoplasmin, coccidioidin) is used in screening procedures to identify people who have been exposed to a specific disease or who may have an active disease, such as tuberculosis.

In special circumstances, certain biologic agents (for example, gamma globulins) may be useful to modify a disease process in the previously unimmunized person.

ADVERSE REACTIONS

In general, mild adverse effects are common and include localized pain and swelling that are mild and of short duration. There are many unfounded reports that these immunizations are linked to other health problems. Although it is true that there are rare instances of more serious problems, the risk of complications from the disease far outweighs the risk of adverse effects for all biologic products. Adverse effects occasionally seen include altered levels of consciousness, headaches, lethargy (sleepiness), rash, urticaria (hives), vesiculation (blistering), diarrhea, increased respiratory rate, shortness of breath, arthralgia (joint pain), fever, lymphadenopathy, and malaise (weakness).

Most states have laws requiring infants and children to be properly immunized before starting school. To reduce the liability faced by pharmaceutical companies, a special fund has been established by the federal government that pays for the medical costs incurred if a patient has a serious adverse effect from required immunizations. A certain percentage of the fee paid by the patient for each immunization goes toward this fund, called the National Vaccine Injury Compensation Program. The fund is administered by the Public Health Service, a division of the U.S. Department of Health and Human Services (DHHS).

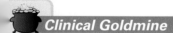
Clinical Goldmine

Adverse Effects of Immunization

Although some parents are afraid of adverse effects from immunizations, their children are statistically more likely to have complications from disease than they are to experience serious side effects from the immunization.

DRUG INTERACTIONS

When several vaccines are given at the same time—for example, when cholera, plague, and typhoid vaccines are given together—the potential for adverse effects is increased. Someone who has passive immunity to a disease (has received antibodies from a maternal or a

vaccine source or through blood products) may not have an adequate active antibody response to the administration of a live, attenuated vaccine.

Nursing Implications and Patient Teaching

Assessment

You should find out as much as you can about the patient's health history, including the patient's previous immunization status and reaction to biologic agents; history of allergy, especially to eggs or feathers; results of any known allergy testing; the presence of underlying disease or concurrent infections; the use of immunosuppressant drugs, immune serums, blood, or blood products; or the possibility of pregnancy.

The patient may have a history of exposure to a specific organism or might plan to travel to areas where disease may be common. You should assess whether the person is at risk for infection, as well as if there are children who require primary immunizations. The U.S. State Department regularly issues travelers' warnings, and you can call the embassy of a foreign government to see if certain immunizations are required for entry into that country.

Diagnosis

You need to determine whether you believe the patient will return for scheduled follow-up immunizations so that you can decide what immunizations to give on the first visit. National health authorities recommend that you give a person several injections at different sites if you think that the patient is not likely to return for follow-up shots.

Planning

The best policy is that immunizations should not be given to patients with active infection, severe febrile illness, or a history of serious side effects from previous vaccinations. Live, attenuated vaccine is usually contraindicated in pregnancy. To be safe, clinicians often do not provide immunizations to children who are being seen for minor illnesses. However, because many children are taken to the health care provider only when they are ill, clinicians may have to give the immunizations then. Otherwise, they may lose a very valuable opportunity to provide increased protection to the child.

Many biologic agents are prepared with animal serum or in chick embryos. Thus people with known allergies may have sensitivity reactions to these preparations. Live, attenuated virus vaccine should not be given if there is a recent history of acquired passive antibodies (immune globulins).

Patients should be screened for current illness. There is an increased risk in using immunologic agents in any person with a compromised immune status (for example, neonates, elderly patients, patients on immunosuppressive therapy, patients with acquired immunodeficiency syndrome [AIDS], or patients with chronic disease).

All vaccines should be used with caution in women who are pregnant or breastfeeding.

Implementation

It is important to follow specific protocols and schedules for administration. There are usually specialized storage instructions, modes of administration, sites, and site preparation techniques for each vaccine. It is also important to consult the package insert for each manufacturer's product information because these products often differ in some ways.

Figure 21-2 shows the dosage schedule recommended for primary immunization of infants, children, and adolescents.

Uncomfortable reactions to active vaccines are frequent and generally range from localized irritation and soreness to a systemic response with fever, malaise, and anorexia (lack of appetite). Specific biologic agents may predispose the patient to a variety of allergic reactions. These range from a localized rash, pruritus (itching), or urticaria to an anaphylactic (shock) reaction.

A record of the patient's immunizations should be kept, and the patient should be provided with a copy of the record to take home for her personal file.

Occasionally, determining antibody blood titers before vaccine administration is helpful to assess antibody development. This is particularly true for rubella.

Table 21-1 provides a summary of agents used for immunity.

Evaluation

Patients receiving immune serums should be evaluated for suppression of the disease. Other patients should be monitored for adverse effects. Adverse effects may occur immediately or be delayed for some time after the preparation has been administered. On all visits, patients should be asked whether or not their immunizations are current. There has been a decrease in the number of children who are getting the recommended immunizations over the past few years. In addition, few adults obtain the booster immunizations they need unless they are in the military, travel to foreign countries, or work in the food industry.

Vaccine ▼ / Age ▶	Birth	1 month	2 months	4 months	6 months	12 months	15 months	18 months	24 months	4–6 years	11–12 years	13–18 years
Hepatitis B[1]	HepB #1	HepB #2				HepB #3				HepB Series		
Diphtheria, Tetanus, Pertussis[2]			DTaP	DTaP	DTaP		DTaP			DTaP	Td	Td
Haemophilus influenzae type b[3]			Hib	Hib	Hib	Hib						
Inactivated Poliovirus			IPV	IPV		IPV				IPV		
Measles, Mumps, Rubella[4]						MMR #1				MMR #2	MMR #2	
Varicella[5]						Varicella				Varicella		
Pneumococcal[6]			PCV	PCV	PCV	PCV				PCV	PPV	
Influenza[7]						Influenza (Yearly)				Influenza (Yearly)		
Hepatitis A[8]										Hepatitis A Series		

Vaccines below red line are for selected populations

This schedule indicates the recommended ages for routine administration of currently licensed childhood vaccines, as of December 1, 2004, for children through age 18 years. Any dose not administered at the recommended age should be administered at any subsequent visit when indicated and feasible.

▨ Indicates age groups that warrant special effort to administer those vaccines not previously administered. Additional vaccines may be licensed and recommended during the year. Licensed combination vaccines may be used whenever any components of the combination are indicated and other components of the vaccine are not contraindicated. Providers should consult the manufacturers' package inserts for detailed recommendations. Clinically significant adverse events that follow immunization should be reported to the Vaccine Adverse Event Reporting System (VAERS). Guidance about how to obtain and complete a VAERS form are available at www.vaers.org or by telephone, 800-822-7967.

▨ Range of recommended ages   ▨ Only if mother HBsAg(–)
▨ Preadolescent assessment   ▨ Catch-up immunization

The Childhood and Adolescent Immunization Schedule is approved by:
Advisory Committee on Immunization Practices www.cdc.gov/nip/acip
American Academy of Pediatrics www.aap.org
American Academy of Family Physicians www.aafp.org

DEPARTMENT OF HEALTH AND HUMAN SERVICES
CENTERS FOR DISEASE CONTROL AND PREVENTION

FIGURE **21-2** Recommended childhood and adolescent immunization schedule, United States, 2005.
Continued

Footnotes
Recommended Childhood and Adolescent Immunization Schedule
UNITED STATES 2005

1. **Hepatitis B (HepB) vaccine.** All infants should receive the first dose of HepB vaccine soon after birth and before hospital discharge; the first dose may also be administered by age 2 months if the mother is hepatitis B surface antigen (HBsAg) negative. Only monovalent HepB may be used for the birth dose. Monovalent or combination vaccine containing HepB may be used to complete the series. Four doses of vaccine may be administered when a birth dose is given. The second dose should be administered at least 4 weeks after the first dose, except for combination vaccines which cannot be administered before age 6 weeks. The third dose should be given at least 16 weeks after the first dose and at least 8 weeks after the second dose. The last dose in the vaccination series (third or fourth dose) should not be administered before age 24 weeks.

   Infants born to HBsAg-positive mothers should receive HepB and 0.5 mL of hepatitis B immune globulin (HBIG) at separate sites within 12 hours of birth. The second dose is recommended at age 1–2 months. The final dose in the immunization series should not be administered before age 24 weeks. These infants should be tested for HBsAg and antibody to HBsAg (anti-HBs) at age 9–15 months.

   Infants born to mothers whose HBsAg status is unknown should receive the first dose of the HepB series within 12 hours of birth. Maternal blood should be drawn as soon as possible to determine the mother's HBsAg status; if the HBsAg test is positive, the infant should receive HBIG as soon as possible (no later than age 1 week). The second dose is recommended at age 1–2 months. The last dose in the immunization series should not be administered before age 24 weeks.

2. **Diphtheria and tetanus toxoids and acellular pertussis (DTaP) vaccine.** The fourth dose of DTaP may be administered as early as age 12 months, provided 6 months have elapsed since the third dose and the child is unlikely to return at age 15–18 months. The final dose in the series should be given at age 4 years. Tetanus and diphtheria toxoids (Td) is recommended at age 11–12 years if at least 5 years have elapsed since the last dose of tetanus and diphtheria toxoid-containing vaccine. Subsequent routine Td boosters are recommended every 10 years.

3. *Haemophilus influenzae* **type b (Hib) conjugate vaccine.** Three Hib conjugate vaccines are licensed for infant use. If PRP-OMP (PedvaxHIB® or ComVax® [Merck]) is administered at ages 2 and 4 months, a dose at age 6 months is not required. DTaP/Hib combination products should not be used for primary immunization in infants at ages 2, 4 or 6 months but can be used as boosters after any Hib vaccine. The final dose in the series should be administered at age 12 months.

4. **Measles, mumps, and rubella vaccine (MMR).** The second dose of MMR is recommended routinely at age 4–6 years but may be administered during any visit, provided at least 4 weeks have elapsed since the first dose and both doses are administered beginning at or after age 12 months. Those who have not previously received the second dose should complete the schedule by age 11–12 years.

5. **Varicella vaccine.** Varicella vaccine is recommended at any visit at or after age 12 months for susceptible children (i.e., those who lack a reliable history of chickenpox). Susceptible persons aged 13 years should receive 2 doses administered at least 4 weeks apart.

6. **Pneumococcal vaccine.** The heptavalent pneumococcal conjugate vaccine (PCV) is recommended for all children aged 2–23 months and for certain children aged 24–59 months. The final dose in the series should be given at age 12 months. **Pneumococcal polysaccharide vaccine (PPV)** is recommended in addition to PCV for certain high-risk groups. See *MMWR* 2000;49(RR-9):1-35.

7. **Influenza vaccine.** Influenza vaccine is recommended annually for children aged 6 months with certain risk factors (including, but not limited to, asthma, cardiac disease, sickle cell disease, human immunodeficiency virus [HIV], and diabetes), healthcare workers, and other persons (including household members) in close contact with persons in groups at high risk (see *MMWR* 2004;53(RR-1):1-40). In addition, healthy children aged 6–23 months and close contacts of healthy children aged 0–23 months are recommended to receive influenza vaccine because children in this age group are at substantially increased risk for influenza-related hospitalizations. For healthy persons aged 5–49 years, the intranasally administered, live, attenuated influenza vaccine (LAIV) is an acceptable alternative to the intramuscular trivalent inactivated influenza vaccine (TIV). See *MMWR* 2004;53(RR-6):1-40. Children receiving TIV should be administered a dosage appropriate for their age (0.25 mL if aged 6–35 months or 0.5 mL if aged 3 years). Children aged 8 years who are receiving influenza vaccine for the first time should receive 2 doses (separated by at least 4 weeks for TIV and at least 6 weeks for LAIV).

8. **Hepatitis A vaccine.** Hepatitis A vaccine is recommended for children and adolescents in selected states and regions and for certain high-risk groups; consult your local public health authority. Children and adolescents in these states, regions, and high-risk groups who have not been immunized against hepatitis A can begin the hepatitis A immunization series during any visit. The 2 doses in the series should be administered at least 6 months apart. See *MMWR* 1999;48(RR-12):1-37.

FIGURE **21-2—cont'd** Recommended childhood and adolescent immunization schedule, United States, 2005.

Patient and Family Teaching

You should tell the patient and family the following:

1. Localized discomfort may be relieved by treating the symptoms: use warm compresses on the area, acetaminophen, rest, and sometimes antihistamines.
2. The patient (or family member) should record the immunization in a personal health file.
3. The patient should notify the nurse, physician, or other health care provider immediately if fever, rash, itching, or difficulty breathing develops.
4. The patient or family should periodically discuss immunizations with the nurse, physician, or other health care provider to make certain that they have adequate immunity.

Key Points

- Immunologic agents provide active or passive immunity to specific diseases.
- Types of immunologic agents are vaccines, toxoids, and other serologic agents used to prevent or modify disease.
- Immunity can be either naturally acquired or artificially acquired.
- It is important to follow specific protocols and schedules for administering these products.
- Adults are commonly underimmunized because they do not realize that their immunity has expired.

Go to the free CD-ROM for an Audio Glossary, animations, video clips, and Review Questions for the NCLEX-PN® Examination.

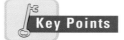 Be sure to visit the companion Evolve website at http://evolve.elsevier.com/Edmunds/LPN/ for WebLinks, a link to the top 200 drugs by prescription, and sign-up pages for newsletter drug updates.

Table 21-1

Agents for Immunity

PRODUCT	COMMENTS AND DOSAGE
AGENTS FOR ACTIVE IMMUNITY	
Toxoids	
Diphtheria and tetanus toxoids and pertussis vaccine, adsorbed	Immunization for infants and children younger than 6 yr. Produces local reactions, fever, malaise, generalized aches, and pain.
Diphtheria and tetanus toxoids, combined	*Primary immunizations:* 2 doses of 0.5 mL IM at 2, 4, and 6 mo, again at 12 mo, and no later than 11-12 yr.
Diphtheria, tetanus toxoid, and acellular pertussis	*Booster:* 0.5 mL IM at 5- to 10-yr intervals. Vaccine is different for children and adults.
Diphtheria, tetanus toxoid, whole cell pertussis, and *Haemophilus influenzae* type b	
Diphtheria toxoid, adsorbed	
Tetanus toxoid	Immunization in adults and children. May produce local reactions, fever, chills, malaise, and myalgia (widespread muscle pain).
	Tetanus toxoid, adsorbed: 2 doses of 0.5 mL IM at 2, 4, and 6 mo, again at 12 mo, and no later than 11-12 yr.
	Booster: every 10 yr.
	Tetanus toxoid, fluid: 3 doses of 0.5 mL IM or subcutaneously at 4- to 8-wk intervals and fourth dose 6-12 mo after third dose.
	Booster: every 5-10 yr, depending on risk of wound.
Bacterial Vaccines	
Bacille Calmette-Guérin (BCG) vaccine	For tuberculosis protection in international travelers to high-risk areas, high-risk infants and children. Place 0.2-0.3 mL on skin. Use multiple-puncture disk.
Cholera vaccine	Required for travel to certain areas. May produce brief local reactions, fever, headache, and malaise. Give 2 doses of 0.5 mL subcutaneously or IM 1 wk to 1 mo apart.
H. influenzae b conjugate vaccine	Routine immunization. Number of doses and amount injected vary by patient age.

Meningococcal polysaccharide vaccine
  Group A, Group C
  Groups A and C
  Groups A, C, Y, and W-135
	Induces formation of antibodies, leading to immunity to specific organisms. Does not provide immunity against all varieties. Give 0.5 mL subcutaneously only. Revaccination may be required in some individuals at high risk, but standards are not specific.

Plague vaccine	Reduces incidence and severity of disease. Give 2 doses 1 mo apart, follow with third dose 1-3 mo later. See dosage schedule in package insert.
Pneumococcal vaccine, polyvalent	Produces immunity against a variety of pneumococcal infections. Give 0.5 mL IM or subcutaneously. Revaccinations necessary in 3 or more yr.
Pneumococcal 7-valent conjugate vaccine (Prevnar)	Provides active immunization for infants and children against *Streptococcus pneumoniae.* Give 3 doses of 0.5 mL administered as IM injection at 2-mo intervals, followed by a fourth dose of 0.5 mL at 12-15 mo of age. Shake suspension vigorously immediately before use.
Typhoid vaccine	Give when there has been exposure to a known carrier or foreign travel to area where typhoid is endemic. May produce local reactions, fever, chills, malaise, and myalgia.
	Primary immunization: 2 doses of 0.5 mL subcutaneously 4 or more wk apart; 0.25 mL for children.
	Booster: 0.3 ml subcutaneously or 0.1 mL intradermal every 3 yr; for children younger than age 10, the dose is 0.25 mL subcutaneously or 0.1 mL intradermally.

Continue

Table 21-1

Agents for Immunity—cont'd

PRODUCT	COMMENTS AND DOSAGE
AGENTS FOR ACTIVE IMMUNITY—cont'd	
Bacterial Vaccines—cont'd	
Lyme disease vaccine	Give to patients at high risk who live or work in *Borrelia burgdorferi*–infected grassy or wooded areas. *Primary immunization:* give a 30-mcg/0.5-mL dose of vaccine, repeat in 1 and 12 mo. Vaccination with all three doses is required to achieve optimal protection. Shake container well before drawing dose. Vaccine is a turbid white suspension. Administer by IM injection only in the deltoid region.
Viral Vaccines	
Hepatitis A vaccine (Havrix)	Give primary dose and then booster 6-12 mo later. Give in deltoid muscle only. Number of doses and amount injected vary by patient age.
Hepatitis B vaccine (Hepavax-B)	For immunization against all known subtypes of hepatitis B virus. May produce local reactions, malaise, fatigue, nausea, myalgia, and headache. *Adults:* 1 mL IM, repeat in 1 and 6 mo. *Children under 10 yr:* 0.5 mL; repeat in 1 and 6 mo.
Influenza virus vaccine	Annual vaccination of high-risk persons. May produce localized reactions, fever, malaise, and myalgia. Dosage schedule varies from year to year.
Measles, mumps, and rubella virus vaccine, live	Same as measles virus vaccine, live attenuated.
Measles, rubeola, and rubella virus vaccine, live	Immunization for children 15 mo to puberty. Give booster at 4-6 yr and 11-12 yr. Give 1 ampule subcutaneously.
Measles virus vaccine, live attenuated	Give before or immediately after exposure to measles or as immunization for children 15 mo or older. May develop fever and rash between 5th and 12th day after injection. Give 1 ampule subcutaneously.
Mumps virus vaccine, live	Give to children 15 mo or older and adults. May develop fever or parotitis. Give 1 ampule subcutaneously.
Pertussis vaccine (in combination)	See diphtheria (earlier in table).
Poliomyelitis vaccine, inactivated (IPV), Salk	Immunization for those with compromised immune systems. May provoke allergic reactions. Give 3 doses of 1 mL each subcutaneously at 4- to 6-wk intervals, then 1 dose of 1 mL 6-12 mo after the third dose. *Booster:* 1 mL subcutaneously every 2-3 yr.
Poliovirus vaccine, live, oral, trivalent (TOPV), Sabin	Prevention of polio in infants and children up to 18 yr. May provoke rare vaccine-related paralysis. Give 3 doses of 0.5 mL PO: first dose at 6-12 wk of age, second dose 6-8 wk later, third dose 8-12 mo after second dose. *Booster:* On entering school.
Rotavirus	Suggested to be given at 2, 4, and 6 mo as protection against gastrointestinal disease caused by rotavirus. Give 2.5 mL PO.
Rubella and mumps virus vaccine, live	Immunization for children 15 mo to puberty. Give 1 ampule subcutaneously.
Rubella virus vaccine, live	Immunization for children 15 mo to puberty. May produce rash, sore throat, fever, headache, and urticaria. Give 1 ampule subcutaneously.
Varicella (Varivax)	Give primary immunization at 12-18 mo, with a booster at 11-12 yr. Give 0.5 mL subcutaneously and repeat 4-8 wk later.
Yellow fever vaccine	Given only at approved World Health Organization centers for people traveling abroad. Give 0.5 mL subcutaneously with revaccination in 10 yr as needed.

Table 21-1

Agents for Immunity—cont'd

PRODUCT	COMMENTS AND DOSAGE
AGENTS FOR PASSIVE IMMUNITY	
Antitoxins and Antivenins	
Black widow spider species antivenin	*Adults and children:* Inject 1 vial IM, preferably in the region of the anterolateral thigh so that a tourniquet may be applied in the event of a systemic reaction. Symptoms usually subside in 1-3 hr.
Diphtheria antitoxin	For prevention and treatment of diphtheria. Give 20,000-120,000 units IM, IV as therapy; 10,000 units IM for prophylaxis.
Immune Serums	
Cytomegalovirus immune globulin (CMV-IGIV)	For the attenuation of primary CMV disease associated with kidney transplantation. Usually give 15 mg/kg/hr IV.
Hepatitis B immune globulin (human)	For postexposure or high-risk patient prophylaxis. Produces local reactions, urticaria, and fever. Give 0.06 mg/kg IM as soon as possible and repeat 28-30 days after exposure.
Immune globulin IV (IGIV)	For the maintenance treatment of patients who are unable to produce sufficient amounts of immunoglobulin G antibodies. Used in patients with immunodeficiency syndrome, idiopathic thrombocytopenic purpura, and beta-cell chronic lymphocytic leukemia. Usually, give 200 mg/kg IV once a month.
Immune serum globulin, human (HISG)	For hepatitis A, rubeola prophylaxis; immunoglobulin deficiency; passive immunization for varicella in immunosuppressed patients. Give 0.02-1.2 mL/kg IM, depending on reason for use.
Lymphocyte immune globulin, antithymocyte globulin	Used in management of allograft rejection in patients who have undergone renal transplant. Give 5-30 mg/kg/day IV.
Rh_0(D) immune globulin	Effectively suppresses the immune response of nonsensitized Rh-negative mothers after delivery of an Rh-positive infant. Give 1 vial IM.
Respiratory syncytial virus (RSV) immune globulin (RespiGam)	Used in prevention of serious lower respiratory tract infection caused by RSV in children less than 24 mo of age with bronchopulmonary dysplasia or a history of premature birth. Give by IV infusion based on body mass.
Tetanus immune globulin, human (HTIG)	For temporary postexposure prophylaxis. Give 4 units/kg IM.
Varicella-zoster immune globulin, human (VZIG)	For temporary passive immunity to varicella. Give deep IM, according to dosage schedule on package insert.
Rabies Prophylaxis Products	
Rabies immune globulin, human (RIG)	Immunization for those thought to be exposed to rabies. May produce fever and soreness at injection site. Give 20 International Units/kg IM; half the dose may be used to infiltrate the wound.
Rabies vaccine, human diploid cell cultures (HDCV)	For prophylaxis and postexposure treatment. May produce nausea, headache, muscle aches, abdominal pain, and local reactions. See package insert for dosage schedule.
IN VIVO DIAGNOSTIC BIOLOGIC AGENTS	
Candida and *Trichophyton*	Give 0.1 mL by shallow subcutaneous injection to detect sensitivity.
Coccidioidin	Used to identify people with exposure to the fungus *Coccidioides* or with active disease (coccidioidomycosis). Give lowest possible dose by intradermal injection and evaluate 24-48 hr later. Positive reaction is area of erythema (redness) and induration (hardening) 5 mm or greater in size.
Histoplasmin	Used to identify people with exposure to the fungus *Histoplasma* or with active disease (histoplasmosis). Give 0.1 mL by intradermal injection and evaluate 24-48 hr later. Positive reaction is area of erythema and induration 5 mm or greater in size.

Continued

Table 21-1

Agents for Immunity—cont'd

PRODUCT	COMMENTS AND DOSAGE
IN VIVO DIAGNOSTIC BIOLOGIC AGENTS—cont'd	
Mumps skin test antigen	Demonstrates cutaneous hypersensitivity to mumps virus. Give 0.1 mL antigen by intradermal injection and evaluate 24-48 hr later. Positive reaction is area of erythema and induration 5 mm or greater in size.
Tuberculin Old, multiple-puncture device	Same as tuberculin PPD multiple-puncture device.
Tuberculin PPD multiple-puncture device	Used to identify persons with active tuberculosis, with exposure to tuberculosis, or needing further testing.
Tuberculin purified protein derivative (Mantoux)	Designed to identify persons with active tuberculosis, with exposure to tuberculosis, or needing further testing. Give 0.1 mL of intermediate-strength PPD by intradermal injection and evaluate in 24-48 hr. Positive reaction must have erythema and induration 9 mm or more in size; areas 5 to 9 mm are questionable; areas under 5 mm are negative.

CASE STUDY

Mr. John Phillips, 53, a state highway patrol officer, discovered an injured raccoon along the highway. As he attempted to remove it from the road, the raccoon scratched and bit him. The raccoon was taken to the local animal control department, where it was discovered to be infected with rabies.

1. What treatment should Mr. Phillips receive?
2. Mr. Phillips tells you he has had prophylactic rabies injections. Does this make a difference in the treatment?
3. What treatments may be required?
4. Administering rabies vaccine to Mr. Phillips is an example of what type of immunity?
5. Which groups of people would commonly be considered at high risk for rabies and thus should receive prophylactic therapy?

DRUG CALCULATION REVIEW

1. Order: Immune globulin IV (IGIV) 14,000 mg IV over 2 hours

   Supply: Immune globulin 14,000 mg in 100 mL of 5% dextrose in water (D₅W)

   Question: How many milliliters per hour should the IV infusion device be set for?

2. Order: Diphtheria antitoxin 20,000 units intramuscular

   Supply: Diphtheria antitoxin 100,000 units/mL

   Question: How many milliliters of diphtheria antitoxin are needed for each dose?

3. Order: Lymphocyte immune globulin 20 mg/kg/day

   Question: How many milligrams of lymphocyte immune globulin are needed each day for a person weighing 65 kg?

CRITICAL THINKING ?

1. Outline the benefits versus the risks of immunizations and their potential adverse effects.

2. You are asked to give immunizations to four children of various ages who are visiting your clinic this afternoon. Draw up a general list of assessment, planning, and implementation strategies that can be used for all four children.

3. Suggest appropriate actions the nurse and patient can take in response to hypersensitivity or allergic reactions commonly seen with immunologic agents.

4. Give examples of the process or development of each of the following types of immunity: (a) artificially acquired active immunity, (b) artificially acquired passive immunity, (c) naturally acquired active immunity, and (d) naturally acquired passive immunity.

5. Identify and suggest ways to counteract the most common side effects of immunologic agents.

6. After giving him an immunization, you explain to Mr. Stavros that he will need a booster later. Mr. Stavros has never heard of a booster. Explain what a booster is, along with the rationale for getting one.

7. When might a patient exhibit extra sensitivity to an immunologic agent?

8. Why is it important to know if someone is allergic to eggs or feathers before immunizing them?

9. Alicia, who is 5 years old, comes to her appointment for her school physical with her mother. As you are preparing to administer her immunizations for school entry, you ask her mother if she has any concerns about Alicia starting school in a few months. Her mother tells you, "Well, I am a little worried. Alicia is very close to my mother, you know. She's been sick with cancer, and Alicia has been spending a lot of time with her, keeping her company. I think my mother's going to be a little lonely when Alicia goes to school every day." Why is this information significant?

22 Antiinflammatory, Musculoskeletal, and Antiarthritis Medications

Objectives

After reading and studying this chapter, you should be able to do the following:

1. List medications commonly used for the treatment of minor musculoskeletal pain and inflammation.
2. Identify the appropriate use for musculoskeletal relaxants.
3. Explain the mechanisms of action for different antiarthritis medications.
4. Describe the clinical situations in which uricosuric therapy may be indicated.
5. Compare the actions of various antiinflammatory and muscle relaxant agents.
6. Describe adverse reactions frequently found in the use of antiarthritis medications.

Key Terms

Be sure to check out the bonus material on the free CD-ROM, including selected audio pronunciations.

arthritis (ărth-RĪ-tĭs, p. 423)
gold compounds (p. 424)
gout (gowt, p. 428)
nonsteroidal antiinflammatory drugs (NSAIDs) (p. 418)
osteoarthritis (ŏs-tē-ō-ărth-RĪ-tĭs, p. 423)
rheumatoid arthritis (RŪ-mă-tŏyd, p. 423)
salicylates (să-LĬS-ĭl-āts, p. 413)
skeletal muscle relaxants (p. 420)
slow-acting antirheumatic drugs (SAARDs) (p. 424)
uric acid (Ū-rĭk, p. 428)
uricosuric agents (Ū-rĭ-kō-SŪR-ĭk, p. 428)

OVERVIEW

This chapter includes the medications helpful in treating problems affecting the bones, joints, muscles, and ligaments. There are a variety of musculoskeletal disorders that cause varying degrees of pain, disability, and deformity. The drugs used to treat these problems are selected on the basis of the severity of the problem and the pathologic mechanisms causing the disorder. Many acute problems, such as sprains, fractures, or tears, require only short-term therapy. Some disorders, such as arthritis, may require long-term therapy with a variety of medications, with more powerful drugs required as the disability increases. Many of these products have serious adverse reactions, and patients must be closely monitored to determine their response to therapy.

This chapter is divided into four sections. Section One deals with antiinflammatory and analgesic medications such as the salicylates and nonsteroidal antiinflammatory drugs (NSAIDs), which are used to treat both severe pain and common orthopedic problems. Section Two presents skeletal muscle relaxants. Section Three introduces a variety of medications used to treat arthritis: the slow-acting antirheumatic drugs (SAARDs). Agents used to treat high uric acid levels found in gout are presented in Section Four.

MUSCULAR AND SKELETAL SYSTEMS

The muscular and skeletal systems work together to provide support and movement for the body (Figures 22-1 and 22-2). The skeletal system is composed of the bones, cartilage, and joints, and the muscular system involves those muscles attached to the skeleton.

The skeleton protects, supports, and allows body movement; produces blood cells in the long bones; and stores minerals. The muscular system provides movement of body parts, maintains posture, and produces body heat.

Pathologic conditions may arise within the body as a whole or in the muscular or ligament attachments. Often injuries are due to trauma or to long-term wear or overuse. Although some traumatic skeletal injuries heal well and the patient has no remaining problems, some injuries may be the site for continuing pain and deformity.

THE INFLAMMATORY RESPONSE

The inflammatory response is necessary for the body's survival when faced with stressors from the environment. A number of things can trigger the inflammatory

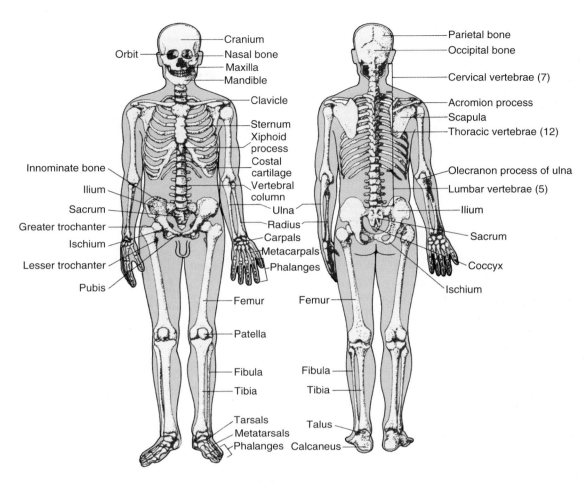

FIGURE 22-1 The skeletal system.

response. These include infectious agents, ischemia (lack of blood supply to a tissue), antigen-antibody interactions, and thermal (heat) or other injury. The inflammatory response has three phases:

1. Acute, brief, local vasodilation (opening up of the blood vessels) and increased capillary permeability
2. A delayed, subacute infiltration (movement) of leukocytes and phagocytic cells into the tissue
3. Chronic proliferative tissue degeneration (breakdown) and fibrosis

The inflammatory response of the body produces the symptoms of erythema (redness or irritation), edema (fluid buildup in the body tissues), tenderness, and pain. This happens when the affected blood cells release a variety of inflammatory mediators (substances that continue the inflammatory response). The inflammatory mediators act to increase blood flow to the area and increase capillary permeability, allowing movement of large molecules across cell walls into the site. One of the most important inflammatory mediators is histamine, which causes vasodilation to increase blood flow to the area. Cytokines help control the inflammatory

process. Prostaglandins also have a role in the inflammatory reaction.

Prostaglandins have several actions in the body. The useful functions of prostaglandins have to do with "housekeeping" actions in the tissues, especially in protecting the mucosa of the gastrointestinal (GI) tract. They also maintain normal renal function, platelet aggregation (clumping together), consciousness and mental functions in the brain, and temperature. Prostaglandins also cause erythema and an increase in local blood flow, and they can remove the vasoconstrictor effects of substances such as norepinephrine and angiotensin. These harmful actions of prostaglandins are controlled by a series of reactions at sites of tissue injury and inflammation.

When circulating proteins and blood cells contact an area where there is tissue disruption or tearing of a cell membrane, phospholipids are released. Phospholipase acts on those phospholipids, leading to the release of arachidonic acid. This chemical reaction is proinflammatory (before the inflammatory stage) and occurs before the development of prostaglandins.

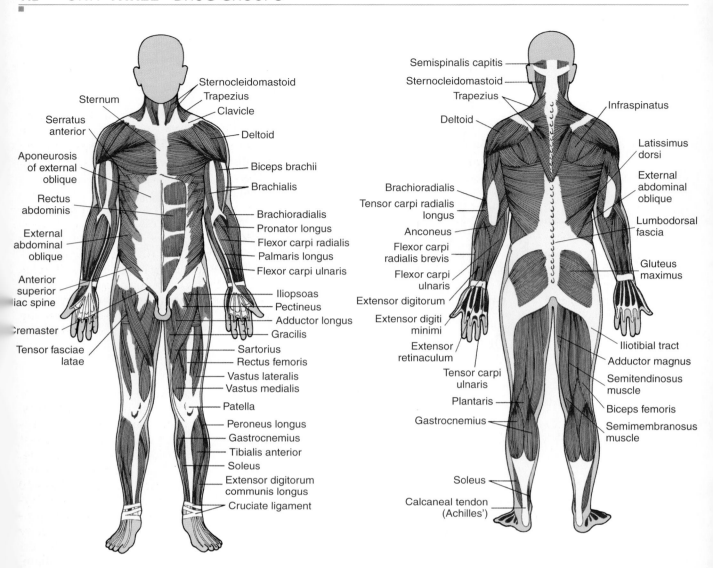

FIGURE **23-1** The muscular system.

In the synthesis or production of prostaglandins, the first enzyme is cyclooxygenase, which converts arachidonic acid into prostaglandins. There are two forms of cyclooxygenase: cyclooxygenase-1 (COX-1) and cyclooxygenase-2 (COX-2). COX-1 is found in blood vessels, the stomach, and the kidneys. The housekeeping functions of prostaglandins are controlled by COX-1. COX-2 is created where there is inflammation caused by cytokines and other inflammatory mediators. It is also found in the brain, where it plays a role in fever and perception of pain. COX-2 is an active participant in the inflammatory process and produces harmful results in the body if not controlled.

Although it is important to have medications that can block the harmful actions of prostaglandins, the important physiologic functions of prostaglandins that are helpful in the body must be preserved. Most antiinflammatory drugs block the actions of both COX-1 and COX-2. A group of drugs known as COX-2 inhibitors or blockers was developed to reduce the inflammatory response in some tissues without destroying the tissue of the GI tract. Although these drugs reduce the incidence of gastric bleeding, current research suggests that they may do so at the expense of the heart—leaving the patient who takes them for a long time at greater risk for heart attack and stroke. Some of the COX-2 inhibitors have been pulled from the market, and the others are now being carefully checked to determine whether they are safe for patients to use.

SECTION ONE

Antiinflammatory and Analgesic Agents

OVERVIEW

Aspirin is one of the most commonly taken medications. The ease with which it can be bought and the fact that people decide when and if they need it should not decrease the importance given to this drug in treating common and significant musculoskeletal problems. Aspirin (acetylsalicylic acid [ASA]) has greater antiinflammatory action than other salicylates and is preferred in the treatment of many problems. Acetaminophen is also used for analgesia in generalized pain and arthritis because of its safety. The NSAIDs are powerful agents to help decrease pain and inflammation. Interest in and research on NSAIDs is expanding. Both salicylates and NSAIDs are thought to limit the production of prostaglandins, which may make peripheral pain receptors more sensitive to painful stimuli.

SALICYLATES

ACTION

Salicylates have analgesic, antipyretic (temperature reducing), and antiinflammatory effects. Salicylates stop the production of prostaglandins, which affects the pain and inflammatory processes through a depressant effect on the central and peripheral pain receptors. They do this by blocking the production of cyclooxygenase, an enzyme that is necessary for the production of prostaglandins.

USES

Aspirin is stronger or more potent in stopping prostaglandin synthesis than are other salicylates, and it has greater antiinflammatory effects. Aspirin is used in the treatment of mild to moderate pain. Aspirin also has an action on the blood. It is the only drug in this category to irreversibly limit platelet aggregation or for the life of the platelet (7 to 10 days). It also interferes with factor III of the clotting mechanism. This makes it useful in reducing the risk for strokes or for additional transient ischemic attacks (TIAs) in men who have had TIAs because of fibrin platelet emboli. However, it is of no benefit for men who have already had strokes. Aspirin does not seem to prevent TIAs or strokes in women.

Small daily doses of aspirin are also used to reduce the risk of death or nonfatal myocardial infarction in patients with previous infarction or unstable angina pectoris. Lower doses seem to be more effective than higher doses for this purpose. Unlabeled uses of aspirin in low doses also include prevention of cataract and prevention of toxemia of pregnancy.

Salicylates are used as first-line therapy to treat various forms of arthritis (rheumatoid arthritis, osteoarthritis, degenerative joint disease). They are used to treat systemic fever produced by bacterial illnesses and in therapy for pain arising from trauma to soft tissue or muscle. Pain in the muscles, nerves, and joints (myalgias, neuralgias, and arthralgias), as well as headache and dysmenorrhea, are also treated with salicylates. The antiinflammatory effects are useful in treating systemic lupus erythematosus, acute rheumatic fever, and similar conditions.

ADVERSE REACTIONS

Adverse reactions to antiinflammatory analgesics include tinnitus (ringing in the ears), visual disturbances, edema, urticaria (hives), rashes, anorexia (lack of appetite), epigastric discomfort, and nausea. The greatest concern is the production of GI distress and bleeding. Bleeding may often occur suddenly and without pain. It is estimated that a normal person taking ASA loses 10 mL of blood every day from minor GI irritation. Hypersensitivity (allergy) is also common and may produce severe symptoms. In overdosage, symptoms may progress from mild to severe, beginning with hyperventilation, diaphoresis (sweating), thirst, headache, drowsiness, skin eruptions, and electrolyte imbalance and progressing to central nervous system (CNS) depression, stupor, convulsions and coma, tachycardia (rapid heartbeat), and respiratory insufficiency. Respiratory and metabolic acidosis are most often seen in children.

DRUG INTERACTIONS

Alcohol taken with any of the antiinflammatory analgesics increases the chance of GI bleeding. Decreased excretion by the kidneys or decreased protein binding may produce an increased *para*-aminosalicylic acid effect. There is an increased effect of anticoagulants, sulfonylureas, and sulfonamides if they are used at the same time as salicylates. Ascorbic acid increases the effect of salicylates by increasing renal tubular reabsorption. Salicylates interact with NSAIDs to increase effects, side effects, and toxicities. Salicylates also increase or potentiate the effects of phenytoin and inhibit hyperuricemia produced by pyrazinamide. Salicylates can affect many laboratory test results.

Nursing Implications and Patient Teaching

Assessment

You should learn all you can about the patient's health history. Check for the presence of hypersensitivity to aspirin or other NSAIDs, history of asthma or nasal polyps, GI problems or ulcer disease, current use of other drugs that may cause interactions, or other hepatic or renal disease. These conditions are precautions or contraindications to the use of salicylates.

The health care provider may ask you to check for occult blood in the patient's stool before beginning the medication. This will help determine whether or not the patient had bleeding in the stool before the medication was started.

Antiinflammatory analgesics are effective for mild to moderate pain of a musculoskeletal nature and in conditions causing mild fever. They are useful for many of the same conditions in which NSAIDs are used.

Diagnosis

Careful attention should be paid to other medications and disease processes of the patient. Are there conditions that would make the use of NSAIDs or salicylates dangerous? What is the risk for GI bleeding in this patient? How much caffeine, alcohol, or tobacco does this patient use? Are there other problems related to weight, mobility, safety, or nutrition?

Planning

Antiinflammatory analgesics should not be used in patients with hepatic disease. Patients on anticoagulant therapy or with abnormalities of clotting must be very careful when they use these products. These drugs also should not be used before surgery, because of their effect on platelet aggregation, or before labor, because bleeding may increase. They should be used with caution in patients with symptoms suggesting TIAs. In patients with musculoskeletal pain that persists for more than 10 days, further evaluation of the pain is needed.

Antiinflammatory analgesics should not be used during pregnancy, especially during the third trimester, because they may have adverse effects on the fetus. Salicylates are excreted in breast milk.

These drugs should be used cautiously in the presence of gastric irritation, especially in patients with a past history of upper GI problems. They should also be used with caution in patients with blood dyscrasias or decreased renal function.

Hydration (supply of fluids) should be monitored carefully in children, because they seem to be more prone to salicylate intoxication or overdose.

Reye's syndrome is an acute, life-threatening problem that produces vomiting and lethargy that may go to delirium and coma with permanent brain damage and possible death. Use of aspirin after influenza,

chickenpox, or other viral conditions in children seems to be closely related to the development of Reye's syndrome and should be avoided.

Many salicylate products are not recommended for use in children younger than 12 years of age. When salicylates are ordered for children, you should check the individual agent to make certain that the product is safe for children.

Clinical Landmine

Reye's Syndrome

Children who have repeated instances of viral upper respiratory tract infection symptoms within a short time span or who have disorientation should not be given salicylates because these drugs have been linked to the development of Reye's syndrome in such conditions.

Implementation

The administration and dosage for each of the salicylate products vary. There are tablets, capsules, drops, chewable preparations, suppositories, and injectable forms of these products. Aspirin is the most active agent and has the greatest amount of salicylate per unit. Individual products should be checked for dosing specifics by age.

Patients with diabetes who are testing their urine with Benedict's Clinitest may get incorrect readings. They may need to switch to another form of urine testing while using salicylate products. Salicylates also increase the action of oral hypoglycemic agents, and diabetic patients should be alert to signs of hypoglycemia (low blood sugar level).

A summary of dosing information for the salicylates is provided in Table 22-1.

Evaluation

The patient should be monitored for the therapeutic effect: subjective relief of pain and reduction in temperature to 101° F or below. The dosage should be reduced or the drug discontinued if tinnitus develops. You should observe for fever that does not resolve or other symptoms that suggest the patient is getting worse and notify the health care provider.

For arthritis, higher dosages are usually needed to control pain and stiffness. The dosage should be slowly increased as necessary while the patient is watched not only for pain relief, but for improvement in such things as increased strength of grip, increased mobility, and improved ability to carry on normal activities of daily living. Patients taking medication over a long time should be monitored for signs of occult (hidden) bleeding with regular blood counts and stool checks. You

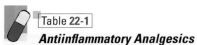

Table 22-1

Antiinflammatory Analgesics

GENERIC NAME	TRADE NAME	COMMENTS AND DOSAGE
SALICYLATES AND ACETAMINOPHEN		
acetaminophen	Acephen Aceta Acetaminophen Apacet Feverall Panadol Tempra 3 Tylenol	Used as an analgesic-antipyretic in the presence of aspirin allergy, and for patients with blood coagulation disorders who are being treated with oral anticoagulants, bleeding diatheses, upper GI disease, gastritis, hiatal hernia, and gouty arthritis. Also used for a variety of soft tissue injuries and for acute pain relief. *Adults:* 325-650 mg q4-6h. *Children:* 320-650 mg, depending on age. Also available in suppository form.
acetylsalicylic acid (ASA, aspirin)	Aspergum Bayer Ecotrin Empirin	The most commonly used antiinflammatory agent. It is the standard against which all other agents are compared. Hypersensitivity often exists. • *Mild to moderate pain:* 325-650 mg PO initially, then repeat q4h. • *Arthritis:* 2.6-5.2 gm/day PO in divided doses. • *Acute rheumatic fever:* Up to 7.8 gm/day in divided doses. *Children:* 65 mg/kg/day in divided doses.

acetylsalicylic acid
  (ASA) buffered
choline
  salicylate
	Alka-Seltzer
	Ascriptin
	Bufferin
	
	choline salicylate
		Aspirin-antacid combinations are used in patients who experience GI distress from plain aspirin.
		Give 325-850 mg q4h prn.
		Dosage and administration are the same as for plain aspirin (above).

	Arthropan	

This is a liquid form of salicylate with fewer GI side effects than aspirin. Used if sodium restriction is necessary. It has an unpleasant aftertaste that may be reduced by giving it in water.
Adults and children over 12 yr: 870 mg PO initially; repeat q3-4h; give no more than 6 times daily.

diflunisal	Dolobid	A salicylic acid nonsteroidal derivative. Give 1 gm PO, then 500 mg q8-12h.
magnesium salicylate	Doan's pills Magan Mobidin	A sodium-free salicylate with a lower incidence of GI problems than ASA. *Adults and children over 12 yr:* 600 mg PO 3 to 4 times daily. May be increased to 3.6 or 4.8 gm PO daily at 3- to 6-hr intervals.
salsalate	Amigesic Salsitab	*Adults:* 3000 mg/day in divided doses.
sodium salicylate	Sodium Salicylate	Give 325- to 650-mg enteric-coated tablet q4h.
sodium thiosalicylate	Rexolate	• *Acute gout:* 100 mg q3-4h IM for 2 days, then 100 mg daily. • *Rheumatic fever:* 100-150 mg IM q4-6h for 3 days, then 100 mg 3 times daily until patient is without symptoms.
NONSTEROIDAL ANTIINFLAMMATORY DRUGS		
diclofenac	Cataflam Voltaren 🍁	Used for chronic long-term therapy. Give 100-150 mg/day in divided doses. Do not exceed dosages of 200 mg/day. Also comes in a delayed-release tablet.
etodolac	Lodine	Give 800-1200 mg/day in divided doses.
fenoprofen	Nalfon	Administer medication 30 min before or 2 hr after meals because food interferes with absorption. • *Mild to moderate pain:* 200 mg PO q4-6h on empty stomach. • *Chronic pain:* 300-600 mg q6-8h on empty stomach; maximum dose 3200 mg/24 hr.
flurbiprofen	Ansaid	Used in rheumatoid arthritis and osteoarthritis. Give 100 mg 2 or 3 times daily.

Continued

Table 22-1

Antiinflammatory Analgesics—cont'd

GENERIC NAME	TRADE NAME	COMMENTS AND DOSAGE
NONSTEROIDAL ANTIINFLAMMATORY DRUGS—cont'd		
ibuprofen	Advil Motrin Nuprin	Approved for use in the treatment of dysmenorrhea. • *Mild to moderate pain:* 400 mg PO q4-6h. • *Chronic pain and acute exacerbations:* 300-600 mg PO q6-8h. • *Antiinflammatory response:* 800 mg q6-8h.
indomethacin	Indocid Indocin 🍁	A *potent* prostaglandin synthesis inhibitor with significant toxic side effects; many adverse reactions (including blood dyscrasias) and drug interactions. • *Acute gouty arthritis:* 50 mg 3 times daily for 3-5 days, then reduce to 25 mg 3 times daily. Gradually wean patient off medication as soon as possible.
ketoprofen	Orudis	Give 25-50 mg q6-8h for primary dysmenorrhea; higher doses in arthritis.
ketorolac	Toradol	Use IM for short-term management of pain. Use orally also for short duration. Give 10 mg q4-6h. May give 30-60 mg IM as loading dose, followed by half the loading dose q6h prn.
meclofenamate	—	Has the ability to block the action of prostaglandins and inhibit their synthesis, as opposed to the other NSAIDs that only inhibit prostaglandin synthesis. *Adults:* 50-100 mg PO q4-6h. Maximum dose 400 mg/day.
mefenamic acid	Ponstan Ponstel 🍁	Recommended for the treatment of dysmenorrhea rather than arthritis or other acute musculoskeletal problems. Give 500 mg, then 250 mg q6h.
meloxicam	Mobic	Give 7.5 mg daily with or without food. May require 15 mg daily.
nabumetone	Relafen	Give 1000 mg as single daily dose with or without food.
naproxen	Aleve Anaprox Naprosyn	• *Mild to moderate pain:* 500 mg initially, followed by 250 mg q6-8h, or 550 mg naproxen sodium, followed by 275 mg naproxen sodium q6-8h. For short-term use. • *Rheumatoid arthritis, osteoarthritis, ankylosing spondylitis:* 250-375 mg PO q12h. Doses do not have to be equal. Long-term therapy may require the higher dosage range. If there is no symptomatic effect in 2 wk, continue trial for 2 more wk before discontinuing the agent. • *Acute gout:* 750 mg (825 mg naproxen sodium), followed by 250 mg (275 mg naproxen sodium) q8h until attack ends.
oxaprozin	Daypro	Give 1200 mg PO once a day.
piroxicam	Feldene	Indicated in the treatment of acute exacerbations and long-term management of rheumatoid arthritis and osteoarthritis. Give 20 mg daily. No therapeutic effects may be seen for 2 wk.
sulindac	Clinoril	• *Arthritis and ankylosing spondylitis:* 150-200 mg twice daily with food. Maximum dose 400 mg/day. • *Acute painful shoulder or gout:* 200 mg twice daily with food. Use for 7 days in gout, 7-14 days for painful shoulder.
tolmetin	Tolectin	One of the few NSAIDs approved for the treatment of juvenile rheumatoid arthritis in children over age 2. • *Osteoarthritis:* 400 mg PO 3 times daily with meals. • *Rheumatoid arthritis:* 600-1600 mg/day in 3 to 4 divided doses with meals; maximum of 2 gm/day PO. *Children over 2 yr:* 15-20 mg/kg/day in 3 to 4 divided doses with meals; dosages higher than 30 mg/kg/day not recommended.
Cyclooxygenase-2 Inhibitor		
celecoxib	Celebrex	Used in osteoarthritis, rheumatoid arthritis, acute pain, and dysmenorrhea. Give 200 mg/day or 150 mg twice daily. Do not use in patients who are allergic to sulfa.

should check for signs of aspirin toxicity, especially tinnitus. Periodic checks of serum salicylate levels may be helpful if the dosage is reaching maximum levels or if there is a question of patient compliance.

Patient and Family Teaching

You should tell the patient and family the following:

1. These drugs may cause stomach upset because they are so strong. This symptom may be reduced by taking medicine with food, milk, or a full glass of water. Patients should never take the medication without adequate liquid because it is very hard on the stomach.
2. The patient should contact the nurse, physician, or other health care provider right away if he notices any ringing in the ears, any abnormal bleeding or bruising, or bloody or black, tarry stools.
3. Chronic problems may require taking the medicine for more than a week before the patient notices any decrease in symptoms.
4. The medication should be taken regularly to reduce inflammation. If the medication is taken regularly, a high level is maintained in the blood and symptoms can be reduced more easily.
5. The patient should not take any other medications without the knowledge of the nurse, physician, or other health care provider. This includes drugs that the patient may purchase over the counter.
6. The nurse, physician, or other health care provider should be contacted if the patient is taking the medicine for a fever and the fever does not come down in 24 to 48 hours or if the patient becomes lethargic (sleepy) or hard to awaken.
7. This medication should be kept out of the reach of children and all others for whom it is not prescribed. Even small doses may be fatal to small children.
8. If the patient is unable to take the medication in the form prescribed, she should contact the nurse, physician, or other health care provider so another form may be ordered. Medication is available in chewable tablets and in suppositories to make it easier for some patients to take.

ACETAMINOPHEN

OVERVIEW

Acetaminophen is an over-the-counter (OTC) medication commonly used to decrease fever and mild pain. It can be used in patients who have experienced gastric irritation with aspirin or other NSAIDs. Acetaminophen is similar to aspirin in its effectiveness in treating fever and pain. It is the drug of choice for relief of minor pain in children. Acetaminophen is different from aspirin in

that it does not have an antiinflammatory effect or an impact on platelet aggregation.

Acetaminophen is a metabolite of phenacetin, a product that was taken off the market because of a link with nephropathy.

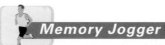

Memory Jogger

Combining Acetaminophen with Codeine

When acetaminophen is given in combination with products such as codeine, it is important to monitor the daily intake of acetaminophen to avoid an overdose.

ACTION

Acetaminophen works as an antipyretic by direct action on the hypothalamic heat-regulating center, lowering the set point to normal. It does this by blocking the action of pyrogenic cytokines on the heat-regulating center. This helps get rid of body heat via vasodilation and sweating.

The mechanism of analgesic action is not clear. It may be due to inhibition of prostaglandin synthetase in the CNS. Acetaminophen differs from ASA in that it does not inhibit peripheral prostaglandin synthesis. This may account for the absence of inflammatory and platelet-inhibiting effects. Acetaminophen is a very effective medication for treating chronic pain of both malignant and nonmalignant origin. Other medications are often combined with acetaminophen to enhance their effectiveness.

Acetaminophen is the initial drug of choice for treatment of osteoarthritis. It is effective in pain relief and has fewer adverse reactions than aspirin or NSAIDs.

ADVERSE REACTIONS

If used as directed, adverse reactions are rare. The symptoms of hypersensitivity are skin eruptions, urticaria and erythema, and fever. Extremely rare hematologic reactions include hemolytic anemia, leukopenia, neutropenia, and pancytopenia. Other reactions are hypoglycemia, liver toxicity, and jaundice (yellow color of skin, eyes, and mucous membranes). Overdosage is possible and may be fatal.

DRUG INTERACTIONS

Use with the following drugs may increase the risk of hepatotoxicity (damage to the liver): barbiturates, hydantoin, carbamazepine, rifampin, sulfinpyrazone, and ethanol.

Activated charcoal reduces acetaminophen absorption. Acetylcysteine (Mucomyst) is used as an antidote in acetaminophen overdose.

Nursing Implications and Patient Teaching

Assessment

You should learn as much as possible about the patient's health history. Ask questions to learn about other problems the patient may have that might have produced fever or pain. Does the patient have any risk factors for drug interactions or bleeding?

Diagnosis

Does the patient have excessive coffee, alcohol, or smoking habits that would increase the risk for bleeding?

Planning

Acetaminophen is available OTC, and many patients decide when and how much medicine to take. Ask specifically about acetaminophen when taking a medication history. Generic acetaminophen is equally effective and less expensive than brand-name products.

Implementation

Acetaminophen is the drug of choice for reduction of fever. Treatment of minor fever is not indicated unless the fever is making the patient uncomfortable. Symptomatic relief of a temperature greater than 40° C is usually required. Treatment of a temperature higher than 41° C or 105° F to 106° F is a medical emergency.

Dosing information for acetaminophen is provided in Table 21-1.

Evaluation

Monitor fever or pain control. Watch for symptoms of gastric distress, nausea, or bleeding.

Patient and Family Teaching

You should tell the patient and family the following:
1. The patient should not exceed the recommended dosage.
2. This medication should be kept out of the reach of children.
3. The patient should stop using this medication if a sensitivity reaction occurs.
4. Severe pain or high fever may indicate serious illness. If symptoms persist, the patient should contact the nurse, physician, or other health care provider.
5. The patient should avoid consumption of large amounts of alcohol while taking this medication because of increased risk of liver damage.

NONSTEROIDAL ANTIINFLAMMATORY DRUGS

ACTION

Nonsteroidal antiinflammatory drugs (NSAIDs) have analgesic, antiinflammatory, and antipyretic effects and are used to treat rheumatic diseases, degenerative joint disease, osteoarthritis, and acute musculoskeletal problems. The exact mode of action of NSAIDs is not known, although it is believed that they work by inhibiting the production of prostaglandins. These agents also inhibit platelet aggregation, but this effect appears to be dose related.

The analgesic and antiinflammatory effects of NSAIDs are largely the result of their ability to stop the production of prostaglandins. All NSAIDs inhibit cyclooxygenase, thus blocking the production of prostaglandins. Some NSAIDs specifically work to inhibit COX-2, the chemical created at sites of inflammation by cytokines and inflammatory mediators.

USES

When the patient's history and physical examination have diagnosed a disease process that has a major effect on the person's normal pattern of living (because of changes in mobility or pain), the use of NSAIDs may be indicated.

Most NSAIDs are used in the treatment of both rheumatoid arthritis and osteoarthritis. They are used specifically in the relief of arthritic signs and symptoms, in treatment of acute inflammatory flare-ups and worsening of symptoms, and for long-term management of arthritis. NSAIDs are also used in treatment of pain associated with dental extraction, minor surgery, and soft-tissue athletic injuries. Ibuprofen has been approved for use in dysmenorrhea because of its inhibition of prostaglandin production.

ADVERSE REACTIONS

Adverse reactions to NSAIDs include asthma, fluid retention, hypertension (high blood pressure), confusion, dizziness, blurred or decreased vision, malaise (weakness), sleepiness, tinnitus, pruritus, skin irritation or rash related to sun exposure, abdominal pain, anorexia, bloating, constipation, diarrhea, dyspepsia (stomach discomfort after eating), excessive gas in the GI tract, GI bleeding (upper or lower), heartburn, nausea, vomiting, hematuria (blood in the urine; occurs with some NSAIDs or with worsened renal failure), and many forms of blood cell changes.

DRUG INTERACTIONS

Because the various NSAIDs are structurally somewhat differently, their specific drug interactions vary. Therefore, each specific agent should be checked for drug interactions that should be monitored. Most products have many significant drug interactions.

Nursing Implications and Patient Teaching

Assessment

You should learn as much as possible about the health history of the patient, including sensitivity to aspirin or any of the products within this group, GI problems,

Geriatric Considerations

NSAIDs

The incidence of perforated peptic ulcers or bleeding is more common in elderly patients taking an NSAID than in younger adults. Serious consequences occur more often in this age group.

Elderly patients with renal impairment may be at higher risk for NSAID-induced hepatotoxicity or nephrotoxicity (damage to the kidney) and often require a lower dose to prevent drug levels from building up.

Clinicians have recommended that patients 70 years or older be started at one half of the usual adult dose, with close monitoring and careful dosage increases. A dosage increase would be based on the patient's therapeutic response and lack of signs and symptoms of toxicity. Specific drug warnings include the following:

- Flurbiprofen (Ansaid) may result in increased peak serum levels in women between 74 and 94 years old. This increased serum level has not been seen in elderly male patients. Therefore, elderly women may need a lower dose to produce a therapeutic response.
- Indomethacin (Indocin) is responsible for a higher incidence of CNS side effects, especially confusion, in elderly patients.
- Naproxen (Naprosyn) administration in the elderly population results in a higher proportion of unbound (free) naproxen, which may be reflected by the total serum level. The concentration of unbound naproxen may be nearly double that in a younger adult, which may result in an increase in side/adverse/toxic effects, even with a normal serum level range. You should be aware of this potential because the physician or other health care provider may need to be notified about the possible need for a dosage reduction.

Modified from McKenry LM, Salerno E: *Mosby's pharmacology in nursing*, ed 21, St Louis, 2003, Mosby.

renal dysfunction, history of asthma or allergic respiratory problems, anticoagulant therapy, bleeding problems, other drugs that are being taken that may cause drug interactions, and the possibility of pregnancy or breastfeeding.

Low doses of ibuprofen are often the first choice for pain relief in the elderly patient. The patient may complain of musculoskeletal pain or tenderness of involved areas, inflammation, stiffness, and an alteration in the normal activities of life. The onset may be gradual—the patient may show only tiredness—or it may be sudden or may occur after a change in activity or minor trauma, depending on the type of arthritic problem. The individual history of onset, duration, and location are important factors in diagnosing which arthritic condition

exists. You should evaluate the patient for signs of inflammation: tenderness, erythema, increased warmth, and swelling. Joint stiffness, decreased range of motion, or crepitus (a clicking sound) may also be present. Distribution, location, pattern (for example, on one side of the body or on both sides), and number of involved joints must be determined.

NSAIDs are contraindicated in patients with past sensitivity to the drug. They are also not to be used in patients who have allergy or hypersensitivity to aspirin, because all of the specific agents are closely related to aspirin and there is a potential for cross-sensitivity. (That is, a patient who is sensitive to aspirin may be sensitive to NSAIDs also.) Other agents in this category should not be given to patients who have had symptoms of bronchospasm, asthma, rhinitis, urticaria, nasal polyps, or angioedema (swelling of the skin and mucous membranes) after using any agents within this group.

Diagnosis

What other medical problems or risk factors does the patient have that might make taking this drug a problem? Does the patient have concerns about weight, nutrition, safety, or mobility? Is the patient suffering from depression?

Planning

Some agents should be used only for short-term therapy because of their toxic side effects. The length of therapy should be considered when a particular drug is selected for treating chronic arthritis.

In problems that occur in only one joint, all infectious processes should be ruled out. This is because NSAIDs may relieve symptoms but will not affect any infectious agent. That would allow greater damage to take place if the patient continues to take NSAIDs.

Implementation

NSAIDs are first-line drugs in the treatment and control of the various forms of arthritis and in many of the single-joint inflammatory processes (for example, bursitis). Because the chemical structure of these agents varies somewhat, if symptoms fail to improve with the use of one agent, this does not mean there will be no improvement with another. Because of the low cost, efficacy, and low toxicity of salicylates, all NSAIDs are compared with them in terms of their therapeutic benefits and side effects (see Table 22-1).

Evaluation

You should watch the patient for therapeutic effects: reduction of symptoms and ability of the patient to return to previous activities without pain. The patient should be evaluated 3 to 4 weeks after starting the medication for the first signs of improvement. If there is no reduction in symptoms or if side effects develop, another drug in the NSAID group can be tried.

The patient should be asked about adverse effects, particularly GI and CNS symptoms. Periodic laboratory analysis should also be carried out while the patient is taking this medication. Collect stool specimens to check for occult bleeding. Complete blood cell counts (CBCs) with indices for anemia, hematologic problems, and ability to fight infection should be done at least twice a year.

Clinical Landmine

Gastrointestinal Upset

Gastrointestinal upset is the most common complication of NSAID use and should be reported to the health care provider. Bowel movements should also be checked for the presence of blood or tarry stools, which result from excessive irritation. This should not be confused with black stools in patients taking iron preparations.

Patient and Family Teaching

You should tell the patient and family the following:
1. These medications should be taken exactly as ordered. The dosage should not be increased or decreased unless the patient is told to do so by the nurse, physician, or other health care provider. Evaluation of the action of these drugs requires returning to the health care provider regularly for checkups.

2. These medications should be taken with meals or with milk to minimize gastric irritation. The patient may use an antacid with the medicine, unless she is told not to do so.
3. Patients who have chronic arthritic problems may need to take the medication for 1 to 2 weeks before noting any improvement. The medication should be taken regularly during this time to evaluate fairly whether or not it is effective.
4. A certain level of medication must be maintained within the body at all times to maintain the antiinflammatory effect of the drug. If the patient does not take the medication regularly, the drug level may become too low to be effective.
5. If a dose is missed, it should be taken as soon as possible. If the patient remembers the missed dose close to the time when the next dose is to be taken, only the regular dose should be taken and the missed dose should be skipped. An increased amount of medication should not be taken to make up for a missed dose.
6. Blurred vision or any other eye problems, ringing in the ears, and rashes should be reported immediately to the nurse, physician, or other health care provider.
7. Some patients have drowsiness, light-headedness, or less alertness when taking this medication. Patients should not drive or perform tasks requiring alertness until they know their reaction to this drug.
8. The patient should not take aspirin or any other antiinflammatory drug while using this product.

SECTION TWO

Skeletal Muscle Relaxants

ACTION

The main action of **skeletal muscle relaxants** is to reduce muscle tone and involuntary (uncontrolled) movement without loss of voluntary (controlled) motor function. These drugs limit the transmission or movement of impulses in the motor pathways at the level of the spinal cord and the brainstem (centrally acting), or they interfere with the mechanism that shortens skeletal muscle fibers (direct myotrophic blocking) so that they contract. Other actions include mild sedation, reduction of anxiety and tension, and changes in pain perception.

USES

Skeletal muscle relaxants are used to relieve pain in musculoskeletal and neurologic disorders involving peripheral injury and inflammation, such as muscle strain or sprain, arthritis, bursitis, low back syndrome, cervical syndrome, tension headaches, cerebral palsy, and multiple sclerosis. They are often used following trauma, such as a motor vehicle or sporting accidents, when muscles throughout the whole body may be aching.

ADVERSE REACTIONS

Adverse reactions to skeletal muscle relaxants include flushing (red color in the face and neck), hypotension, syncope (light-headedness and fainting), tachycardia, ataxia (poor coordination), blurred vision, confusion, drowsiness, headache, insomnia (inability to sleep), irritability, abdominal pain, anorexia, bleeding, diarrhea, hiccups, nausea, many blood cell disorders, anaphylactic (shock) reactions, asthma-like reaction, dermatoses, erythema, fever, pruritus, rash, dysuria (painful urination), incontinence, urinary retention, dyspnea (uncomfortable breathing), nasal congestion, shortness of breath, wheezing, dyspepsia, euphoria (excessive happiness), metallic taste, pain or sloughing at injection site, and tremors.

Clinical Landmine

Skeletal Muscle Relaxants

Skeletal muscle relaxants, like other CNS depressants, can become habit forming. Their long-term use is not recommended.

DRUG INTERACTIONS

Skeletal muscle relaxants are known to increase the effect of CNS depressants, including sedatives, narcotic analgesics, antianxiety agents, hypnotics, and alcohol. They also increase the effects of general anesthetics, monoamine oxidase (MAO) inhibitors, and tricyclic antidepressants. Cyclobenzaprine and orphenadrine have the same effects as anticholinergic drugs. Cyclobenzaprine may interfere with the antihypertensive activity of the alpha-adrenergic blockers.

Nursing Implications and Patient Teaching

Assessment

You should learn as much as possible about the patient's health history, including the presence of hypersensitivity, use of other drugs that might produce drug interactions, and history of respiratory, renal, hepatic, or cardiac dysfunction. These drugs also should not be given to women who are pregnant or breastfeeding or to persons with a history of drug dependency.

The patient may have a history of pain caused by acute muscular trauma or inflammation (sprains or strains), low back syndrome, arthritis, multiple sclerosis, muscular tension with or without intermittent relief, headache, and muscle rigidity.

Diagnosis

Does this patient have other problems that you should be concerned about? Is the patient able to take care of activities of daily living, including personal hygiene and eating? Is the patient able to travel, or is he confined at home? Is depression a problem? Has the problem made a significant difference in the patient's activity level? All of these things may require nursing intervention. Will the patient be involved in a lawsuit or criminal inquiry as a result of the trauma? Are there legal or financial issues to consider?

Planning

Using a skeletal muscle relaxant with other CNS drugs, including alcohol, increases the sedative actions of this drug. Therefore, these drugs are not recommended for persons with a history of alcoholism or alcohol abuse.

The efficacy and safe use of these drugs have not been established in children.

Implementation

Skeletal muscle relaxants are available in both tablet and injectable forms. Although many muscle relaxants are given orally (PO), research suggests these drugs may not always be effective when given by this route. The oral dose would have to be 5 to 10 times greater than the parenteral dose to obtain true muscle relaxation. For this reason, the parenteral form of these drugs is recommended over the oral form. However, the parenteral form of the drug can cause local tissue irritation with injection.

In rare instances, the first dose of skeletal muscle relaxants produces an idiosyncratic (unique and unknown cause) reaction within minutes or hours. Symptoms include extreme weakness, transient quadriplegia, dizziness, ataxia, temporary loss of vision, diplopia (double vision), mydriasis, dysarthria, agitation, euphoria, confusion, and disorientation.

Table 22-2 provides a summary of skeletal muscle relaxants.

Evaluation

Hepatotoxicity, nephrotoxicity, and blood dyscrasias have been reported with the use of skeletal muscle relaxants. Signs of hepatotoxicity include abdominal pain, high fever, nausea, and diarrhea. Signs of blood dyscrasias include fever, sore throat, mucosal irritation, malaise, and petechiae (tiny red spots on the skin). Side effects that occur most commonly include drowsiness, diplopia, dizziness, weakness, mild muscular incoordination, anorexia, nausea, vomiting, syncope, and hypotension.

The lowest dosage possible should be used, and the patient should be monitored for signs and symptoms of hepatotoxicity, blood dyscrasias, dependence, and adverse drug reactions. The drug should be stopped if no improvement occurs after 45 days, because the risk of hepatotoxicity increases with long-term use of these drugs.

The acuteness of the musculoskeletal disorder or type of neurologic impairment dictates the duration of drug use. Stopping the drugs suddenly can cause withdrawal symptoms after long-term use, so the dosage should be gradually reduced before being stopped.

The patient should be observed for signs and symptoms of therapeutic effect, such as increased range of motion, relief from muscle spasm, and pain relief.

Table 22-2

Skeletal Muscle Relaxants

GENERIC NAME	TRADE NAME	COMMENTS AND DOSAGE
CENTRALLY ACTING		
baclofen	Lioresal	• *Muscle relaxant, antispastic:* Begin dosage regimen with 5 mg 3 times daily for 3 days. Thereafter, increase the dosage in increments of 5 mg per dose every 3 days until the desired response is obtained. The dosage is adjusted according to the reversal of spasticity symptoms. The maximum daily dose is 80 mg.
carisoprodol	Soma	• *Muscle relaxant:* 350 mg PO 3 times daily and at bedtime. Administration with meals will help reduce gastric distress.
chlorphenesin carbamate	Maolate Myci1	• *Muscle relaxation:* 800 mg 3 times daily until a therapeutic effect is achieved; then give maintenance dose of 400 mg 3 times daily. Treatment should not exceed 8 wk.
chlorzoxazone	Paraflex Parafon Forte DSC Remular-S	*Adults:* 250-750 mg 3 times daily. Initial dose for painful musculoskeletal conditions should be 500 mg 3 times daily. If adequate response is not obtained, the dosage may be increased to 750 mg 3 to 4 times daily and then gradually reduced to a maintenance dose of 250 mg 3 times daily once the therapeutic effect is achieved. Administration with meals may help avoid GI irritation. *Children:* Give 20 mg/kg 3 times daily, not to exceed 125-500 mg. The tablets may be crushed and mixed with food.
cyclobenzaprine	Flexeril	Relieves acute skeletal muscle spasm of local origin without interfering with muscle function. • *Local muscle spasm:* 10 mg 3 to 4 times daily. Do not administer for longer than 2-3 wk.
diazepam	Valium	*Adults:* 2-10 mg PO 2 to 4 times daily. Give sustained-release capsules 15-30 mg daily. *Geriatric or debilitated patients:* 2-2.5 mg PO daily or twice daily. Gradually increase dose as needed. • *Parenteral therapy:* Inject IV medication slowly only into large veins, 1 min for each 5 mg. *Adults:* 5-10 mg IV initially, repeated prn at 10- to 15-min intervals. Maximum IV dose is 30 mg. Therapy may be repeated in 2-4 hr as needed.

Patient and Family Teaching

You should tell the patient and family the following:

1. The patient should take this medication as advised and not stop taking it suddenly or increase the dosage without knowledge of the nurse, physician, or other health care provider.

2. The patient should avoid driving, operating heavy machinery, or doing tasks requiring alertness while taking skeletal muscle relaxants.

3. The patient should avoid taking other medications that depress CNS functions at the same time. These include antihistamines, allergy or cold medications, sedatives, tranquilizers, sleeping medications, anticonvulsants, narcotic analgesics, and tricyclic antidepressants.

4. If a dose of medication is missed, it may be taken within an hour of when it was scheduled. If the patient remembers the missed dose close to the time when the next dose is to be taken, only the regular dose should be taken and the missed dose should be skipped.

5. The nurse, physician, or other health care provider should be contacted immediately if any of the following side effects occur: dizziness or fainting, mental depression, unusually fast heartbeat, wheezing, shortness of breath, difficult breathing, abdominal pain, high fever, nausea, diarrhea, sore throat, malaise, mucosal ulceration, or petechiae.

6. The patient should take the last dose at bedtime so that drowsiness will help her go to sleep.

7. This medication must be kept out of the reach of children and all others for whom it is not prescribed.

Table 22-2

Skeletal Muscle Relaxants—cont'd

GENERIC NAME	TRADE NAME	COMMENTS AND DOSAGE
CENTRALLY ACTING—cont'd		
metaxalone	Skelaxin	• *Muscle relaxation:* 800 mg PO 3 times daily in patients 12 yr and older.
methocarbamol	Robaxin	*Adults:* 500- or 750-mg tablets 3 to 4 times daily. The drug may change the color of standing urine to green or black. • Relief of muscle spasm: 1.5 gm PO 4 times daily as initial loading dose for the first 3-4 days of treatment. The maintenance dose is 750-1000 mg qd in 4 divided doses. IV and IM dosage should not exceed 30 mg (3 vials) per day for more than 3 days, except in the treatment of tetanus. Specifically for IV dosage, do not exceed a rate of 3 mL (300 mg)/min.
orphenadrine citrate	Norflex Flexoject	• *Muscle spasm:* Administer 100-mg tablet in the morning and evening; or give 60 mg IM or IV q12h.
quinine sulfate	Legatrin (OTC)	• *Relief of leg muscle cramps:* 1 tablet at bedtime; increase the dose to add 1 tablet at the evening meal when necessary.
tizanidine	Zanaflex	Give a single oral dose of 8 mg. Effect peaks in 1-2 hr and recedes over 3-6 hr. Effects are dose related.
DIRECT ACTING		
dantrolene	Dantrium	• *Spasticity* *Adults:* Begin therapy with 25 mg daily; increase to 25 mg 2 to 4 times daily; and then by increments up to as high as 100 mg 2 to 4 times daily if necessary. Doses higher than 400 mg/day are not recommended. Each dosage should be maintained for 4-7 days to determine the patient's response. *Children >5 yr only:* Begin with 1 mg/kg daily and increase by 0.5-mg/kg increments to a maximum of 3 mg/kg 2 to 4 times daily.
COMBINATION PRODUCTS		
carisoprodol and aspirin (also comes with codeine)	Soma Compound	Combination centrally acting skeletal muscle relaxant. Used to treat acute muscle spasms and to relieve pain associated with musculoskeletal conditions. Has CNS depressant effects and physical and psychologic addictive effects, and withdrawal effects occur if the drug is abruptly stopped. • *Relief of muscle spasm and pain:* 1-2 tablets 3 to 4 times daily.
methocarbamol and aspirin	Robaxisal	A centrally acting skeletal muscle relaxant. • *Relief of muscle spasm and for analgesia:* 2 tablets 3 to 4 times daily; in severe conditions, 3 tablets 3 to 4 times daily for 1-3 days.
orphenadrine citrate, aspirin, and caffeine	Norgesic	Combination centrally acting skeletal muscle relaxant indicated for the relief of mild to moderate pain and muscle spasms of acute musculoskeletal conditions. • *Relief from pain and muscle spasms:* 1-2 tablets 3 to 4 times daily.

SECTION THREE

Antiarthritis Medications

OVERVIEW

The term **arthritis** covers more than 100 different types of joint disease in which inflammation or destruction is present. The most common types are rheumatoid arthri- tis and osteoarthritis. **Rheumatoid arthritis** is a sys- temic disease that involves an autoimmune respons caused by failure of the body to recognize its own tissue and results in destruction of the joint. **Osteoarthritis** a more local form of joint destruction, particularly i weight-bearing joints or stressed joints, that results gradually over time from overuse and increasing age.

Symptoms of arthritis include swelling, pain, and stiffness in one or more joints. In rheumatoid arthritis, as the disease progresses, there is degeneration and destruction of the joint with permanent changes that produce deformities and immobility.

Arthritis is one of the most common disorders. Patients often do not get good relief from any of the medicines they try, so they may turn to alternative medicine and herbal products to reduce arthritic symptoms and reduce pain. These herbal products have many possible interactions with other medications (see the Complementary and Alternative Therapies box).

SLOW-ACTING ANTIRHEUMATIC DRUGS

Salicylates and NSAIDs are first-line drugs for the treatment of arthritis. The antiarthritis medications are used only in confirmed cases of rheumatoid arthritis that has been getting worse despite other methods of therapy, including high doses of NSAIDs. None of these agents is without significant risk and toxic effects. Patients taking these drugs need constant follow-up and regular evaluation.

The **slow-acting antirheumatic drugs (SAARDs)** that are useful in treating significant cases of rheumatoid arthritis include hydroxychloroquine sulfate, penicillamine, methotrexate, and gold compounds. Most of these medications are designed to reduce pain, swelling, and inflammation; these drugs cannot stop the arthritic process. Gold compounds and penicillamine are used to help slow or halt joint destruction and so may prevent greater deformity. Each is briefly described.

GOLD COMPOUNDS

Action and Uses

Therapy with **gold compounds** (gold salts) is also called *chrysotherapy*. The exact mechanism of action of gold is not known. Gold is a heavy metal that interferes with a wide range of biochemical reactions on a cellular level. It is thought that it may inhibit lysosomal enzyme activity in macrophages and decrease their phagocytic activity. It is also believed that it in some way affects the antigen formation in the autoimmune response of patients with rheumatoid arthritis. It appears to stop the synovitis (inflammation of the joint synovium) of active rheumatoid disease and therefore reduce the amount of damage done.

These drugs have many contraindications and precautions to their use. They also have many toxic effects,

---

✿ Complementary and Alternative Therapies

Arthritis

PRODUCTS	COMMENTS
OSTEOARTHRITIS	
Grape seed	Potential interaction with anticoagulants, aspirin, NSAIDs, antiplatelet agents, methotrexate
Ginger	Potential interaction with anticoagulants, aspirin, NSAIDs, antiplatelet agents, cardiac glycosides
Cat's claw	Potential interaction with anticoagulants, aspirin, NSAIDs, antiplatelet agents
Tumeric	Potential interaction with anticoagulants, aspirin, NSAIDs, antiplatelet agents
Boswellia	No reported interactions
Chondroitin sulfate	No reported interactions
Glucosamine sulfate	No reported interactions
RHEUMATOID ARTHRITIS	
Cat's claw	Potential interaction with anticoagulants, aspirin, NSAIDs, antiplatelet agents
Boswellia	No reported interactions
Devil's claw	No reported interactions
Evening primrose	Potential interaction with anticoagulants, aspirin, NSAIDs, antiplatelet agents
Tumeric	Potential interaction with anticoagulants, aspirin, NSAIDs, antiplatelet agents
Bromelain	Potential interaction with anticoagulants, aspirin, NSAIDs, antiplatelet agents
Chondroitin sulfate	No reported interactions
Glucosamine sulfate	No reported interactions

Modified from Krinsky DL, Lavella JB, Hawkins EB, et al: *Natural therapeutics pocket guide*, ed 2, Hudson, Ohio, 2003, Lexi-Comp, Inc.

and only 30% to 35% of patients gain benefit from their use. The patient should be warned of this before starting on these agents.

The most common side effects, which are mucocutaneous (in the skin and mucous membranes), occur in about 15% of all patients. Gold dermatitis has a variety of appearances but is always pruritic. Often this pruritus occurs before a rash is seen and is most commonly periorbitally (around the eyes) and on the palms and dorsa of the hands. Stomatitis (inflammation of the mouth) may be seen, with painful ulcers on the buccal mucosa, tongue, palate, or pharynx. These may be preceded by a metallic taste.

A number of patients have what is known as the "nitritoid-like response" with the use of gold sodium thiomalate (Myochrysine). This is a mild and benign reaction caused by the aqueous (water) medium of the gold. It causes the patient to feel flushed and light-headed and occasionally leads to fainting. These symptoms occur right after the injection. For this reason, patients getting Myochrysine injections should lie down for 10 to 15 minutes after the injection. This problem is self-limiting and requires no other treatment.

The dosage regimen for the use of gold has three phases: (1) a 2- or 3-week period of injections that increase gradually to test for severe reactions or unusual problems; (2) a "loading period" of weekly injections, until a total dose of 1 gm of injected gold is reached; and (3) a gradual decrease in dose until a maintenance dosage is found. Follow the very specific dosage schedule included in the package insert.

Gold salts come in two solution forms for injection: one in an oil medium and the other in an aqueous medium. They are both painful injections and should be given only in the gluteus maximus muscle. There is also an oral form of gold on the market.

HYDROXYCHLOROQUINE SULFATE

Action

The mechanism of action of hydroxychloroquine sulfate is not understood. This is an antimalarial drug that in some way stops the formation of antigens in the body. These antigens produce the hypersensitivity reactions leading to the physiologic changes of rheumatoid arthritis and systemic lupus erythematosus.

 Clinical Landmine

Hydroxychloroquine Sulfate

The most serious side effect of hydroxychloroquine sulfate is damage to the eyes, which usually appears in two forms: (1) retinopathy with irreversible visual loss and (2) corneal infiltration that may be somewhat reversible when the medication is stopped.

Uses

Hydroxychloroquine sulfate is used in confirmed cases of rheumatoid arthritis that have been getting worse despite other methods of therapy, including high doses of NSAIDs. This agent is not without significant risk and toxic effects. Patients taking this drug need constant follow-up and regular evaluation. This drug may also be used in confirmed diagnosis of systemic or discoid lupus erythematosus.

Adverse Reactions

This medication requires 4 to 12 weeks of therapy before improvement is seen. If there is no improvement after 6 months, the drug should be stopped.

If the drug is stopped while the patient is feeling relief from the symptoms, the agent can be reintroduced if the disease flares up again. Corticosteroids or NSAIDs may be used with this drug until the effects of this slow-acting drug become apparent.

Retinopathy is a serious adverse effect. The retinopathy does appear to be dose related, so patients should have an expert ophthalmologic evaluation before beginning the drug and periodic checkups every 3 to 6 months throughout therapy. The drug should be stopped if there are any visual complaints or symptoms, such as seeing flashes or streaks of light, because the retinal damage may progress even after the drug is stopped.

This product must not be used with other SAARDs, especially gold, because combined use will greatly increase the chance of dermatologic reactions.

INFLIXIMAB

Action and Uses

This drug is used in combination with methotrexate to reduce the signs and symptoms of rheumatoid arthritis and limiting the worsening of damage to joints. This leads to improved physical function in patients with moderate to severe active rheumatoid arthritis who have had an inadequate response to methotrexate alone. It is also used in Crohn's disease and some other orthopedic inflammatory or destructive processes.

Adverse Reactions

The Food and Drug Administration (FDA) requires a warning that this drug may activate tuberculosis, invasive fungal infections, and other opportunistic infections. (A test for tuberculosis should be given and any latent tuberculosis treated prior to beginning the patient on this therapy.) There is a high rate of mortality in patients who have preexisting congestive heart failure. Watch for hypersensitivity and infusion-related reactions (for example, dyspnea, flushing, headache, and rash that may occur within 1 to 2 hours of the infusion).

LEFLUNOMIDE

Action and Uses

This product is a pyrimidine synthesis inhibitor that has an antiinflammatory effect. It is used in treatment of active rheumatoid arthritis in adults to reduce signs and symptoms and to slow structural damage in joints. Therapy is started with a single oral 100 mg/day dose for 3 days. The usual maintenance dose is 20 mg/day.

Adverse Reactions

The FDA requires a warning label that pregnancy must be ruled out and avoided in all women who are of childbearing age while they are taking this drug. This is a category X drug that is contraindicated during pregnancy. Leflunomide may produce hepatotoxicity, and there is some evidence of increased risk of cancer of the lymph system.

METHOTREXATE

ACTION AND USES

Methotrexate (Amethopterin) is a medication that has been used for years to treat various cancerous and psoriatic conditions. The mechanism of action in rheumatoid arthritis is unknown. It may affect immune function. It reduces joint swelling and tenderness in 3 to 6 weeks, but there is no evidence that it causes remission of the disease or limits bone erosions.

Methotrexate is used in cases of severe rheumatoid arthritis that are unresponsive to other treatment. This product has a high possibility of severe adverse reactions, including death. It is most toxic to the bone marrow, liver, kidney, and lungs. It has many contraindications to use, drug interactions, and dosage precautions. Consult the package insert for specific information.

PENICILLAMINE

ACTION AND USES

Penicillamine is a chemical breakdown product of penicillin. It is a chelating agent that is used to bind heavy metals in conditions such as lead and copper poisoning. Its mode of action in the treatment of rheumatoid arthritis is not understood. It is known to be effective in relieving the symptoms of arthritis and in some way stops the disease progression. However, only about 30% of patients who are prescribed this agent get any benefit from its use. The patient should be warned of this before starting the agent.

This drug requires excellent patient compliance, because it is an oral preparation that patients must administer themselves. The special dosage schedule enclosed as a package insert should be followed. Maintenance dosage is that dose at which clinical improvement begins to occur. When a maintenance dosage is reached, the blood and urine follow-up should continue every 2 weeks for 6 months and then monthly thereafter for as long as the patient receives the medication. If a worsening of disease occurs during therapy, the use of NSAIDs is indicated rather than a rapid increase in the penicillamine dosage. No therapeutic effect may be seen for 3 to 6 months.

ADVERSE REACTIONS

This drug has many toxic side effects. Patients with a history of renal impairment or active renal impairment should not receive this drug because of its risk for toxic effects on the kidneys. Blood dyscrasias and skin reactions are particularly dangerous. Use of penicillamine along with other drugs that could potentiate blood dyscrasias, such as gold compounds or cytotoxic drugs, is contraindicated.

 Clinical Landmine

Adverse Reactions with Penicillamine

About 50% of patients taking penicillamine have adverse reactions, some of which are fatal.

Nursing Implications and Patient Teaching

Assessment

After reading specific information from the package insert about the medication, you should learn as much as you can about the patient's health history, including the treatment history of the patient's arthritis; presence of drug sensitivities; underlying diseases such as renal, liver, cardiovascular, or hematopoietic diseases that would contraindicate any of these products; the possibility of pregnancy; and other drugs taken at the same time that might cause drug interactions.

Diagnosis

What is the patient's general level of mobility? Is the patient depressed about his disease state? Is he able to comply with the treatment regimen? Does the patient experience side effects from his medications? Do deformities interfere with his ability to perform activities of daily living or perform required tasks in his job?

Planning

Only 30% to 35% of patients may benefit from these drugs. The patient should be counseled not to develop unrealistic hopes and should be made aware of the potential risk of many serious adverse reactions associated with these products.

Implementation

Gold compounds are very painful on injection and must be given in the gluteus maximus muscle. Patients receiving Myochrysine injections should remain lying down for 15 minutes after the injection and should then be helped carefully to their feet. They should be monitored for any symptoms of nitritoid-like reaction. The vial should be shaken well before administering the injection, and the concentration of the medication should be checked. The color of the medication should be checked; if it is darker than pale yellow, it should not be used.

A summary of dosage information concerning antiarthritis medications is provided in Table 22-3.

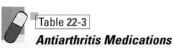

Table 22-3
Antiarthritis Medications

GENERIC NAME	TRADE NAME	COMMENTS AND DOSAGE
SLOW-ACTING ANTIRHEUMATIC DRUGS		
hydroxychloroquine	Plaquenil	• *Rheumatoid arthritis:* 400-600 mg PO daily with meals or food to prevent GI upset. *Maintenance dose:* Continue 400-600 mg PO daily for 4-12 wk, until patient has symptomatic improvements. Then reduce dosage to 200-400 mg PO daily and maintain that dosage.
methotrexate	Amethopterin Rheumatrex 🍁	Therapy generally begins with 7.5 mg/wk. An initial test dose is usually given before beginning a regular dosage schedule to detect any extreme sensitivity reactions. See the package insert for specific guidelines. Therapeutic response is generally seen in 3-6 wk, and the patient may continue to improve for another 12 wk. Optimal duration of therapy is unknown. Arthritis may worsen within 3-5 wk of ending therapy.
penicillamine	Cuprimine Depen	This product has a very specific dosage schedule that covers three specific phases. The format should be followed as closely as possible. See the package insert for details.
GOLD COMPOUNDS		
auranofin	Ridaura	Comes as a capsule to be taken PO. Contains 29% gold. Give 6 mg daily in 1 or 2 doses. If response is inadequate after 6 mo, increase dosage to 9 mg/day. If no response after 3 more mo, stop the drug.
aurothioglucose	Solganal	There appear to be fewer skin eruptions and a greater incidence of stomatitis and albuminuria with this preparation. Oil and aqueous preparations may be alternated. This injection is painful and should be given deep into the gluteus maximus muscle. Contains 50% gold.
gold sodium thiomalate	Aurolate	This injection is painful and should be given only in the gluteus maximus muscle. This preparation is also responsible for producing a "nitritoid-like response" in some patients, and patient must remain lying down for 10-15 min after injection to decrease possibility of fainting. Shake vial well before injection and make certain proper concentration of medication is used. Contains 50% gold.
OTHER		
infliximab	Remicade	Give 3 mg/kg as an IV infusion followed with similar doses at 2 and 6 wk after the first infusion and then every 8 wk. The dose may be adjusted up to 10 mg/kg or treatment as often as every 4 wk. Watch for postinfusion reactions within 1-2 hr after infusion is finished.
leflunomide	Arava	Begin therapy with 100 mg PO daily for 3 days; maintenance dose is usually about 20 mg/day. Check liver enzymes prior to beginning therapy.
sulfasalazine	Azulfidine EN Tablets	Give 2 gm daily in divided doses to patients with rheumatoid arthritis who have not responded to salicylates or other standard forms of treatment.

Evaluation

The nurse should observe for the therapeutic effect and monitor closely for the numerous and serious adverse effects that may develop.

Patient and Family Teaching

You should tell the patient and family the following:

1. These drugs are very potent and slow acting. They may be helpful in some patients in reducing symptoms or actually halting joint destruction caused by arthritis. They do not help all patients, and a thorough trial will take 12 to 20 weeks before response to the drug can be determined.

2. There are serious toxic effects that can occur with this drug. The patient must work closely with the nurse, physician, or other health care provider, keep appointments, and have laboratory work performed.

3. The patient and the nurse, physician, or other health care provider should be alert for problems that may develop in the kidneys, lungs, liver, skin, or blood.

4. This medication requires frequent response and dosage monitoring.

5. Some patients experience a brief increase in pain and joint achiness for 1 to 2 days after receiving an injection, but these problems usually disappear. The patient should contact the nurse, physician, or other health care provider if she continues to experience great discomfort after 2 days.

6. The most common adverse effects are skin rashes, itching, ulcers or sores in the mouth, and easy bruising or bleeding.

7. The nurse, physician, or other health care provider should be contacted if the patient notes a metallic taste in the mouth, purple blotches, bruising, or problems with bleeding.

SECTION FOUR
Antigout Medications

OVERVIEW

Uric acid, a metabolite of protein, is present in the blood within a very specific range. Several pathologic processes, metabolic changes, or drug interactions may be responsible for increasing the uric acid level of the blood above an acceptable amount. High uric acid levels cause the excess uric acid to form crystals, usually in the kidneys and in joint spaces. These crystals have very long, sharp, and jagged edges. These crystals tear and bruise the tissues with which they come in contact. The result is swelling, heat, inflammation, and severe pain—the syndrome called **gout.** Gout is a form of arthritis caused when the body makes too much (overproduction) or does not get rid of (underexcretion) uric acid.

The drugs used to treat gout vary in their method of action. Those used to treat acute attacks act to relieve pain and inflammation. Other drugs, called uricosurics, alter the body's response to, production of, or distribution of uric acid.

ACTION

Uricosuric agents increase the excretion of urate salts in the urine by blocking tubular reabsorption of these salts in the kidney. They also decrease the amount of circulating urate and the deposition of urate and promote reabsorption of urate deposits. Sulfinpyrazone also has platelet inhibitory and antithrombotic effects. Uricosuric agents do not have significant antiinflammatory or analgesic properties and therefore are of little help during an acute episode of gout.

Colchicine is a special drug used to treat acute gouty attacks. It is not an antiinflammatory, analgesic, or uricosuric agent. The mechanism of action of colchicine in relieving gouty attacks is not completely known. It is believed to be involved in the inhibition of leukocyte migration and phagocytosis that causes the inflammatory response in gout. It also decreases uric acid deposits in the tissues. In addition to use in the acute stage, it may also be used with allopurinol or other uricosuric agents to prevent an acute attack.

Probenecid inhibits tubular reabsorption of urate, increasing uric acid excretion.

Allopurinol inhibits the production of uric acid by decreasing the production of xanthine oxidase, an enzyme that metabolizes purine hypoxanthine to xanthine and xanthine to uric acid. This drug has no analgesic or antiinflammatory properties and therefore is not beneficial in the treatment of acute gout. Instead, it is used in prophylactic (preventive) therapy for repeated or chronic gout. It is also used in patients with renal failure that is severe enough to increase their uric acid levels to a point where they may develop gouty attacks.

USES

Usually the patient comes in with an acute attack and the diagnosis of gout is made. Colchicine is used when the diagnosis of gout is either confirmed or suspected by the patient's history and physical examination and when examination of joint fluid is not possible. It relieves the pain of acute attacks. It is also used along with allopurinol or uricosuric agents to prevent a gouty attack until the serum uric acid level is reduced to normal and stabilized. It has no effect on uric acid levels itself. It may be used prophylactically to prevent recurrent attacks, but only in combination with a uricosuric agent.

Uricosuric agents are primarily used to reduce uric acid levels in patients who do not excrete enough uric acid. The diagnosis of gout is confirmed by serum uric acid levels greater than 7 mg/100 mL and a 24-hour urine test for uric acid of less than 800 mg/day. The patient has usually had more than one acute episode before being started on these agents.

Sulfinpyrazone is used only in patients who do not respond to all other drugs.

Allopurinol usually is used when objective findings show any of the following conditions:

- Overproduction of uric acid on a general diet (24-hour urine test shows uric acid excretion greater than 700 mg/day).
- Uric acid nephropathy with impaired renal function (creatinine clearance less than 80 mL/min).
- Tophi, or small masses of crystals, on bony prominences (often the elbow or ankle).
- Documentation of kidney stones by flat plate x-ray study of the abdomen.
- Primary or secondary hyperuricemia associated with blood dyscrasias and their treatment.
- Gout not controlled by uricosuric drugs alone, caused by the patient's intolerance of the drug or when the drug is not effective.
- A need for prophylactic therapy in patients with lymphomas, leukemias, or other malignancies requiring chemotherapy or radiation therapy that results in an increase in the serum uric acid level as tissue is broken down.

Probenecid is also often used with penicillin preparations to treat venereal diseases because of its ability to increase the plasma level of penicillin. Levels may increase two to four times normal, irrespective of the route of penicillin administration.

ADVERSE REACTIONS

Uricosuric agents may produce drug fever, dizziness, pruritus, rashes, anorexia, constipation, diarrhea, nausea, vomiting, and exacerbation of acute attacks of gout. Rarely, anaphylaxis, nephrotic syndrome, hepatic necrosis, and aplastic anemia are seen.

Colchicine may cause abdominal pain, severe diarrhea, nausea, and vomiting. Prolonged use may cause bone marrow depression, peripheral neuritis, purpura (bruising), myopathy, and alopecia (hair loss). There is

usually a delay between overdosage and onset of symptoms. Deaths have been reported with as little as 7 mg.

Allopurinol may produce drowsiness, alopecia, rash (even up to several months after therapy is started), purpura, diarrhea, abdominal pain, nausea, vomiting, and blood dyscrasias. It may also produce idiosyncratic drug reactions with fever, chills, arthralgias (joint pain), skin rash, pruritus, nausea, vomiting, interstitial nephritis, occasional development of cataracts, and vasculitis that may lead to hepatotoxicity and death.

DRUG INTERACTIONS

Salicylates antagonize (interfere with) the uricosuric action of these drugs. Uricosurics increase the effects of the following drugs by decreasing renal tubular excretion: sulfonamides, sulfonylureas, naproxen, indomethacin, rifampin, dapsone, pantothenic acid, aminosalicylic acid, and methotrexate. Additionally, sulfinpyrazone affects anticoagulants by increasing their platelet aggregation effects.

The effects of colchicine are blocked by acidifying agents and increased by alkalinizing agents. Patients taking this drug may have an increased sensitivity to CNS depressants. Colchicine also decreases gut absorption of vitamin B_{12}. The effects of sympathomimetics are increased by colchicine.

Hypersensitivity may occur in patients with renal compromise who are taking thiazides and allopurinol at the same time. Use at the same time as ampicillin may increase the chance for skin rashes. Allopurinol increases the half-life of anticoagulants and many other drugs.

Nursing Implications and Patient Teaching

Assessment

You should learn as much as possible about the patient's health history, including the presence of hypersensitivity, other drugs being taken that could cause drug interactions, history of other disease, or the possibility of pregnancy. These conditions are precautions or contraindications to the use of antigout medications. The frequency and severity of the attacks should be recorded to help determine whether therapy with colchicine is indicated.

The patient may complain of an initial or recurrent attack of inflammation, erythema, swelling, extreme tenderness, and pain, usually in a single joint. At least 50% of initial attacks occur in the great toe at the metatarsal phalangeal joint (podagra). This disease usually develops in the lower extremities. Joints affected may be in the instep, ankles, heels, or knees, although some patients are also bothered in wrists, fingers, and elbows. In patients with a severe or worsening form of the disease, additional joints may be involved. These symptoms are sudden in onset, and the patient may complain of being unable to tolerate clothing, shoes, or even bed coverings touching the site of inflammation. In some cases, there is a history of minor trauma to the involved joint, obesity, alcohol intake, use of a new drug such as hydrochlorothiazide, or low-dose aspirin consumption.

Diagnosis

In addition to the medical diagnosis, what other problems exist for the patient? Are there general concerns about weight, diet, stress, or conditions that would limit the use of medication? How can you help the patient prevent other attacks? What does this patient need to learn about gout and its treatment?

Planning

You can assist in collecting a 24-hour urine test for uric acid level and creatinine clearance and baseline laboratory tests as ordered by the health care provider.

Uricosuric agents are to be started only after the acute attack has resolved. Prophylactic therapy is recommended in patients having more than one acute attack per year. If affected less often than that, the patient should try to control attacks by having colchicine on hand and beginning treatment as soon as symptoms develop.

Initiation of therapy with uricosuric agents may cause an acute attack of gout, and so colchicine is often given also to prevent such an attack.

The use of salicylates in small or large doses is contraindicated in patients taking probenecid, because salicylates antagonize the uricosuric action of this drug. Patients needing mild pain relief for other conditions should be told to use only acetaminophen products.

Allopurinol may also cause a gouty attack during the initial treatment phase. This is easily prevented by prophylactic use of colchicine 0.5 mg twice daily PO for 2 weeks to 1 month. Good fluid intake and neutral or alkaline pH of the urine are important to prevent the possibility of xanthine stone or calculi forming. Patients with poor renal function require smaller doses, and renal function should be carefully watched.

In switching patients from uricosuric agents to allopurinol, a gradual increase of allopurinol with a gradual decrease of the other agent should be made over a period of several weeks. The patient should be watched and blood work should be done to maintain a normal serum uric acid level.

Implementation

The patient's urine should be alkalinized to prevent hematuria or formation of urate stones, especially during the initial stages of therapy. Injectable doses of colchicine are not to be given intramuscularly (IM) or subcutaneously but must be given only intravenously (IV).

With an acute attack, colchicine should be given immediately and then a dose should be given every hour until either symptoms go away or the patient develops signs of toxicity.

Table 22-4 provides a summary of dosage information concerning some common antigout medications.

Evaluation

Colchicine must be started immediately, and you should observe for therapeutic effects and adverse reactions. The patient being treated for acute attacks with a loading dose can usually reach a maximum dose level before the onset of GI side effects. The patient should be checked frequently for weakness, anorexia, nausea, vomiting, or diarrhea, because these are the first indications of toxicity. If these symptoms appear, the dosage should be reduced. If the patient has taken colchicine for a long time, vitamin B_{12} deficiency may develop.

If you are seeing the patient over several months, you should watch for the therapeutic effects (decrease in frequency and severity of gouty attacks) of these drugs and watch for symptoms of the arthritis process (joint deformity, destruction, or formation of tophi).

The effect of allopurinol is seen 5 to 10 days after therapy is started. The dosage should be adjusted to maintain a serum uric acid level of less than 7 mg/100 mL. Levels as low as 2 to 3 mg/100 mL are not harmful. Adverse reactions such as rash, appearance of tophi, and change in joint deformities should be monitored.

If a maculopapular rash develops in the patient taking allopurinol at any time during therapy, the drug should be stopped immediately and it should not be restarted.

Patient and Family Teaching

You should tell the patient and family the following:
1. The uricosuric drugs do not have an effect on acute gouty attacks, but they help prevent attacks if they are taken regularly. After the initial dose, an acute attack may be precipitated, but the medicine will decrease future chances of severe attacks. These drugs do not cure gout, but they should help control it.
2. Uricosuric medication should be taken as outlined by the health care provider. It should be taken with meals to help decrease GI upset.
3. The patient should drink at least 8 glasses of fluid (especially water or citrus juices) every day while taking uricosuric medication to prevent kidney stones from developing. Although not stressed as much as in the past, low-purine diets are still recommended for patients who have experienced acute gouty attacks.
4. The patient should observe stools and urine for blood.

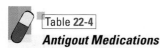

Table 22-4

Antigout Medications

GENERIC NAME	TRADE NAME	COMMENTS AND DOSAGE
URICOSURIC AGENTS		
probenecid	Benemid Benuryl Probenecid	Increases urate excretion. Often used with penicillin to treat venereal disease. There is cross-sensitivity to phenylbutazone and other pyrazoles. *Initial dosage:* 250 mg twice daily for 1 wk. *Maintenance:* 500 mg twice daily.
sulfinpyrazone	Anturane	This drug is reserved for patients who are refractory to all other modalities of therapy. *Initial dose:* 200-400 mg/day in 2 divided doses; take with meals. *Maintenance dose:* 400 mg/day in divided doses; may be increased to 800 mg/day or reduced to as low as 200 mg/day as long as serum uric acid level remains normal. Therapy should be continued even during acute episodes, and patient may be switched from other uricosuric agents to this drug at full maintenance dose.
ANTIGOUT ANALGESIC PREPARATIONS		
allopurinol	Purinol Zyloprim	Gastrointestinal side effects are usually reduced if taken with meals. The dosage to control gout and hyperuricemia is variable. The average is 200-300 mg for patients with mild gout, 400-600 mg for those with moderately severe or tophaceous gout. Dosages of 300 mg or more should be given in divided doses; less than that can be given once daily.
colchicine	Colchicine	• *Acute attack of gout:* Begin therapy at first warning of an acute attack. The delay of only a few hours greatly reduces the therapeutic effectiveness. *PO:* 0.6-1.25 mg initially, followed by 1 tablet q1-2h until pain is relieved or nausea, vomiting, or diarrhea develops. Total dose is 4-8 mg. Pain is usually relieved in 12 hr and gone in 24-48 hr. *IV:* 1-2 mg initially, then 0.5 mg q3-6h until pain is relieved; total dose is 4 mg. • *Prophylactic therapy:* 0.5-1 mg/day in single or divided doses, usually in combination with a uricosuric agent.

5. The nurse, physician, or other health care provider should be contacted immediately if any rash, stomach problems, or new or troublesome symptoms develop.

6. This medication must be kept out of the reach of children and all others for whom it is not prescribed.

7. Colchicine should be kept on hand in case the patient develops an attack of gout. At the first sign of gout, the patient should take two tablets, and then one tablet every hour or every 2 hours until the symptoms are relieved or until he develops nausea, diarrhea, or vomiting. The patient should not take more than 12 tablets.

8. If the patient is taking colchicine regularly with other drugs, it should be taken with meals to reduce GI upset.

9. Colchicine must be taken regularly as ordered if it is to help prevent gouty attacks.

10. While the patient is taking colchicine on a daily basis, the drug should be stopped if the patient notices symptoms of nausea, vomiting, or diarrhea. In this situation, the patient should contact the nurse, physician, or other health care provider. The patient should also report any skin rash, fever, sore throat, unusual bleeding, or bruising.

11. The patient should not take any other medications without the knowledge of the nurse, physician, or other health care provider. Some drugs interact adversely with allopurinol because it can block the action of the P-450 enzyme system.

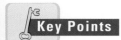

Key Points

- This chapter discussed musculoskeletal and antiarthritis medications, which are used to treat problems affecting bones, joints, muscles, and ligaments.
- The specific drug used to treat the disorder is selected based on the severity of the problem and the mechanism causing the problem.
- Many acute problems require only short-term therapy. Some disorders, such as arthritis, may require long-term therapy with a variety of medications, including more powerful medications as the disease gets worse.
- Many of these products have significant side effects and therefore require close monitoring.

Go to the free CD-ROM for an Audio Glossary, animations, video clips, and Review Questions for the NCLEX-PN® Examination.

evolve Be sure to visit the companion Evolve website at http://evolve.elsevier.com/Edmunds/LPN/ for WebLinks, a link to the top 200 drugs by prescription, and sign-up pages for newsletter drug updates.

CASE STUDY

Larry Stephenson is a 43-year-old Air Force colonel. He comes into the medical clinic complaining of severe back pain from a ruptured vertebral disc. The pain starts in his left buttock and travels down his left leg. He is sent home with the following medications:
- Ibuprofen 800 mg q8h PO
- Medrol Dose Pack as ordered for 7 days
- Hydrocodone 5 mg q6h prn

1. Describe why each of these medications is ordered for this problem.
2. The dose of ibuprofen is very high. Why is this dose ordered? Mr. Stephenson returns to the clinic in 1 week. He is not feeling any better. He continues to have severe buttocks pain and has trouble sleeping. He also complains of severe itching.
3. The health care provider discontinues the hydrocodone and orders acetaminophen #2 with codeine. Why do you think she did this?

4. The health care provider also started the patient on orphenadrine (Norflex). Why was this medication ordered?
5. Does this patient have any contraindications to the use of this product?
6. Mr. Stephenson develops slight tachycardia, headache, dizziness, and blurred vision. Under questioning, he also reports increasing problems with constipation. Are these serious problems related to any of his medications?
7. Mr. Stephenson also reports that he has been having a lot of gastric burning. What is happening, and what can be done about it?
8. After a month, Mr. Stephenson still reports a little pain, particularly at night. He is feeling a little discouraged that he has not made a complete recovery. The health care provider starts him on amitriptyline. Why is this medication ordered?

DRUG CALCULATION REVIEW

Order: Acetaminophen 280 mg oral every 4 hours prn T >100.6.

Supply: Acetaminophen 80 mg/0.8 mL

Question: How many milliliters of acetaminophen should be given with each dose?

Order: Toradol 15 mg IV every 6 hours (maximum of 6 doses)

Supply: Toradol 30 mg/mL

Question: How many milliliters of Toradol will be given with each dose?

3. Order: Aspirin 5 gr by mouth daily

Supply: Aspirin 300 mg/tablet

Question: How many aspirin tablets should be given with each dose?

CRITICAL THINKING ?

1. Mr. Lionhart has started taking a salicylate for his arthritis. He says he has a sister with lupus who is also taking a salicylate. Mr. Lionhart wonders about the discrepancy in their dosages, despite the fact that he and his sister are similar in body weight and size. Explain the importance of different dosages depending on the problem.

2. In assessing Mr. Lionhart, his health care provider asks you to test for "occult blood." What is that, and how do you test for it?

3. Mr. Franklin is being evaluated for progression of his gout, which was diagnosed 3 years ago. He tells you he "doesn't think the doctor knows what he's doing, because the pills he told me to take don't help the pain at all." How would you address this with Mr. Franklin?

4. Ms. French is receiving an NSAID for her rheumatoid arthritis. Why might this drug be preferred over ASA or salicylate therapy? What adverse reactions should Ms. French be told to watch out for?

5. Mr. Henson has been prescribed an oral skeletal muscle relaxant. Mr. Henson asks, "Wouldn't an injection or something be more helpful?" What is a possible rationale for the oral form?

6. Because oral skeletal muscle relaxants pose serious risks to patients, carefully prepare a teaching plan that includes a discussion of the high incidence of serious and potentially fatal adverse effects. This plan should stress the importance of excellent patient compliance.

7. Discuss the two etiologies of high uric acid levels, comparing the signs and symptoms of each.

8. When managing pain associated with orthopedic injuries, what nursing interventions can be implemented for increasing patient comfort in addition to analgesics?

CHAPTER 23

Topical Preparations

Objectives

After reading and studying this chapter, you should be able to do the following:

1. Identify major categories of medications used topically.
2. List at least three preparations used to treat eye, ear, and skin problems.
3. Describe specific administration techniques for topical products.

Key Terms

Be sure to check out the bonus material on the free CD-ROM, including selected audio pronunciations.

anorectal preparations (ā-nō-RĔK-tăl, p. 434)
antiglaucoma agents (ĂN-tī-glăw-KŌ-mă, p. 436)
antipsoriatics (ĂN-tī-SŌ-rē-ĂT-ĭks, p. 441)
antiseptics (ăn-tī-SĔP-tĭks, p. 436)
mydriasis (mĭ-DRĪ-ă-sĭs, p. 436)
pediculicides (pĕ-DĬK-ū-lĭ-sīdz, p. 441)
scabicides (SKĂB-ĭ-sīdz, p. 441)
vasoconstrictors (vās-ō-kŏn-STRĬK-tŏrz, p. 441)

OVERVIEW

This chapter presents a brief overview of the many products that may be used topically somewhere on the skin. Many of these products are purchased over the counter (OTC). Because hundreds of preparations are available and new products come onto the market very quickly, only a few selected examples of drugs in the major categories can be presented. As a nurse, you may play a major role in teaching the patient the proper administration of these medications and precautions for their use. Side effects are usually local unless systemic sensitization (allergic reaction) develops.

INTEGUMENTARY SYSTEM

The integumentary system is made up of the skin, hair, nails, and sweat glands (Figure 23-1). The skin provides the most important barrier to infection and protects the body, regulates temperature, prevents water loss, and produces the chemicals that develop into vitamin D.

The skin, the mucous membranes, and the surfaces of the eye, ear, nose, mouth, and vagina are often the site of minor infections. Medications are frequently used to treat disease in these areas. Special preparations and procedures are required to allow medication to go deep within these tissues.

TOPICAL MEDICATIONS

ANORECTAL PREPARATIONS

Action and Uses

Anorectal preparations include emollients, foams, and gels for topical anesthesia or healing of the rectal area. They are used for symptomatic relief of discomfort from hemorrhoids. They may be used on a long-term basis or briefly for hemorrhoids associated with pregnancy, prolonged sitting, or other temporary problems. Table 23-1 presents a summary of these preparations.

Adverse Reactions

The patient may have sensitization to the product.

MOUTH AND THROAT PREPARATIONS

Action and Uses

These miscellaneous products are used to soothe minor inflammation in the mouth. Some release oxygen to provide cleansing, whereas others contain an anesthetic property to reduce pain. These preparations are used for minor oral inflammation, such as canker sores, dental irritation, and pain after dental procedures; for relief of dryness of the mouth and throat; or for treatment of minor sore throat discomfort and control of cough caused by colds.

Products are available in mouthwashes, sprays, solutions, troches, lozenges, and disks. The patient should be taught the appropriate administration technique for the drug form that is being used. Patients should not take these products for longer than 3 or 4 days for normal therapy. Table 23-2 presents a summary of these products.

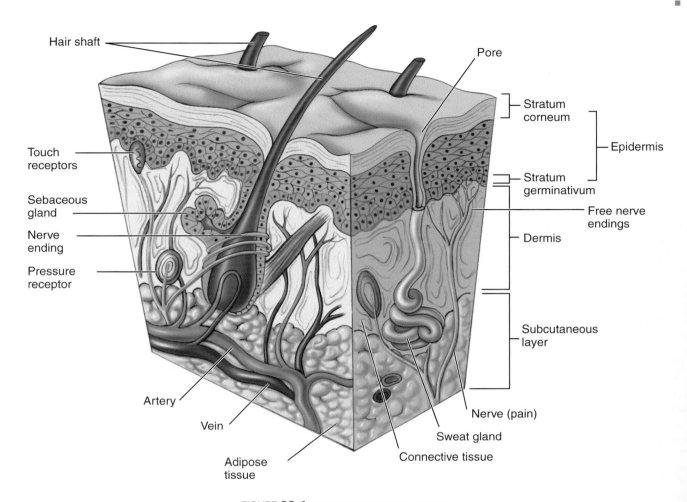

FIGURE **23-1** The integumentary system.

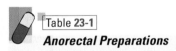

Table **23-1**

Anorectal Preparations

GENERIC NAME	TRADE NAME	COMMENTS AND DOSAGE
dibucaine	Nupercainal (OTC)	Apply ointment morning and night and after each bowel movement. For suppositories, insert one after each bowel movement.
hydrocortisone acetate	Anusol-HC	Contains hydrocortisone. Insert suppository in the morning and at bedtime for 3-6 days or until inflammation subsides. Apply cream
zinc sulfate monohydrate	Anusol (OTC)	to anal area and gently rub in 3 to 4 times daily for 3-6 days.
—	Preparation H (OTC)	
hydrocortisone foam	ProctoFoam-HC	Steroid used for antiinflammatory treatment of ulcerative proctitis and distal ulcerative colitis. Contains hydrocortisone. Insert one applicatorful per rectum daily or twice daily for 2-3 wk, then every other day. Decrease therapy gradually.

Table 23-2

Mouth and Throat Preparations

GENERIC NAME	TRADE NAME	COMMENTS AND DOSAGE
ORAL PREPARATIONS		
carbamide peroxide	Orajel Proxigel	Do not dilute. Apply directly to affected area 4 times daily, spit out after 2-3 min.
LOZENGES AND TROCHES		
—	Cepacol Cepastat Robitussin Sucrets	For mouth pain. Dissolve 1 lozenge in mouth up to qh if needed. Take no more than 12 lozenges daily.
clotrimazole	Mycelex	For oral thrush. Take 1 troche 5 times/day for 14 days. Dissolve slowly in mouth.
GARGLES, GELS, MOUTHWASHES, AND SPRAYS		
—	Cepacol Chloraseptic	For mouth pain. Follow directions on bottle or package. Wide variation among products.
nystatin	Mycostatin Nilstat	Antifungal; for oral thrush. Take 400,000-600,000 units for 10-14 days. Dissolve slowly in mouth.
SALIVA SUBSTITUTES		
—	Optimoist Salivart	Used to relieve dry mouth and throat; spray into mouth as needed.

OPHTHALMIC DRUGS

Action and Uses

A wide variety of preparations are used for eye problems (Table 23-3). Local anesthetics are useful in procedures such as tonometry, gonioscopy, cataract surgery, and removal of foreign bodies from the cornea. **Antiseptics** are compounds that are capable of preventing infection. They are used for the prevention of gonorrheal ophthalmia neonatorum when babies are born or any time germicidal or astringent (tissue constricting) action is needed. Antiinfectives are used to treat common eye infections caused by bacteria, fungi, or viruses. Artificial tears provide tearlike lubrication to relieve dry eyes, eye irritation secondary to wearing contact lenses, or deficient tear production caused by a wide variety of disorders. Diagnostic products include topical fluorescein stains, which are used to detect foreign bodies or scratches.

Increased intraocular pressure is a sign of the eye condition called *glaucoma*. This condition results from either excess production or reduced outflow of aqueous humor (ocular fluid). There are three major forms of glaucoma. Primary glaucoma includes narrow-angle glaucoma and wide-angle glaucoma. Patients with narrow-angle glaucoma have a shallow anterior chamber, possibly because of the anatomy or physiologic action with which they were born. Drugs are used to control the acute problem before there is a permanent surgical solution. Wide-angle glaucoma has a gradual onset, and its control depends on permanent drug therapy. Secondary glaucoma may result from other eye problems such as cataract extraction and is treated with medication. Congenital glaucoma is a birth defect requiring surgical correction. Medications for treating glaucoma use a variety of mechanisms to increase outflow of aqueous humor.

Antiglaucoma agents make up a large class of medications with a variety of actions. Mydriatic-cycloplegics block the action of acetylcholine. The sphincter of the iris is paralyzed, causing **mydriasis**, or abnormal dilation (opening) of the pupil, and the ciliary muscles are paralyzed, blocking accommodation (the ability to switch from near to far vision and back), or adjustment of the focus of the eye. These agents are used in some tests for glaucoma. Atropine and scopolamine are long-acting agents that produce complete cycloplegia, or paralysis. Homatropine, cyclopentolate, and tropicamide have shorter durations of action and are most useful for diagnostic procedures. Long-acting cholinesterase inhibitors include miotic-antiglaucoma agents that inactivate acetylcholinesterase. This provides iris sphincter contraction, leading to miosis (small pupils), and ciliary muscle constriction, which leads to increased aqueous humor outflow. Parasympathomimetic or miotic drugs, such as carbachol, act as cholinergic agonists to reduce intraocular pressure by causing iris sphincter contraction, leading to miosis. This leads to an increased outflow of aqueous humor by opening up the anterior chamber angle. Cholinesterase inhibitors such as physostigmine salicylate briefly

Table 23-3

Ophthalmic Preparations

GENERIC NAME	TRADE NAME	COMMENTS AND DOSAGE
LOCAL ANESTHETICS		
benoxinate	Fluress	Often used when suturing of eye is required. Instill 1-2 drops before procedure.
proparacaine	Alcaine Ophthaine	Use 1-2 drops immediately before tonometry, 2-3 min before suture removal or removal of foreign body.
tetracaine	Pontocaine	Instill 1-2 drops or ½-1 inch of ointment to lower conjunctival area.
ANTISEPTIC OINTMENTS		
silver nitrate	Silver Nitrate	After birth, clean infant's eyes with cotton ball and instill 2 gtt 1% solution qh.
OPHTHALMIC ANTIINFECTIVES (Preparations must be labeled "ophthalmic")		
Alpha₂-Adrenergic Agonist		
brimonidine	Alphagan	Instill 1 drop in the affected eye(s) q8h.
Antibiotics		
bacitracin	AK-Tracin	Apply sparingly into conjunctival sac 2 to 3 times daily.
chloramphenicol	Chloroptic AK-Chlor	Apply small amount of ointment to the lower conjunctival sac, or instill 2 drops of solution q3h for the first 48 hr, then prn. Continue for at least 48 hr after the eye appears to be normal.
ciprofloxacin	Ciloxan	Instill 1-3 gtt into conjunctival sac, close eyes, and apply light pressure over lacrimal sac for 1 minute after instillation.
erythromycin	Ilotycin	Apply to affected eye 3 times daily or more often, depending on severity of infection.
gentamicin	Garamycin Genoptic Gentacidin	Instill 1-2 drops into affected eye q4h. In severe infections, dosage may be increased to as much as 2 drops hourly. Apply ointment sparingly 2 to 3 times daily.
levofloxacin	Quixin	Instill 1-2 drops in the affected eye(s) q2h while awake, up to 8 times/day for 2 days. Then instill 1-2 drops in the affected eye(s) q4h while awake, up to 4 times/day for days 3 through 7.
norfloxacin	Chibroxin	Instill 1-3 gtt into conjunctival sac, close eyes, and apply light pressure over lacrimal sac for 1 min after instillation.
ofloxacin	Ocuflox	Instill 1-3 gtt into conjunctival sac, close eyes, and apply light pressure over lacrimal sac for 1 min after instillation.
polymyxin B	Polymyxin-B	Instill 1-2 drops of 0.1%-0.25% qh; increase prn.
sulfacetamide sodium	AK-Sulf Sodium sulamyd	Instill 1-2 drops q2-3h during day, less at night. May also apply ½- to 1-inch ribbon of ointment in lower conjunctival sac at night.
tobramycin	Tobrex AK-Tob Defy	Instill 1-2 drops 4 to 6 times daily.
Antiviral Agents		
fomivirsen	Vitravene	Use 330 mcg as a single intravitreal injection every other week for 2 doses followed by maintenance doses of 330 mcg once every 4 wk in treatment of cytomegalovirus retinitis.
ganciclovir	Vitrasert	Used in treating cytomegalovirus retinitis in patients with AIDS. Use 4.5-mg insert that is designed to release the drug over a 5- to 8-mo period. May be repeated as needed.
idoxuridine	Herplex Stoxil 🍁	Saturate tissue for best results. Instill 1 drop in infected eye qh during day. At night, instill 1 drop qoh.
trifluridine	Viroptic	Instill 1 drop onto the cornea of eye with corneal ulcers q2h while awake for a maximum of 9 drops/day. Continue until reepithelialization, then for 7 days give 1 drop q4h while awake.

Table 23-3

Ophthalmic Preparations—cont'd

GENERIC NAME	TRADE NAME	COMMENTS AND DOSAGE
OPHTHALMIC ANTIINFECTIVES (Preparations must be labeled "ophthalmic")—cont'd		
Antiviral Agents—cont'd		
vidarabine	Vira-A	Apply ½ inch of ointment to the lower conjunctival sac 5 times daily at 3-hr intervals.
Artificial Tears		
—	Isopto alkaline Liquifilm Forte Refresh Endura Systane Tearisol Tears Plus	1-3 drops may be instilled in the eyes 3 to 4 times daily or prn. Some of these preparations, such as Tearisol, are not to be used with soft contact lenses. Keep the solution free from contamination.
—	Lacrisert	Insert once a day into inferior cul-de-sac beneath base of tarsus.
ANTIGLAUCOMA AGENTS		
Sympathomimetics		
apraclonidine	Iopidine	Instill 1 drop 1% solution before laser surgery.
dipivefrin	Propine	Instill 1 drop 0.1% solution into eyes q12h.
epinephrine	Epifrin	Instill 1-2 drops into affected eyes daily to twice daily.
	Glaucon	Instill 1 drop daily or twice daily.
Beta Blockers		
betaxolol	Betoptic	Instill 1 drop twice daily.
carteolol	Ocupress	Instill 1 drop 1% solution twice daily.
levobetaxolol	Betaxon	Instill 1 drop twice daily.
levobunolol	Betagan	Instill 1 drop 0.25% solution daily.
metipranolol	OptiPranolol	Instill 1 drop 0.3% solution twice daily.
timolol	Timoptic	Instill 1 drop 0.25% solution twice daily.
Miotics, Direct-Acting		
acetylcholine Cl	Miochol-E	Instill 0.5-2 mL 3 times daily.
carbachol	Isopto-carbachol	Instill 1-2 drops up to 3 times daily.
pilocarpine	Pilocar Pilostat	Instill 1-2 drops up to 6 times daily.
pilocarpine ocular therapeutic system	Ocusert	The system is placed in and removed from the eye by the patient, according to instructions in the package. Releases 20 or 40 mcg pilocarpine per hour for 1 wk.
Miotics, Cholinesterase Inhibitors		
demecarium	Humorsol	Instill 1-2 drops into eyes daily.
echothiophate	Phospholine Iodide	Instill 1-2 drops daily.
Carbonic Anhydrase Inhibitors		
brinzolamide	Azopt	Give 1 gtt 3 times daily.
dorzolamide	Trusopt	Give 1 gtt 3 times daily.
Cholinergic Blocking Agents		
Mydriatic-Cycloplegics		
atropine	Atropisol	1 drop of 0.5% or 1% solution daily to 3 times daily, or 0.3-0.5 gm of 1% ointment daily to 3 times daily.
cyclopentolate	Cyclogyl	Give 1 drop of 1% or 2% solution; repeat in 5 min. Refraction can occur in 40-50 min.
homatropine	Isopto-Homatropine	Give 1 drop of 2% or 5% solution; repeat 2 to 5 times until desired results occur.
scopolamine	IsoptoHyoscine	Give 1 drop of 0.25% solution daily to 3 times daily.
tropicamide	Mydriacyl	Give 1 drop of 1% solution; repeat in 5 min.

Table 23-3
Ophthalmic Preparations—cont'd

GENERIC NAME	TRADE NAME	COMMENTS AND DOSAGE
OPHTHALMIC ANTIINFECTIVES (Preparations must be labeled "ophthalmic")—cont'd		
Mydriatic		
phenylephrine	Neo-Synephrine	• *Mydriasis:* 1 drop of 2.5%-10% solution topically on conjunctiva. Repeat in 5 min prn. • *Vasoconstriction:* 1 drop of 0.02%-0.15% solution topically to conjunctiva 3 to 4 times daily prn. • *Conjunctivitis:* 1-2 drops qh until condition improves, and then 1 drop 3 to 4 times daily.
OTHER OPHTHALMIC PREPARATIONS		
Alpha-Adrenergic Blocking Agent		
dapiprazole	Rev-Eyes	Instill 2 drops, followed 5 min later by an additional 2 drops.
Prostaglandin Agonists		
bimatoprost	Lumigao	1 drop daily in the evening to reduce IOP.
latanoprost	Xalatan	Instill 1 drop in affected eye(s) once daily in the evening. Do not exceed this dose.
travoprost	Travatan	1 drop daily in the evening to reduce IOP.
unoprostone	Rescula	1 drop twice daily. May be used with other drops if administered at least 5 min apart.
Antihistamines		
azelastine	Optivar	1 drop twice daily to reduce itching from allergic conjunctivitis.
emedastine	Emadine	Instill 1 drop in affected eye(s) 4 times daily. Do not use if patient is wearing contact lenses.
olopatadine	Patanol	1-2 drops twice daily at intervals of 6-8 hr.
Vasoconstrictors/Mydriatics		
hydroxy-amphetamine	Paredrine	Instill 1-2 drops in conjunctival sac.
naphazoline	Allerest Degest 2 Vasocon	Use 1-2 drops 2 to 3 times daily prn to relieve irritation or redness. Mydriasis occurs within 1 hr, recedes within 6 hr of administration. Do not give to patients with angle-closure glaucoma or narrow anterior angle.
oxymetazoline	OcuClear	Instill 1-2 drops q6h.
tetrahydrozoline	Murine Plus Tetrazine Visine	Use 1-2 drops in each eye 2 to 3 times daily prn. Mydriasis occurs in 1 hr, recedes within 6 hr. Do not give to patients with narrow-angle glaucoma.
Eye Diagnostic Products		
fluorescein	Fluor-I-Strip Ophthfluor Fluorescite AK-Fluor Ful-Glo	For examination of corneal and conjunctival epithelium, pour 1 drop sterile water on strip, touch to cornea, and close lid for 60 sec. Use Wood's lamp to visualize. Add drops; patient should blink. Examine the eye under fluorescing light, and areas of foreign body or abrasion should fluoresce bright green or yellow.
Nonsteroidal Antiinflammatory Drugs		
diclofenac	Voltaren	Give 1 drop to affected eye 4 times daily beginning 24 hr after cataract surgery and continuing throughout the first 2 wk of the postoperative period.
flurbiprofen	Ocufen	For inhibition of intraoperative miosis, for inflammation after cataract, glaucoma, or laser surgery and uveitis syndromes. Give 1 gtt every 30 min beginning 2 hr before surgery.

Continu

Table 23-3

Ophthalmic Preparations—cont'd

GENERIC NAME	TRADE NAME	COMMENTS AND DOSAGE
OTHER OPHTHALMIC PREPARATIONS—cont'd		
Nonsteroidal Antiinflammatory Drugs—cont'd		
ketorolac	Acular	For relief of ocular itching caused by seasonal allergic conjunctivitis, treatment of postoperative inflammation of postcataract extraction. Instill 1 drop to the affected eye(s) 4 times daily beginning 24 hr after cataract surgery and continuing for 2 wk.
suprofen	Profenal	For treatment of postoperative inflammation after cataract extraction. On the day before surgery, instill 2 drops into conjunctival sac every 4 hr while awake; on the day of surgery use 2 drops 3, 2, and 1 hr before surgery.
Mast Cell Stabilizers		
nedocromil	Alocril	Use 1 or 2 drops in each eye twice daily to treat itching of allergic conjunctivitis.
pemirolast	Alamast	Use 1-2 drops in each eye 4 times daily to prevent itching from allergic conjunctivitis.
Ophthalmic Decongestants		
cromolyn sodium	Crolom	Instill 1 or 2 drops 4 to 6 times/day.
iodoxamide	Alomide	Instill 1-2 drops in each eye 4 times daily for up to 3 mo in patients with vernal conjunctivitis or vernal keratitis.
ketotifen	Zaditor	Instill 1 drop q8-12h to prevent itching of eye from allergic conjunctivitis.
levocabastine	Livostin	Instill 1 drop in affected eye(s) 4 times daily for up to 2 wk.
Ophthalmic Corticosteroids		
dexamethasone	AK-Dex Maxidex	*Sol:* Instill 1-2 drops qh during the day and q2h at night until symptoms reduce; then q4h.
fluorometholone	Flarex Fluor-Op	*Suspension:* Shake well and instill 1-2 drops in conjunctival sac 2 to 4 times daily. *Ointment:* Apply ½-inch ribbon into conjunctival sac 1 to 3 times daily.
loteprednol	Lotemax Alrex	Use 1 drop 4 times daily. Shake well before using.
medrysone	HMS	Shake well and instill 1 drop into conjunctival sac up to every 4 hr.
prednisolone	AK-Pred Pred Forte Pred Mild Inflamase	Shake well and instill 1-2 drops in conjunctival sac 2 to 4 times daily.
rimexolone	Vexol	1-2 drops in affected eye 4 times daily beginning 24 hr after ocular surgery and for 2 wk.

IDS, Acquired immunodeficiency syndrome; *IOP,* intraocular pressure.

inactivate acetylcholinesterase to allow acetylcholine to accumulate, which increases parasympathetic tone. This causes iris sphincter contraction, resulting in miosis, increased ciliary muscle constriction, and an increase in aqueous humor outflow. Timolol is a beta blocker that reduces intraocular pressure, probably by reducing the formation of aqueous humor. Sympathomimetic agents such as epinephrine produce vasoconstriction (narrowing of the blood vessels) and decreased intraocular pressure in open-angle glaucoma, probably as a result of decreased production of aqueous humor. Phenylephrine acts as a mydriatic, causing constriction of the dilator muscles of the pupil, leading to mydriasis and

Clinical Goldmine

Ophthalmic Preparations

Ophthalmic preparations are the mildest chemicals used in the body. If something is safe enough to put in the eye, it should be safe enough for use anywhere else. Each of these preparations has numerous precautions, contraindications, and minor adverse effects. You should check the package inserts for more detailed information and Table 23-3 for a summary.

Table 23-4 *Otic Preparations*

OTIC PREPARATIONS (Preparations must be labeled "otic")

benzocaine	Americaine	Swab ear with solution; instill 4-5 drops of warmed solution. Insert cotton pledget in meatus. Patient should remain on side for a few minutes.
carbamide peroxide	Debrox	To remove ear wax, instill 5-10 drops, keeping head tilted so that solution stays in. Maintain position for a few minutes. Repeat twice daily for 3-4 days. May use before irrigation with bulb syringe.
chloramphenicol	Chloromycetin	Effective against many gram-positive and gram-negative organisms. *Adults and children:* Instill 2-3 drops into the ear 3 times daily.
desonide, acetic acid	Tridesilon	Useful in superficial infections of the external canal. Instill 3-4 drops into affected ear 3 to 4 times daily.
triethanolamine polypeptide oleate-condensate	Cerumenex	To remove cerumen. May be given as drops to loosen cerumen. Use patch test to check for sensitivity 24 hr before use. Tilt patient's head to 45-degree angle and fill ear canal with solution. Insert cotton plug for 30 min. Gently flush ear with warm water using a soft, rubber syringe.

OTIC STEROID AND ANTIBIOTIC COMBINATIONS

ciprofloxacin, hydrocortisone	Cipro HC Otic	Instill 4 drops 3 or 4 times daily.
hydrocortisone, neomycin	Cortisporin-TC	Instill 4 drops 3 or 4 times daily.
hydrocortisone, neomycin, and polymyxin B	Cortisporin Otocort	Instill 4 drops 3 or 4 times daily.

vasoconstriction of the arterioles of the conjunctiva. **Vasoconstrictors** such as naphazoline cause direct stimulation of the alpha receptors of vascular smooth muscle, leading to vasoconstriction. This action lasts for several hours.

It is especially important for you to avoid dilating the pupils of a patient who may have glaucoma, because angle closure could be provoked, leading to a surgical emergency.

OTIC PREPARATIONS

Action and Uses

Topical antibiotics are used to control superficial infections of the ear through bactericidal or bacteriostatic mechanisms. Other products may be used in prophylaxis of infections for swimmers, and for removing cerumen (earwax) plugs. There are also some steroid products available for ear problems. You should check the package inserts of individual products for precautions, contraindications, and adverse effects. Table 23-4 presents a summary of otic preparations.

TOPICAL SKIN PREPARATIONS

Action and Uses

Topical preparations for the skin may include medicated bar soaps and foams, sulfur preparations, topi-cal antibiotics, and medications used for acne. A wide variety of steroids are also available for topical use in a variety of dermatologic disorders. These preparations come in mild, intermediate, and strong concentrations. Fluorinated products should not be used on the face, because they may cause thinning of the skin and may leave scars. Steroids also should not be used if there is strong indication of bacterial or fungal infections.

Antipsoriatics accelerate scaling and healing of dry lesions in chronic psoriasis. Antiseborrheic shampoos promote shedding and softening of the horny cell layer and inhibit the growth of microorganisms in seborrhea and dandruff. There are now antiviral agents used to treat herpes simplex. These agents helps reduce the severity of symptoms and lengthen the time between outbreaks. **Scabicides** are applied to the skin and in the hair to treat scabies. **Pediculicides** are used to treat pediculosis, an infection of the dermis seen mostly in children. There are also a variety of burn preparations, cauterizing agents, emollients, keratolytics, and wet dressings and soaks on the market. These agents all have their own specific precautions, adverse reactions, and drug interactions. The specific product information should be consulted. These preparations are summarized in Table 23-5. Any of the chemicals in these products may interact with other medications the patient may be taking.

Table 23-5

Topical Skin Products

GENERIC NAME	TRADE NAME	COMMENTS AND DOSAGE
ACNE PRODUCTS		
adapalene	Differin	Wash face and then apply a thin film of the gel once daily to affected areas. An exacerbation of acne may initially be seen; therapeutic results usually seen in 8-12 wk.
azelaic	Azelex	Wash face and dry thoroughly. Then apply thin film twice daily to affected areas and gently massage into skin. Results usually seen in 4 wk.
benzoyl peroxide bars and soaps	Clearasil Desquam-X Oxy-10	Apply daily to affected areas after cleansing skin. After 3-4 days, if redness, dryness, and peeling do not occur, increase application to twice daily. Use instead of soap. These products promote drying of skin and provide a gentle abrasive action when applied. If undue skin irritation develops, stop use and contact nurse, physician, or other health care provider. Available OTC.
isotretinoin	Accutane ❦	This product must not be taken by women who are pregnant, because severe fetal abnormalities may be produced. Women in childbearing years should be protected by adequate contraception methods during the course of therapy. • *Cystic acne:* 1-2 mg/kg/day divided into 2 doses for 2 wk. Dosage may then be adjusted for individual weight and severity of disease.
sulfur preparations	Liquimat	Thin film of medication should be applied daily or twice daily to clean skin. Used to treat oily skin and mild acne.
tazarotene	Tazorac	Wash face and then apply a thin film to affected areas once daily.
tretinoin	Retin-A Vesanoid ❦	Apply to affected area, on clean skin only, daily at bedtime. Start with low doses; may irritate skin initially. Makes individuals more sensitive to the sun, and they must wear sunscreen. Also evidence that this product restores skin collagen and turgor, reversing fine wrinkles. Do not use in pregnant women.
TOPICAL ANTIINFECTIVES		
bacitracin	Baciguent	Apply small amount to infected area 3 times daily; comes as cream.
chloramphenicol	Chloromycetin	Apply small amount to infected area 3 times daily; comes as cream.
clindamycin	Cleocin T	Apply small amount to infected area twice daily.
erythromycin	Akne-mycin	Apply small amount to infected area 3 times daily; comes as cream.
gentamicin	Garamycin	Apply small amount to infected area 3 times daily; comes as cream.
mupirocin	Bactroban	New topical antibiotic. Used to treat impetigo; may produce superinfection. Apply small amount to affected area 3 times daily. May cover with gauze. Must be reevaluated within 3 days.
neomycin sulfate	Myciguent	Apply small amount to infected area 3 times daily; comes as cream.
Combination Products		
polymyxin B, neomycin, and bacitracin	Neosporin	Apply small amount to infected area 3 times daily; comes as ointment.
polymyxin B and bacitracin	Polysporin	Apply small amount to infected area 3 times daily; comes as ointment.
TOPICAL CORTICOSTEROIDS		
alclometasone	Aclovate	For relief of inflammatory and pruritic manifestations of corticosteroid-responsive dermatoses. Apply sparingly to affected areas 2 to 4 times daily.
amcinonide	Cyclocort	Apply sparingly to affected areas 2 to 4 times daily.
betamethasone dipropionate	Diprolene Diprosone	Fluorinated product, relatively expensive. Comes as cream, lotion, ointment, or topical aerosol. Use sparingly for dermatoses needing antiinflammatory medication.

Table 23-5

Topical Skin Products—cont'd

GENERIC NAME	TRADE NAME	COMMENTS AND DOSAGE
TOPICAL CORTICOSTEROIDS—cont'd		
betamethasone valerate	Beta-Val Valisone	Fluorinated product that may be used with occlusive dressings; comes as cream, lotion, or ointment. Apply sparingly daily to 3 times daily for adults.
desonide	Tridesilon	Gently rub in medication 2 to 4 times daily.
desoximetasone	Topicort	Do not use near eyes; apply sparingly daily to twice daily.
diflorasone	Maxiflor	Apply sparingly to affected areas 2 to 4 times daily.
fluocinolone acetonide	Flurosyn Synalar	Rub cream in gently, 2 to 4 times daily. Apply very sparingly; use less frequent applications for children.
fluocinonide	Lidex	Comes as cream, gel, or ointment; apply 3 to 4 times daily.
flurandrenolide	Cordran	Shake lotion well; protect from light, heat, and freezing. Also comes as a film tape. Apply sparingly 2 to 3 times daily.
halcinonide	Halog	Ointment, cream, solution; protect ointment from light. Apply sparingly 2 to 3 times daily.
hydrocortisone	Cortizone Hycort	One of the few steroids that can be used safely on the face, axilla, and groin, and under the breasts. Comes as ointment, cream, or lotion. Apply thin coat once daily to 4 times daily; increase strength as indicated by condition.
hydrocortisone acetate	Cortaid Lanacort-5	This form is more expensive. Apply thin coat of ointment or apply the cream gently and sparingly. Apply once daily to 4 times daily as needed by condition. The lowest doses are available without a prescription.
hydrocortisone plus antibiotics	Cortisporin	Comes with neomycin sulfate and polymyxin B. Apply to affected area 2 to 3 times daily; withdraw gradually if medication has been used for a long time.
methyl-prednisolone	Medrol	Very expensive; apply ointment once daily to 4 times daily.
triamcinolone acetonide	Aristocort Kenalog	Fluorinated steroid, highest potency; has many precautions to use. Apply to affected area 2 to 4 times daily. Do not use on face.
triamcinolone plus antifungals	Mycolog II	Many precautions and warnings. Apply ointment to affected areas 2 to 3 times daily. Ototoxicity (damage to the ear) and nephrotoxicity (damage to the kidney) have been reported if preparation is overused.
ANESTHETICS FOR MUCOUS MEMBRANES AND SKIN		
benzocaine	Solarcaine Teething syrup 🍁	Used for toothaches, wounds, ulcers, and lesions of oral mucosa. Apply 20% aerosol or gel to affected areas 2 to 3 times daily.
butamben picrate	Butesin Picrate	Temporary relief of pain caused by minor burns. Apply sparingly to small areas as needed.
dibucaine	Nupercainal	For abrasions, minor burns, sunburn, and hemorrhoids. Apply ointment or cream sparingly to affected area 2 to 3 times daily.
tetracaine	Pontocaine	Used in treating hemorrhoids and minor skin disorders. Apply sparingly 3 to 4 times daily.
ANTIPSORIATICS		
acitretin	Soriatane	This systemic psoriasis therapy is for severe disease. Give 25-50 mg/day once daily with main meal, continue with 25-50 mg/day as maintenance dose.
anthralin	Anthra Forte Anthra-Derm	Apply thin layer of 0.1% ointment once to twice daily for 2 wk.

Continu

Table 23-5

Topical Skin Products—cont'd

GENERIC NAME	TRADE NAME	COMMENTS AND DOSAGE
ANTIPSORIATICS—cont'd		
calcipotriene	Dovonex	A synthetic vitamin D_3 derivative indicated for the topical treatment of moderate plaque psoriasis. Calcipotriene is similar to vitamin D_3 in its effects on keratinocyte proliferation and differentiation, yet it has a less potent effect on calcium metabolism. It also modifies the immune activity of monocytes, macrophages, and T lymphocytes. In clinical trials, improvement in psoriasis has been noted within 2 wk of initiating topical therapy (twice-daily application). Approximately 70% of patients have shown marked improvement after 8 wk of therapy, with 10% showing complete clearing. Apply thin layer twice daily and rub in completely.
etretinate	Tegison	Initiate doses at 0.75-1 mg/kg/day in divided doses. Maintenance doses of 0.5-0.75 mg/kg/day generally begin after 8-16 wk of therapy.
tazarotene	Tazorac	For topical treatment of patients with stable plaque psoriasis with approximately 20% body surface area involvement. The 0.1% gel also is indicated for mild to moderately severe facial acne vulgaris.
ANTISEBORRHEIC PRODUCTS		
povidone-iodine	Betadine	Shampoo with 2 tsp to hair and scalp. Lather with warm water and rinse. Repeat application and allow to remain on scalp 5 min; rinse thoroughly. Use twice weekly until improvement, then once weekly.
selenium	Selsun Selsun Blue	Massage 1-2 tsp into wet scalp. Allow medicated shampoo to remain on scalp for 2-3 min; rinse thoroughly; repeat application and rinse. Use twice weekly for 2 wk, then weekly for 2 wk.
sulfacetamide	Sebizon	Shampoo hair and rinse. Then apply medication at bedtime and allow it to remain on scalp overnight.
ANTIVIRAL AGENTS		
acyclovir	Zovirax	For treatment of herpes simplex. Cover all lesions q3h, 6 times per day for 6 days. Approximately ½-inch ribbon of ointment per 4 square inches of surface area should be used. Oral forms are available for treatment of herpes labialis (cold sores).
penciclovir	Denavir	Apply cream q2h while awake for 4 days. Start treatment as early as possible to reduce symptoms.
BURN PREPARATIONS		
mafenide	Sulfamylon	Apply once or twice daily to a thickness of approximately ¹⁄₁₆ inch. No dressing is required.
nitrofurazone	Furacin	Soluble dressing: apply directly to lesions daily; topical cream: apply directly to lesion once daily or every few days.
silver nitrate	Silver Nitrate	Saturate dressing with warmed solution and apply to burn wound. Mold dressing to body surface and cover with dry dressing. Reapply solution q2h. Change dressing at least once daily.
silver sulfadiazine	Silvadene	Apply once or twice daily to a thickness of approximately ¹⁄₁₆ inch. Dressing not required.
SCABICIDES/PEDICULICIDES		
crotamiton	Eurax	Used in scabies and very pruritic skin conditions. Massage into skin of the whole body; apply a second coating 24 hr later. Clothing and bed linen should be changed after 24 hr. Bath should be taken 48 hr after the last application.
gamma benzene hexachloride (Lindane)	G-Well	Lotion or shampoo. Bathe, dry skin. Apply thin layer over body (not face). Leave on 8-12 hr and then wash off.

Table 23-5

Topical Skin Products—cont'd

GENERIC NAME	TRADE NAME	COMMENTS AND DOSAGE
SCABICIDES/PEDICULICIDES—cont'd		
malathion	Ovide	Apply to hair and let hair dry naturally. Wash after 8-12 hr and comb hair. Repeat in 7-9 days, if necessary. Massage into skin from scalp to soles of feet. Wash off after 8-14 hr. For pediculosis capitis in infants, wet hair, shampoo, and then apply medication to hairline, neck, scalp, temple, and forehead, and wash off after 10 min.
permethrin	Elimite Nix Acticin	Sprinkle lotion on dry hair and rub into scalp.
MISCELLANEOUS SKIN PREPARATIONS		
Cauterizing Agents		
dichloroacetic acid	Bichloracetic Acid	Apply petrolatum to tissue surrounding area to be treated. Solution should then be carefully applied to lesion. A kit is provided with detailed instructions.
monochloroacetic acid	Mono Chlor	Used for removing verrucae or warts. Do not drip solution on normal tissue or mucous membranes. Apply solution with cotton-tipped applicator or capillary tube. Cover with bandage and allow to remain in place for 4-6 days. May require more than one application.
podofilox	Condylox	Apply solution or gel morning and evening to venereal warts with a cotton-tipped applicator.
podophyllum resin	Podofin Podocon-25	Applied to venereal warts only by health care provider. Cleanse area and then apply sparingly to lesion. Leave on 30-40 min to check sensitivity, and no longer than 4 hr. Remove with alcohol or soap and water.
silver nitrate solution or sticks	—	Apply to local area as needed.
trichloroacetic acid	Tri-Chlor	Use on débrided skin to remove verruca. Apply to wart, then cover for 5-6 days. Peel off wart tissue.
Emollients		
colloidal baths	Alpha Keri Aveeno	Bath additives for treating widespread eruptions. Limit bath time to 30 min; patient should be aware that preparations often make tub slippery. Follow directions on packet or bottle.
dexpanthenol	Panthoderm	Stimulates epithelization and granulation. Aids in the healing of skin lesions and relieves pruritus. Apply directly to clean skin once to twice daily.
salicylic acid	Mediplast-Salacid Wart-Off	Use creams for corns and calluses. Apply directly to area daily for 2 wk. Cut out piece of plaster to fit callus, or apply gels to well-hydrated skin. Check callus q24h; discontinue if irritation develops.
urea	Aquacare Nutraplus	Hydrates skin and aids in removing scales and crusts. Apply directly to clean skin 2 to 3 times daily, affected area only.
vitamin E	Vite E Cream Vitec	Apply cream or ointment to skin to hydrate.
vitamins A, D, and E	Retinol Comfortine Clocream	Apply cream or ointment to skin.
Smoking Cessation Products		
—	Habitrol Nicoderm CQ Nicotrol	Used to decrease withdrawal symptoms as part of smoking cessation program. Do not have serious side effects. In association with behavior modification programs, use patch daily. Use 2 wk at each of 3 strengths in decreasing order of strength.

Continu

Table 23-5

Topical Skin Products—cont'd

GENERIC NAME	TRADE NAME	COMMENTS AND DOSAGE
MISCELLANEOUS SKIN PREPARATIONS—cont'd		
Smoking Cessation Products—cont'd		
nicotine gum	Nicorette	Use 2- or 4-mg gum to reduce cravings. Chew gum steadily and then place gum against buccal membranes.
nicotine inhalation system	Nicotrol Inhaler	4-mg inhaler. Use as part of withdrawal system.
nicotine nasal spray	Nicotrol NS	Spray 0.5 mg into nostril to reduce symptoms of withdrawal.
Wet Dressings and Soaks		
Burow's solution	Domeboro	Used for open wet dressings in inflammatory conditions of skin. They cool and dry through evaporation, which causes local vasoconstriction. Moisten dressing and apply multiple layers to prevent rapid drying and cooling. Reapply every 15-30 min as indicated for 4-8 hr.

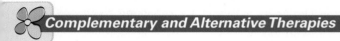

Complementary and Alternative Therapies

Oral or Topical Products for Eye, Ear, and Skin Problems

PRODUCTS	COMMENTS
ACNE	
Chasteberry/Vitex	Potential interaction with hormonal replacements or oral contraceptives
Tea tree	No known interactions
Olive leaf	No known interactions
ATHLETE'S FOOT	
Cat's claw	Potential interaction with anticoagulants, aspirin, NSAIDs, antiplatelet agents
Tea tree	No reported interactions
Olive leaf	No reported interactions
Garlic	Potential interaction with anticoagulants, aspirin, NSAIDs, antiplatelet agents, hypolipidemics, antihypertensives
CONTACT DERMATITIS/ECZEMA	
Milk thistle	No reported interactions
Evening primrose	Potential interactions with anticoagulants, aspirin, NSAIDs, antiplatelet agents
Grapefruit seed extract	Avoid terfenadine, astemizole, cisapride, or other medications metabolized by cytochrome P-450 3A4 subsystem
Olive leaf	No reported interactions
Artichoke	No reported interactions
Aloe	No known interactions
Calendula	No known interactions
Echinacea	No known interactions
GLAUCOMA	
Bilberry	Potential interaction with anticoagulants, aspirin, NSAIDs, antiplatelet agents
Grape seed	Potential interaction with anticoagulants, aspirin, NSAIDs, antiplatelet agents, methotrexate

Complementary and Alternative Therapies—cont'd

PRODUCTS	COMMENTS
OTITIS MEDIA	
Echinacea	Potential interaction with therapeutic immunosuppressants and corticosteroids
Astragalus	May interact with immune stimulants or immunosuppressants
Olive leaf	No reported interactions
PSORIASIS	
Coleus (PO)	Potential interaction with anticoagulants, aspirin, NSAIDs, antiplatelet agents, antihistamines, decongestants, anticoagulants, antihypertensives
Milk thistle (PO)	No known interactions
Gotu kola	Application may cause dermatitis
Evening primrose	Potential interaction with anticoagulants, aspirin, NSAIDs, antiplatelet agents
ROSACEA	
Cat's claw	Potential interaction with anticoagulants, aspirin, NSAIDs, antiplatelet agents
Chasteberry/Vitex (PO)	Potential interaction with hormonal replacements or oral contraceptives
Milk thistle (PO)	No known interactions
Grapefruit seed extract (PO)	Avoid terfenadine, astemizole, cisapride, or other medications metabolized by cytochrome P-450 3A4 subsystem
Evening primrose	Potential interaction with anticoagulants, aspirin, NSAIDs, antiplatelet agents
SUNBURN	
Aloe	No known interactions
Lavender	No known interactions
St. John's wort	No known interactions if used topically

Modified from Krinsky DL, Lavella JB, Hawkins EB, et al: *Natural therapeutics pocket guide,* ed 2, Hudson, Ohio, 2003, Lexi-Comp, Inc.
NSAIDs, Nonsteroidal antiinflammatory drugs.

COMPLEMENTARY AND ALTERNATIVE PRODUCTS

Patients use a wide variety of topical herbal products. The Complementary and Alternative Therapies box summarizes common herbal preparations and their potential for interactions with other medications.

Go to the free CD-ROM for an Audio Glossary, animations, video clips, and Review Questions for the NCLEX-PN® Examination.

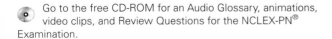 Be sure to visit the companion Evolve website at http://evolve.elsevier.com/Edmunds/LPN/ for WebLinks, a link to the top 200 drugs by prescription, and sign-up pages for newsletter drug updates.

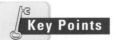 **Key Points**

- This chapter presented a brief overview of the wide variety of topical preparations available, many of which are OTC products.
- Even though the dose of medication in these products is usually small, they may still interact with other medications the patient is taking.
- Your role in the use of these medications often is one of teaching the patient how to apply or administer the products.
- Review the material on topical drug administration in Chapter 7.
- Side effects are usually localized unless systemic sensitization develops.

CASE STUDY

Jenny Hawkes has worn contacts for over 30 years. She has ophthalmic examinations about every 2 years and has been relatively free of problems. When she had her last visit, the doctor told her she had a little conjunctivitis and ordered an antibiotic.

1. What are some topical antiinfectives that might be ordered?
2. On her yearly visits, the ophthalmologist measures the intraocular pressure and dilates her eyes to view the retina. This year, there is some evidence that Jenny is developing glaucoma. Is there any concern about dilating her eyes if she might be developing glaucoma?
3. Why are there different categories of drugs used in the treatment of glaucoma?
4. After several follow-up visits, Jenny is started on Timoptic. What kind of a medication is this, and what are some of the anticipated reactions to the drug?

5. After a number of years taking Timoptic, the intraocular pressure again begins to rise. Is the disease process worsening? What is causing the change?
6. What other antiglaucoma products might Jenny take?
7. Do antiglaucoma products interfere with wearing contact lenses?
8. Jenny wakes up one morning with sharp, scratchy pains in her left eye. Her eye is tearing, and she is unable to keep it open. The eye doctor puts fluorescein sodium in her eye. Why?
9. The doctor discovers a small foreign body lodged in the cornea. It is removed with a needle, Jenny's eye is patched, and she is sent home. What types of medications might be required?

DRUG CALCULATION REVIEW

1. Order: Nystatin 500,000 units, swish and swallow 4 times per day

   Supply: Nystatin 100,000 units/mL

   Question: How many milliliters of nystatin are needed with each dose?

2. Order: Accutane 40 mg by mouth twice a day

   Supply: Accutane 20 mg per tablet

   Question: How many tablets of Accutane are needed with each dose?

3. Order: Wash hair daily with selenium 10 mL

   Question: How many teaspoons of selenium are needed for each wash?

CRITICAL THINKING ?

1. Mr. Samms comes to the clinic for an eye examination. His pupils must be dilated first. Describe the precautions you must take in dilating his pupils.

2. Mr. Samms' physician has recommended an OTC ophthalmic product for control of mild glaucoma. Explain glaucoma to Mr. Samms, along with the actions and effects of the antiglaucoma agents.

. While waiting for his prescription, Mr. Samms asks you what exactly his new medication is called. Name at least three types of medications he might take for glaucoma.

. Mr. Samms also has to take medication in the form of eye drops for 1 week for a separate, minor disorder. He has never needed eye drops until now. He tells you that he is nervous about being able to self-administer these. Develop a teaching plan for describing or demonstrating this process to Mr. Samms.

Why are there differences between administration of eye ointments and that of eye drops?

6. Mrs. Johnson and her 4-year-old son come into the clinic needing treatment for swimmer's ear. Why is the administration of ear drops different for each of these patients?

7. The physician also discovers that Mrs. Johnson's ears are filled with wax. What medication is the doctor most likely to order for this?

8. Conduct an informal investigation at your nearest pharmacy or drugstore: compare administration instructions on the labels or (if you can get access to them) the package inserts of several OTC skin products. Are some more specific in their instructions than others? Why might that be?

9. You are the school nurse in an elementary school. Daniel, who is in the third grade, comes in to your office scratching his head and complaining his head "itches." Upon checking his scalp, you realize he has pediculosis, or head lice. What instructions should you give to his parents?

After reading and studying this chapter, you should be able to do the following:

1. Identify the actions and indications for vitamins and minerals.
2. List at least six products used to treat vitamin or mineral deficiencies.
3. Present a teaching plan for patients who require vitamin or mineral supplements.

Key Terms

Be sure to check out the bonus material on the free CD-ROM, including selected audio pronunciations.

ascorbic acid (ă-SKŌR-bĭk, p. 454)
minerals (MĬN-ĕr-ălz, p. 458)
niacin (NĪ-ă-sĭn, p. 451)
riboflavin (RĪ-bō-flā-vĭn, p. 451)
thiamine (THĪ-ă-mĕn, p. 451)
vitamin A (VĬT-ă-mĭn, p. 450)
vitamins (p. 449)

OVERVIEW

This chapter discusses the uses of vitamins and minerals. An overview of their actions, indications for use, and common adverse effects and drug interactions is presented. Brief comments are included of importance to you as a nurse. Summaries of a sample of medications available on the market are included in tables at the ends of each major discussion. These over-the-counter (OTC) products change quickly, and the latest information should always be obtained for specific products. See Chapter 15 for additional related information about fluid and electrolyte products.

SECTION ONE

Vitamins

OVERVIEW

Vitamins are chemical compounds found naturally in plant and animal tissues but not made in the human body. They are necessary for life and essential to normal metabolism. They can act as coenzymes to regulate the creation of compounds in the body. Vitamins are classified into two types: fat soluble (which are stored in the body), and water soluble (which are excreted in the urine). Usually, patients get enough vitamins from a well-balanced, nutritious diet, except when certain conditions prevent them from swallowing (such as intravenous therapy when a patient is taking nothing by mouth) or prevent their metabolism (as in disorders that

block fat metabolism). Such conditions may require vitamin supplement until a normal diet can be resumed or the underlying problem corrected.

In accepting that many people in the United States eat poorly, the American Medical Association has for the first time recently recommended the use of a daily vitamin if patients do not eat a well-balanced diet and eat lots of high-fat or "empty calorie" foods. Supplements or vitamins cannot make up for a poor diet or other unhealthful lifestyle practices such as smoking or lack of exercise. If patients cannot tolerate certain foods such as dairy products, they may need to supplement their diet to ensure they are getting the nutrients provided by that food group.

A deficiency of one vitamin in a diet that is otherwise adequate is rare. Deficiency signs and symptoms in a patient may point to a lack of one vitamin, but usually a deficiency of several vitamins will be found. Because of the vast number of multiple-vitamin preparations that are easily available to consumers, as well as television and magazine advertisements, hypervitaminosis (excess amounts of several vitamins) is more likely to occur than are deficiencies of single vitamins.

Although controversy exists over natural versus synthetic vitamin preparations, vitamins are still vitamins, and the least-expensive vitamin preparation is most likely as good therapeutically as a more expensive version. There are still many mysteries about the action of various vitamins in the body, but it is clear that taking large amounts of vitamins is unnecessary, may be harmful, and should be avoided.

There is a lot of literature now about antioxidant vitamins and nutritional supplements. The major antioxidants are vitamin E (alpha-tocopherol); beta-carotene (a precursor, or forerunner, to vitamin A); vitamin C (ascorbic acid); and the mineral selenium. All of these are found in fruits and vegetables. Many research studies are looking at the mechanism of action of antioxidants. Current research suggests that, when low-density lipoprotein (LDL) cholesterol is oxidized, often incomplete oxidation takes place, producing free radicals that lead to atherosclerotic plaques. (An analogy has been made to wood that burns incompletely in a fireplace and "pops," sending sparks against the screen.) It is thought that antioxidants retard or prevent LDL oxidation because they are oxidized in preference over LDL. This slows or eliminates the progression of atherosclerosis. It is also believed that antioxidants may slow the process that may cause cancer in a cell. This has resulted in a large market for antioxidants to reduce cardiovascular disease and cancer.

Although many major research studies have looked at antioxidants after the fact and have suggested major benefits from increased use for many disease states, there are at present no intervention studies that support the role of antioxidants in cancer prevention. Epidemiologic evidence does indicate that those who eat fruits and vegetables regularly have less risk of cancer, although there is no conclusive evidence that this is the result of antioxidants. Therefore, supplementation with vitamin antioxidants may be beneficial; however, in certain populations, such as smokers, research has found that it may actually be harmful. Nonetheless, the U.S. Department of Agriculture and the U.S. Department of Health and Human Services released a new version of the food pyramid in early 2005 in which there is even more emphasis on eating fruits and vegetables and whole-grain products, and on taking in fewer calories and getting more exercise in order to reverse widespread obesity in all age groups.

VITAMIN A

ACTION AND USES

Vitamin A is a fat-soluble, long-chain alcohol that comes in several isometric forms: retinol, retinene, carotene, and retinoic acid. Its best understood action is helping the eye adjust to changes from light to darkness. Less understood actions include helping to stabilize and maintain the cell membrane structure, especially of epithelial cell membranes, and therefore helping the body to resist infection; affecting the synthesis of protein, which affects growth of skeletal and soft tissue; and playing an essential role in reproduction. A quantity sufficient to meet a 2-year requirement is stored in the normal adult Kupffer cells of the liver.

Vitamin A is used to treat deficiency that may be provoked by sprue, colitis, regional enteritis, biliary tract or pancreatic disease, or partial gastrectomy. It is also used for the treatment of specific eye diseases and night blindness.

ADVERSE REACTIONS

If vitamin A is given in high doses for a long time, the treatment should be stopped at times to avoid hypervitaminosis. Any patient receiving 25,000 International Units (IU) or more should be closely supervised. Pregnant women should not receive more than 6000 IU daily, or they may risk fetal abnormalities.

DRUG INTERACTIONS

Women taking oral contraceptives often show very high elevation in plasma vitamin A levels and should be closely monitored for hypervitaminosis. Mineral oil interferes with the absorption of fat-soluble vitamins. Certain antihyperlipidemic agents may also affect absorption of this product.

Nursing Implications and Patient Teaching

One IU of vitamin A is equivalent to 0.6 mcg of beta-carotene or 0.3 mcg of retinol. This medication may be given orally (PO), intravenously (IV), or intramuscularly (IM), depending on the rapidity of needed replacement.

Recommended daily allowances (RDAs) are as follows:

Children 0 to 9 years: 300 to 450 mcg/day
Children 9 to 18 years: 575 to 750 mcg/day
Adults 18 to 75 years and older: 750 mcg/day
Pregnant women (second and third trimesters): 750 mcg/day
Lactating women: 1200 mcg/day

Some foods rich in vitamin A are animal products such as dairy products, eggs, and organ meats (all contain preformed vitamin A) and deep orange, yellow, and green fruits and vegetables (these contain carotene). In addition, some fortified sources of vitamin A are infant formula, skim milk, margarine, and some cereals.

VITAMIN B₁ (THIAMINE)

ACTION AND USES

Vitamin B₁, or **thiamine,** is water soluble and functions as a coenzyme that is closely involved with carbohydrate metabolism. Thiamine is involved in 24 different reactions, including the citric acid cycle. It also has been thought to have a role in neurophysiology. Thiamine is excreted in the urine.

Vitamin B₁ is used to treat beriberi, which is rare in the United States but does sometimes occur. It is usually found in patients with alcoholism, gastric lesions, or hyperemesis of pregnancy. Symptoms include anorexia (lack of appetite), vomiting, fatigability, aching muscles, ataxia (poor coordination) of gait, and emotional disturbances such as moodiness or depression.

ADVERSE REACTIONS

Adverse reactions to thiamine include sensitivity (allergy) reactions, particularly after parenteral administration, which can be of a severe type, including anaphylaxis (shock). Fatalities may occur. Sensitivity tests should be done before the therapeutic dose is given. IV doses should be given very slowly. Feelings of warmth, pruritus (itching), urticaria (hives), nausea, angioneurotic edema, pulmonary edema, sweating, tightness of the throat, malaise (weakness), and cyanosis (blue color to the skin) are also seen.

DRUG INTERACTIONS

Neutral or alkaline solutions will produce poor stability of thiamine preparations.

Nursing Implications and Patient Teaching

Thiamine is easily leached (lost) out of food and is destroyed when food is heated over 100° C, fried in hot pans, or cooked for a long time under pressure. There is some loss of thiamine during dehydration of vegetables. The product is also sensitive to ultraviolet light. Foods rich in thiamine include pork, whole grains, enriched breads, cereals, and legumes. Satisfactory sources include green vegetables, fish, meats, fruits, and milk.

VITAMIN B₂ (RIBOFLAVIN)

ACTION AND USES

Vitamin B₂, or **riboflavin,** is water soluble and acts as a precursor of two essential enzymes that deal with metabolism of proteins, fats, and carbohydrates. It is related to the release of energy to the cells and is active in tissue respiratory systems. It is used for the prophylaxis or treatment of riboflavin deficiency in which there is soreness and burning of the tongue, lips, and mouth; discomfort in eating and swallowing; and photophobia (sensitivity to light), lacrimation (excess tear production), burning and itching of the eyes, visual fatigue, and the loss of visual acuity.

DRUG INTERACTIONS

Riboflavin is only slightly soluble in water. Riboflavin levels in the body can be decreased by oral contraceptives, even in low doses. This loss has been shown through studies to be greater when patients have been taking oral contraceptives over a period of at least 3 years.

Nursing Implications and Patient Teaching

This product should be protected from light by keeping it in a tightly closed, light-resistant container. The medication turns urine a yellow color. Food sources naturally rich in riboflavin include milk; eggs; liver; kidney; heart; green, leafy vegetables; and enriched breads and cereals.

NIACIN

ACTION AND USES

Niacin, previously called vitamin B₃, is water soluble and an essential part of two coenzymes (nicotinamide adenine dinucleotide [NAD] and nicotinamide adenine dinucleotide phosphate [NADP]) that transfer hydrogen in intracellular respiration. These coenzymes convert lactic acid to pyruvic acid and function in energy release and in amino acid metabolism.

Niacin is used to prevent or treat deficiency states. Deficiency can be caused by either a limited dietary intake of niacin, excessive dietary intake of leucine (which increases the daily need for niacin), general anorexia related to disease or other problems, or malabsorption syndrome. The deficiency state is known as pellagra, which is rare but may be more prevalent in geographic regions where corn is the major staple food. Pellagra is usually found along with other vitamin deficiencies.

Pellagra symptoms are seen in mucous membrane, cutaneous, gastrointestinal (GI), and central nervous system (CNS) changes. Anorexia, irritability, anxiety, and mental changes such as hallucinations, lassitude (weariness), apprehension, and depression may be easily noticed.

GI symptoms include glossitis (swollen, beefy, red tongue), stomatitis (inflammation of the mouth), and diarrhea. Dermatitis of different body parts exposed to sun or trauma may develop, as well as lesions on the skin from sun, fire, or heat. Mental changes that are mild early in deficiency may progress to disorientation, loss of memory, confusion, hysteria, and sometimes manic outbursts.

ADVERSE REACTIONS

Adverse reactions to niacin include dry skin, pruritus, skin rash, GI disorders, allergies, feelings of warmth, headache, tingling of the skin, and transient flushing (red color in the face and neck).

DRUG INTERACTIONS

Sympathetic blocking agents (antihypertensives) may increase the vasodilatory effect of niacin, leading to postural hypotension (low blood pressure when a person suddenly stands up).

Nursing Implications and Patient Teaching

Flushing is a frequent side effect of niacin. If patients feel weak or dizzy, they should lie down until they feel better. Usually this reaction does not require stopping the drug. The usual dose is 8 mg/1000 kcal for infants and 6.6 mg/1000 kcal for children and adolescents. Not less than 8 mg/day should be given. The recommended intake for adults is 13 mg/day for women and 18 mg/day for men.

Foods rich in niacin are lean meats, peanuts, yeast, and cereal (especially bran and wheat germ). Other good sources include eggs, liver, red meat, whole grains, and enriched bread.

PANTOTHENIC ACID

ACTION AND USES

Pantothenic acid, previously known as vitamin B_5, is essential for the synthesis of coenzyme A, which has a role in the release of energy in fats, proteins, and carbohydrates. This vitamin has been used to treat paralytic ileus after surgery, possibly acting to stimulate GI motility. Deficiency states are produced only in the laboratory.

Nursing Implications and Patient Teaching

When food is cooked above the boiling point, considerable loss of pantothenic acid occurs. The loss is smaller when food is moderately cooked or baked.

This vitamin is available naturally in all plant and animal tissues. Much of the original vitamin content is lost from frozen meat in the liquid that drips off during thawing. Rich sources include yeast, liver, kidney, egg yolk, wheat bran, and fresh vegetables. Human milk contains 2.2 mg/L and cow's milk contains 3.4 mg/L.

VITAMIN B_6

ACTION AND USES

Vitamin B_6, or pyridoxine hydrochloride, is water soluble and functions as a coenzyme in the metabolism of protein, carbohydrates, and fat.

Pyridoxine is used to treat pyridoxine deficiency seen in patients with inborn errors of metabolism, such as vitamin B_6 dependency; vitamin B_6-responsive chronic anemia; and other rare vitamin problems.

Pyridoxine deficiency is most likely to develop in the elderly population and in women of childbearing age, especially those who are pregnant or breastfeeding. Women taking oral contraceptives, alcoholics, and those whose diets are of poor quality and quantity or are rich in refined foods are also at risk.

Symptoms of deficiency include malaise, nervousness, irritability, and difficulty in walking. There may also be personality changes in adults, such as depression and a loss of sense of responsibility. High doses of pyridoxine may produce neurotoxicity—ataxia, numb feet, and clumsiness.

ADVERSE REACTIONS

No adverse effects are usually seen in patients taking pyridoxine. Pyridoxine dependency (a state of conditioned need) may develop in adults taking doses exceeding 200 mg/day for a month.

DRUG INTERACTIONS

Oral contraceptives may induce pyridoxine deficiency. Concurrent use with levodopa will neutralize CNS effects. Pyridoxine may prevent chloramphenicol-induced optic neuritis. Some drugs interfere with vitamin activity enough to block action and produce symptoms of deficiency.

Nursing Implications and Patient Teaching

Pyridoxine should be kept in a tightly sealed, light-resistant container. Good food sources of vitamin B_6 include yeast, wheat, corn, egg yolk, liver, kidney, and muscle meats; limited amounts are available from milk and vegetables. It is also found in liver, whole-grain breads and cereals, and soybeans.

Appropriate food preparation is important in preserving this vitamin. Freezing of vegetables results in a 20% loss of pyridoxine, and the milling of wheat results in a 90% loss.

FOLIC ACID

ACTION AND USES

Folic acid (also known as vitamin B_9) is required for normal erythropoiesis, or red blood cell formation, and nucleoprotein synthesis. It is metabolized in the liver, where it is changed to its more active form. Folic acid is used to treat anemias caused by folic acid deficiency; it is also used in alcoholism, hepatic disease, hemolytic anemia, infancy (especially for infants receiving artificial formulas), lactation, oral contraceptive use, and pregnancy. Folic acid supplements may be needed in low-birth-weight infants, infants nursed by mothers deficient in folic acid, or infants with infections or prolonged diarrhea. Recent guidelines have emphasized the importance of increased folic acid intake by women intending to get pregnant and in early pregnancy to help prevent spinal cord malformations in the fetus. The folic acid additives in commercial bread and grain products have been increased in an attempt to provide more adequate supplies of this important vitamin.

Research has suggested that homocysteine concentrations increase with age and with low levels of folate and vitamins B_6 and B_{12}. High homocysteine levels may be involved in the development of occlusive vascular disease, which may increase the risk of myocardial infarction. Therefore, the level of folate in persons under 65 years of age should be measured.

ADVERSE REACTIONS

Folic acid is not toxic. An allergic reaction may produce bronchospasm, erythema (redness or irritation), malaise, pruritus, and rash; large amounts may discolor the urine.

DRUG INTERACTIONS

Chloramphenicol and methotrexate are folate antagonists, and they may cause decreased folic acid activity. *Para*-aminosalicylic acid and sulfasalazine may cause symptoms of folic acid deficiency. Use with many anticonvulsants may decrease the anticonvulsant effect, leading to increased seizure activity. Use of oral contraceptives may lead to folic acid deficiency.

Nursing Implications and Patient Teaching

The RDAs of folic acid are as follows:
Adult men: 0.15 to 0.2 mg/day
Adult women: 0.15 to 0.18 mg/day
Pregnant and lactating women: 0.4 mg/day
These RDAs are usually provided by an adequate diet.

Folic acid for parenteral use must be protected from light.

Proper nutrition is essential, and dietary measures are preferable to drug therapy. The patient should be counseled to eat foods high in folic acid to prevent a deficiency problem in the future.

Blood for hematologic laboratory tests should be drawn before beginning therapy. Drug therapy should improve the blood test results within 2 to 5 days.

You should talk to the patient about the importance of remaining under medical supervision while receiving therapy. The patient may need to have the dose increased or decreased. Patients often fail to return for follow-up visits when they begin to feel better.

Diet is important in restoring proper folic acid levels and in preventing deficiencies in the future. The patient should eat foods high in folate, including fresh, leafy green vegetables; other vegetables and fruits; yeast; and organ meats.

VITAMIN B_{12}

ACTION AND USES

Vitamin B_{12} is water soluble and contains cobalt. It is produced by the bacterium *Streptomyces griseus*. It functions in many metabolic processes in protein, fat, and carbohydrate metabolism. The coenzymes of B_{12} are also part of the erythrocyte-maturing factor of the liver and are required in the synthesis of deoxyribonucleic acid (DNA). Vitamin B_{12} has a hemopoietic activity identical to the antianemia factor of the liver, and it is essential for growth, cell reproduction, and nucleoprotein and myelin synthesis. Intrinsic factor must be present in the stomach and small intestine to absorb B_{12}. Vitamin B_{12} interacts with folate in metabolic functions, and a deficiency in B_{12} makes folate useless in the body.

Vitamin B_{12} is used to treat all B_{12} deficiency conditions, including pernicious anemia (with or without neurologic symptoms), certain other anemias, malabsorption syndromes, hemorrhage, blind loop syndrome, pregnancy, chronic liver disease complicated by deficiency of vitamin B_{12}, malignancy, thyrotoxicosis, and renal disorders. Vitamin B_{12} is also used as the flushing dose in Schilling's test. Symptoms of deficiency are rare, occurring mainly in people on strict vegetarian diets, because vitamin B_{12} is found only in animal products. Symptoms include dyspepsia, sore tongue, breathlessness, and a characteristic stiff back, often dubbed a "poker" or "vegan" back.

Nascobal is a vitamin B_{12} nasal spray that is used as a maintenance drug for persons in remission after undergoing IM therapy for pernicious anemia. The dose is usually 500 mcg intranasally once weekly. If the patient develops adverse effects such as infection, headache, glossitis, nausea, and rhinitis after taking the nasal spray, it is often necessary to start IM vitamin B_{12} again.

ADVERSE REACTIONS

Allergy to vitamin B_{12} is rare. The patient may report pruritus, feeling of swelling of the entire body, or a severe anaphylactic reaction. A few patients may experience mild pain, localized skin irritation, or mild transient diarrhea after an injection of cyanocobalamin.

DRUG INTERACTIONS

Alcohol, colchicine, and *para*-aminosalicylic acid lower the absorption of vitamin B_{12}. Some antibiotics lower the response to vitamin B_{12} therapy.

Nursing Implications and Patient Teaching

Irreparable neurologic damage may occur if a deficiency state continues longer than 3 months or when treatment for pernicious anemia includes only folic acid. If colchicine, *para*-aminosalicylic acid, or excessive alcohol intake occurs for more than 2 weeks, malabsorption of vitamin B_{12} may occur.

The recommended daily intake of cyanocobalamin for adults is 3 mcg. The best food sources of B_{12} include organ meats; bivalves such as clams and oysters; nonfat dry milk; seafood such as lobster, scallops, flounder, haddock, swordfish, and tuna; and fermented cheese such as Camembert and Limburger.

VITAMIN C

ACTION AND USES

Vitamin C, or **ascorbic acid,** has multiple functions, some of which are understood more than others. Vitamin C functions in a number of enzyme systems and is involved in intracellular oxidation-reduction potentials. It aids in the change of folic acid and the metabolism of certain amino acids, assists the absorption of iron and calcium, and blocks the absorption of copper in the GI tract. Ascorbic acid protects vitamins A and E and polyunsaturated fatty acids. It is also necessary for the formation of the ground substance of bones, teeth, connective tissue, and capillaries and for the synthesis of collagen. Ascorbic acid aids in wound healing and may be involved in blood clotting.

Ascorbic acid is used to treat debilitated (weak) patients, especially after surgery in elderly patients with fractures, and as a supplement for burn victims or patients undergoing severe stress. Infection, smoking, chronic illness, and febrile states may increase the need for vitamin C. It is used along with iron therapy and in patients on prolonged IV therapy. Premature infants require relatively large doses. It is also used for the prophylaxis and treatment of scurvy, the deficiency state.

With modern refrigeration and processing methods of citrus fruits, scurvy is rarely seen in the United States, but it may be found when other vitamin deficiencies are present. Symptoms include tender, painful muscles, joints, and bones; muscle cramps; anorexia; fatigue; malaise; and sore gums. Wound healing is impaired, and hemorrhagic manifestations are demonstrated by subperiosteal bleeding and petechial hemorrhages. Vasomotor instability, bruising, faulty bone and tooth development, loosened teeth, and gingivitis also may develop.

ADVERSE REACTIONS

The patient may experience mild, brief soreness at injection sites if the medication is given IM or subcutaneously. Patients may also experience brief episodes of faintness or dizziness when IV injections are given too rapidly. Excessive doses are usually rapidly excreted into the urine. Doses in excess of 1 to 3 gm daily may result in GI complaints, glycosuria, oxaluria, and development of renal stones, especially in patients prone to these problems. Patients who chronically overuse vitamins may develop dependency.

DRUG INTERACTIONS

Ascorbic acid may have varying effects on anticoagulants, blocking the action of some and prolonging the intensity and duration of others. Ascorbic acid increases the effect of salicylates through increased renal tubular reabsorption. There is also an increased chance of crystallization of sulfonamides in the urine when ascorbic acid is given at the same time. Ascorbic acid decreases the effect of tricyclic antidepressants by decreasing renal tubular reabsorption. Calcium ascorbate may cause cardiac dysrhythmias (irregular heartbeats) in patients receiving digitalis. Ascorbic acid is chemically incompatible with potassium penicillin G and should not be mixed in the same syringe. Smoking may lead to an increased need for vitamin C by decreasing ascorbic acid serum levels. Intermittent use of ascorbic acid in patients taking ethinyl estradiol may increase the risk of contraceptive failure. Large doses of vitamin C may interfere with urine testing in some diabetic testing methods.

Nursing Implications and Patient Teaching

Vitamin C comes in three major forms that may be given orally or parenterally: ascorbic acid, sodium ascorbate, and calcium ascorbate. The recommended daily intake is 60 mg for adults.

Vitamin C is easily destroyed by air, heat, and light. This medication should be kept tightly capped in its own container. Foods high in vitamin C should not be boiled for long periods of time or left uncovered in the refrigerator.

Good food sources of vitamin C include green, leafy vegetables; oranges; grapefruit; strawberries; cauliflower; cantaloupe; beef liver; asparagus; and potatoes.

VITAMIN D

ACTION AND USES

"Vitamin D" is a label used for a group of fat-soluble, chemically similar sterols. The three main categories within this group are:

1. Ergocalciferol (vitamin D_2), which is very limited in nature in both distribution and concentration but can be artificially manufactured by ultraviolet irradiation on ergot and yeasts.
2. Cholecalciferol (vitamin D_3), which occurs naturally in fish liver oils and can be formed in animals and humans by ultraviolet irradiation on the skin.
3. Other lesser compounds (vitamins D_4, D_5, D_6, and D_7), which are formed by irradiation of sterols.

Therefore, the term *vitamin D* has become rather ambiguous.

The main action of this group of sterols is the movement of calcium and phosphorus ions into three main sites: the small intestine (to promote absorption of calcium and phosphorus from the gut); the kidneys (to cause phosphate reabsorption in the proximal convoluted tubules and, to a lesser extent, to stimulate calcium and sodium reabsorption); and bone (to help increase the mineralization of newly formed bone). Vitamin D_3 has been shown to inhibit the spread of fibroblasts and keratinocytes in the skin and to promote epidermal keratinocyte differentiation. It is used in the treatment of some skin disorders.

Vitamin D preparations are used to treat childhood rickets and adult osteomalacia, hypoparathyroidism, and familial hypophosphatemia. In childhood, rickets may be diagnosed by complaints of excessive sweating and GI disturbances. These may be the first symptoms, appearing before any objective findings. In adult cases of osteomalacia, patients may complain of skeletal pain and progressive muscular weakness.

ADVERSE REACTIONS

Symptoms of vitamin D toxicity include anorexia, nausea, malaise, weight loss, vague aches and stiffness, constipation, diarrhea, convulsions, anemia, mild acidosis, and impairment of renal function. The renal effects are usually reversible. A variety of more serious systemic effects may all be seen in adults. Dwarfism may be present in infants and children. Most toxic effects persist for several months in adults at doses of 100,000 IU or more daily or in children at doses of 20,000 IU or more daily. Reactions gradually disappear if treatment is discontinued at the first sign of symptoms.

DRUG INTERACTIONS

Mineral oil and some of the antihyperlipidemic agents may interfere with the absorption of fat-soluble vitamins. Thiazide diuretics and vitamin D together contribute to hypercalcemia. There is a possible connection between Dilantin and phenobarbital use leading to hypocalcemia, which, in turn, may contribute to rickets or osteomalacia.

Nursing Implications and Patient Teaching

The dosage of vitamin D must be planned for each patient and given under close supervision, because the range between the therapeutic and the toxic levels is narrow. Calcium intake should be enough to give a serum calcium level between 9 and 10 mg/dL. In rickets, 12,000 to 500,000 IU/day can be taken. In hypoparathyroidism, initially give 50,000 to 200,000 IU/day, with a maintenance dosage of 50,000 to 400,000 IU/day. Most people obtain all the vitamin D they need from the food in their diet. Natural sources of vitamin D are few, and the majority of vitamin D must be obtained from fortified sources. Fortified foods high in this vitamin are milk, evaporated milk, infant formula, powdered skim milk, and human milk. Cereals, margarine, and diet foods also contain vitamin D supplements. Vitamin D should be protected from light in a light-resistant container.

VITAMIN E

ACTION AND USES

Vitamin E is fat soluble and consists of naturally occurring tocopherols. Vitamin E is considered an essential nutrient for humans even though its specific functions are not yet understood. Vitamin E may function as an antioxidant, to prevent damage to cell membranes. It stabilizes red blood cell walls and protects them from hemolysis or destruction. It may also increase vitamin A use and stop platelet aggregation.

Many suggested uses of vitamin E are controversial and unproved. The only established use is to prevent or treat vitamin E deficiency. Vitamin E has been touted as a powerful antioxidant. New evidence suggests that vitamin E supplements do not reduce the risk of cancer or major cardiovascular disease and may even increase the risk of heart failure. High intake of vitamin E from food as tocopherol may be inversely related to Alzheimer's disease. Vitamin E in supplements is usually present as alpha-tocopherol and is less helpful in decreasing risk.

ADVERSE REACTIONS AND DRUG INTERACTIONS

Vitamin E appears to be the least toxic of the fat-soluble vitamins. No signs and symptoms of toxicity or hypervitaminosis have been identified as yet in humans. However, results of a 2004 metaanalysis of research studies suggests that doses over 150 IU/day increase the risk of all-cause mortality. The higher the dose taken, the higher the mortality rate. The most common marketed dose in the United States is 400 IU. Many individuals take up to 2000 IU/day.

Nursing Implications and Patient Teaching

Food sources of vitamin E are primarily from plants. The highest amounts are found in vegetable oils such as soybean and corn; nuts; green, leafy vegetables; wheat germ; and rice germ. Meat and dairy products provide less. An accurate assessment of tocopherol levels in food is difficult to obtain. The amount in the body depends on the initial concentration of vitamin E and the processing, storage, and preparation of the food. Vitamin E products should be stored in tightly closed, light-resistant containers.

VITAMIN K

ACTION AND USES

Vitamin K helps hepatic formation of active prothrombin (factor II), proconvertin (factor VII), plasma thromboplastin component (factor IX), and the Stuart factor (factor X), which are essential for normal blood clotting.

The exact mechanism is unknown. Menadione (K_3) and phytonadione (K_1) are synthetic lipid-soluble forms of vitamin K. Menadiol sodium diphosphate (K_4) is changed in the body to menadione. Menadione is not commonly available now.

Vitamin K is used to treat or prevent various blood clotting disorders that result in damaged formation of factors II, VII, IX, and X. The American Academy of Pediatrics recommends routine phytonadione (K_1) injection at birth to prevent hemorrhagic disease of the newborn. Vitamin K does not counteract the anticoagulant activity of heparin, although it is helpful in reversing the effects of warfarin (Coumadin) overdosage.

ADVERSE REACTIONS

Specific adverse reactions to menadione (K_3)/menadiol sodium diphosphate (K_4) include headache, rash, urticaria, gastric upset, redness, and pain or swelling at injection site. Specific adverse reactions to phytonadione (K_1) include brief hypotension (low blood pressure), rapid and weak pulse, dizziness, flushing, sweating, unusual taste sensations, redness, and pain or

Table 24-1

Vitamins

GENERIC NAME	TRADE NAME	COMMENTS AND DOSAGE
vitamin A	Aquasol A Palmitate	Give 50,000-100,000 IU/day for 3 days to 2 wk; follow by 10,000-20,000 IU/day for 2 mo.
vitamin B₁ (thiamine)	Thiamilate	Medications may be given PO, IM, or IV. Daily average dose is 0.5 mg/1000 kcal intake, or usually 1-1.4 mg/day PO. Usual dosage is 50 mg IM for deficiency states, and 5-10 mg PO daily as dietary supplement for adults and children over 12 yr of age.
vitamin B₂ (riboflavin)	Riboflavin	Give 0.4-0.6 mg for infants; 0.8-1.2 mg for children; 1.4-1.6 mg for males and 1.1-1.3 mg for females. For deficiency states, usually give 50 mg IM and 5-10 mg daily as dietary supplements for adults and children older than 12 yr of age.
niacin (vitamin B₃) nicotinic acid	Niacor Novonacin 🍁	May be given IM, subcutaneously, or IV; the IV route with slow drip is preferred when parenteral medication is necessary. • *Deficiency states:* 50-100 mg daily. • *Pellagra:* Up to 500 mg/day. • *Hyperlipidemia:* 1-2 gm 3 times daily; maximum dosage is 6 gm/day.
niacinamide	Nicotinamide	500 mg PO daily, or may give 100-200 mg 1 to 5 times daily parenterally, depending on the severity of the symptoms.
calcium pantothenate (vitamin B₅)	Calcium Pantothenate	A daily intake of 5-10 mg is thought to be adequate, with the lower level suggested for children and the upper level suggested for pregnant and breastfeeding women. A dosage of 2 mg/day has been suggested for infants and 4-7 mg/day for adolescents. Usual dosage is 10 mg/day.
vitamin B₆ (pyridoxine)	Hexa-Betalin 🍁 Nestrex Aminovin	Recommended daily allowances range from 2 to 2.2 mg. Preparation may be given PO, IM, or IV. • *Dietary deficiency:* 10-20 mg/day for 3 wk, then 2-5 mg/day for several weeks. • *Vitamin B₆ dependency states:* May give up to 600 mg/day initially, dropping to 50 mg/day for life.
		folic acid and derivatives (vitamin B₉)
folic acid and derivatives (vitamin B₉) folic acid	Folvite	• *Dietary supplement:* 100 mcg (0.1 mg)/day (up to 1 mg/day in pregnancy); may be increased to 500 mcg (0.5 mg) to 1 mg daily or more if underlying condition causes increased requirements (for example, in tropical sprue, 3-15 mg daily may be needed). • *Treatment of deficiency:* Initially give 250 mcg (0.25 mg) to 1 mg daily PO, IM, IV, or deep subcutaneous until hematologic response occurs; for maintenance, give 400 mcg (0.4 mg) to 1 mg daily. • *Pregnant and lactating women:* 800 mcg (0.8 mg) daily.
leucovorin calcium (folinic acid)	Wellcovorin	Megaloblastic anemia: Give approximately 1 mg daily IM or PO; greater doses do not lead to increased efficacy.

swelling at injection site. Severe reactions, including fatalities, have occurred with the use of IV phytonadione, even when caution is used (dilution of drug, slow infusion).

DRUG INTERACTIONS

Concurrent use of vitamin K with oral anticoagulants may decrease the effects of the anticoagulant. Mineral oil and cholestyramine inhibit GI absorption of oral vitamin K.

Nursing Implications and Patient Teaching

The preferred routes of administration of vitamin K are subcutaneous or IM. IV administration is not recommended because of the risk of anaphylaxis. Naturally occurring vitamin K is found in liver and green, leafy vegetables.

A summary of selected vitamin preparations on the market is presented in Table 24-1.

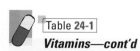

| Table 24-1 |
| *Vitamins—cont'd* |

GENERIC NAME	TRADE NAME	COMMENTS AND DOSAGE

vitamin B$_{12}$ (cyanocobalamin)	Crystamine Rubesol-1000	• *Nutritional deficiency:* Give 100-250 mcg/day PO.
		• *Vitamin B$_{12}$ deficiency:*
		  PO: 1000 mcg/day
		  IM, subcutaneously: If patients have normal gastrointestinal absorption, give 15 mcg/day along with other multiple vitamins. In other cases, give 30 mcg daily for 5-10 days, and then 100-200 mcg monthly for life.
		• *Schilling test:* 1000 mcg IM as a flushing dose.

	Big Shot B-12	2 mcg/day RDA for adults. Give 100-5000 mcg/day PO in deficiency states. Not used for pernicious anemia.
	Nascobal	Intranasal spray with 500 mcg once weekly.

vitamin C
  ascorbic acid
  calcium
  ascorbate
	Cevi-Bid
	Cecon
	Apo-C 🍁
		• *Prophylactically:* 50-100 mg as indicated.
		• *Therapeutically:* 100 mg or more as needed.
		• *Parenterally:* 100-250 mg given slowly once or twice daily up to a maximum of 1-2 gm daily.

vitamin D
  calcifediol
  calcitriol
	Calcifedrol 🍁
	Calderol
	Calcijex 🍁
	D-Tabs 🍁
	Rocaltrol
		Usually can give 20-50 mcg/day or 100-200 mcg every other day.
		Give 300-350 mcg/wk administered daily or every other day.
		Initially give 0.25 mcg/day. May increase by 0.25 mcg/day at 2- to 4-wk intervals until satisfactory response is obtained. Some patients may respond to doses of 0.25 mcg every other day. Patients undergoing hemodialysis may require doses of 0.5-1 mcg/day.

cholecalciferol (D$_3$)	DHT Hytakerol	*Initial:* 0.75-2.5 mg daily for several days. *Maintenance:* 0.2-1 mg daily, titrated by serum calcium levels. Average dose is 0.6 mg.
ergocalciferol (D$_2$)	Calciferol drops	• *Vitamin D–resistant rickets:* 50,000-500,000 IU daily. • *Hypoparathyroidism:* 50,000-400,000 IU of vitamin D daily plus 4 gm of calcium lactate, administered 6 times daily.
vitamin E	DryE 400 Aquavit-E	A range of 10-20 IU of vitamin E should provide adequate levels for an adult diet. Do not give more than 150-400 IU/day.
vitamin K phytonadione	AquaMEPHYTON Mephyton	• *Anticoagulant-induced prothrombin deficiency:* 2.5-10 mg or up to 25 mg initially. Frequency and dosage of subsequent therapy are determined by prothrombin time response. See package insert for other uses.
para-aminobenzoic acid	Potaba	Accessory food factor. *Adults:* 12 gm daily in divided doses.

IU, International units.

SECTION TWO
Minerals

OVERVIEW

There are 19 inorganic substances called **minerals** present in the body, at least 13 of which are essential to normal metabolism and function. These minerals are present as ions with positive and negative charges, leading to the formation of salts. They act as catalysts to speed up various biochemical reactions. Minerals are obtained from a diet varied in animal and vegetable products that meets the energy and protein needs of the body. The Food and Nutrition Board of the National Research Council has established recommended daily intakes for calcium and iron. Calcium, iron, and iodine are the three elements most frequently missing in the diet. Zinc, iron, copper, magnesium, and potassium are the five minerals most frequently involved in disturbances of metabolism. As electrolytes, these preparations are commonly infused to critically ill patients unable to take food orally.

CALCIUM

ACTION AND USES

Calcium is a major mineral in the body and is essential for muscular and neurologic activity, especially in the cardiac system. Calcium functions in the formation and repair of skeletal tissues (bones and teeth); activates several enzymes that influence cell membrane permeability and muscle contraction; aids in blood clotting by stimulating the release of thromboplastin and the conversion of fibrinogen to fibrin; activates pancreatic lipase; influences the intestinal absorption of cobalamin; and, in extracellular fluids, is involved in the transmission of neurotransmitters and in metabolic processes. Calcium is also involved in the regulation of lymphocyte and phagocyte function through interaction with calmodulin.

Calcium is used as a supplement when dietary levels of calcium are not adequate. Calcium requirements may be increased during pregnancy, breastfeeding, and adolescence and for postmenopausal women. Calcium is also used to treat neonatal hypocalcemia and to prevent and treat postmenopausal and senile osteoporosis. It may also be used as a supplement to parenterally administered vitamin D in cases of hypoparathyroidism, pseudohypoparathyroidism, rickets, and osteomalacia.

ADVERSE REACTIONS

You should watch for symptoms of hypercalcemia, such as polyuria (excretion of a large amount of urine), constipation, abdominal pain, dryness of mouth, anorexia, nausea, and vomiting.

DRUG INTERACTIONS

Vitamin D is essential for the absorption of calcium in the body. Calcium status is affected by the calcium-to-phosphorus ratio in the body and by the level of protein in the diet. Phytic acid (found in bran and whole-grain cereals) and oxalic acid (found in spinach and rhubarb) may interfere with calcium absorption by combining with calcium to form insoluble salts in the intestine. Calcium compounds and calcium-rich substances such as milk interfere with the absorption of oral tetracycline, and use together should be avoided. Use of corticosteroids may also decrease the absorption of calcium.

Nursing Implications and Patient Teaching

In patients with low calcium levels, carpal spasm may be elicited by compressing the upper arm with a blood pressure cuff, causing ischemia (decreased blood supply) to the distal nerves. The patient may report a tingling sensation and may inadvertently flex her arm. Excessive amounts of calcium may lead to hypercalcemia and hypercalciuria, especially in hyperthyroid patients. Serum and renal calcium levels should be followed to detect the development of renal stones; calcium should not be given to patients who already have renal stones.

Calcium products come in combination with various other chemicals, with a concentration of between 6% and 40%. Preparations come in both parenteral and oral forms. The antacid Tums is composed of calcium carbonate, the most elemental form of calcium. It is better absorbed than many calcium products and is a smaller tablet than many other calcium products, making administration easier.

The recommended daily intake of calcium is 800 mg/day for adults, 1200 mg/day for adolescents, 800 mg/day for children, 360 to 540 mg/day for infants from birth to 1 year, and 1500 mg/day for nursing mothers. Milk and dairy products are the richest sources of calcium. Egg yolks and most dark green, leafy vegetables are also good sources.

FLUORIDE

ACTION AND USES

Fluoride is concentrated in bones and teeth and is present in soft tissues only in very small amounts. It is an essential trace element but has not been proven to be essential to life. Fluoride is taken into the surface enamel of teeth in higher concentrations than in deeper layers.

This strengthening of the enamel provides greater resistance to damage by acids produced in dental plaque. Fluoride has therefore been found useful in reducing dental caries.

Fluoride is recommended for the prevention of dental caries in all age groups. It may be used topically or systemically. It is primarily administered in places without fluoride in the water supply or to individuals with a genetic tendency for dental caries.

ADVERSE REACTIONS

Gastric distress, headache, urticaria, and malaise may be seen in hypersensitive individuals. Excessive salivation, mottling of teeth, GI disturbances, and nausea are seen in acute overdosage.

DRUG INTERACTIONS

Fluoride in the water supply may produce calcium fluoride, a poorly absorbed product, when taken with dairy foods.

Nursing Implications and Patient Teaching

Fluoride is available in gels, pastes, drops, tablets, capsules, and mouth rinses. The preparation and quantity chosen should be adjusted to the fluoride level of the local water supply. The county water commissioner may be contacted for this information. Fluoride products should be taken as ordered. Tablets and drops may be dissolved in water used for making infant formula or added to food or juices. Tablets may also be swallowed, chewed, or allowed to dissolve slowly in the mouth. Products are best taken after meals. For rinses and gels, teeth should be brushed thoroughly, and then the coating should be applied to clean teeth. The fluoride coating should not be swallowed. The patient should not rinse the mouth, eat, or drink for 30 minutes after treatment. Plastic containers should be used for diluting fluoride drops or rinses, and glass should be avoided. Milk may decrease absorption of oral fluoride products, so the patient should avoid taking fluoride with milk or dairy products.

IRON

ACTION AND USES

Iron is an essential mineral for the synthesis of myoglobin and hemoglobin. It stimulates the hematopoietic system and increases hemoglobin to correct iron deficiency.

Iron is used to treat symptomatic iron deficiency anemia only after the cause of the anemia has been identified, and it is used to prevent hypochromic anemia during infancy, childhood, pregnancy, and breastfeeding; in patients recovering from other anemias; and after some GI surgeries.

ADVERSE REACTIONS

Adverse reactions to iron supplements include constipation, cramping, diarrhea, epigastric or abdominal pain, GI irritation, and allergic reactions to any component of the iron preparation. Symptoms of overdosage may occur after 30 minutes to several hours and include lethargy (sleepiness), nausea, vomiting, abdominal pain, diarrhea, melena, and dyspnea (uncomfortable breathing). Coma and metabolic acidosis may occur, as well as symptoms of systemic absorption.

DRUG INTERACTIONS

Large iron doses may cause a false-positive test result for occult blood using the toluidine test (Hematest, Occultist, Clinistix). Absorption of oral iron is inhibited by antacids (particularly magnesium trisilicate–containing antacids), milk, and eggs. Patients receiving chloramphenicol concurrently with iron may show a delayed response to iron therapy. Absorption of iron increases when given with ascorbic acid in doses of 200 mg per 30 mg of iron. Iron interferes with absorption of oral tetracycline. Vitamin E decreases the response to iron therapy. Many other medications may have interactions.

Nursing Implications and Patient Teaching

The cause of the anemia must be identified and treated. You should help get stools for occult blood tests after the patient has been on a red meat–free diet for at least 3 days. Although dietary lack may contribute to iron deficiency, especially in those older than 75 years of age, blood loss is the primary cause. Heavy menstrual periods and multiple pregnancies in women may produce anemia. Hematologic laboratory values are often normally lower in the elderly, leading to overprescribing of iron for geriatric patients. Liquid preparations can discolor teeth and should be taken through a straw after dilution with liquid.

Replacement of iron in iron deficiency anemia requires 90 to 300 mg of elemental iron daily in divided doses (6 mg/kg/day). Symptoms should go away within 2 weeks and laboratory studies should be normal within 2 months if diagnosis and treatment are adequate. Therapy for 4 to 6 months after the anemia has been corrected is advised to replenish iron stores. More iron is absorbed if the iron is taken on an empty stomach with water or in an acid environment, although taking it after meals can reduce stomach irritation. Taking iron after a meal can reduce the absorption by 40% to 50%. Different oral preparations vary in cost and percentage of elemental iron. Product selection must be based on how well it is absorbed, how well it is tolerated, and the individual needs of the patient. All simple oral iron preparations are available over the counter. The absorption of iron taken orally or through dietary foods is generally about 10%. The body does have the capability to increase iron absorption during times of physiologic stress, such as pregnancy and severe blood loss.

The recommended daily intake of elemental iron in adult males is 10 mg; in adult women, 18 mg (with an additional 10 mg during pregnancy or lactation); and in children, 10 to 15 mg. A diet high in natural iron should be encouraged to meet these needs. Fish, meat, and dried fruits are the best sources of dietary iron.

Iron can cause dark green or black stools. The patient should report constipation, diarrhea, nausea, or abdominal pain to the health care provider.

MAGNESIUM

ACTION AND USES

Magnesium is an electrolyte that is essential to several enzyme systems. It is important in maintaining osmotic pressure, ion balance, bone structure, muscular contraction, and nerve conduction. This mineral has been determined to be especially important in cardiac function, and only slight deficiencies may prolong the Q-T interval and lead to a very dangerous form of ventricular tachycardia (rapid heartbeat) called *torsades de pointes.*

ADVERSE REACTIONS

Excessive magnesium intake may produce diarrhea.

Nursing Implications and Patient Teaching

Magnesium deficiencies are seen primarily when malabsorption syndromes are present. Magnesium is usually used with other vitamins as a general dietary supplement when multiple deficiencies are suspected. Deficiency states have been associated with convulsions, slowing of growth, digestive disturbances, spasticity of muscles and nerves, accelerated heartbeat, dysrhythmias, nervous conditions, and vasodilation opening of blood vessels). Magnesium is available in adequate quantities in meat, milk, fruits, and vegetables, and special dietary planning is unnecessary.

MANGANESE

ACTION AND USES

Manganese activates many enzymes, assists in normal skeletal and connective tissue development, helps in the initiation of protein synthesis, and plays a part in the synthesis of cholesterol and fatty acids. It is found throughout all body tissues and fluids. No precise RDA has been established.

Manganese is used in dietary supplements. Usually it used with other vitamins when multiple deficiencies

are suspected. Research subjects with manganese deficiency experienced weight loss, changes in beard and hair growth (usually slowing of growth), and occasional nausea and vomiting. There are no known adverse effects or drug interactions.

Nuts, whole-wheat cereals, and grains are the foods richest in manganese. Tea and cloves are exceptionally rich. Meat, fish, and dairy products have low amounts of manganese.

POTASSIUM

ACTION AND USES

Potassium is the principal intracellular cation of most body tissues, acting in the maintenance of normal renal function, contraction of muscle, and transmission of nerve impulses. It is found in the body within a very narrow range.

Potassium may be taken prophylactically (for prevention) when the patient has nephrotic syndrome, in hepatic cirrhosis with ascites, and in patients with hyperaldosteronism who have normal renal function. Potassium products are used prophylactically or to replace potassium that may be lost as a result of long-term diuretic therapy, digitalis intoxication, or low dietary intake of potassium; or for deficits resulting from vomiting and diarrhea, diabetic acidosis, metabolic alkalosis, or corticosteroid therapy; or to counteract increased renal excretion of potassium because of acidosis, certain renal tubular disorders, or diseases that produce increased secretion of glucocorticoids or aldosterone.

ADVERSE REACTIONS

Either excess or deficit of potassium causes symptoms. Adverse reactions to potassium supplements include nausea, vomiting, diarrhea, abdominal discomfort, and GI bleeding. Potassium intoxication or hyperkalemia (increased potassium in the blood) may result from overdosage of potassium or from a change in the patient's underlying condition, which may make potassium buildup possible. Signs and symptoms of potassium intoxication include flaccid paralysis, paresthesias (numbness and tingling) of the hands and feet, mental confusion, restlessness, listlessness, malaise, and heaviness of the legs. Hypotension and cardiac dysrhythmias leading to heart block may also develop. Potentially fatal dysrhythmias may develop if potassium cannot be excreted (or if it is administered too rapidly IV). When it is detected, hyperkalemia requires immediate treatment because lethal levels of potassium may be reached in a few hours in untreated patients. Potentially lethal dysrhythmias may also occur with hypokalemia (decreased potassium in the blood).

DRUG INTERACTIONS

Potassium should not be used in patients receiving potassium-sparing agents such as aldosterone antagonists or triamterene because overdosage may develop.

Nursing Implications and Patient Teaching

All potassium supplements must be diluted properly or taken with plenty of liquid to avoid producing GI ulcers. The usual adult dietary intake of potassium ranges between 40 and 60 mEq/day. The loss of 200 or more mEq of potassium from the total body store is enough to produce hypokalemia.

The dosage must be titrated (increased or decreased slowly) based on the individual's needs, and the patient should be closely watched during therapy, especially in the initial stages of therapy. For patients receiving diuretic therapy, 20 mEq/day is usually adequate for the prevention of hypokalemia. In cases of potassium depletion, 40 to 100 mEq/day or more may be required for replacement. Blood levels must be monitored closely.

Potassium comes in various salt combinations; potassium chloride is the form most frequently prescribed. It may be ordered either by percentage of potassium chloride or in milliequivalents of potassium chloride, with 10 mEq KCl per 15 mL equivalent to 5% KCl. Other salt combinations are potassium gluconate, potassium citrate, potassium acetate, and potassium bicarbonate. Potassium is also available in combination with vitamin C, ammonium chloride, citric acid, betaine HCl, and L-lysine monohydrochloride.

Many health care providers tell patients to eat a potassium-rich diet, as well as a potassium supplement. A potassium-rich diet includes food such as bananas, citrus fruits (especially tomatoes and oranges), apricots, and dried fruits such as raisins, prunes, and dates. Cantaloupe and watermelon (in season), nuts, dried beans, beef, and fowl also contain ample quantities of potassium.

ZINC

ACTION AND USES

Zinc is a part of many enzymes and is essential for normal growth and tissue repair. Zinc functions in the mineralization of bone and in the detoxification and oxidation of methanol and ethylene glycol. It plays a role in the creation of DNA and the synthesis of protein from amino acids. It is important in wound healing and functions in moving vitamin A from liver stores.

Zinc is used to prevent zinc deficiency and to treat delayed wound healing. It has been tested for use in rheumatoid arthritis and acne.

Patients taking zinc may complain of abnormalities of taste and smell, rough skin, and anorexia with profound disinterest in food. Patients who lack zinc may demonstrate sexual immaturity, delayed wound healing, and decreased absorption of dietary folate.

ADVERSE REACTIONS

Adverse reactions to zinc supplements include gastric ulceration, nausea, and vomiting. Doses in excess of 2 gm produce emesis (vomiting). Acute zinc intoxication produces drowsiness, lethargy, light-headedness, staggering gait, restlessness, and vomiting leading to dehydration.

DRUG INTERACTIONS

Calcium competes with zinc for absorption. Phytates form insoluble complexes with zinc and interfere with its absorption. Zinc impairs the absorption of tetracycline derivatives.

Nursing Implications and Patient Teaching

The minimum daily requirements of zinc include the following: infants to 1 year, 3 to 5 mg/day; children 1 to 10 years, 10 mg/day; adolescents 11 to 18 years, 15 mg/day; adults, 15 mg/day; pregnant women, 20 mg/day; and lactating women, 25 mg/day. Seafood and meats are rich sources of natural zinc; cereals and legumes also have significant amounts of this mineral.

Table 24-2 presents a summary of minerals.

VITAMIN AND MINERAL DEFICIENCIES

Nursing Implications and Patient Teaching

Assessment

You should try to learn as much as possible about the patient's health history, including the presence of hypersensitivity, pregnancy, breastfeeding, underlying systemic disease, hereditary disorders, and use of other medications that may cause drug interactions. The patient should be assessed for symptoms of multiple deficiency or disease states.

Diagnosis

In addition to the medical problems resulting in the need for vitamin or mineral products, does the patient have financial, cultural, or nutritional problems or attitudes that contribute to the problem? Does the patient have lack of knowledge about how to prepare, store, or use water- or fat-soluble vitamins? Does the patient do things that would interfere with getting the vitamins from the food he eats? Does the patient try to make up for poor diets by taking vitamins or nutritional supplements?

Planning

Many medications require baseline laboratory assessment before starting therapy so that progress may be monitored.

Table 24-2

Minerals

GENERIC NAME	TRADE NAME	COMMENTS AND DOSAGE
CALCIUM		
calcium acetate	Phos-Ex Calphron	Has 25% calcium. Give 1200-1800 mg qd.
calcium carbonate	Os-Cal 500 Caltrate	Has 40% concentration of calcium, the largest of any calcium product. Give 1-1.5 gm PO daily with meal.
calcium citrate	Citracal	Has 21% calcium. Give 1200-1800 mg qd.
calcium glubionate	Neo-Calglucon	Oral preparation contains 6% calcium. Administer before meals to increase absorption. *Adults (including pregnant and breastfeeding women) and children 4 yr or older:* 15 mL 3 times daily. *Children under 4 yr:* 5-10 mL 3 times daily.
calcium gluconate	Calcium Gluconate	Comes in both oral and parenteral forms. IV infusion is preferred over IM injection and is used frequently in emergency situations. Check equivalency of all oral products, because they vary from preparation to preparation. In parenteral forms, 10 mL contains 90 mg (4.5 mEq) calcium. *Orally:* Give 1-2 gm PO daily. *Parenterally:* 1-15 gm daily IV for adults; 500 mg/kg/day in divided doses for children.
calcium lactate	Calcium Lactate	Contains 13% calcium and is given orally. It is available without prescription. Give 325 mg to 1.3 gm PO 3 times daily with meals.
tricalcium phosphate	Posture	Has 39% calcium. Give 1200-1800 mg qd.
FLUORIDE		
fluoride (oral)	Fluoritab Flura	Adjust dosage according to local water fluoride level. • *General oral dosages:* 1 gm daily. *Children 3 yr old and younger:* 0.5 mg daily.
fluoride (topical)	Dermalar 🍁 Fluonicle 🍁 Fluorigard Fluorinase Prevident	Products used between professional dental fluoride treatments for patients who have excessive problems with tooth decay. After brushing, hold preparation in mouth for at least 1 min, then spit out. Do not swallow; do not eat, drink, smoke, or rinse mouth for at least 15-30 min after treatment to obtain maximum benefit. *Adults and children over 12 yr:* 10 mL daily. *Children 6-12 yr:* 5-10 mL daily.
IRON-CONTAINING PRODUCTS		
ferrous fumarate	Femiron Feostat	Few reported side effects with this product. It is better tolerated than sulfate or gluconate. Contains 33% elemental iron. *Adults:* 600-800 mg/day PO in divided doses. *Children under 5 yr:* 100-300 mg/day PO in 3 to 4 divided doses.
ferrous gluconate	Fergon	Less corrosive than ferrous sulfate. Indicated for those patients who cannot tolerate sulfate because of gastric irritation. It contains 11.6% elemental iron. *Adults:* 320-640 mg PO 3 times daily. *Children 6-12 yr:* 100-300 mg PO 3 times daily. *Children under 6 yr:* 120-300 mg PO daily.
ferrous sulfate	Feosol Fer-in-sol Fer-Iron	Ferrous sulfate is the standard preparation against which all other iron salts are compared. Optimal compound because it is the least expensive and contains 20% elemental iron. Timed-release capsules are more expensive and less well absorbed but reportedly have fewer side effects. *Adults:* 300-1200 mg PO daily in divided doses. *Children:* 600 mg PO daily in divided doses.

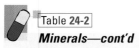

Table 24-2
Minerals—cont'd

GENERIC NAME	TRADE NAME	COMMENTS AND DOSAGE
IRON-CONTAINING PRODUCTS—cont'd		
ferrous sulfate exsiccated	Feosol Feratab Slow FE	This product contains more elemental iron per milligram of compound than other products. It is more expensive than plain ferrous sulfate. The liquid preparation of Feosol cannot be mixed with juice. *Iron deficiency states:* 30-90 mg elemental iron daily.
iron dextran	DexFerrum InFeD 🍁 Infufur 🍁	Used in cases in which oral iron administration is impossible or unsatisfactory. Parenteral iron has caused fatal anaphylactic-type reactions and must be used with care. *Test dose:* 0.5 mL IV or IM 1 hr before the therapeutic dose, to rule out hypersensitivity. Calculate the total dose required to return hemoglobin and iron stores to normal using the following formula: $$0.3 \times \text{Weight in lb} \times \left(\frac{100 - \text{hemoglobin gm/dl} \times 100}{14.8} \right) = \text{mg iron}$$ For patients weighing less than 30 lb, reduce to 80% total calculated. The Z-track method should be used for injection into the gluteus maximus muscle only. Inject deeply using a 2- or 3-inch needle of 19-20 gauge.
MAGNESIUM		
magnesium	Maglucate Magonate 🍁 Magtrate Slow Mag	RDA for adult men is 350 mg; adult women, 330 mg. As a dietary supplement, give 27-133 mg daily to 3 times daily.
MANGANESE		
manganese	Chelated Manganese	No RDA has been determined. Suggested daily intakes include 0.5-0.7 mg PO for infants, 2.5-5.0 mg PO for adolescents, and 3-7 mg PO for adults.
PHOSPHORUS		
phosphorus	Neutra-Phos Uro-KP-Neutral	*Adults:* 800-1200 mg. May have mild laxative effect.
POTASSIUM		
potassium chloride liquid powder tablets	Cena-K Kaon K-Lor K-Lyte Slow-K	Wide variation in concentration, price, flavor. Make certain medication is diluted with water or juice or is taken with adequate quantities of liquid. Titrate to individual requirements. Usual dosage is 20 mEq/day for prophylaxis and 40-100 mEq/day for treatment of potassium depletion.
Combinations of Potassium Gluconate, Potassium Citrate, Potassium Acetate, Potassium Bicarbonate		
effervescent tablets liquids powders	Effer-K K-Lyte Cena-K Kaon Kaylixir Klorvess Kolyum	These products, most of which require prescriptions, are used primarily in patients in whom chloride is restricted. Because some of these products do contain chloride, it is important to carefully choose the potassium salt desired. There is wide variability in the cost of these products, with most tending to be more expensive than potassium chloride products. Effervescent tablets must be dissolved completely in water before administration. Dosage should be titrated to individual needs. Usual dosage is 20 mEq/day for prophylaxis and 40-100 mEq/day for treatment of potassium depletion.
SODIUM CHLORIDE		
sodium chloride	Slo-Salt	Supplementation on rare occasions.
ZINC		
zinc	Orazinc	Give 10-20 mg/day.

You should make certain that the medication is stored properly, protected from light and heat to avoid destruction of the medication.

Implementation

You should make certain that the way you are giving the medicine is appropriate before you give it. Many products must be given very slowly or only by certain routes.

Evaluation

You should watch for the therapeutic effect or to see if the patient has adverse effects. You may need to help the patient get follow-up laboratory studies to measure improvement.

Patient and Family Teaching

You should tell the patient and family the following:

1. The patient should take the medication exactly as ordered. If a dose is missed, the patient should take it as soon as he or she remembers but should not take it if it is almost time for the next dose. The doses should not be doubled. The nurse, physician, or other health care provider should be informed if doses of vitamin K are missed.
2. The patient will need to make regular return visits to see the nurse, physician, or other health care provider while taking some vitamins. The patient should inform all physicians and dentists about vitamin and mineral products he or she is taking.
3. The patient must not take other medications, including OTC drugs, without first discussing them with the nurse, physician, or other health care provider.
4. Some forms of the drugs may cause unusual taste sensations, must be protected from light and heat, or have special storage instructions. The patient must be taught how to store and use the medications.

5. The patient should avoid overdosage of the medication. Taking too much of a vitamin is not helpful and may lead to toxicity or dependency on the vitamin, or to waste when the excess vitamin passes into the urine.
6. The patient should eat well-balanced meals. The nurse, physician, or other health care provider should teach the patient about foods that contain naturally occurring vitamins.
7. Vitamin and mineral preparations should be kept out of the reach of children and all others for whom they are not prescribed.
8. Vitamins and minerals sold as special products in health food stores may not demonstrate any nutritional superiority over less expensive products sold elsewhere.

Key Points

- Vitamins and minerals are essential for the body to function properly.
- They are often taken as supplements when dietary levels are inadequate.
- There is still much to be learned about the action of vitamins and minerals in the body.
- It is important to note that overconsumption can create as many problems as deficiency and should be avoided.

Go to the free CD-ROM for an Audio Glossary, animations, video clips, and Review Questions for the NCLEX-PN® Examination.

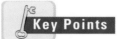 Be sure to visit the companion Evolve website at http://evolve.elsevier.com/Edmunds/LPN/ for WebLinks, a link to the top 200 drugs by prescription, and sign-up pages for newsletter drug updates.

 ## CASE STUDY

Mrs. Casper, 77, has been in a nursing home for several years. She suffers from a variety of chronic diseases. When she was recently admitted to the hospital for pneumonia, the physician discovered that she was mildly anemic. She was prescribed the following:

Ferrous sulfate: 300 mg 3 times daily PO
Vitamin C: 1000 mcg daily
Ciprofloxacin: 750 mg PO q12h
Why is the ferrous sulfate ordered?
Why is vitamin C given?

3. Why is ciprofloxacin given?
4. After several days of therapy, the patient does not seem to be getting any better. Can you determine any reason why this might be so?
5. The patient is switched to another antibiotic and eventually goes home to stay with her son and grandchildren. Her 4-year-old granddaughter opens her ferrous sulfate and swallows 8 tablets. What should be done? Why?

DRUG CALCULATION REVIEW

1. Order: Vitamin B_{12} 200 mcg IM every month

   Supply: Vitamin B_{12} 1000 mcg/mL

   Question: How many milliliters of vitamin B_{12} is needed with each dose?

2. Order: Iron dextran 100 mg IV over 6 hours

   Supply: Iron dextran 100 mg/250 mL 0.9% normal saline

   Question: How many milliliters per hour should the IV infusion device be set for? (Round to the nearest whole number.)

3. Order: Potassium chloride 60 mEq in 200 mL 0.9% normal saline

   Facility's Policy: Infuse potassium at a maximum rate of 10 mEq/hr

   Question: How many milliliters per hour should the IV infusion device be set for? (Round to the nearest whole number.)

CRITICAL THINKING ?

1. What are the two types of vitamins? How does each type react differently, overall, within the body?

2. What are two circumstances under which a patient may be unable to obtain sufficient amounts of vitamins, despite having a well-balanced, nutritious diet?

3. Explain the difference between vitamins and minerals.

4. Mr. Baker leads a very athletic life and is proud of his strict diet and voluminous intake of vitamins, which he says he "keeps on the kitchen counter so [he] won't forget them." He comes to your clinic feeling "a little under the weather." He is surprised and confused when he is told that he has developed hypervitaminosis. After listening to your explanation of hypervitaminosis, its causes, and its effects, Mr. Baker remains confused, insisting that "A vitamin is a vitamin, and more is better when it comes to vitamins . . . and minerals, too, as far as that goes." What would be an appropriate approach to use for educating Mr. Baker?

5. Create a nutrition chart to show Mr. Baker how he can get adequate amounts of vitamins and minerals by eating a well-balanced diet. Be prepared to counteract Mr. Baker's frequent protest: "A vitamin is a vitamin!"

6. What three minerals are most often missing from our diets? Why is that?

7. Ms. Mariani stops to talk to you after seeing her doctor for a physical exam. She is upset because the doctor told her she "has anemia, and now I have to get a needle once a week. Why can't I just eat more red meat or liver to build up my blood?" What should you tell her about her anemia?

CATEGORY	DESCRIPTION
A	Adequate, well-controlled studies in pregnant women have not shown an increased risk of fetal abnormalities.
B	Animal studies have revealed no evidence of harm to the fetus; however, there are no adequate and well-controlled studies in pregnant women. **OR** Animal studies have shown an adverse effect, but adequate and well-controlled studies in pregnant women have failed to demonstrate a risk to the fetus.
C	Animal studies have shown an adverse effect and there are no adequate and well-controlled studies in pregnant women. **OR** No animal studies have been conducted and there are no adequate and well-controlled studies in pregnant women.
D	Studies, adequate well-controlled or observational, in pregnant women have demonstrated a risk to the fetus. However, the benefits of therapy may outweigh the potential risk.
X	Studies, adequate well-controlled or observational, in animals or pregnant women have demonstrated positive evidence of fetal abnormalities. The use of the product is contraindicated in women who are or may become pregnant.

From Meadows M: Pregnancy and the drug dilemma, *FDA Consumer Magazine,* 2001. Available at www.fda.gov/fdac/features/2001/301_preg.html#categories, accessed June 2005.

B Nursing Mothers Risk Categories

Hale's Lactation Risk Categories

L1: SAFEST

This drug has been taken by a large number of breastfeeding mothers without any observed increase in adverse effects in the infant. Controlled studies in breastfeeding women fail to demonstrate a risk to the infant, *and* the possibility of harm to the breastfeeding infant is remote; *or* the product is not orally bioavailable in an infant.

L2: SAFER

This drug has been studied in a limited number of breastfeeding women without an increase in adverse effects in the infant; *and/or,* the evidence of a demonstrated risk that is likely to follow use of this medication in a breastfeeding woman is remote.

L3: MODERATELY SAFE

There are no controlled studies in breastfeeding women, but the risk of untoward effects to a breastfed infant is possible; *or,* controlled studies show only minimal nonthreatening adverse effects. Drugs should be given only if the potential benefit justifies the potential risk to the infant.

L4: POSSIBLY HAZARDOUS

There is positive evidence of risk to the breastfed infant or to breast milk production, but the benefits from use in breastfeeding mothers may be acceptable despite the risk to the infant (for example, if the drug is needed in a life-threatening situation or for a serious disease for which safer drugs cannot be used or are ineffective).

L5: CONTRAINDICATED

Studies in breastfeeding mothers have demonstrated that there is significant and documented risk to the infant based on human experience, or it is a medication that has a high risk of causing significant damage to an infant. The risk of using the drug in breastfeeding women clearly outweighs any possible benefit. The drug is contraindicated in women who are breastfeeding an infant.

Data from Hale, 2002, http://neonatal.ttuhsc.edu/lact/html/drug_entry.html; and Hale, 2002, http://neonatal.ama.ttuhsc.edu/lact/html/radio.html.

C Special Medication Precautions

Drugs Associated With Serious Adverse Effects

Hepatotoxic Drugs	Nephrotoxic Drugs	Other Toxicities
acetaminophen	acyclovir	*Anaphylaxis:* penicillins, heparin, aspirin, parenteral iron, dextran
4-aminoquinoline	aminoglycoside antibiotics	*Asthma:* aspirin, ibuprofen
amiodarone	amphotericin B	*Blood dyscrasias:* chloramphenicol, anticonvulsants, penicillins, hydralazine, sulfonamides, anticancer drugs
Anabolic steroid agents	analgesic combinations	
Antithyroid agents	capreomycin	
asparaginase	captopril	
azlocillin	cisplatin	
carbamazepine	cyclosporine	*Damage to eighth cranial nerve:* furosemide, aspirin and other salicylates, Vibramycin, gentamicin
carmustine	demeclocycline	
Contraceptives (estrogen)	edetate calcium disodium	
dantrolene	enalapril	*Eye damage:* topical corticosteroids, ethambutol, Thorazine, chloroquine
daunorubicin	gold compounds	
disulfiram	lithium	*Peripheral neuritis:* isoniazid, vincristine, hydralazine, ethambutol
divalproex	methotrexate	
erythromycin	methoxyflurane	
estrogen, conjugated	neomycin	
etretinate	NSAIDs	
gold compounds	penicillamine	
halothane	pentamidine	
isoniazid	plicamycin	
ketoconazole	rifampin	
mercaptopurine	streptozocin	
methotrexate	sulfonamides	
methyldopa	tetracycline	
mezlocillin	vancomycin	
naltrexone		
phenothiazine		
phenytoin		
piperacillin		
plicamycin		
rifampin		
sulfonamides		
tetracycline		
valproic acid		

ta from McKenry LM, Salerno E, *Mosby's pharmacology in nursing*, ed 21, St Louis, 2003, Mosby; Hardman JG, Limbird LW et al, editors. *Goodman and man's pharmacological basis of therapeutics*, ed 10, New York, 2001, McGraw-Hill; and Katzung BG: *Basic and clinical pharmacology*, ed 8, Norwalk, Conn, 2000, pleton & Lange.
AIDs, Nonsteroidal antiinflammatory drugs.

Answers to Drug Calculation Review Questions

CHAPTER 9: CALCULATING DRUG DOSAGES

1. $? \text{ days} = \dfrac{1 \text{ day}}{} \left| \dfrac{\overset{1}{\cancel{\text{tablespoon}}}}{3 \text{ teaspoons}} \right| \dfrac{\overset{1}{\cancel{\text{teaspoon}}}}{5 \text{ mL}} \left| 500 \text{ mL} \right. = \dfrac{500}{3(5)} = \dfrac{500}{15} = 33 \text{ days}$

2. $?\text{mL} = \dfrac{1 \text{ mL}}{100 \text{ units}} \left| 30 \text{ units} \right. = \dfrac{3}{10} = 0.3 \text{ mL}$

3. $?\text{mL} = \dfrac{1 \text{ mL}}{330 \text{ mg}} \left| 500 \text{ mg} \right. = \dfrac{50}{33} = 1.5 \text{ mL}$

4. $?\dfrac{\text{gtt}}{\text{min}} = \dfrac{10 \text{ gtt}}{1 \text{ mL}} \left| \dfrac{2500 \text{ mL}}{24 \text{ hr}} \right| \dfrac{1 \text{ hr}}{60 \text{ min}} = \dfrac{10(25)}{24(6)} = \dfrac{2500}{144} = 17 \text{ gtt/min}$

5. $?\dfrac{\text{mg}}{\text{kg/min}} = \dfrac{\overset{10}{\cancel{500} \text{ mg}}}{\underset{5}{\cancel{250} \text{ mL}}} \left| \dfrac{1 \text{ mL}}{60 \text{ megtt}} \right| \dfrac{\overset{3}{\cancel{150} \text{ megtt}}}{\underset{1}{\cancel{50} \text{ kg/min}}} = \dfrac{10(3)}{5(60)} = \dfrac{30}{300} = 0.1 \text{ mg/kg/min}$

6. $?\text{mL} = \dfrac{1 \text{ mL}}{5000 \text{ units}} \left| 7500 \text{ units} \right. = \dfrac{75}{50} = 1.5 \text{ mL}$

7. $?\text{mL} = \dfrac{1 \text{ mL}}{\text{gr } \frac{1}{150}} \left| \text{gr } \frac{1}{300} \right. = \dfrac{\frac{1}{300}}{\frac{1}{150}} = \dfrac{1}{300} \times \dfrac{150}{1} = \dfrac{150}{300} = 0.5 \text{ mL}$

8. $?\text{tablets} = \dfrac{1 \text{ tablet}}{0.1 \text{ g}} \left| \dfrac{1 \text{ g}}{\underset{20}{\cancel{1000} \text{ mg}}} \right| \overset{1}{\cancel{50} \text{ mg}} = \dfrac{1}{0.1(20)} = \dfrac{1}{2} \text{ tablet}$

9. $?\text{mL} = \dfrac{1 \text{ mL}}{\underset{1}{\cancel{0.05} \text{ mg}}} \left| \overset{5}{\cancel{0.25} \text{ mg}} \right. = \dfrac{5}{1} = 5 \text{ mL}$

10. $?\text{tablets} = \dfrac{1 \text{ tablet}}{400 \text{ mg}} \left| \dfrac{1000 \text{ mg}}{1 \text{ g}} \right| 1 \text{ g} = \dfrac{10}{4} = 2.5 \text{ tablets}$

CHAPTER 11: ALLERGY AND RESPIRATORY MEDICATIONS

1. *Fraction:* $\dfrac{300 \text{ mg}}{100 \text{ mg}} \times 1 \text{ tablet} = \dfrac{300}{100} = 3 \text{ tablets}$

Ratio-proportion: 100 mg : 1 tablet :: 300 mg : x tablets

$100x = 300$

$$\frac{100x}{100} = \frac{300}{100} = 3$$

$x = 3$ tablets

Dimensional analysis: ?tablets $= \dfrac{1 \text{ tablet}}{100 \text{ mg}} \Bigg| \dfrac{300 \text{ mg}}{1} = \dfrac{3}{1} = 3$ tablets

2. *Fraction:* $\dfrac{4 \text{ mg}}{2 \text{ mg}} \times 1$ tablet $= \dfrac{4}{2} = 2$ tablets

Ratio-proportion: 2 mg : 1 tablet :: 4 mg : x tablets

$2x = 4$

$$\frac{2x}{2} = \frac{4}{2} = 2$$

$x = 2$ tablets

Dimensional analysis: ?tablets $= \dfrac{1 \text{ tablet}}{2 \text{ mg}} \Bigg| \dfrac{4 \text{ mg}}{1} = \dfrac{4}{2} = 2$ tablets

3. *Fraction:* $\dfrac{25 \text{ mg}}{50 \text{ mg}} \times 1$ mL $= \dfrac{25}{50} = \dfrac{1}{2} = 0.5$ mL

Ratio-proportion: 50 mg : 1 mL :: 25 mg : x mL

$50x = 25$

$$\frac{50x}{50} = \frac{25}{50} = 0.5$$

$x = 0.5$ mL

Dimensional analysis: ?mL $= \dfrac{1 \text{ mL}}{\overset{}{\underset{2}{50 \text{ mg}}}} \Bigg| \dfrac{\overset{1}{25 \text{ mg}}}{} = \dfrac{1}{2} = 0.5$ mL

CHAPTER 12: ANTIINFECTIVE MEDICATIONS

. *Fraction:* $\dfrac{600 \text{ mg}}{100 \text{ mg}} \times 1$ mL $= \dfrac{600}{100} = 6$ mL

Ratio-proportion: 100 mg : 1 mL :: 600 mg : x mL

$100x = 600$

$$\frac{100x}{100} = \frac{600}{100} = 6$$

$x = 6$ mL

A. ?mL $= \dfrac{1 \text{ mL}}{100 \text{ mg}} \Bigg| \dfrac{600 \text{ mg}}{1} = \dfrac{6}{1} = 6$ mL

B. Dorsal or ventral gluteal

C. This injection needs to be divided into two doses of 3 mL each.

Fraction: $\dfrac{1,000,000 \text{ units}}{600,000 \text{ units}} \times 1$ mL $= \dfrac{1,000,000}{600,000} = 1.67$ mL

Ratio-proportion: 600,000 units : 1 mL :: 1,000,000 units : x mL

$600,000x = 1,000,000$

$$\frac{600,000x}{600,000} = \frac{1,000,000}{600,000} = 1.67 \text{ mL}$$

$x = 1.67$ mL

$$\text{Dimensional analysis: } ?mL = \frac{1 \text{ mL}}{600,000 \text{ units}} \left| \frac{1,000,000 \text{ units}}{1} \right. = \frac{10}{6} = 1.67 \text{ mL}$$

3. $\text{Fraction: } \dfrac{1 \text{ gm}}{1.5 \text{ gm}} \times 150 \text{ mL/hr} = \dfrac{150}{1.5} = 100 \text{ mL/hr}$

$\text{Ratio-proportion: } 1.5 \text{ gm} : 150 \text{ mL/hr} = 1 \text{ gm} : x \text{ mL/hr}$
$1.5x = 150$
$\dfrac{1.5x}{1.5} = \dfrac{150}{1.5} = 100$
$x = 100 \text{ mL/hr}$

$$\text{Dimensional analysis: } ?mL/hr = \frac{150 \text{ mL}}{1.5 \text{ gm}} \left| \frac{1 \text{ gm}}{1 \text{ hr}} \right. = \frac{150}{1.5} = 100 \text{ mL/hr}$$

4. $\text{Fraction: } \dfrac{400 \text{ mg}}{500 \text{ mg}} \times 2.2 \text{ mL} = \dfrac{400(2.2)}{500} = \dfrac{880}{500} = 1.76 \text{ mL} = 1.8 \text{ mL}$

$\text{Ratio-proportion: } 500 \text{ mg} : 2.2 \text{ mL} :: 400 \text{ mg} : x \text{ mL}$
$500x = 2.2(400) = 880$
$\dfrac{500x}{500} = \dfrac{880}{500} = 1.76$
$x = 1.76 \text{ or } 1.8 \text{ mL}$

$$\text{Dimensional analysis: } ?mL = \frac{2.2 \text{ mL}}{500 \text{ mg}} \left| \frac{400 \text{ mg}}{1} \right. = \frac{2.2(4)}{5} = \frac{8.8}{5} = 1.76 \text{ mL} = 1.8 \text{ mL}$$

CHAPTER 13: ANTIVIRALS, ANTIRETROVIRALS, AND ANTIFUNGAL MEDICATIONS

1. *For fraction and ratio-proportion, first convert pounds to kilograms:*
$2.2 \text{ lbs} : 1 \text{ kg} :: 110 \text{ lbs} : x \text{ kg}$
$2.2x = 110$
$\dfrac{2.2x}{2.2} = \dfrac{110}{2.2} = 50$
$x = 50 \text{ kg}$

$\text{Fraction: } \dfrac{50 \text{ kg}}{1 \text{ kg}} \times 10 \text{ mg} = \dfrac{50(10)}{1} = \dfrac{500}{1} = 500 \text{ mg}$

$\text{Ratio-proportion: } 1 \text{ kg} : 10 \text{ mg} :: 50 \text{ kg} : x \text{ mg}$
$1x = 10(50) = 500$
$x = 500 \text{ mg}$

$$\text{Dimensional analysis: } ?mg = \frac{10 \text{ mg}}{1 \text{ kg}} \left| \frac{1 \text{ kg}}{2.2 \text{ lbs}} \right| \frac{110 \text{ lbs}}{1} = \frac{10(110)}{2.2} = \frac{1100}{2.2} = 500 \text{ mg}$$

2. $\text{Fraction: } \dfrac{60 \text{ min}}{30 \text{ min}} \times 100 \text{ mL/hr} = \dfrac{60(100)}{30} = \dfrac{6000}{30} = 200 \text{ mL/hr}$

$\text{Ratio-proportion: } 30 \text{ min} : 100 \text{ mL/hr} :: 60 \text{ min} : x \text{ mL/hr}$
$30x = 60(100) = 6000$
$\dfrac{30x}{30} = \dfrac{6000}{30} = 200$
$x = 200 \text{ mL/hr}$

$$\text{Dimensional analysis: } ?mL/hr = \frac{100 \text{ mL}}{30 \text{ min} \atop 1} \left| \frac{\overset{2}{60 \text{ min}}}{1 \text{ hr}} \right. = \frac{100(2)}{1} = \frac{200}{1} = 200 \text{ mL/hr}$$

CHAPTER 14: ANTINEOPLASTIC MEDICATIONS

1. *Dimensional analysis**: $?\dfrac{\text{gtt}}{\text{min}} = \dfrac{20\ \text{gtt}}{1\ \text{mL}} \left| \dfrac{1000\ \text{mL}}{10\ \text{mg}} \right| \dfrac{1.25\ \text{mg}}{1\ \text{hr}} \left| \dfrac{1\ \text{hr}}{60\ \text{min}} \right. = \dfrac{2(100)(1.25)}{6} = \dfrac{250}{6} = 42\ \text{gtt/min}$

2. *Fraction:* $\dfrac{45\ \text{units}}{15\ \text{units}} \times 1\ \text{vial} = \dfrac{45}{15} = 3\ \text{vials}$

   Ratio-proportion: 15 units : 1 vial :: 45 units : x vials
   $15x = 45$
   $\dfrac{15x}{15} = \dfrac{45}{15} = 3$
   $x = 3\ \text{vials}$

   Dimensional analysis: $?\text{vials} = \dfrac{1\ \text{vial}}{15\ \text{units}} \times \dfrac{45\ \text{units}}{1} = \dfrac{45}{15} = 3\ \text{vials}$

3. *Fraction:* $\dfrac{65\ \text{kg}}{1\ \text{kg}} \times 10\ \text{mg} = \dfrac{65(10)}{1} = \dfrac{650}{1} = 650\ \text{mg}$

   Ratio-proportion: 1 kg : 10 mg :: 65 kg : x mg
   $1x = 65(10) = 650$
   $x = 650\ \text{mg}$

   Dimensional analysis: $?\text{mg} = \dfrac{10\ \text{mg}}{1\ \text{kg}} \times \dfrac{65\ \text{kg}}{1} = \dfrac{10(65)}{1} = 650\ \text{mg}$

4. *Fraction:* $\dfrac{3,000,000\ \text{IU}}{6,000,000\ \text{IU}} \times 1\ \text{mL} = \dfrac{3,000,000}{6,000,000} = 0.5\ \text{mL}$

   Ratio-proportion: 6,000,000 IU : 1 mL :: 3,000,000 IU : x mL
   $6,000,000x = 3,000,000$
   $\dfrac{6,000,000x}{6,000,000} = \dfrac{3,000,000}{6,000,000} = 0.5$
   $x = 0.5\ \text{mL}$

   Dimensional analysis: $?\text{mL} = \dfrac{1\ \text{mL}}{\underset{2}{\cancel{6}}\ \text{IU}} \left| \dfrac{\overset{1}{\cancel{3}}\ \text{IU}}{1} \right. = \dfrac{1}{2} = 0.5\ \text{mL}$

CHAPTER 15: CARDIOVASCULAR AND RENAL MEDICATIONS

For fraction and ratio-proportion, first convert grams to milligrams:
1 gm : 1000 mg :: 0.1 gm : x mg
$1x = 1000(0.1) = 100$
$x = 100\ \text{mg}$

Fraction: $\dfrac{100\ \text{mg}}{200\ \text{mg}} \times 1\ \text{mL} = 0.5\ \text{mL}$

Ratio-proportion: 200 mg : 1 mL :: 100 mg : x mL
$200x = 100$
$\dfrac{200x}{200} = \dfrac{100}{200}$
$x = 0.5\ \text{mL}$

*Only dimensional analysis is shown because it is the most efficient method for solving this problem.

Dimensional analysis: $?\text{mL} = \dfrac{1\ \text{mL}}{\cancel{200\ \text{mg}}_{1}} \bigg| \dfrac{\overset{5}{\cancel{1000\ \text{mg}}}}{\cancel{1\ \text{g}}} \bigg| 0.1\ \cancel{\text{g}} = \dfrac{5(0.1)}{1} = \dfrac{0.5}{1} = 0.5\ \text{mL}$

2. *Fraction:* $\dfrac{30\ \text{mg}}{20\ \text{mg}} \times 1\ \text{tablet} = \dfrac{30}{20} = 1.5\ \text{tablets}$

   Ratio-proportion: 20 mg : 1 tablet :: 30 mg : x tablet
   $20x = 30$
   $\dfrac{20x}{20} = \dfrac{30}{20} = 1.5$
   $x = 1.5\ \text{tablets}$

   Dimensional analysis: $?\text{tablets} = \dfrac{1\ \text{tablet}}{20\ \cancel{\text{mg}}} \bigg| \dfrac{30\ \cancel{\text{mg}}}{1} = \dfrac{3}{2} = 1.5\ \text{tablets}$

3. *Fraction:* $\dfrac{60\ \text{mg}}{20\ \text{mg}} \times 5\ \text{mL} = \dfrac{60(5)}{20} = \dfrac{300}{20} = 15\ \text{mL}$

   Ratio-proportion: 20 mg : 5 mL :: 60 mg : x mL
   $20x = 5(60) = 300$
   $\dfrac{20x}{20} = \dfrac{300}{20}$
   $x = 15\ \text{mL}$

   Dimensional analysis: $?\text{mL} = \dfrac{5\ \text{mL}}{\cancel{20\ \text{mg}}_{1}} \bigg| \dfrac{\overset{3}{\cancel{60\ \text{mg}}}}{1} = \dfrac{5(3)}{1} = \dfrac{15}{1} = 15\ \text{mL}$

CHAPTER 16: CENTRAL AND PERIPHERAL NERVOUS SYSTEM MEDICATIONS

1. *For fraction and ratio-proportion, first convert pounds to kilograms:*
   2.2 lb : 1 kg :: 150 lbs : x kg
   $2.2x = 150$
   $\dfrac{2.2x}{2.2} \times \dfrac{150}{2.2} = 68.18$
   $x = 68.18\ \text{kg}$

   Fraction: $\dfrac{15\ \text{mg}}{1\ \text{kg}} \times 68.18\ \text{kg} = \dfrac{15(68.18)}{1} = \dfrac{1023}{1} = 1023\ \text{mg}$

   Ratio-proportion: 1 kg : 15 mg :: 68.18 kg : x mg
   $1x = 15(68.18) = 1023$
   $x = 1023\ \text{mg}$

   Dimensional analysis: $?\text{mg} = \dfrac{15\ \text{mg}}{1\ \cancel{\text{kg}}} \bigg| \dfrac{1\ \cancel{\text{kg}}}{2.2\ \cancel{\text{lbs}}} \bigg| \dfrac{150\ \cancel{\text{lbs}}}{1} = \dfrac{15(150)}{2.2} = \dfrac{2250}{2.2} = 1023\ \text{mg}$

2. *Fraction:* $\dfrac{200\ \text{mg}}{125\ \text{mg}} \times 5\ \text{mL} = \dfrac{200(5)}{125} = \dfrac{1000}{125} = 8\ \text{mL}$

   Ratio-proportion: 125 mg : 5 mL :: 200 mg : x mL
   $125x = 5(200) = 1000$
   $\dfrac{125x}{125} = \dfrac{1000}{125} = 8$
   $x = 8\ \text{mL}$

   Dimensional analysis: $?\text{mL} = \dfrac{\overset{1}{\cancel{5}}\ \text{mL}}{\cancel{125\ \text{mg}}_{25}} \bigg| \dfrac{200\ \cancel{\text{mg}}}{1} = \dfrac{200}{25} = 8\ \text{mL}$

3. *Fraction:* $\dfrac{0.5 \text{ mg}}{2 \text{ mg}} \times 1 \text{ mL} = \dfrac{0.5}{2} = 0.25 \text{ mL}$

Ratio-proportion: 2 mg : 1 mL :: 0.5 mg : x mL
$2x = 0.5$
$\dfrac{2x}{2} = \dfrac{0.5}{2} = 0.25$
$x = 0.25 \text{ mL}$

Dimensional analysis: $?\text{mL} = \dfrac{1 \text{ mL}}{2 \text{ mg}} \bigg| \dfrac{0.5 \text{ mg}}{1} = \dfrac{0.5}{2} = 0.25 \text{ mL}$

CHAPTER 17: MEDICATIONS FOR PAIN MANAGEMENT

1. *For fraction and ratio-proportion, first convert grains to milligrams:*
1 gr : 60 mg :: gr¼ : x mg
$1x = 60(\frac{1}{4}) = \dfrac{60}{4} = 15 \text{ mg}$

Fraction: $\dfrac{15 \text{ mg}}{10 \text{ mg}} \times 1 \text{ mL} = \dfrac{15}{10} = 1.5 \text{ mL}$

Ratio-proportion: 10 mg : 1 mL :: 15 mg : x mL
$10x = 15$
$\dfrac{10x}{10} = \dfrac{15}{10} = 1.5$
$x = 1.5 \text{ mL}$

Dimensional analysis: $?\text{mL} = \dfrac{1 \text{ mL}}{10 \text{ mg}} \bigg| \dfrac{60 \text{ mg}}{1 \text{ gr}} \bigg| \dfrac{\text{gr} \frac{1}{4}}{1} = \dfrac{60\left(\frac{1}{4}\right)}{10} = \dfrac{15}{10} = 1.5 \text{ mL}$

2. *Fraction:* $\dfrac{0.5 \text{ mg}}{20 \text{ mg}} \times 200 \text{ mL} = \dfrac{0.5(200)}{20} = \dfrac{100}{20} = 5 \text{ mL/hr}$

Ratio-proportion: 20 mg : 200 mL :: 0.5 mg : x mL
$20x = 200(0.5) = 100$
$\dfrac{20x}{20} = \dfrac{100}{20} = 5$
$x = 5 \text{ mL/hr}$

Dimensional analysis: $?\text{mL/hr} = \dfrac{\overset{10}{200} \text{ mL}}{20 \text{ mg}} \bigg| \dfrac{0.5 \text{ mg}}{1 \text{ hr}} = \dfrac{10(0.5)}{1} = \dfrac{5}{1} = 5 \text{ mL/hr}$

Fraction: $\dfrac{0.4 \text{ mg}}{0.2 \text{ mg}} \times 1 \text{ mL} = \dfrac{0.4}{0.2} = 2 \text{ mL}$

Ratio-proportion: 0.2 mg : 1 mL :: 0.4 mg : x mL
$0.2x = 0.4$
$\dfrac{0.2x}{0.2} = \dfrac{0.4}{0.2} = 2$
$x = 2 \text{ mL}$

Dimensional analysis: $?\text{mL} = \dfrac{1 \text{ mL}}{0.2 \text{ mg}} \bigg| \dfrac{\overset{2}{0.4} \text{ mg}}{1} = \dfrac{2}{1} = 2 \text{ mL}$

CHAPTER 18: GASTROINTESTINAL MEDICATIONS

Fraction: $\dfrac{20 \text{ mg}}{40 \text{ mg}} \times 5 \text{ mL} = \dfrac{20(5)}{40} = \dfrac{100}{40} = 2.5 \text{ mL}$

Ratio-proportion: 40 mg : 5 mL :: 20 mg : x mL

$40x = 5(20) = 100$

$\dfrac{40x}{40} = \dfrac{100}{40} = 2.5$

$x = 2.5$ mL

Dimensional analysis: $?\text{mL} = \dfrac{5\text{ mL}}{\overset{2}{\cancel{40\text{ mg}}}} \left| \dfrac{\overset{1}{\cancel{20\text{ mg}}}}{1} \right. = \dfrac{5}{2} = 2.5$ mL

2. *For fraction and ratio-proportion, first convert pounds to kilograms:*

2.2 lbs : 1 kg :: 143 lbs : x kg

$2.2x = 143$

$\dfrac{2.2x}{2.2} = \dfrac{143}{2.2} = 65$

$x = 65$ kg

Fraction: $\dfrac{65\text{ kg}}{1\text{ kg}} \times 1.8\text{ mg} = \dfrac{65(1.8)}{1} = 117$ mg

Ratio-proportion: 1 kg : 1.8 mg :: 65 kg : x mg

$1x = 1.8(65) = 117$

$x = 117$ mg

Dimensional analysis: $?\text{mg} = \dfrac{1.8\text{ mg}}{\cancel{1\text{ kg}}} \left| \dfrac{\cancel{1\text{ kg}}}{2.2\text{ lbs}} \right| \dfrac{143\cancel{\text{ lbs}}}{1} = \dfrac{1.8(143)}{2.2} = \dfrac{257.4}{2.2} = 117$ mg

3. *Fraction:* $\dfrac{1.5\text{ gm}}{1\text{ gm}} \times 10\text{ mL} = \dfrac{1.5(10)}{1} = \dfrac{15}{1} = 15$ mL

Ratio-proportion: 1 gm : 10 mL :: 1.5 gm : x mL

$1x = 10(1.5) = 15$

$x = 15$ mL

Dimensional analysis: $?\text{mL} = \dfrac{10\text{ mL}}{\cancel{1\text{ gr}}} \left| \dfrac{1.5\cancel{\text{ gr}}}{1} \right. = \dfrac{10(1.5)}{1} = \dfrac{15}{1} = 15$ mL

CHAPTER 19: HEMATOLOGIC PRODUCTS

1. *Fraction:* $\dfrac{7500\text{ units}}{20{,}000\text{ units}} \times 1\text{ mL} = \dfrac{7500}{20{,}000} = 0.375$ or 0.38 mL

Ratio-proportion: 20,000 units : 1 mL :: 7500 units : x mL

$20{,}000x = 7500$

$\dfrac{20{,}000x}{20{,}000} = \dfrac{7500}{20{,}000} = 0.375$

$x = 0.375$ or 0.38 mL

Dimensional analysis: $?\text{mL} = \dfrac{1\text{ mL}}{20{,}000\ \cancel{\text{units}}} \left| \dfrac{7500\ \cancel{\text{units}}}{1} \right. = \dfrac{75}{200} = 0.375$ or 0.38 mL

2. *Dimensional analysis*:* $?\text{mL/hr} = \dfrac{500\text{ mL}}{24\text{ hr}} = 20.8$ or 21 mL/hr

---

*Only dimensional analysis is shown because it is the most efficient method for solving this problem.

3. *Fraction:* $\dfrac{30 \text{ mg}}{150 \text{ mg}} \times 1 \text{ mL} = \dfrac{30}{150} = 0.2 \text{ mL}$

Ratio-proportion: 150 mg : 1 mL :: 30 mg : x mL
$150x = 30$
$\dfrac{150x}{150} = \dfrac{30}{150} = 0.2$
$x = 0.2 \text{ mL}$

Dimensional analysis: $?\text{mL} = \dfrac{1 \text{ mL}}{\underset{5}{\cancel{150 \text{ mg}}}} \;\Bigg|\; \dfrac{\overset{1}{\cancel{30 \text{ mg}}}}{} = \dfrac{1}{5} = 0.2 \text{ mL}$

CHAPTER 20: HORMONES AND STEROIDS

1. *Fraction:* $\dfrac{6 \text{ mg}}{4 \text{ mg}} \times 1 \text{ mL} = \dfrac{6}{4} = 1.5 \text{ mL}$

Ratio-proportion: 4 mg : 1 mL :: 6 mg : x mL
$4x = 6$
$\dfrac{4x}{4} = \dfrac{6}{4} = 1.5$
$x = 1.5 \text{ mL}$

Dimensional analysis: $?\text{mL} = \dfrac{1 \text{ mL}}{\underset{2}{\cancel{4 \text{ mg}}}} \;\Bigg|\; \dfrac{\overset{3}{\cancel{6 \text{ mg}}}}{1} = \dfrac{3}{2} = 1.5 \text{ mL}$

2. *For fraction and ratio-proportion, first convert micrograms to milligrams:*
1000 mcg : 1 mg :: 125 mcg : x mg
$1000x = 125$
$\dfrac{1000x}{1000} = \dfrac{125}{1000} = 0.125$
$x = 0.125 \text{ mg}$

Fraction: $\dfrac{0.125 \text{ mg}}{0.25 \text{ mg}} \times 1 \text{ tablet} = \dfrac{0.125}{0.25} = 0.5 \text{ tablet}$

Ratio-proportion: 0.25 mg : 1 tablet :: 0.125 mg : x tablet
$0.25x = 0.125$
$\dfrac{0.25x}{0.25} = \dfrac{0.125}{0.25} = 0.5$
$x = 0.5 \text{ tablet}$

Dimensional analysis: $?\text{tablets} = \dfrac{1 \text{ tablet}}{0.25 \text{ mg}} \;\Bigg|\; \dfrac{125 \text{ mcg}}{1} \;\Bigg|\; \dfrac{1 \text{ mg}}{1000 \text{ mcg}} = \dfrac{125}{0.25(1000)} = \dfrac{125}{250} = 0.5 \text{ tablet}$

Fraction: $\dfrac{60 \text{ mg}}{125 \text{ mg}} \times 1 \text{ mL} = \dfrac{60}{125} = 0.48 \text{ or } 0.5 \text{ mL}$

Ratio-proportion: 125 mg : 1 mL :: 60 mg : x mL
$125x = 60$
$\dfrac{125x}{125} = \dfrac{60}{125} = 0.48$
$x = 0.48 \text{ or } 0.5 \text{ mL}$

Dimensional analysis: $?\text{mL} = \dfrac{1 \text{ mL}}{125 \text{ mg}} \;\Bigg|\; \dfrac{60 \text{ mg}}{1} = \dfrac{60}{125} = 0.48 \text{ or } 0.5 \text{ mL}$

CHAPTER 21: IMMUNOLOGIC MEDICATIONS

1. *Dimensional analysis*:* $?mL/hr = \dfrac{\overset{50}{\cancel{100}}\,mL}{\underset{1}{\cancel{2}}\,hr} = \dfrac{50}{1} = 50\ mL/hr$

2. *Fraction:* $\dfrac{20{,}000\ units}{100{,}000\ units} \times 1\ mL = \dfrac{20{,}000}{100{,}000} = 0.2\ mL$

   Ratio-proportion: 100,000 units : 1 mL :: 20,000 units : x mL
   $100{,}000x = 20{,}000$
   $\dfrac{100{,}000x}{100{,}000} = \dfrac{20{,}000}{100{,}000} = 0.2$
   $x = 0.2\ mL$

   Dimensional analysis: $?mL = \dfrac{1\ mL}{\underset{5}{\cancel{100{,}000}\ units}}\ \bigg|\ \dfrac{\overset{1}{\cancel{20{,}000}\ units}}{1} = \dfrac{1}{5} = 0.2\ mL$

3. *Fraction:* $\dfrac{65\ kg}{1\ kg} \times 20\ mg = \dfrac{20(65)}{1} = 1300\ mg$

   Ratio-proportion: 1 kg : 20 mg :: 65 kg : x mg
   $1x = 1300$
   $x = 1300\ mg$

   Dimensional analysis: $?mg = \dfrac{20\ mg}{1\ \cancel{kg}}\ \bigg|\ \dfrac{65\ \cancel{kg}}{1} = \dfrac{20(65)}{1} = 1300\ mg$

CHAPTER 22: ANTIINFLAMMATORY, MUSCULOSKELETAL, AND ANTIARTHRITIS MEDICATIONS

1. *Fraction:* $\dfrac{280\ mg}{80\ mg} \times 0.8\ mL = \dfrac{280(0.8)}{80} = \dfrac{224}{80} = 2.8\ mL$

   Ratio-proportion: 80 mg : 0.8 mL :: 280 mg : x mL
   $80x = 0.8(280) = 224$
   $\dfrac{80x}{80} = \dfrac{224}{80} = 2.8$
   $x = 2.8\ mL$

   Dimensional analysis: $?mL = \dfrac{0.8\ mL}{\underset{2}{\cancel{80\ mg}}}\ \bigg|\ \dfrac{\overset{7}{\cancel{280\ mg}}}{1} = \dfrac{0.8(7)}{2} = \dfrac{5.6}{2} = 2.8\ mL$

2. *Fraction:* $\dfrac{15\ mg}{30\ mg} \times 1\ mL = \dfrac{15}{30} = 0.5\ mL$

   Ratio-proportion: 30 mg : 1 mL :: 15 mg : x mL
   $30x = 15$
   $\dfrac{30x}{30} = \dfrac{15}{30} = 0.5$
   $x = 0.5\ mL$

   Dimensional analysis: $?mL = \dfrac{1\ mL}{\underset{2}{\cancel{30\ mg}}}\ \bigg|\ \dfrac{\overset{1}{\cancel{15\ mg}}}{1} = \dfrac{1}{2} = 0.5\ mL$

---

*Only dimensional analysis is shown because it is the most efficient method for solving this problem.

3. *Fraction:* $\dfrac{5 \text{ gr}}{1 \text{ gr}} \times 60 \text{ mg} = 300 \text{ mg} = 1 \text{ tablet}$

Ratio-proportion: 1 gr : 60 mg :: 5 gr : x mg
$1x = 60(5) = 300$
$x = 300 \text{ mg} = 1 \text{ tablet}$

Dimensional analysis: $?\text{tablets} = \dfrac{1 \text{ tablet}}{300 \text{ mg}} \bigg| \dfrac{60 \text{ mg}}{1 \text{ gr}} \bigg| \dfrac{5 \text{ gr}}{1} = \dfrac{60(5)}{300} = \dfrac{300}{300} = 1 \text{ tablet}$

CHAPTER 23: TOPICAL PREPARATIONS

1. *Fraction:* $\dfrac{500,000 \text{ units}}{100,000 \text{ units}} \times 1 \text{ mL} = \dfrac{500,000}{100,000} = 5 \text{ mL}$

Ratio-proportion: 100,000 units : 1 mL :: 500,000 units : x mL
$100,000x = 500,000$
$\dfrac{100,000x}{100,000} = \dfrac{500,000}{100,000} = 5$
$x = 5 \text{ mL}$

Dimensional analysis: $?\text{mL} = \dfrac{1 \text{ mL}}{100,000 \text{ units}} \bigg| \dfrac{500,000 \text{ units}}{1} = \dfrac{5}{1} = 5 \text{ mL}$

2. *Fraction:* $\dfrac{40 \text{ mg}}{20 \text{ mg}} \times 1 \text{ tablet} = \dfrac{40}{20} = 2 \text{ tablets}$

Ratio-proportion: 20 mg : 1 tablet :: 40 mg : x tablet
$20x = 40$
$\dfrac{20x}{20} = \dfrac{40}{20} = 2$
$x = 2 \text{ tablets}$

Dimensional analysis: $?\text{tablets} = \dfrac{1 \text{ tablet}}{20 \text{ mg}} \bigg| \dfrac{\overset{2}{40 \text{ mg}}}{1} = \dfrac{2}{1} = 2 \text{ tablets}$

. *Fraction:* $\dfrac{10 \text{ mL}}{5 \text{ mL}} \times 1 \text{ teaspoon} = \dfrac{10}{5} = 2 \text{ teaspoons}$

Ratio-proportion: 5 mL : 1 teaspoon :: 10 mL : x teaspoons
$5x = 10$
$\dfrac{5x}{5} = \dfrac{10}{5} = 2$
$x = 2 \text{ teaspoons}$

Dimensional analysis: $?\text{teaspoons} = \dfrac{1 \text{ teaspoon}}{5 \text{ mL}} \bigg| \dfrac{\overset{2}{10 \text{ mL}}}{1} = \dfrac{2}{1} = 2 \text{ teaspoons}$

CHAPTER 24: VITAMINS AND MINERALS

Fraction: $\dfrac{200 \text{ mcg}}{1000 \text{ mcg}} \times 1 \text{ mL} = \dfrac{200}{1000} = 0.2 \text{ mL}$

Ratio-proportion: 1000 mcg : 1 mL :: 200 mcg : x mL
$1000x = 200$
$\dfrac{1000x}{1000} = \dfrac{200}{1000} = 0.2$
$x = 0.2 \text{ mL}$

Dimensional analysis: $?\text{mL} = \dfrac{1\ \text{mL}}{\underset{5}{\cancel{1000}}\ \cancel{\text{mcg}}} \left| \dfrac{\overset{1}{\cancel{200}}\ \cancel{\text{mcg}}}{1} = \dfrac{1}{5} = 0.2\ \text{mL}\right.$

2. *Dimensional analysis*:* $?\text{mL/hr} = \dfrac{250\ \text{mL}}{6\ \text{hr}} = 41.66\ \text{or}\ 42\ \text{mL/hr}$

3. *Fraction:* $\dfrac{10\ \text{mEq}}{60\ \text{mEq}} \times 200\ \text{mL} = \dfrac{10(200)}{60} = \dfrac{2000}{60} = 33.3\ \text{or}\ 33\ \text{mL/hr}$

Ratio-proportion: 60 mEq : 200 mL :: 10 mEq : x mL
$60x = 200(10) = 2000$
$\dfrac{60x}{60} \times \dfrac{2000}{60} = 33.3$
$x = 33.3\ \text{or}\ 33\ \text{mL/hr}$

Dimensional analysis: $?\text{mL/hr} = \dfrac{200\ \text{mL}}{\cancel{60}\ \cancel{\text{mEq}}} \left| \dfrac{\overset{}{\cancel{10}}\ \cancel{\text{mEq}}}{1\ \text{hr}} = \dfrac{200}{6} = 33.3\ \text{or}\ 33\ \text{mL/hr}\right.$

---

*Only dimensional analysis is shown because it is the most efficient method for solving this problem.

Bibliography

Alcohol-medication interaction, Alcohol Alert No 27 PH 355, Washington, DC, 1995, National Institute on Alcohol Abuse and Alcoholism.

American Diabetes Association: Consensus statement: type 2 diabetes in children and adolescents, *Diabetes Care* 23(3):381–9.

American Psychiatric Association: *Diagnostic and statistical manual of mental disorders,* ed 4, text revision, Washington, DC, 2000, American Psychiatric Press.

Barker LR, Burton JR, Zieve PD: *Principles of ambulatory medicine,* ed 4, Baltimore, 1995, Williams & Wilkins, pp 25–49.

Bennett PN, Brown MJ: *Clinical pharmacology,* ed 9, St Louis, 2003, Mosby.

Carter BL: Patient education and disease monitoring. In Herfindal ER, Gourley DR, Hart LL, editors. *Clinical pharmacy and therapeutics,* ed 5, Baltimore, 1992, Williams & Wilkins.

Culbertson VL et al: Consumer preferences for verbal and written medication information, *Drug Intell Clin Pharm* 22(5):390–6, 1988.

DiPiro JT et al: *Pharmacotherapy: a pathophysiologic approach,* ed 5, Norwalk, CT, 2002, McGraw Hill/Appleton & Lange.

Dison N: *Simplified drugs and solutions for health care professionals,* ed 11, St Louis, 1997, Mosby.

Edmunds MW, Mayhew MS: *Pharmacology for the primary care provider,* ed 2, St Louis, 2004, Mosby.

Hardman J, Limbird I, editors: *Goodman & Gilman's the pharmacological basis of therapeutics,* ed 10, New York, 2001, McGraw-Hill.

Herlihy B, Maebius NK: *The human body in health and illness,* ed 2, Philadelphia, 2003, WB Saunders.

Institute of Medicine: *To err is human: building a safer health system,* Washington, DC, 2000, National Academy of Science.

Janney C, Timpke J: *Calculation of drug dosages,* ed 6, Penn Valley, VA, 2001, TJ Designs.

Kastrup EK et al, editors: *Facts and comparisons,* St Louis, 2005, Wolters Kluwer.

Katzung BG: *Basic and clinical pharmacology,* ed 9, Norwalk, CT, 2004, Appleton & Lange.

Kirsch IS et al: *Adult literacy in America: a first look at the results of the National Adult Literacy Survey,* Washington, DC, 1993, National Center for Education Statistics. Available at http://nces.ed.gov/pubsearch/pubsinfo.asp?pubid=93275.

Krinsky DL et al: *Natural therapeutics pocket guide,* ed 2, Hudson, Ohio, 2003, Lexi-Comp, Inc.

Lonn E et al: Effects of long-term vitamin E supplementation on cardiovascular events and cancer: a randomized controlled trial, *JAMA* 293(11):1338–41, 2005.

MarketLetter: *From compliance to concordance,* Washington, DC, March 24, 1997.

McCance KL, Huether SE: *Pathophysiology: the biological basis for disease in adults and children,* ed 2, St Louis, 1994, Mosby.

McEvoy GK: *The American hospital formulary service,* Bethesda, MD, 1997, American Society of Hospital Pharmacists.

McKenry LM, Salerno E: *Mosby's pharmacology in nursing,* ed 21, St Louis, 2003, Mosby.

Medication teaching manual: the guide to patient drug information, ed 5, Bethesda, MD, 1998, American Society of Hospital Pharmacists.

Miller ER 3rd et al: Meta-analysis: high-dosage vitamin E supplementation may increase all-cause mortality, *Ann Intern Med* 142(1):37–46, 2005.

Morris LA et al: A segmentational analysis of prescription drug information seeking, *Med Care* 25:953–64, 1987.

Morris MC et al: Relation of the tocopherol forms to incident Alzheimer disease and to cognitive change, *Am J Clin Nutr* 81(2):508–14, 2005.

Mosby's 2006 Drug consult for nurses, ed 2, St Louis, 2005, Mosby.

National Heart, Lung, and Blood Institutes, National High Blood Pressure Education Program: *The seventh report of the Joint National Committee on the Prevention, Detection, Evaluation, and Treatment of High Blood Pressure,* Bethesda, MD, 2003, National Institutes of Health.

Ogden SJ: *Calculation of drug dosages,* ed 7, St Louis, 2003, Mosby.

Physicians' Desk Reference, ed 59, Montvale, NJ, 2005, Medical Economics.

Rang HP et al: *Pharmacology,* ed 5, St Louis, 2003, Mosby.

Rankin SH, Stallings KD: *Patient education in health and illness,* ed 5, Philadelphia, 1990, Lippincott.

Saxton D et al: *Math and meds for nurses,* ed 2, Albany, NY, 2005, Delmar.

Slater MD et al: Hypermedia use by the disadvantaged: assessing a health information program, *Hypermedia* 6(2):67–86, 1994.

Steckel SB: *Patient contracting,* Norwalk, CT, 1982, Appleton-Century-Crofts.

Tierney LM, McPhee SJ, Papadakis MA: *Current medical diagnosis & treatment 2005,* ed 44, New York, 2005, McGraw-Hill Medical.

United States Pharmacopeia Dispensing Information: *Drug information for the health care provider,* vol 1; *Advice for the patient,* vol 2; ed 19, Rockville, MD, 1999, United States Pharmacopeial Convention.

Illustration Credits

Chapter 5

Figure 5-1: From Moore KL, Persaud TVN: *The developing human: clinically oriented embryology,* ed 7, Philadelphia, 2002, WB Saunders.

Chapter 9

Figure 9-5: From Lilley LL, Harrington S, Snyder JS: *Pharmacology and the nursing process,* ed 4, St Louis, 2005, Mosby; modified from data by Boyd E, West CD. In Behrman RE, Kleigman RM, Jensen HB: *Nelson textbook of pediatrics,* ed 17, Philadelphia, 2004, WB Saunders.

Chapter 10

Figures 10-6, A, 10-25, 10-26, 10-27, 10-28: Copyright Baxter Healthcare Corporation, Deerfield, IL.
Figure 10-6, B: From Potter PA, Perry AG: *Fundamentals of nursing,* ed 6, St Louis, 2005, Mosby.
Figure 10-10, B, C, D, E: Courtesy Hospira, Inc., Lake Forest, IL.

Chapter 11

Figure 11-1: From Herlihy B, Maebius NK: *The human body in health and illness,* ed 2, Philadelphia, 2003, WB Saunders.

Chapter 13

Figure 13-1: Redrawn from McCance KL, Huether SE: *Pathophysiology: the biological basis for disease in adults and children,* ed 2, St Louis, 1994, Mosby.
Figure 13-2: Redrawn from McCance KL, Huether SE: *Pathophysiology: the biological basis for disease in adults and children,* ed 2, St Louis, 1994, Mosby; modified from Yarcoan R, Metsuya H, Broder S: *AIDS therapies, the science of AIDS, readings from Scientific American,* New York, 1989, WH Freeman.

Chapter 15

Figures 15-1, 15-2, 15-5, A, 15-9, 15-10: From Herlihy B, Maebius NK: *The human body in health and illness,* ed 2, Philadelphia, 2003, WB Saunders.
Figure 15-3: From Thibodeau GA, Patton KT: *Anatomy & physiology,* ed 5, St Louis, 2003, Mosby.
Figure 15-5, B: Modified from Herlihy B, Maebius NK: *The human body in health and illness,* ed 2, Philadelphia, 2003, WB Saunders.
Figure 15-7, B: From Damjanov I, Linder J, editors: *Anderson's pathology,* ed 10, St Louis, 1996, Mosby.
Figure 15-12: From Brundage DJ: *Renal disorders,* St Louis, 1992, Mosby.

Figure 15-13: Redrawn from McCance KL, Huether SE: *Pathophysiology: the biological basis for disease in adults and children,* ed 2, St Louis, 1994, Mosby.
Figure 15-14: Redrawn from National Heart, Lung, and Blood Institute, National High Blood Pressure Education Program: *The seventh report of the Joint National Committee on the Prevention, Detection, Evaluation and Treatment of High Blood Pressure,* Bethesda, MD, 2003, National Institutes of Health.

Chapter 17

Figure 17-1: From Black JM, Hawks JH: *Medical-surgical nursing: clinical management for positive outcomes,* ed 7, Philadelphia, 2005, WB Saunders.
Figure 17-2: From Wong DL, Hockenberry-Eaton M, Wilson D et al: *Wong's essentials of pediatric nursing,* ed 6, St Louis, 2001, p 1301. Copyrighted by Mosby, Inc. Reprinted by permission.
Figure 17-3, A: Copyright Baxter Healthcare Corporation, Deerfield, IL.
Figure 17-3, B: From deWit S: *Fundamental concepts and skills for nursing,* ed 2, Philadelphia, 2005, WB Saunders.

Chapter 18

Figure 18-1: From Herlihy B, Maebius NK: *The human body in health and illness,* ed 2, Philadelphia, 2003, WB Saunders.

Chapter 20

Figures 20-1, 20-2: From Herlihy B, Maebius NK: *The human body in health and illness,* ed 2, Philadelphia, 2003, WB Saunders.
Figure 20-3: From Harkreader H, Hogan MA: *Fundamentals of nursing: caring and clinical judgment,* ed 2, Philadelphia, 2004, WB Saunders.

Chapter 21

Figure 21-1: From Thibodeau GA, Patton KT: *Anatomy & physiology,* ed 5, St Louis, 2003, Mosby.
Figure 21-2: From Centers for Disease Control and Prevention: *Recommended childhood and adolescent immunization schedule,* United States, 2005.

Chapter 23

Figure 23-1: From Herlihy B, Maebius NK: *The human body in health and illness,* ed 2, Philadelphia, 2003, WB Saunders.

Glossary

A

abortifacients Drugs used to stimulate uterine contractions and cause the uterus to empty (p. 372).

absorption The process by which a drug enters the body and passes into the body fluids and tissues; occurs through diffusion, filtration, or osmosis (p. 32).

acetylcholine One of two major neurotransmitters in the body; acts on the parasympathetic nerves (p. 265).

acquired immunodeficiency syndrome (AIDS) A disease caused by the human immunodeficiency virus, which enters the body through mucous membranes or infected blood and produces a defect in the ability of the immune system to fight infection. AIDS is associated with a long course marked by increasing weakness and is manifested by various opportunistic infections (p. 197).

action potential duration Length of time for one cell to electrically fire (depolarize) and recover (repolarize) (p. 230).

acute pain Pain related to an injury such as recent surgery, trauma, or infection; ends within an expected time (p. 313).

addiction The desperate need to have and use a drug for a nonmedical reason (p. 314).

additive effect When two drugs are given together, the combined effect of the drugs is equal to either that of the more active drug or the sum of the effects of the individual drugs (p. 36).

adolescence The period in development between the onset of puberty and adulthood. For calculation of drug dosage, it generally refers to the ages between 12 and 16 (p. 43).

adrenergic blocking agents Agents that block the release of epinephrine and norepinephrine at the postganglionic nerve endings of the sympathetic nervous system, producing dilation of the blood vessels and a decrease in cardiac output (p. 265).

From Chabner D: *The language of medicine*, ed 7, Philadelphia, 2004, Saunders.

adrenergic drugs Drugs that produce sympathetic nervous system effects; also called *sympathomimetics* or *catecholamines* (p.265).

adrenergic fibers Sympathetic nerve fibers that release epinephrine at a synapse when a nerve impulse passes (p. 265).

adverse reactions Unexpected and undesirable symptoms or problems that arise because of a medication. The more severe reactions often require hospitalization and may cause death. Also called *adverse effects* (p. 34).

agonists Drugs that bond well with receptor sites in the patient's body and activate the receptor, producing an action similar to that of the body's own chemicals (p. 31).

alkylating agents Synthetic compounds that combine readily with other molecules and interfere with the normal process of cell division; used in chemotherapy (p. 211).

allergy Acquired sensitivity or heightened immune response to a drug or a foreign substance (antigen) (p. 35).

alternative medicine Health practices that are either scientifically untested or lacking in supportive data. Some alternative therapies are herbal therapies, aromatherapy, chiropractic, acupuncture, massage, and homeotherapy (p. 59).

ampules Small, breakable glass containers that contain one dose of medication in each; used for intramuscular injections or intravenous infusions (p. 108).

anaphylactic reaction Life-threatening allergic reaction to medication so severe that the patient has difficulty breathing and may have cardiovascular collapse (p. 35).

androgens The male hormone testosterone and its related hormones; help develop and maintain the male sex organs at puberty and develop secondary sex characteristics in men (p. 382).

anorectal preparations Emollients, foams, or gels used for topical anesthesia or healing of the rectal area; used for symptomatic relief of discomfort associated with hemorrhoids (p. 434).

antacids Drugs that neutralize hydrochloric acid and increase gastric pH, thus inhibiting pepsin (p. 329).

antagonistic effect When two drugs are given together, one drug interferes with the action of the other (p. 36).

antagonists Agents that attach at a receptor site but then produce no new chemical reaction; prevent the activation of the receptor, stopping other chemical reactions from occurring (p. 31).

antibiotic preparations Antimicrobial agents used therapeutically not for their antiinfective properties but to delay or prevent cell division of malignant cells (p. 211).

antibiotics Antimicrobial chemicals that are produced from other living microorganisms and that are antagonistic to some other forms of life. Their actions are classified as bactericidal or bacteriostatic (p. 166).

anticholinergics Agents that block the release of acetylcholine and inhibit cholinergic activity; they reduce gastrointestinal tract spasm and intestinal motility, acid production, and gastric motility, which reduces the associated pain (p. 265).

anticoagulants Agents that inhibit the blood clotting mechanism and increase the time it takes for blood to clot (p. 349).

antidiarrheals Agents that reduce the fluid content of the stool or decrease peristalsis and motility of the intestinal tract (p. 334).

antiflatulents Agents that break up and prevent mucus-surrounded pockets of gas from forming in the intestine (p. 342).

antifungal medications Medications used to treat mycotic infections (p. 205).

antigen-antibody response Response that occurs when foreign substances (antigens) that invade the body cause the immune system to make proteins (antibodies) that react specifically with the foreign substances to help neutralize their effects. This response is seen in allergies and in infectious disease (p. 400).

antiglaucoma agents Medications used to reduce the secretion of aqueous humor in the eye, block the action of acetylcholine, produce complete paralysis, aid in diagnostic procedures, provide iris sphincter contraction, and act as cholinergic agonists to reduce intraocular pressure (p. 436).

antihistamines Drugs given to relieve the effects of histamine on body organs and structures. Histamine is responsible for the signs and symptoms of allergic reactions (p. 142).

antimetabolites Agents that disrupt normal cell functions by interfering with various metabolic functions of the cells (p. 212).

antimicrobials Chemicals that kill or damage pathogenic organisms (p. 166).

antipsoriatics Agents that accelerate scaling and healing of dry lesions in chronic psoriasis (p. 441).

antiretrovirals Drugs used to slow growth or prevent duplication of retroviruses (for example, human immunodeficiency virus) (p. 197).

antiseptics Compounds that are capable of preventing infection (p. 436).

antiserums Serums made up of concentrated antibodies (immune globulins) obtained from humans or animals that have developed these antibodies in response to a specific antigen (p. 401).

antitussives Drugs used to relieve coughing (p. 146).

apothecaries' system System used in England for measuring and weighing drugs and solutions. Uses whole numbers and fractions; basic units are grains for solids and minims for liquids (p. 76).

arthritis Painful, swollen, and stiffened joints caused by more than 100 types of joint disease in which destruction or inflammation is present (p. 423).

artificially acquired active immunity Resistance to disease that is developed in individuals by giving them laboratory-produced vaccines that contain either live, attenuated (weakened) or killed antigens (p. 400).

ascorbic acid An essential vitamin that is found in fresh fruits and vegetables, especially citrus fruits; also called *vitamin C*. Has multiple functions and is important in wound healing and for increasing resistance to disease (p. 454).

asepsis Freedom from contaminated or infectious material; prevention of infection (p. 97).

assessment Process of gathering information about the patient, the patient's problem, and any factors that may influence the choice of drug to be given (p. 1).

auscultation One of the four standard physical assessment techniques; generally involves using a stethoscope to listen to heart, lung, or bowel sounds (p. 2).

B

bactericidal Drug that kills bacteria (p. 167).

bacteriostatic Drug that limits or slows the growth of bacteria (p. 167).

barbiturates Primary category of anticonvulsants used for their sedative effect on the brain (p. 269).

barrel Portion of a syringe that is the container for holding medication; it is marked by calibrations (printed numbers) to indicate the volume of medication inside it (p. 106).

bioequivalent Products that are chemically identical and so are interchangeable (p. 35).

biotransformation Metabolic process by which medication is gradually broken down, primarily in the liver, through complex chemical reactions until it becomes chemically inactive (p. 33).

body surface area (BSA) A formula used to calculate the total tissue area; used to determine pediatric dosages of medication. It is calculated in square meters by using charts constructed from height and weight data (p. 90).

broad-spectrum drugs Antiinfective medications that are effective against a wide variety of organisms (p. 167).

bronchodilators Drugs used in patients with asthma or chronic obstructive pulmonary disease to open the bronchi and allow air to pass out more freely (p. 150).

bronchospasm A narrowing or collapse of bronchial airways, often associated with increased mucus production. Irritation of the reduced airway often causes the patient to cough (p. 148).

buccal administration Applying medication directly against the buccal or mucous membranes of the cheek, where it is rapidly absorbed into the bloodstream, bypassing the liver (p. 133).

C

capsules Gelatin containers that hold powder or liquid medicine (p. 97).

catecholamines Drugs that produce effects in the body similar to those produced by norepinephrine; also called *adrenergic* or *sympathomimetic* drugs (p. 265).

Celsius Scale that measures temperature; boiling point is 100° and freezing point is 0° (p. 80).

central nervous system The portion of the nervous system consisting of the brain and spinal cord (p. 264).

chemical name The name for a drug that describes the chemical composition and the atomic or molecular structure (p. 31).

chemotherapeutic agents Drugs used to treat malignant diseases by slowing cell growth or delaying the spread the malignant cells throughout the body (p. 211).

cholinergic drugs Agents whose action is similar to acetylcholine; also called *parasympathomimetics* (p. 265).

cholinergic fibers Parasympathetic nerve fibers that release acetylcholine at a synapse when a nerve impulse passes (p. 265).

chronic heart failure (CHF) A syndrome of weak or inadequate heart action caused by many different factors. Signs and symptoms include a decrease in cardiac output, less effective removal of waste products by the kidneys, and pooling of fluid between the cells or organs or in other dependent tissues (p. 241).

chronic pain Any pain that continues beyond the usual course of an acute injury process (p. 313).

chronotropic Affects the rate of rhythmic movements, such as the heartbeat (p. 241).

Clark's rule A method for determining the pediatric dosage of medication based on the child's body weight; calculated by ratios and proportions (p. 89).

common denominator A denominator (the bottom number of a fraction) that is the same number for each fraction used in a calculation. Needed when the calculation involves fractions with different denominators; can be found by multiplying the denominators of each fraction by one another (p. 70).

compelling indications Other diseases for which a specific class of drugs that was developed for a disease has been shown to improve the patient's condition (p. 250).

complementary medicine Alternative (nontraditional) therapies used in addition to standard medical care (p. 59).

complex fraction A fraction that contains a fraction in its numerator (top number in the fraction), its denominator (bottom number in the fraction), or both (p. 69).

compliant Term that describes a patient who follows a prescribed plan of care (p. 9).

concordance Partnership between the nurse, patient, family, and pharmacist in which all work together to reduce problems with taking drugs (p. 9).

contraindications Factors that rule out the use of a particular drug or class of drugs to treat a medical condition (p. 143).

controlled substances Category of drugs that are most heavily regulated by U.S. federal legislation because of their high potential for abuse; includes major pain killers (narcotics) and some sedatives or tranquilizers (p. 16).

corticosteroids Substances manufactured by the adrenal cortex, which influence many organs, structures, and life processes of the body; composed of glucocorticoids and mineralocorticoids (p. 375).

culture The shared values, beliefs, customs, and behavior of the members of a specific group; learned through both formal teaching and informal life experiences (p. 52).

D

database Information about a patient's level of health, health care practices, past and present illnesses, and physical examination that is combined to serve as the basis for the plan of care (p. 2).

dehydration Loss of a large amount of water from the body tissues, along with loss of electrolytes (p. 260).

delegation When the responsibility for performing a task is passed from one person to another, but the accountability for what happens, or the outcome, remains with the original person (p. 20).

denominator Number in the bottom part of a fraction, below the line (p. 68).

dependence A state in which the body shows withdrawal symptoms when the drug is stopped or a reversing drug (antagonist) is given (p. 314).

depolarization The movement of electrolytes into and out of the cell as it prepares to send another electrical message (p. 231).

desired action The expected response of a medication (p. 34).

diabetes mellitus Disorder of carbohydrate metabolism that may result from a relative lack of insulin or an insensitivity of the body to the available insulin. Abnormalities in fat and protein metabolism also result from serious carbohydrate metabolism disruptions (p. 362).

diagnosis Conclusion about what the patient's problems are; made by the health care team after critically assessing the patient's condition through history, physical examination, and laboratory testing (p. 3).

digestive enzymes Substances that promote digestion by acting as replacement therapy when the body's natural pancreatic enzymes are lacking, not secreted, or not properly absorbed (p. 344).

digitalis toxicity A life-threatening condition in which a patient shows gradual onset of uncomfortable and harmful reactions to digitalis. High concentration of medication results in gradual poisoning of tissues (p. 241).

digitalizing dose Frequent, high doses of digitalis given when a patient begins taking digitalis; done so that a specific level of medication can be quickly achieved in the blood to improve cardiac function or control dysrhythmias or other adverse conditions (p. 243).

dimensional analysis A mathematical procedure often used in biology, physics, chemistry, and pharmacology to solve problems by using a grid to establish proportional relationships; reduces the chance of errors in conversion of units (p. 90).

displacement When two drugs are given together, one drug replaces another at the drug receptor site, increasing the effect of the first drug (p. 36).

distribution The extent to which drugs have moved from circulating body fluids to their sites of action in the body (p. 33).

disulfiram reaction Immediate and severe nausea, vomiting, and diarrhea, as well as many other adverse reactions, caused when a patient mixes disulfiram with alcohol. Some medications, such as Flagyl (used to treat vaginal infections), can produce a similar reaction (p. 345).

dromotropic Influences the speed of the passage of an electrical impulse in nerve or cardiac muscle fibers (p. 241).

drop factor The number of drops per milliliter of liquid in an intravenous solution; determined by the size of the drops (p. 88).

drug interaction A change in the effect of a drug when it is administered with food or another drug; may increase or decrease the action of the drug (p. 35).

dysrhythmia Irregular beating of the heart (p. 228).

E

ectopic beats Irregular or premature beats of the heart caused by increased sensitivity of electrical cells (p. 230).

edema Abnormal pooling of fluid in the spaces between cells or organs or in other dependent tissues (p. 241).

effective refractory period Time period during which the muscle cells cannot discharge their electrical activity (p. 230).

electrocardiogram (ECG) A graphic record of the electrical activity of the heart produced by an electrocardiograph (p. 229).

elixirs Clear liquid made up of drugs dissolved in alcohol and water; may have coloring and flavoring agents added (p. 97).

emetics Drugs used in emergency situations to cause vomiting so as to remove poisons from the stomach before they can be absorbed (p. 346).

emulsions Solutions that have small droplets of water and medication dispersed in oil, or oil and medication dispersed in water (p. 97).

end-organ damage Damage to the vascular tissues of the heart, kidneys, brain, eyes, and other organs caused by a continuing increase in systolic and diastolic blood pressure (p. 250).

engineering controls Safety features built into equipment to reduce risk of infection and other hazards in health care institutions (p. 28).

enteral (route) Administration of drug directly into the gastrointestinal tract through the mouth, nasogastric tube, or rectum (p. 33).

estrogen Principal female sex hormone, manufactured in the ovaries; responsible for development of the female reproductive organs and secondary sex characteristics and involved with ovulation, pregnancy, and menstruation (p. 382).

evaluation Process of looking at the results when a plan is implemented and determining if the results are what is intended. The plan is modified until the desired results are obtained (p. 7).

excretion Process by which inactive chemicals, chemical by-products, and waste are removed from the body. The kidney is the most important organ of excretion, but feces, tears, and the respiratory tract are also locations of excretion (p. 33).

expectorants Agents that decrease the thickness of respiratory secretions and aid in their removal (p. 160).

F

Fahrenheit Scale that measures temperature; boiling point is 212° and freezing point is 32° (p. 80).

fibrin A netlike substance in the blood that traps red and white blood cells and platelets and forms the matrix of a blood clot (p. 349).

fibrinogen A protein found in the blood plasma that is converted to fibrin by the action of thrombin; also known as *clotting factor I* (p. 349).

first-pass (effect) The percentage of medication that is inactivated after it goes through the liver the first time (p. 33).

flow rate The rate at which intravenous fluids are given; measured in drops per minute (p. 88).

fluid and electrolyte mixtures Solutions of water and calories in the form of carbohydrates, with minerals and electrolytes such as sodium, potassium, chloride, calcium, and phosphorus. These are given when oral food intake has been stopped or to prevent dehydration (p. 260).

fraction One or more equal parts of a unit; written as two numbers separated by a line, such as ½ (p. 68).

Fried's rule Method for calculating pediatric dosages that is used for infants and children under age 2. Dosage is found by dividing the infant's age in months by 150 and then multiplying by the adult dose (p. 90).

G

generation Term used to describe a group of drugs based on their development from other similar medications. Later generations of drugs are often more specific in action but may also have more adverse effects (p. 166).

generic name Assigned name for a drug; not licensed and can be used by any manufacturer (p. 30).

geriatric Pertaining to the physiology of aging and the diagnosis and treatment of diseases affecting the elderly population; also refers to older adult and elderly people (p. 46).

glucometers Hand-held machines used to measure the blood glucose level (p. 365).

gold compounds Gold salts that, when used as a drug, interfere with a wide range of biochemical reactions on a cellular level (also called *chrysotherapy*); used primarily in preventing joint destruction in rheumatoid arthritis (p. 424).

gout A form of arthritis caused by overproduction or underexcretion of uric acid (p. 428).

gram Unit of weight used in the metric system of measurement (p. 77).

H

half-life The time it takes to remove 50% of a drug from the body (p. 34).

health disparity When the inability to read and write puts a person at higher risk for disease and disability (p. 10).

health literacy The ability to understand and use information that is important in keeping oneself healthy (p. 10).

health promotion Performing specific activities intended to maintain or improve one's health and well-being (p. 64).

helminthiasis Infestation by worms (p. 188).

hepatotoxic Having the potential to damage the liver (p. 34).

herbal Compounds made from plant sources that are used in alternative or complementary medical practice to relieve symptoms. Often prepared as teas, poultices, or wraps (p. 60).

histamine Chemical produced by the body that is responsible for the inflammatory response. When the body is injured or sensitized to an allergen, histamine is released (p. 142).

histamine H$_2$-receptor antagonists Agents that promote healing of ulcers and act with antacids to produce more alkaline conditions in the gastrointestinal tract (p. 329).

hormones Chemicals that are made in an organ or gland and are carried through the bloodstream to another part of the body, where they stimulate that part of the body to increase its activity or secretion (p. 360).

human immunodeficiency virus (HIV) A type of retrovirus that causes acquired immunodeficiency syndrome (AIDS). It is transmitted through contact with an infected individual's blood, semen, cervical secretions, cerebrospinal fluid, or synovial fluid. It produces defects in cellular immunity (p. 197).

hydration The amount of fluid in body tissue (p. 321).

hyperglycemia Condition seen with fasting blood glucose levels greater than 150 mg/dL. Signs include glycosuria, ketonuria, Kussmaul's respiration, tachycardia, and acetone breath. People may have hyperglycemia for a variety of reasons; chronic high blood glucose levels are usually associated with diabetes mellitus (p. 364).

hyperlipidemia An increase in levels of one or more of the types of lipoproteins in the blood. This may mean that there are high amounts of cholesterol, triglycerides, or both (p. 236).

hyperlipoproteinemia An increase in the lipoprotein concentration in the blood, usually caused by defects in lipoprotein transport or metabolism (p. 235).

hypersensitivity Increased reaction to a drug; often used to describe an allergy (p. 35).

hyperthyroidism Overproduction of thyroid hormone. Symptoms include weight loss, decreased or absent menstruation, rapid or pounding heart, heat intolerance, nervousness, irritability, diarrhea, sweaty skin, inability to fall asleep, fever, and chest pain (p. 393).

hypnotic agent Drug that produces sleep, relaxation, or loss of memory in a patient (p. 306).

hypoglycemia Condition in which serum glucose levels are less than 60 mg/dL. Produces sudden onset of nervousness; hunger; weakness; cold, clammy, skin; lethargy; no urine glucose or acetone; pallor; diaphoresis; change in level of consciousness; and shallow respirations. May be caused by excessive doses of insulin (p. 364).

hypothyroidism Condition in which there is a decrease in production of thyroid hormone. Symptoms include fatigue, weakness, lethargy, moderate weight gain with minimal appetite, cold intolerance, menorrhagia, dry skin, coarse hair, hoarseness, impaired memory, and constipation (p. 393).

I

idiopathic Of an unknown cause; for example, most hypertension is idiopathic in origin (p. 269).

idiosyncratic response Strange, unique, or unpredicted response to a drug (p. 34).

immunity Resistance to invading proteins and diseases that is produced by either having a disease and recovering from it or being immunized to prevent getting the disease (p. 400).

implementation Performance of the nursing care plan; involves administering therapeutic agents, helping with feeding or activities of daily living, providing dressing changes, or giving teaching and counseling (p. 5).

improper fraction Fraction that has a numerator (top number in the fraction) the same as or larger than the denominator (bottom number in the fraction) (p. 69).

incompatibility When two drugs do not mix well chemically; an attempt to combine them in a syringe causes a chemical reaction so that neither can be used (p. 36).

infants Children from the first month after birth to approximately 12 months of age, when babies are able to assume an erect posture; some extend the period to 24 months of age (p. 44).

initial insomnia Difficulty falling asleep (p. 306).

inspection One of the four traditional physical assessment techniques; involves the nurse looking closely for physical findings or observing the patient (p. 2).

insulin Hormone necessary for the metabolism and use of glucose in the body; produced by the beta cells of the pancreas (p. 362).

insulin-dependent diabetes mellitus (IDDM) Former name for type 1 diabetes (p. 363).

integrative practices Health care utilizing both alternative (nontraditional) and traditional practices and products (p. 59).

interference When two drugs are given together, one drug promotes the rapid excretion of the other drug, thus reducing its activity (p. 36).

intermittent insomnia Inability to stay asleep (p. 306).

intramuscular (IM) injections Injections that deposit the medication deep into the muscle mass, past the dermis and subcutaneous tissue, where the rich blood supply allows for rapid and complete absorption (p. 116).

intravenous (IV) route Route used to administer a drug directly into the bloodstream via a needle (p. 119).

L

laxatives Drugs that help draw fluid into the intestine to promote fecal softening, speed the passage of feces through the colon, or increase peristalsis to aid in the elimination of stool from the rectum (p. 338).

legal responsibility A nurse's authority as clearly defined by the nurse practice act of each state. Involves a nurse's judgment and actions while performing professional duties. Because of the variability of practice in different states, it is mandatory that each nurse learn what is legally authorized with regard to medications and ensure that the rules are clearly followed (p. 20).

leukotriene receptor inhibitors Drugs that block receptors for the leukotriene bronchoconstrictors; used in the treatment of asthma (p. 156).

lipodystrophy Shrinkage and loss of the fatty tissue when medication, particularly insulin, is given in the same spot too frequently (p. 363).

liter Unit of volume used in the metric system of measurement (p. 77).

literacy The ability to read, write, and speak in English; to do math; and to solve problems at the level necessary to function on the job and in society (p. 10).

lozenges Medicine mixed with a sugar base to produce small, hard preparations of various sizes or shapes. They are sucked to obtain the medication (p. 97).

M

male or female hormones Chemicals produced by sex glands that are responsible for secondary sex characteristics, fertility, and reproduction (p. 212).

malignancy Refers to rapid and uncontrolled growth of abnormal or cancerous cells that can travel throughout the body, spread into other areas, occupy space, and rob tissues of the nutrients required to maintain normal health (p. 211).

metastasis Movement of uncontrolled, rapidly growing cells from their point of origin (primary site) into other tissues adjacent to or far removed from the primary site (for example, a lung tumor that metastasizes to the brain) (p. 211).

meter Unit of length used in the metric system of measurement (p. 77).

metric system System of measurement developed in France and based on the decimal system. Built on multiples of 10; basic units are meter for length, liter for volume, and gram for weight (p. 77).

minerals Inorganic elements essential to normal metabolism and function because of their role in speeding up biochemical reactions (p. 458).

miosis Constriction of the pupil of the eye (p. 314).

mitotic inhibitors Group of medications that interfere with or stop cell division directly (p. 212).

mixed number A number that consists of a whole number and a proper fraction (p. 69).

Mix-o-vial A two-compartment vial that contains a sterile solution in one compartment and medication powder in the other, separated by a rubber stopper; solution and powder are mixed together immediately before use (p. 111).

motility Spontaneous, unconscious or involuntary movement; may apply to food moving through the gastrointestinal tract or to muscular activity (p. 334).

mycotic infections Yeastlike or moldlike diseases in humans that are produced by a fungus (p. 205).

mydriasis Abnormal dilation of the pupil (p. 436).

myocardial infarction Death of cardiac muscle cells resulting from decreased blood supply through the coronary artery, as in coronary thrombosis (p. 237).

myocardium Middle layer of the heart wall; made up of special muscle cells (p. 228).

myxedema Severe form of hypothyroidism. Skin changes include nonpitting edema, doughy skin, puffy face, large tongue, decreased body hair, and cool, dry skin. May lead to coma and death (p. 394).

N

narcotic Any substance that produces stupor associated with analgesia (p. 312).

narrow-spectrum drugs Antiinfective medications that are useful against only a few organisms (p. 167).

nasogastric (NG) tube An enteral route for medication; tube that goes through the nose and opens directly into the stomach (p. 100).

naturally acquired active immunity Immunity obtained by the development of antibodies when a person gets an infectious disease (p. 400).

needle Instrument used with a syringe to deliver medication; made up of the hub, which attaches to the syringe; the shaft, which is the hollow part through which the medication passes; and the beveled tip, which pierces the skin (p. 106).

neonates The newborn or initial stage of life from birth to 1 month of age (p. 43).

neoplasms Tumors or abnormal growths; may be benign or malignant (p. 211).

nephrotoxic Having the potential to damage the kidney (p. 34).

neurotransmitters Chemical messengers released at the nerve synapse that take part in the transmission of impulses from one nerve ending to another; convey information from the brain to other body parts and produce physiologic responses (p. 265).

niacin Water-soluble and essential B complex vitamin that is a component of two coenzymes that transfer hydrogen in intracellular respiration (p. 451).

nomogram Chart that displays relationships between two types of data; used so that complex mathematical calculations are not necessary. In pharmacology, an example would be a chart used to calculate body surface area (p. 90).

noncompliance A decision or action on the part of the patient not to adhere to a therapeutic suggestion. This may be because of a health belief, a cultural or spiritual value, misunderstanding, failure to appreciate risk, or a problem in the relationship between the provider of the recommendation and the patient. Also refers to the inappropriate use of medications (p. 54).

noncompliant Term used to describe a patient who does not follow a prescribed plan of care (p. 9).

non–insulin-dependent diabetes mellitus (NIDDM) Former name for type 2 diabetes (p. 363).

nonsteroidal antiinflammatory drugs (NSAIDs) Agents that have analgesic, antiinflammatory, and antipyretic effects; used in treating rheumatic diseases, degenerative joint disease, osteoarthritis, and acute musculoskeletal problems (p. 418).

norepinephrine One of two major neurotransmitters in the body; acts on the sympathetic nerves (p. 265).

normal sinus rhythm The regular beating of the heart using the usual path of electrical communication throughout the heart. The electrical stimuli in the cardiac muscle originate in the sinoatrial node, pass through the atrium to the atrioventricular node, through the bundle of His, through the right and left bundle branches, and out through the Purkinje fibers of the myocardium. The heart will then contract, forcing blood out into the arteries. Then the cycle begins again (p. 229).

numerator Number in the top part of a fraction, above the line (p. 68).

nurse practice act State law passed to license practical nurses, registered nurses, nurse practitioners, nurse-midwives, and nurse anesthetists. Describes minimal requirements the individual must have that will protect the public safety. Provides title protection to those who can document their educational preparation and show willingness to accept professional responsibility. Describes what functions the nurse is authorized to perform, including drug prescription or administration (p. 20).

nursing process Plan developed over the years that organizes and coordinates the nurse's activities. Its five major parts are assessment, diagnosis, planning, implementation, and evaluation (p. 1).

O

objective data Information obtained from documentation that patients may bring with them, such as electrocardiogram results or x-rays, or information that can be directly observed during a physical examination or obtained from laboratory tests and diagnostic procedures (p. 2).

official name Name given to a drug by the Food and Drug Administration; may be similar to the brand or trade name (p. 31).

opioids Narcotics used for treating severe pain (p. 312).

opportunistic infections Infections caused by normally nonpathogenic organisms in a person whose resistance has been decreased by such disorders as diabetes mellitus, acquired immunodeficiency syndrome (AIDS), or cancer; by a surgical procedure such as a cerebrospinal fluid shunt or a cardiac or urinary tract catheterization; or by immunosuppressive drugs (p. 202).

oral hypoglycemics Products that stimulate insulin release by the beta cells of the pancreas (p. 369).

osteoarthritis Common form of arthritis with localized joint destruction, particularly in weight-bearing joints or stressed joints, resulting gradually from overuse and increasing age (p. 423).

ototoxic Drug that may damage hearing (p. 143).

over-the-counter (OTC) medications Category of drugs identified by federal legislation as having low risk to patients and that may be purchased without a prescription; have low risk for abuse and are safe if directions are followed (p. 16).

oxytocic agents Drugs that cause the uterus to contract, produce narrowing of the blood vessels, and stimulate the flow of breast milk; used to help labor move on to delivery (p. 372).

P

pacemaker Special group of nerve fibers located in the sinoatrial node that starts the spread of electrical impulses throughout the other muscle cells in the heart, causing the heart to pump (p. 228).

pain An unpleasant sensation or emotion that produces or might produce tissue damage (p. 313).

palpation One of the four standard physical assessment techniques; involves use of the hands and the sense of touch to gather data about the patient's physical condition (p. 2).

parenteral route Administration of drug by injection directly into dermal, subcutaneous, or intramuscular tissue, or epidurally into the cerebrospinal fluid, or through intravenous injection into the bloodstream (pp. 33, 104).

Parkinson's disease Paralysis agitans; a chronic disorder of the central nervous system that is thought to involve an imbalance or relative decrease in chemical neurotransmitters within the brain (p. 282).

partial agonists Drugs that attach at the receptor site, but produce only a small chemical response (p. 31).

passive immunity Short-term resistance to invading proteins and diseases that is produced in two ways: (1) by taking immune globulins from a person who has had a specific antigen-antibody response and giving them to another person who has not had this response to protect that individual from a specific disease, or (2) when antibodies pass from the mother to the fetus through the placenta or to the nursing infant through the breast milk (p. 401).

pathogen An organism that produces infection (p. 166).

pediatric Pertaining to preventive and primary health care and treatment of children and the study of childhood diseases; also refers to children from infancy to adolescence (p. 45).

pediculicides Agents used to treat pediculosis, an infection of the dermis seen mostly in children (p. 441).

percent Parts per hundred units; symbol: % (p. 72).

percussion One of the four traditional physical assessment techniques. Uses tapping of tissues overlying various body organs and structures to produce vibration and sound to detect underlying abnormalities (p. 2).

percutaneous (route) Administration of drug through topical (skin), sublingual (under the tongue), buccal (against the cheek), or inhalation (breathing) methods (pp. 33, 130).

perennial allergic rhinitis (PAR) Inflammation of the nasal mucous membranes caused by reaction to indoor allergens (for example, animal dander and dust mites) (p. 142).

perennial nonallergic rhinitis (PNAR) Inflammation of the nasal mucous membranes caused by conditions other than allergies (p. 142).

peripheral nervous system The portion of the nervous system that consists of the nerves connecting the brain and spinal cord to other parts of the body (p. 264).

pharmacodynamics The effects of drugs on functions of the body (p. 30).

pharmacokinetics The action of drugs in the body (p. 30).

pharmacotherapeutics The use of drugs in the treatment of disease (p. 30).

physical dependence Physiologic need for a medication to relieve shaking, pain, or other symptoms (p. 18).

piggyback infusion A second intravenous infusion added to allow administration of medication while the original infusion is clamped off. Patient requires only one needle for both infusions (p. 124).

pill Oral, solid medication; may be a tablet or capsule (p. 97).

plunger Inner portion of a syringe that fits into the barrel. When the plunger is pushed into the barrel, the medication is forced out through the needle (p. 106).

positive inotropic action Drug effect that increases the strength of each heartbeat and in turn increases cardiac output (p. 241).

precautions Factors that indicate that a particular drug or class of drugs should be used with great care to treat a medical condition (p. 143).

prescription, or legend, drugs Category of drugs that are regulated by federal legislation because they are dangerous and their use must be controlled; may be purchased only when prescribed by an authorized prescriber. Examples are antibiotics and oral birth control pills (p. 16).

primary hypertension Hypertension (elevation of a patient's blood pressure above normal values for the patient's age) with unknown causes that accounts for 80% to 90% of all cases of high blood pressure; also called *essential hypertension* (p. 246).

problem-oriented medical record (POMR) A format for patient charts developed by Lawrence Weed in 1969. It uses a list of numbered patient problems as an index to the chart and includes a summary sheet, history and physical examination, problem list, physician's orders, progress notes, graphic record, laboratory tests, and consultations (p. 22).

professional responsibility The obligation of nurses to act appropriately, ethically, and to the best of their abilities as health care providers (p. 20).

progesterone Sex steroid hormone produced by the ovaries, by the placenta, and in small amounts by the adrenal cortex that helps prepare the uterus for implantation. Along with estrogen, it helps maintain normal uterine and mammary gland function (p. 382).

proper fraction Part of a whole number, or numbers less than 1. Numerator (top number) is less than denominator (bottom number) in these fractions (p. 69).

prophylaxis Prevention of or protection against disease (p. 148).

proportion A way of expressing a relationship of equality between two ratios. When written, the two ratios are separated by a double colon (p. 73).

psychologic dependence Feeling of anxiety, stress, or tension felt if a patient does not have a medication (p. 18).

R

ratio A way of expressing the relationship of one number to another number, or of expressing a part of a whole number. When written, the numbers are separated by a colon. Term is often used along with *proportion* (p. 72).

rebound effect Increase in symptoms that you are trying to stop; frequently caused by taking too much medication or when medication is suddenly stopped (p. 143).

rebound vasodilation Condition in which a drug that was given to constrict the veins causes them to become dilated instead because of its action on both types of receptors; causes an increase in blood flow that may lead to further symptoms (p. 157).

receptor A structure that acts as a "lock" for a specific chemical ("key") that must fit into the receptor before an action can be produced (p. 265).

receptor site A specific site in the body where a medication bonds chemically (p. 31).

refractoriness Lack of response to a drug that a patient has used before with good effectiveness (p. 151).

regimen A specific medication plan or a therapeutic plan such as a diet or exercise schedule (p. 48).

retrovirus A virus that contains RNA rather than DNA as its genetic material. Retroviruses produce the enzyme reverse transcriptase, which allows transcription of the viral genome onto the DNA of the host cell (p. 197).

rheumatoid arthritis A systemic disease that involves an autoimmune response caused by failure of the body to recognize its own tissue, resulting in destruction of the joint (p. 423).

riboflavin Water-soluble vitamin (B_2) that functions as a precursor of two essential enzymes that deal with metabolism of proteins, fats, and carbohydrates (p. 451).

Roman numeral system System of numbers commonly used as units of the apothecaries' system of weights and measures in writing prescriptions. Consists of seven basic numerals in different combinations: I = 1, V = 5, X = 10, L = 50, C = 100, D = 500, M = 1000 (p. 68).

S

salicylates Agents used to treat mild to moderate pain and reduce fever. They have analgesic, antipyretic, and anti-inflammatory effects (p. 413).

scabicides Agents applied to skin and in hair to kill scabies (p. 441).

scheduled drugs Controlled substances that are highly regulated because they are commonly abused (p. 16).

seasonal allergic rhinitis (SAR) Inflammation of the nasal mucous membranes caused by reaction to outdoor allergens (for example, pollen); also called *hay fever* (p. 142).

secondary hypertension Hypertension resulting from a known disease or other problem, such as coarctation of the aorta (p. 246).

sedative agent Medication that relaxes the patient and allows the patient to sleep (p. 306).

seizures Sudden muscle contractions that happen without conscious control; a symptom of abnormal and excessive discharge of electrical impulses in the brain (p. 269).

sex hormones Substances that influence many organs, structures, and life processes of the body as they prepare the body to reproduce. They are produced in the adrenal cortex and gonads and include androgens and estrogens (p. 375).

side effects Any unintended reactions or consequences that result from a medication; usually mild and may be beneficial or annoying (p. 34).

six "rights" of medication administration Six points to check when administering a drug. These include five points to check before administering medication (the right drug, the right time, the right dose, the right patient, and the right route) and one point to check after administration (the right documentation) (p. 5).

skeletal muscle relaxants Drugs used to decrease muscle tone and involuntary movement without loss of voluntary motor function. They inhibit the transmission of impulses in the motor pathways at the level of the spinal cord and the brainstem or interfere with the mechanism that shortens the skeletal muscle fibers so that they contract (p. 420).

slow-acting antirheumatic drugs (SAARDs) Agents used in limiting joint destruction in significant cases of rheumatoid arthritis (p. 424).

solubility The ability of a medication to dissolve (p. 32).

Somogyi effect Rebound increase in glucose levels that is caused by hypoglycemia (p. 368).

spectrum The variety or number of organisms against which a medication is effective (p. 167).

status epilepticus A condition in which a series of severe grand mal seizures occur one after another without stopping (p. 271).

steroids A group of hormones that have powerful effects on cell sensitization, healing, and development. They are also associated with many adverse effects, particularly in patients who must take them chronically (p. 360).

subcutaneous injections Injections that place no more than 2 mL of fluid into the loose connective tissue between the dermis of the skin and the muscle layer (p. 113).

subjective data Information supplied by the patient or family. It may be felt or known only by the patient and not detectable to anyone else (p. 2).

sublingual administration Applying medication to mucous membranes under the tongue (p. 133).

superinfection Overgrowth of other organisms not sensitive to a prescribed antiinfective medication when the medication kills sensitive organisms that would have ke them under control. Common adverse reaction seen when antibiotics kill all the bacteria in a patient and allow overgrowth of yeast (p. 167).

suspensions Liquids with solid, insoluble drug particles dispersed throughout. Must be shaken before pouring because solids tend to settle out in layers (p. 97).

sympathomimetics Beta-adrenergic agents that dilate the bronchi through their action on beta-adrenergic receptors (p. 150).

synergistic effect When two drugs are given together, the effect is greater than the sum of the effects of each drug given alone (p. 36).

syringes Calibrated containers used for injecting liquids into the body. May be plastic or glass and are available in 1-, 3-, 5-, 10-, 20-, and 50-mL sizes (p. 106).

syrups Liquids with high sugar content designed to disguise the bitter taste of a drug; often used in pediatric patients (p. 97).

systemic acidosis A condition in which the basic fluid and electrolyte balance of the body is disturbed and the blood pH is decreased. Symptoms include nausea, vomiting, and changes in level of consciousness (p. 364).

T

tablets Dried, powdered drugs compressed into shapes small enough to be swallowed whole; may contain coating to increase solubility or absorption (p. 97).

teratogenic Likely to produce malformations or damage in the embryo or fetus (p. 49).

terminal insomnia Early awakening with an inability to return to sleep (p. 306).

therapeutic effects Occur when the drug produces the intended reaction and the therapeutic goal is met (p. 7).

thiamine Water-soluble vitamin (B_1) that functions as a coenzyme that is closely involved with carbohydrate metabolism (p. 451).

thrombi Blood clots made of fibrin, platelets, and cholesterol; often found in large veins. Pieces known as *emboli* may break off and travel to the heart, the brain, or the lung, causing strokes or death (p. 349).

thromboplastin A complex substance that initiates the clotting process by converting prothrombin to thrombin in the presence of calcium ion. It is found in most tissue cells, red cells, and leukocytes; functions as factor III in blood coagulation (p. 349).

tip Portion of a syringe that holds the needle. The needle either screws onto the tip or fits tightly so it does not fall off (p. 106).

tocolytics Agents that stop uterine contractions during labor (p. 373).

tolerance A state in which the same amount of drug produces less effect over time (p. 314).

topical medications Drugs applied directly to the area of skin requiring treatment; most common forms are creams, lotions, and ointments (p. 131).

toxoid A toxin that is attenuated, or weakened (p. 401).

trade name Brand name of a drug; licensed to a certain manufacturer and cannot be used by other manufacturers (p. 31).

type 1 diabetes Insulin-dependent diabetes mellitus or juvenile diabetes; patients usually has little or no production of insulin by the pancreas (p. 363).

type 2 diabetes Non–insulin-dependent diabetes mellitus or late-onset diabetes; patient usually has a functioning pancreas that can be encouraged by medication to produce more insulin (p. 363).

U

uric acid A metabolite of protein that is present in the blood within a very specific range. Increased levels may precipitate as crystals in tissues, causing the condition known as *gout* (p. 428).

uricosuric agents Drugs that increase the excretion of urate salts by blocking their renal tubular reabsorption. Also used to decrease the amount of circulating urate and the deposition of urate and promote reabsorption of urate deposits (p. 428).

uterine relaxants Agents that act on the beta-adrenergic receptors to stop uterine smooth muscle contractions; used in the management of preterm or premature labor (p. 372).

V

vaccines Substances containing weakened or dead antigens given to allow an individual to develop immunity to the antigen (p. 400).

vasoconstrictors Agents that cause direct stimulation of the alpha receptors of vascular smooth muscle, leading to a narrowing of the blood vessels (p. 441).

vials Small single- or multiple-dose glass containers of medication (p. 108).

virions Rudimentary virus particles with a central nucleoid surrounded by a protein sheath or capsid. The complete nucleocapsid with a nucleic acid core may constitute a complete virus, or it may be surrounded by an envelope (p. 197).

vitamin A Fat-soluble, long-chain alcohol that comes in several isometric forms; helps the eye adjust to changes from light to darkness (p. 450).

vitamins Chemical compounds found naturally in plant and animal tissues but not made in the human body; necessary for life and essential to normal metabolism (p. 449).

W

wheezing A musical respiratory sound heard during respiratory expiration when a patient with asthma begins to breathe faster or has a lot of bronchoconstriction (p. 148).

withdrawal symptoms Changes in the body or mind, such as nausea or anxiety, that occur when a drug is stopped or reduced after regular use (p. 314).

X

xanthines Bronchodilators that act directly to relax the smooth muscle cells of the bronchi, thereby dilating the bronchi (p. 150).

Y

Young's rule Method for calculating pediatric dosing that is used for children ages 2 to 12 years. The dosage can be found by dividing the child's age by the child's age plus 12 and then multiplying by the adult dose (p. 90).

Disorders Index

General Index

A

Abacavir, 203t
Abbokinase. *See* **Urokinase.**
Abbreviations
  do-not-use list for, 27t
  pharmacologic, 27t
Abciximab, 354t
Abortifacients, 372–373, 374t
Absorption, drug process of, 32–33, 32b, 34f
Acarbose, 371t
Accolate. *See* **Zafirlukast.**
Accupril. *See* **Quinapril.**
Accutane. *See* **Isotretinoin.**
ACE (angiotensin-converting enzyme) in-
    hibitors, 250, 252t, 256t
Acebutolol, 234t, 251t
Acephen. *See* **Acetaminophen.**
Aceta. *See* **Acetaminophen.**
Acetaminophen, 321t, 323t
  adverse reactions to, 417
  antiinflammatory analgesic use of, 415t,
    417–418
  drug interactions of, 417
  nursing implications of, 418
Acetazolamide, 270t, 276t
Acetylcarbromal, insomnia treated with, 309t
Acetylcholine
  neurotransmitter function of, 265
  ophthalmic use of, 438t
Acetylsalicylic acid
  antiinflammatory analgesic use of, 413–
    417, 415t
  antiplatelet effect of, 354t
Aciphex. *See* **Rabeprazole.**
Acitretin, 443t
Acne, topical agents for, 442t
Acquired immunodeficiency syndrome. *See*
    AIDS (acquired immunodeficiency
    syndrome).
ACTH. *See* **Corticotropin.**
ACTH-80. *See* **Corticotropin repository.**
Acthar. *See* **Corticotropin.**
Acticin. *See* **Permethrin.**
Actigall. *See* **Ursodiol.**
Actiq. *See* **Fentanyl.**
Activase. *See* **Alteplase.**
Activated charcoal, 343t
Actos. *See* **Pioglitazone.**
Acular. *See* **Ketorolac.**
Acyclovir, 199t, 444t
Adapalene, 442t
Addiction, 314
  drug-related, 314
Adenocard. *See* **Adenosine.**
Adenosine, antidysrhythmic role of, 234t
Adrenalin. *See* **Epinephrine.**
Adrenergic inhibitors
  adverse effects of, 255t
  benign prostatic hyperplasia and, 259t
  hypertension treated with, 246, 247–249,
    251t, 255t
Adrenergics, definition of, 265
Adrenocortical hormones, 378–382, 379t,
    381t. *See also* Corticosteroids.
  adverse reactions to, 378, 379t
  drug interactions of, 378

Adrenocortical hormones *(Continued)*
  glucocorticoids as, 381t
  mineralocorticoids as, 381t
  nursing implications of, 378–382
Adriamycin. *See* **Doxorubicin.**
Adrucil. *See* **Fluorouracil.**
Adverse reaction, definition of, 34, 35b
Advil. *See* **Ibuprofen.**
AeroBid. *See* **Flunisolide.**
Aerosols, 136b
Afrin. *See* **Oxymetazoline.**
Age, drug assimilation and metabolism re-
    lated to, 43–52
Agenerase. *See* **Amprenavir.**
Aggrastat. *See* **Tirofiban.**
Agonist, definition of, 312
Agoral. *See* **Senna.**
Agrylin. *See* **Anagrelide.**
AIDS (acquired immunodeficiency
    syndrome)
  overview of, 197, 198f, 201f
  Standard Precautions related to, 104, 105b
Air, in intravenous tubing, 128, 129t
AK-Chlor. *See* **Chloramphenicol.**
AK-Dex. *See* **Dexamethasone.**
AK-Fluor. *See* **Fluorescein.**
Akineton. *See* **Biperiden.**
Akne-mycin. *See* **Erythromycin.**
AK-Pred. *See* **Prednisolone.**
AK-Sulf. *See* **Sulfacetamide.**
AK-Tob. *See* **Tobramycin.**
AK-Tracin. *See* **Bacitracin.**
Alamast. *See* **Pemirolast.**
Albamycin. *See* **Novobiocin.**
Albendazole, 191t
Albenza. *See* **Albendazole.**
Albuterol, 152t
Alcaine. *See* **Proparacaine.**
Alcohol
  disulfiram reaction due to, 343t, 345–346
  drug interaction role of, 35–41, 37t–40t
Aldesleukin, 217t
Aldomet. *See* **Methyldopa.**
Alfenta. *See* **Alfentanil.**
Alfentanil, 318t
Alimentary canal, definition of, 327
Alka-Seltzer. *See* **Acetylsalicylic acid.**
Alkeran. *See* **Melphalan.**
Alkylamines, allergy treated with, 144t
Alkylating agents, 211, 213t–214t
Allegra. *See* **Fexofenadine.**
Allerest. *See* **Naphazoline.**
Allergy
  antihistamine therapy for, 142–146, 144t–
    145t
  insulin causing, 365
  IV medication causing, 129, 129t
  latex vial stopper causing, 111
  medication causing, 35, 35b
  skin test injections in, 112–113, 113f, 114f,
    114t
Alleve. *See* **Naproxen.**
Allopurinol, 214t, 431t
Almotriptan, 268t
Alocril. *See* **Nedocromil.**
Alomide. *See* **Iodoxamide.**
Alpha Keri. *See* **Colloidal baths.**
Alphagan. *See* **Brimonidine.**
Alprazolam, 289t
Altace. *See* **Ramipril.**

Alteplase, 354t
Alternative therapies, 57–60. *See also* Herbal
    therapies.
  over-the-counter products in, 19, 58–59
Altretamine, 213t
Alu-Cap. *See* **Aluminum hydroxide gel.**
Aluminum carbonate gel, 332t
Aluminum hydroxide gel, 332t
Alupent. *See* **Metaproterenol.**
Alurate. *See* **Aprobarbital.**
Alveolus, 141f
Amantadine, 199t, 284t
Amaryl. *See* **Glimepiride.**
Ambien. *See* **Zolpidem.**
Amcinonide, 442t
Amebiasis, 187–188, 189t
  adverse reaction in, 187
  medications for, 187–188, 189t
Amen. *See* **Medroxyprogesterone acetate.**
Amerge. *See* **Naratriptan.**
Americaine. *See* **Benzocaine.**
Amethopterin. *See* **Methotrexate.**
Amigesic. *See* **Salsalate.**
Amikacin, 178t
Amikin. *See* **Amikacin.**
Amiloride, 251t
Aminoglycosides, 175t, 176t
Aminopenicillins, 170t
Aminophylline, 153t
Aminoquinolines, 193t
Aminovin. *See* Pyridoxine (vitamin B6).
Amiodarone, 234t
Amitriptyline, 293t
Amlodipine, 252t
Amobarbital, 270t, 274t, 308t
Amoxapine, 293t
Amoxicillin, 170t
Amoxil. *See* **Amoxicillin.**
Amphojel. *See* **Aluminum hydroxide gel.**
Amphotec. *See* **Amphotericin B.**
Amphotericin B, 208t
Ampicillin, 170t
Amprenavir, 204t
Ampules
  opening of, 108–109, 110f
  parenteral medications packaged in, 108–
    111, 110f
  removing contents of, 108–111, 110f
Amyl nitrite, 226t, 227t
Amytal. *See* **Amobarbital.**
Anacin, 323t
Anafranil. *See* **Clomipramine.**
Anagrelide, 354t
Analgesics. *See also* Acetaminophen;
    Salicylates.
  antiinflammatory applications of, 413–420,
    415t–416t
  food and alcohol interactions with, 37t
  narcotics combined with, 321t
  nonnarcotic, 323–324, 323t, 324t
  nonsteroidal antiinflammatory drugs as,
    415t–416t, 418–420
  urinary tract treated with, 258, 259t
Anaphylactic reaction, 35, 35b
Anaprox. *See* **Naproxen.**
Anaspaz. *See* **Atropine.**
Anastrozole, 215t
Ancef. *See* **Cephazolin.**
Ancobon. *See* **Flucytosine.**
Androderm. *See* **Testosterone transdermal.**